TEXTBOOK OF **Diagnostic ultrasonography**

TEXTBOOK OF
Diagnostic ultrasonography

SANDRA L. HAGEN-ANSERT, B.A., R.D.M.S.

Educational Coordinator, Division of Ultrasound,
Thomas Jefferson University Medical Center,
Philadelphia, Pennsylvania

with **1200** illustrations including drawings by
ERIC P. TEICHMAN, R.D.M.S.

Clinical Instructor, Division of Ultrasound,
Thomas Jefferson University Medical Center,
Philadelphia, Pennsylvania

The C. V. Mosby Company SAINT LOUIS 1978

Copyright © 1978 by The C. V. Mosby Company

All rights reserved. No part of this book may be reproduced in any manner without written permission of the publisher.

Printed in the United States of America

The C. V. Mosby Company
11830 Westline Industrial Drive, St. Louis, Missouri 63141

Library of Congress Cataloging in Publication Data

Hagen-Ansert, Sandra L.
  Textbook of diagnostic ultrasonography.

  Bibliography: p.
  Includes index.
  1. Diagnosis, Ultrasonic. I. Title.
[DNLM: 1. Ultrasonics—Diagnostic use. WB289
H143t]
RC78.7.U4H33   616.07′54   78-4105
ISBN 0-8016-2011-2

CB/CB/B 9 8 7 6 5 4 3 2 1

To my
DAD
who encouraged me to
"Hang in there, baby . . ."

Preface

Medicine has always been a fascinating field. I was introduced to it by Dr. Charles Henkelmann, who provided me with the opportunity to learn radiography. Although x-ray technology was interesting, it was not challenging enough. It did not provide the opportunity to evaluate patient history or to follow through interesting cases, which seemed to be the most intriguing aspect of medicine and my primary concern.

Shortly after I finished my training, I was assigned to the radiation therapy department, where I was introduced to a very quiet and young, dedicated radiologist, whom I would later grow to admire and respect as one of the foremost authorities in diagnostic ultrasound. Convincing George Leopold that he needed another hand to assist him was difficult in the beginning, and it was through the efforts of his resident, Dan MacDonald, that I was able to learn what has eventually developed into a most challenging and exciting new medical modality.

Utilizing high-frequency sound waves, diagnostic ultrasound provides a unique method for visualization of soft tissue anatomic structures. The challenge of identifying such structures and correlating the results with clinical symptoms and patient data offered an ongoing challenge to the sonographer. The state of the art demands expertise in scanning techniques and maneuvers to demonstrate the internal structures; without quality scans, no diagnostic information can be rendered to the physician.

Our initial experience in ultrasound took us through the era of A-mode techniques, identifying aortic aneurysms through pulsatile reflections, trying to separate splenic reflections from upper-pole left renal masses, and, in general, trying to echo every patient with a probable abdominal or pelvic mass. Of course, the one-dimensional A-mode techniques were difficult for me to conceptualize, let alone believe in. However, with repeated success and experience from mistakes, I began to believe in this method. The conviction that Dr. Leopold had about this technique was a strong indicator of its success in our laboratory.

It was when Picker brought our first two-dimensional ultrasound unit to the laboratory that the "skeptics" started to believe a little more in this modality. I must admit that those early images were weather maps to me for a number of months. The repeated times I asked, "What is that?" were enough to try anyone's patience.

I can recall when Seimens installed our real-time unit and we saw our first obstetric case. Such a thrill for us to see the fetus move, wave its hand, and show us fetal heart pulsations.

By this time we were scouting the clinics and various departments in the hospital for interesting cases to scan. With our success rate surpassing our failures, the case load increased so that soon we were involved in all aspects of ultrasound. There was not enough material or reprints for us to read to see the new developments. It was for this reason that excitement in clinical research soared, attracting young physicians throughout the country to develop techniques in diagnostic ultrasound.

Because Dr. Leopold was so intensely interested in ultrasound, it became the diagnostic method of choice for our patients. It was not long before conferences were incomplete without the mention of the technique. Later, local medical meetings and eventually national meetings grew to include discussion of this new modality. A number of visitors were attracted to our laboratory to learn the technique, and thus we became swamped with a continual flow of new physicians, some eager to work with ultrasound and others skeptical at first but believers in the end.

Education progressed slowly at first, with many laboratories offering a one-to-one teaching experience. Commercial companies thought the only way to push the field was to develop their own national training programs, and thus several of the leading manufacturers were the first to put a dedicated effort into the development of ultrasound.

It was through the combined efforts of our laboratory and commercial interests that I became interested in furthering ultrasound education. Seminars, weekly sessions, local and national meetings, and consultations became a vital part of the growth of ultrasound.

Thus, as ultrasound grew in popularity, more intensified training was desperately needed to maintain its initial quality that its pioneers strived for.

Through working with one of the commercial ultrasound companies conducting national short-term training programs, I became acquainted with Barry Goldberg and his enthusiasm for quality education in ultrasound. His organizational efforts and pioneer spirit led me to the east coast to further develop more intensive educational programs in ultrasound.

Through these experiences the need for a diverse ultrasound textbook was shown. Thus this text was written for the sonographer involved in clinical ultrasound, with emphasis on anatomy, physiology, pathology, and ultrasonic techniques and patterns. Clinical medicine and patient evaluation are important parts of the ultrasonic examination and as such are discussed as relevant to pathology demonstrated by ultrasound.

It is my hope that this textbook will not only introduce the reader to the field of ultrasound but also go a step beyond to what I have found to be a very stimulating and challenging experience in diagnostic patient care.

I would like to acknowledge the individual who contributed most to my early interest in diagnostic ultrasound, George R. Leopold, M.D., for his personal perseverance and instruction, as well as for his outstanding clinical research. My thanks also to Dr. Sam Halpern for the encouragement to publish; to Dr. Barry Goldberg for the opportunity to develop training programs in an independent fashion and for his encouragement to stay with it; to Drs. Barbara Gosink, Robert O'Rourke, Mike Crawford, and David Sahn for their encouragement throughout the years at U.C.S.D.; to Drs. Jagdish Patel and Carl Rubin for their continued interest in developing ultrasonic techniques; to Dr. Daniel Yellon for his early hours of anatomy dissection and instruction in clinical cardiology; to Dr. Carson Schneck for his excellent instruction in gross anatomy and sections of "Geraldine"; to Dr. Harvey Watts for his help in the preparation of the gross anatomy pathology photographs from Episcopal Hospital; to Dr. Jacob Zatuchni for the interest, enthusiasm, and understanding he showed me while at Episcopal Hospital; to Drs. Paul Walinski and Edward Sacks for their enthusiastic support in echocardiology; to Rueben Mezrich, David Vilkomberson, Ray Wood, Joe Geck, and Nate Pinkney for their continued support and participation in the physics chapter; to Marcia Lavery for her support with the liver chapter; to John Dietz for the photography of the equipment and patient positions; to Bill Burke, medical illustrator, for his aid in the preparation of the photographs and cardiac illustrations; to Arthur J. Ansert, Jr., who provided the atmosphere of productivity to complete such a book.

The students in diagnostic ultrasound from Episcopal Hospital and Thomas Jefferson University Medical Center continually work toward the development of finer ultrasound techniques and instruction, and for their support I would like to thank them.

A special acknowledgment is made to the many contributors of various chapters within the textbook. Much of this information was accumulated as part of their student participation in the Ultrasound Program at Episcopal Hospital and Thomas Jefferson University Medical Center.

Sandra L. Hagen-Ansert

Contents

PART ONE BASIC PRINCIPLES OF ULTRASOUND

1 □ Physics

RANDY KEMBERLING, R.D.M.S.

Ultrasound is the term used to describe sound frequencies above what the human ear can detect. The earliest application of ultrasound was in sonar (sound navigation and ranging). A Frenchman by the name of P. Langevin applied ultrasound during World War I for the detection of submarines. Following this discovery came the development of flaw-detection devices in industrial materials.

Prior to World War II, researchers began finding medical applications for ultrasound in the hope of detecting internal body structures noninvasively. These initial experiments revealed few positive results and were abandoned. However, with improved techniques in radar and sonar technology after World War II, ultrasound was successfully used for the detection of internal body structures.

In the past two decades ultrasound has become a practical and inexpensive tool with tremendous clinical applications. Such applications include the fields of neurology, ophthalmology, abdominal evaluation, obstetrics, gynecology, and cardiology.

In medical applications a beam of ultrasound is directed into the body. The ultrasonic beam propagates through the tissue by means of vibration. Reflections of the ultrasound occur at various interfaces due to the different biologic makeup of the tissues. These reflections are then processed electronically and displayed in either one- or two-dimensional imaging displays.

The following information will show how ultrasonic energy propagates through tissue and how it is produced, detected, and displayed for use in medical imaging.

AUDIBLE SOUND

Sound waves are mechanical waves that can be made to propagate through solids, liquids, and gases.

Audible waves may originate from vibrating strings such as violins and human vocal cords, or vibrating air columns such as a pipe organ and clarinet, or vibrating membranes such as a drum and loudspeaker. The vibrating elements will in turn cause vibration of the air particles or molecules. The air then transmits these vibrations or disturbances outward from the vibrating sound source as a wave. On entering the human ear these waves produce the sensation known as sound.

Audible sound is confined to a specific range that can stimulate the human ear to the sensation of hearing. Anything above the audible range is termed ultrasound.

Frequency

Frequency (f) is the number of vibrations, or oscillations, that a vibrating particle, for example, an air molecule, performs within a given amount of time.

The vibration of the air molecule back and forth over the same path is termed vibratory, or oscillatory, movement. A vibration, or oscillation, is one round trip of that motion; therefore the period of the motion (T) is the time required for one round-trip motion or one vibration (Fig. 1-1). The frequency of the motion (f) is the number of vibrations per unit time. Therefore frequency (f) can be determined as follows:

$$f = 1/T$$

The number of complete vibrations, or oscillations, and thus the frequency in ultrasound is usually expressed as the number of cycles per second (cps). The unit hertz (Hz) is a standard to indicate cycles per second. Thus 10 cps would be 10 Hz. Other terms in use are the kilohertz (kHz), meaning 1000 cps, and the megahertz (MHz), meaning 1 million cps. One million cycles per second (1,000,000 Hz) can then be written 1000 kHz or 1 MHz.

The frequency for audible sound is in the range of 20 to 20,000 cps. Any frequency above this value is termed ultrasound. In medical applications for ultra-

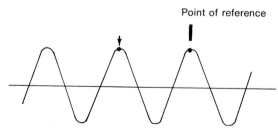

Fig. 1-1. Frequency is the number of times a complete cycle passes the point of reference each second.

Table 1-1. Applications of sound frequency ranges

Frequency range	How produced	Some applications
Infrasound 0 to 25 Hz	Electromagnetic vibrators	Vibration analysis of structures
Audible 20 Hz to 20 kHz	Electromagnetic vibrators, human voice, musical instruments	Communication, signaling
Ultrasound 20 to 100 kHz	Air whistles, electric devices	Biology, sonar
Ultrasound 100 kHz to 1 MHz	Electric devices	Flaw detection, biology
Ultrasound 1 to 20 MHz	Electric devices	Medicine (diagnostic)

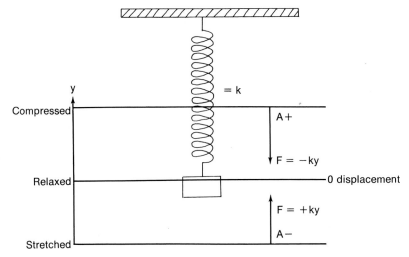

Fig. 1-2. Model for demonstration of simple harmonic motion.

sound the frequency range used is from 1 to 20 MHz. Table 1-1 lists the various sound frequency ranges and their applications.

SIMPLE HARMONIC MOTION

Imagine a particle, such as an air molecule, vibrating about its equilibrium, or resting, position because of the interaction of forces. The distance the particle is moved away from its equilibrium position is proportional to the disturbing force. (Force is the product of the mass of the particle times the acceleration of that particle, or $F = ma$, Newton's second law.) With the particle vibrating about its equilibrium position at a constant rate, we now say that the particle along with the applied forces is in simple harmonic motion.

Let us look at the example in Fig. 1-2. Consider a mass of a certain weight attached to a spring with a specific force constant (k). Assume that the spring and mass are suspended and can move with 0 friction loss. Allow the origin of the mass to be its equilibrium, or relaxed, position and let the motion of the particle be along the y axis. With the particle displaced to point y, the spring exerts a force (F) on the mass so that $F = -ky$, where the negative sign indicates the force toward the equilibrium (0) position as the mass is displaced upward away from its equilibrium position.

By pulling this mass down to a specific displacement (A−) and releasing it, the mass will be forced upward by the spring force (k). Inertia causes the mass to pass its equilibrium position to a point (A+) or maximum displacement in an upward direction. The mass is now forced downward because of the compressed spring force ($F = -ky$).

Without friction loss the mass will continue this vibratory behavior with a constant displacement (A) and a constant frequency. This is called simple harmonic motion.

Medium propagation

Now that simple harmonic motion has been discussed, we can go on to visualize how mechanical sound waves are transmitted through a medium. Consider a vibrating source with a specific displacement and a specific frequency coupled to a medium such as gelatin. The coupling of the source and the medium allows for a pulling and pushing force on the gelatin particles, much the same way the spring (with force k) pulled and pushed on the mass. As the object vibrates against the gelatin, the particles within the gelatin began to oscillate about their equilibrium position in simple harmonic motion (Fig. 1-3). (The term particle is applied to a small volume, in this case gelatin, in which all atoms are considered to be experiencing the same physical forces.) As the particles move about their resting position, orderly oscillations (of displacement A) occur according to the repetition rate (f) of the initial vibratory element. Thus the simple harmonic motion set up from the initial vibratory element is transferred to the gelatin particles, creating the same simple harmonic motion of the same displacement and frequency.

Applying this example to medical ultrasonics, consider the vibrating element to be the ultrasonic transducer emitting sound waves. The gelatin corresponds to the actual tissue over which the transducer was coupled, and the particles would represent actual molecular makeup of the human tissue. Thus sound is transferred through tissue in simple harmonic motion

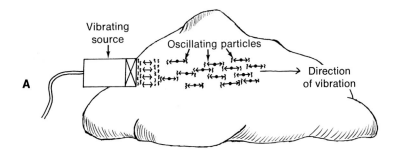

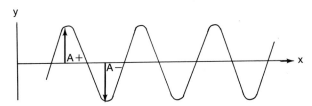

Fig. 1-5. Sinusoidal graph demonstrating variations in particle displacement plotted as a function of amplitude (A).

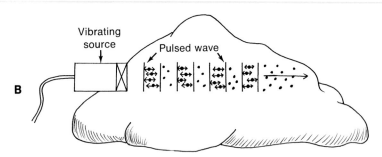

Fig. 1-3. Particle vibrations in continuous waveforms **(A)** and pulsed waveforms **(B)**.

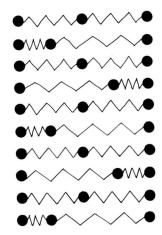

Fig. 1-4. Molecular model demonstrating particle motion about its resting position. (From Goldberg, B. B., Kotler, M. N., Ziskin, M., and Waxham, R. D.: Diagnostic uses of ultrasound, New York, 1975, Grune & Stratton, Inc. Used by permission.)

either in continuous forms or short bursts of energy (Fig. 1-3).

Ultrasonic wave motion cannot exist without some type of medium, whether it is air, liquid, gelatin, or tissue.

Robert Boyle (1627-1691), the outstanding chemist and physicist, discovered that air transmits sound. To prove air carried sound, Boyle put a large ticking clock inside a glass globe and began to extract the air. He witnessed that as the air was withdrawn from the globe, the ticking became fainter and fainter, until it could no longer be heard. As air was again let into the globe, the ticking sound resumed. Thus sound, including ultrasound, must have a medium.

Imagine a medium such as a tissue, composed of black dots with springs connecting these dots (Fig. 1-4). As the ultrasonic force of some source is coupled to this medium model, the vibration from the source begins to create orderly oscillations of the black dots about their resting position. Thus simple harmonic motion is produced.

As the ultrasonic force passes through the medium, one of the molecules is displaced to the left and thus the spring is compressed. The force then, has created compression of the molecular medium. This causes the spring to the right to be displaced and stretched to the left. The resulting force of the spring creates a returning motion toward the black dot's equilibrium position. Due to inertia, however, the black dot moves past its resting position and causes the spring to stretch to the left, initiating return motion of the black dot in the opposite direction, again passing its equilibrium position. This type of simple harmonic motion continues until friction causes it to stop. The compressed areas of the spring, then, are termed compression, and the stretched areas, rarefaction.

It is important to realize that as the vibrating force transmits through the medium there is no net motion of the medium. The total displacement of the motion is confined to the molecular resting position. This will hold true as long as the force causing the compression and rarefaction does not exceed the elastic limit of the medium. This can be demonstrated in Hooke's law, which states that when a solid is deformed, it resists the deformation with a force proportional to the amount of deformation, provided the deformation is not too great. If the spring force is executed beyond its elastic limit, it will remain permanently deformed.

Sinusoidal motion

For ease of representation, consider a graph of the particle displacement (Fig. 1-4) along the y axis being represented in A+ or A− terms. This displacement will be plotted at a constant rate along the x axis (Fig. 1-5). If we consider that all motion in Fig. 1-5 has the same period of oscillation (T) and this is determined by the mass (m) of the vibrating particle and the force

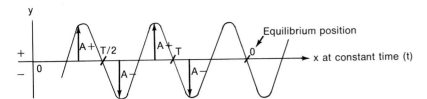

Fig. 1-6. Sinusoidal graph demonstrating changes of amplitude through period *T*.

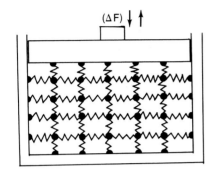

Fig. 1-7. Model demonstrating the effects of varying force on a molecular substance.

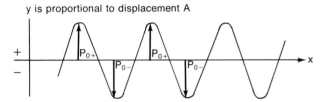

Fig. 1-8. Sinusoidal graph demonstrating variations in pressure as ultrasound propagates through tissue.

constant of the spring (k), we can then plot the graph in Fig. 1-6. This graph may be expressed mathematically with the equation

$$y = A \sin \sqrt{\frac{k}{m}} t$$

where y is the instantaneous displacement of the mass (m), equal to the maximum value (A) multiplied by a sinusoidally varying term related to the spring constant (k), the mass (m), and the time (t) from zero. This graph represents the sinusoidal function of the displacement at a specific frequency.

Pressure representation

Pressure can be described as the force acting on a fluid. In ultrasonic physical parameters, human tissue is considered to have the physical properties of a liquid medium.

Pressure (P) is defined as the magnitude of the normal force per unit surface area.

An oscillating transducer will apply a varying force (ΔF) over its cross-sectional area to the medium (ΔS)

with which it makes contact. This action can be represented as pressure, or force of the transducer (ΔF) displacing the particles of the medium, divided by its cross-sectional area (ΔS) of the medium. In other words

$$P = \frac{\Delta F}{\Delta S}$$

or pressure equals force divided by the area over which that force is applied.

Since tissue is considered to resemble liquid in its physical properties, liquid will be used as an example.

Imagine a container filled with water. The water molecules are bonded together by tiny springs. The fluid is at rest. A flat plunger of cross-sectional area (ΔS) is placed on top of the water within the container and a certain force (ΔF) is applied to it. This compresses the tiny connecting springs between the molecules a specific amount proportional to force ΔF. The water molecules, however, will create an equal and opposite force due to the constant of the compressed springs (Fig. 1-7). This force per unit area is termed pressure. By moving the plunger up and down at a constant rate, the resultant picture of the variation in pressure in the medium can be seen (Fig. 1-8). (NOTE: This applies to the pressure produced by the ultrasonic transducer on tissue particles.) Thus we have plotted a pressure gradient the maximum of which is at P_0+ and the minimum at P_0-. This corresponds to the particle displacement with amplitude (A). (See Fig. 1-6.) Pressure is used to describe sound waves because of its displacement characteristics on the medium.

Another graph can be plotted just below the pressure presentation depicting volume changes with pressure fluctuations (Fig. 1-9). It was stated earlier that as the spring in Fig. 1-4 was compressed, compression occurred, and as the spring was stretched, rarefaction occurred. As pressure propagates through a medium, the particles react to a change in volume according to the pressure gradient. As pressure reaches maximum (P_0+), compression occurs causing a small decrease in volume. As the pressure reaches (P_0-), the volume returns to normal. Pressure variations, then, are accompanied by a small change in the volume occupied by a given group of molecules.

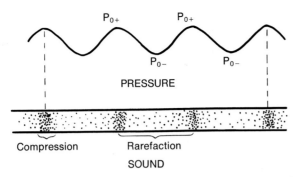

Fig. 1-9. Graph of pressure changes with volume fluctuating accordingly.

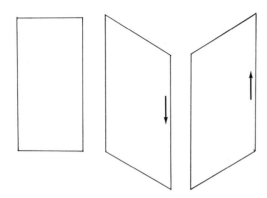

Fig. 1-10. Arrows indicate vectors of distortion in shear waves with the resulting deformation.

Longitudinal waves

It has been demonstrated that the vibrations of the source cause a propagatory wave perpendicular to the plane of the vibrating surface (Fig. 1-5). This then causes corresponding alternating compression and rarefaction of the particles in the direction of wave propagation.

This type of wave is called longitudinal, or compressional. In ultrasonics, where soft tissue is examined, longitudinal waves make up the largest percentage of the wave phenomenon.

Shear waves

It is also possible to propagate wave formations in parallel with the plane of the vibrating surface. This causes a shear stress motion to the particles of the medium rather than a vibrating motion in the longitudinal waveform (Fig. 1-10). Thus the wave phenomenon created here is termed shear wave, or transverse wave. To produce shear waves the medium must have the characteristics of a solid. Since soft tissue properties are considered very close to those of liquid, the shear wave phenomenon is not important to the ultrasonographer except for areas of bone, such as the skull.

ELASTICITY

Sound waves are called mechanical waves because they originate due to the displacement of some portion of an elastic medium from its normal position, causing the particle to oscillate about an equilibrium position. The medium transmitting a mechanical wave must have inertia and elasticity. Because of the elastic properties of the medium, the disturbance is transmitted from one particle to the next. Thus the wave propagates through the medium.

Elasticity is stated to be the ability of an object to return to its original size and shape after compression or stretching has occurred. Force and stress are therefore proportional up to a certain point (Hooke's law), which is $F = ky$. The elastic property of the material itself is known as the elastic modulus. Two types of elastic moduli that are important to the sonographer are Young's modulus and bulk modulus.

Young's modulus (stretch modulus)

The velocity of ultrasound depends on two important properties of the medium through which the ultrasound will travel—the elasticity or the stretch modulus (E) of the medium and the density of the medium, or mass per unit volume.

A change in the length of the spring (ΔL) is caused by a change in force (ΔF). This ratio ($\Delta F/\Delta L$) is a constant for any given spring. This is dependent, however, on the original length of the spring (L) and the cross-sectional area (D). Thus, if we consider springs of the same substance but different in cross section and length, the amount of stretch will be proportional to the original length of the spring, whereas the force required to stretch the spring any given length is proportional to the cross-sectional area.

Therefore stress, which is the change in force (ΔF) divided by the cross-sectional area (D), is equal to the stress modulus (E) times the strain ($\Delta L/L$):

$$\frac{\Delta F}{D} = E \frac{\Delta L}{L}$$

or

$$\text{Stress} = \text{Modulus} \times \text{Strain}$$

Stress is the force per unit of cross-sectional area and has the dimensions of pressure (P_0), whereas strain is the stretch per unit length.

E represents Young's modulus and is calculated by dividing the stretching stress ($\Delta F/D$) over the stretching strain ($\Delta L/L$). Thus Young's modulus (E) equals:

$$\frac{\text{Stretching stress}}{\text{Stretching strain}}$$

or

$$E = \frac{\Delta F/D}{\Delta L/L}$$

Elasticity (E) can be described as the amount of pressure ($\Delta F/D$) divided by the resultant percentage change in length ($\Delta L/L$) of the spring.

Bulk modulus

Consider a sound wave with a specific pressure (P_0). As the sound pressure is transmitted through tissue of specific volume (V), areas of compression occur causing a decrease in volume ($-\Delta V$) over that specific area.

This pressure-induced distortional decrease in volume with the ability to return to normal is known as its elastic modulus, or the bulk modulus.

Bulk modulus is defined as that increment in pressure (P_0) required to produce a corresponding fractional decrease in volume (V). Bulk modulus is determined by the increase in pressure ($+\Delta P_0$) over the decrease in volume ($-\Delta V$) divided by the original volume (V).

$$\text{Bulk modulus} = \frac{\text{Increase in pressure}}{\text{Decrease in volume}}$$

or

$$B = \frac{\Delta P_0}{-\Delta V/V}$$

Thus the elasticity (B) can be described as the amount of increase in pressure ($+\Delta P_0$) needed to change a specified volume ($-\Delta V$) divided by the percentage change in volume ($-\Delta V/V$).

Either of these two forms of elastic modulus, Young's modulus (E) or bulk modulus (B), can be used to describe the changes in length (ΔL) or volume ($-\Delta V$) of a specific material caused by a certain ultrasonic force (P_0). We can see the duality by the following equations:

$$\frac{\Delta F}{D} = \Delta P_0 \text{ and } \Delta L = -\Delta V$$

NOTE:

$$\text{Young's modulus} = \frac{\text{Stretching stress}}{\text{Stretching strain}}$$

whereas

$$\text{Bulk modulus} = \frac{\text{Volume stress}}{\text{Volume strain}}$$

Just as Young's modulus was previously used to describe the effect of the force acting on the spring constant in longitudinal wave propagation, bulk modulus applies to the description of areas of compression and rarefaction in the medium. Both elastic moduli describe physical effects to the medium from wave propagations.

DENSITY

Density is the mass per unit volume given in grams per cubic centimeter (g/cc). Density and elasticity must be considered together when establishing the velocity of ultrasound through a specific medium.

VELOCITY

Velocity of sound is affected by both the elasticity of the medium and the density of that medium.

The greater the elasticity of a medium, the tighter the bonds to the molecules. The strength with which these molecules are bonded together is determined by their connections of constant (k). The stronger the constant, the faster the molecules will oscillate about their resting position—thus the faster the ultrasonic velocity. For instance, consider a piece of plastic in which ultrasound has a velocity of 2500 m/sec and a piece of metal in which the velocity is 5000 m/sec. The elasticity of metal is greater than that of plastic.

Density plays a role in determining velocity as well. The denser the material, the slower the velocity for a given elasticity of the medium. But care must be used when applying these relationships. For instance, water has a density of 1.00×10^3 kilograms per cubic meter (kg/m^3) with a velocity of 1430 m/sec. Iron has a density approximately 7.6×10^3 kg/m^3 with a corresponding velocity of 5130 m/sec. The density of iron is far greater than that of water, which implies that the velocity of ultrasound in water would be faster than in iron; however, because of the elasticity of iron, the stronger the bonds between the molecules, the faster the velocity.

Table 1-2. Sound velocities

Material	Velocity (m/sec)
Air	332
Fat	1450
Human soft tissue (mean value)	1540
Brain	1541
Liver	1549
Vitreous humor of eye	1520
Kidney	1561
Spleen	1566
Blood	1570
Muscle	1585
Lens of eye	1620
Skull bone	4080

NOTE: Skull bone is approximately 3 times faster than soft tissue; air is approximately 4.5 times slower than soft tissue.

Therefore the velocity of sound through a specific medium must be estimated by calculating velocity (c) equal to the square root of the elasticity (E or B) divided by the density (P).

Using Young's modulus (E) for the elasticity, we can calculate $c = \sqrt{\dfrac{E}{P}}$. Thus velocity is a function of elasticity and density.

Table 1-2 gives velocities of ultrasound in various nonbiologic and biologic material at standard atmospheric pressure and temperature between 17° and 25° C.

To know the velocity of tissue is very important to the ultrasonographer for the following reasons.

1. The ultrasonic velocity through a tissue must be known to convert the pulse-echo time into depth of tissue by the machine.

2. Regions of two different velocities within a block of tissue can cause the beam to bend if they are crossed by the beam.

3. Velocity is a property of tissue and is actually a measure of tissue elasticity.

It is important to note that the medium itself does not move as a whole along with the wave motion; the various parts of the medium oscillate only in limited paths along the equilibrium position.

The energy in the waves is the sum of kinetic and potential energy of the matter, and the transmission of this total energy comes about by being passed along one part of the matter to the next. Long-range motion of the matter, however, does not exist.

One more point to consider is that simple harmonic oscillation is a conservative system. No dissipative forces act on the system, so the total mechanical energy is conserved.

The formula for kinetic energy (K) is one half the mass times the velocity squared ($K = \frac{1}{2}mv^2$). If this were plotted along a sinusoidal graph against potential energy (U), which is $U = \frac{1}{2}kx^2$, or one half the force constant times the amount of displacement (x), a graph such as that in Fig. 1-11 would result.

It can be seen that kinetic energy and potential energy are equal and opposite to each other; however, their sum is equal to the total energy of the system and has a value of one half the force constant times the maximum displacement (A).

$$\Sigma E = \frac{1}{2}kA^2$$

and

$$K + U = \frac{1}{2}mv^2 + \frac{1}{2}kx^2 = \frac{1}{2}kA^2$$

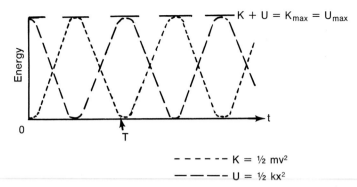

$$K + U = K_{max} = U_{max}$$

$- - - - -$ $K = \frac{1}{2}mv^2$
$- \cdot - \cdot -$ $U = \frac{1}{2}kx^2$

Fig. 1-11. Graph depicting the kinetic energy (short dashes) and the potential energy (long dashes). Note that the two are equal but in opposite phase, making up the sum of total energy.

Therefore the total energy of a particle executing simple harmonic motion is proportional to the square of the amplitude of motion.

WAVELENGTH

The frequency, as stated before, is the number of oscillations a particle performs per unit time with respect to the associated pressure wave (Fig. 1-1).

The wavelength (λ) of ultrasound is defined with respect to the associated pressure wave. It is determined by the distance from one pressure wave peak to the next.

Wavelength plays an important role in determining ultrasonic beam width and pulse length and thus will greatly influence resolving capabilities of the ultrasonic machine.

The relationship of wavelength (λ), frequency (f) and velocity (c) of the ultrasound is represented in the following equation:

$$c = f\lambda$$

Since velocity of ultrasound in soft tissue is a relative constant (mean value 1540 m/sec), the wavelength for a given frequency can be calculated by the following equation:

$$\lambda = \frac{c}{f}$$

Wavelength of a 2 MHz sound source propagating in soft tissue with a mean velocity of 1540 m/sec is calculated as follows:

$$\lambda = c/f$$
$$\lambda = \frac{1540 \text{ m/sec}}{2 \text{ MHz}}$$
$$\lambda = \frac{1540}{2 \times 10^6} \text{ m}$$
$$\lambda = 770 \times 10^{-6} \text{ m}$$
$$\lambda = 770 \times 10^{-3} \text{ mm}$$
$$\lambda = 0.770 \text{ mm}$$

Various wavelengths of given frequencies follow:

2 MHz	$\lambda = 0.77$ mm
5 MHz	$\lambda = 0.31$ mm
10 MHz	$\lambda = 0.15$ mm
15 MHz	$\lambda = 0.10$ mm
20 MHz	$\lambda = 0.08$ mm

Note that as frequency increases the wavelength becomes smaller. This results in better image detail at higher frequencies.

CHARACTERISTIC ACOUSTIC IMPEDANCE

Impedance is a general term used to state the characteristics of a specific elastic medium. Acoustic impedance affects the sound pressure as it propagates through tissue.

The amount of impedance (Z) is governed by two variables: (1) the elasticity and (2) the density. If this seems familiar, it is because velocity is also affected by the same two factors. Their relationship, however, which can be seen in the accompanying equation, is somewhat different.

The characteristic acoustic impedance of a medium can be calculated by taking the square root of the product of the elasticity times the density.

$$Z = \sqrt{EP}$$

Imagine two blocks of a homogeneous isotropic material placed side by side with only a potential space between them. With a change in either the elasticity or the density of either one of the materials there will be a mismatch of impedance of the two media. This means that the sum of the energy ($\frac{1}{2}KA^2$) in the first medium will not be the same under identical factors as it is transferred to the second medium. This results in a transfer of energy with a different pressure value (P_2) than before (P_0). Since energy cannot be destroyed, the difference in energy will be reflected away from the boundary in a direction equal to that of the angle of the original pressure wave.

The amount of reflected wave is said to be the pressure reflection coefficient and occurs when pressure through a specific medium (Z_1) is passed to another medium (Z_2) with either a difference in elasticity or density. This causes a resultant reflected wave (r) with a different pressure wave (P_2).

The reflection coefficient is calculated as the impedance of the second medium minus that of the first medium over the sum of the two impedances.

$$r = \frac{\sqrt{EP_1} - \sqrt{EP_2}}{\sqrt{EP_2} + \sqrt{EP_1}}$$

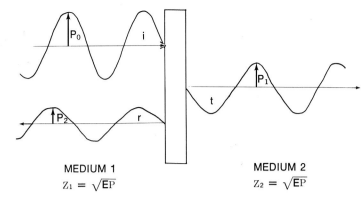

Fig. 1-12. Model demonstrating the reflected (*r*) and transmitted (*t*) waves on hitting and the flat interface with the incident wave (*i*) at 90°. Note variations in pressure.

Table 1-3. Amplitude ratios and percentage energies at tissue interfaces

Reflecting interface	Amplitude ratio (P_2/P_0)	Energy reflected (%)
Fat-muscle	0.10	1.08
Muscle-blood	0.03	0.07
Bone-fat	0.69	48.91
Soft tissue–water	0.05	0.23
Soft tissue–air	0.9995	99.9
Soft tissue–castor oil	0.06	0.43

or

$$r = \frac{Z_2 - Z_1}{Z_2 + Z_1}$$

Thus characteristic acoustic impedance can be evaluated by the equation $Z = \sqrt{EP}$, whereas the effect of the mismatch between the two media can be stated as

$$r = \frac{Z_2 - Z_1}{Z_2 + Z_1}.$$

It can be seen from the previous information that the pressure reflection coefficient is then defined as the ratio of the peak pressure in the reflected wave to the peak pressure in the incident wave.

The type of reflection shown in Fig. 1-12 is specular, or mirrorlike, reflection. This type is seen on the ultrasound machine as a very heavy or dark echo. The interface is examined at right angles to the transducer sound beam.

The possible differences in the acoustic impedance of a particular tissue are important in the detection of disease within a certain organ. Imagine a liver with a lesion deep within the parenchyma. The ability to detect that lesion will depend on the difference in either the elasticity or density from that of normal liver tissue. Without a significant difference in the acoustic impedance this lesion will not be detected with present ultrasonic systems.

In Table 1-3, note the amount of reflection occurring from the interface of air to soft tissue. Virtually all the sound striking the interface is reflected away from it.

The reflection of air causes a tremendous problem in clinical ultrasound. Because of virtually total reflection, air-filled lung and gas-filled intestinal gut cannot be examined. This also demonstrates the need for a coupling agent to prevent air from getting between the sound source and the skin.

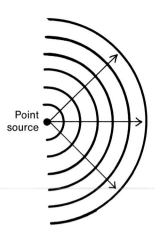

Fig. 1-13. Spherical waves radiating from a point source.

REFLECTION AND REFRACTION
Huygens' principle

As stated before, the amount of reflection (r) will be determined by the difference between the two impedances (Z) of the tissue layers.

Huygens' principle allows prediction of a new wave front when the position of an earlier one is known. Wave front is a generalized term used to describe points on a wave, the phase of motion of which is constant.

Waves in which disturbances are propagated in a single direction are termed plane waves. Plane waves at a given instant are the same everywhere on any plane perpendicular to the direction of propagation.

If the propagation fans out in all directions from a point source, the waves are termed spherical. Here the disturbance created by the wave front radiates in all directions (Fig. 1-13).

Consider every point on the wave front as the source of a small wavelet that spreads in a forward direction away from the original source. By enveloping all the preceding wavelets, a line across them corresponding to a new wave front is created (Fig. 1-14).

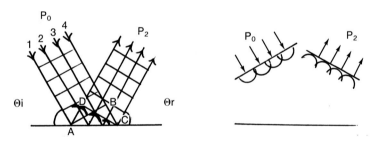

Fig. 1-14. Model demonstrating Huygens' principle.

Huygens' principle states simply that all points on a wave front can be considered as point sources for the production of spherical secondary wavelets.

As stated earlier, if there is reflection from a flat plane with the incident sound beam (P_0) at right angles to the plane surface, the reflected sound wave (P_2) will be reflected in like manner 90° away from the plane surface, with a resultant transmitted wave (P_1) continuing 90° away from the plane surface but in a direction opposite to that of P_2 (Fig. 1-12). Incident wave fronts occurring at a specific angle (Θ), however, will change the angle at which the reflected wave will go.

Consider what will happen to the reflected wave (with angle Θr) as the incident wave (i) strikes the interface at a specific angle (Θi) (Figs. 1-15 and 1-16). Note that the angle of the reflected wave (P_2) is at the same angle (Θi) as the incident wave (P_0). Thus Θi and Θr are equal but opposite in direction. Referring to

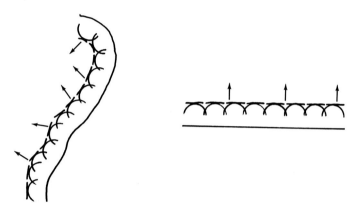

Fig. 1-15. Huygens' principle applied to the incident and reflected sound beams.

Huygens' principle (Fig. 1-15), the wave front A-B is perpendicular to the incoming sound energy 1-2-3-4.

While energy 4 is traveling from B to C, energy 1 spreads out in a sphere with a radius of AD. Hence AD = BC. According to Huygens' principle, the reflected wave front is CD, which is a surface line to all the wavelets in that reflected wave.

Refraction of the sound wave occurs because the velocity is different for each material. As sound is transmitted, the different velocities govern the degree of its angle (Θt) (Fig. 1-17). If the velocity of medium

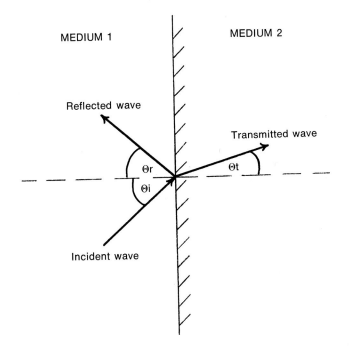

Fig. 1-16. Relationship between the incident, reflected, and transmitted waves. (From Goldberg, B. B., Kotler, M. N., Ziskin, M., and Waxham, R. D.: Diagnostic uses of ultrasound, New York, 1975; Grune & Stratton, Inc. Used by permission.)

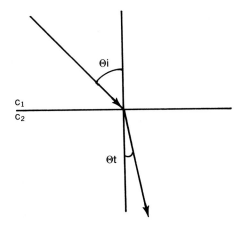

Fig. 1-17. Angular difference of the incident wave to the transmitted wave because of the variations in velocity (c) from one medium to the next.

2 is slower than that of medium 1, the sound, or transmitted wave, will bend in a negative direction $(-\Theta t)$ to that of the incident angle (Θi). With the velocity of medium 1 slower than that of medium 2, the angle of the transmitted wave will be greater $(+\Theta t)$ than the incident angle. Again, Huygens' principle of wavelet theory applies to the transmitted wave as well.

Snell's law

Beam bending occurs if part of the wave crest in medium 2 has a different velocity $(-c$ or $+c)$ from that of the first medium.

We can calculate the angle of the transmitted wave by Snell's law, which follows:

$$\frac{\text{Sin } \Theta t}{\text{Sin } \Theta r} = \frac{c_2}{c_1} = \text{Acoustic refractive index}$$

This demonstrates that the ratio of the angle of the transmitted wave to the reflected wave is equal to the change in velocity between Z_2 and Z_1.

It is important to note that so far all reflecting surfaces discussed have been flat planes, and therefore the reflection and refraction have specular characteristics. For rough and irregular surfaces, however, the situation becomes quite complicated. The total reflection of a wave is then determined by the difference in impedance and the amount of incident angle. Reflection will be greatest at right angles to the plane surface (specular reflection).

ULTRASONIC BEAM PARAMETERS
Cylindrical radiation

In medical ultrasonics the sound source, that is, the active crystal of the transducer, is circular with a specific radius (R). Thus the actual ultrasonic beam is cylindrical in radiation. As the sound is emitted from the source, the beam is a circular cylinder corresponding to the diameter of the crystal propagating further into a diverging cone.

Huygens' principle states that any wave phenomenon can be analyzed by the addition of contributions from some distribution of simple sources properly selected in phase and amplitude to represent the physical situation.

Consider a flat circular piston with radius R vibrating along the z axis and producing ultrasonic radiation of wave pressure (Fig. 1-18). If the crystal is divided into a number of small elements, analysis of the radiation from these elements will show that summation of these sources creates a beam that is approximately cylindrical. However, the sound pressure will become acoustically complex because of the superimposition of wavelets from different wave fronts. This causes pressure to increase (maxima) and decrease (minima) dramatically at specific distances along the z axis.

The actual pressure at a certain point along the z axis is calculated by subdividing the wave front into an infinite number of point sources (Huygens' principle) and superimposing the wave or pressure disturbances at a certain point (x_1) along the z axis. The exact problem is quite complicated, but an understanding of the physical problem can be gained from the following example.

Imagine that as sound leaves the transducer, the cylindrical pressure radiation is not a constant. The

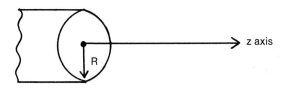

Fig. 1-18. Radius (R) of the circular transducer with the z axis of propagation extending outward.

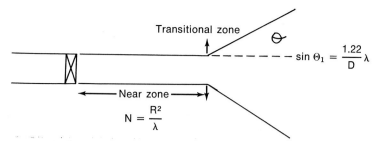

Fig. 1-20. Near and far fields with their corresponding calculations.

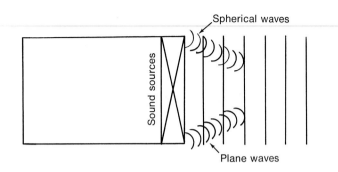

Fig. 1-19. Spherical waves emitted from the transducer edges cause interference of the planar waves.

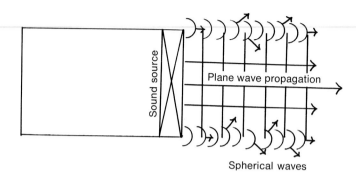

Fig. 1-21. Interference of the spherical waves with planar waves.

plane waves being generated by the central axis of the transducer (z) are affected by spherical waves being emitted from the edges of the transducer. Thus we can imagine a situation occurring similar to that in Fig. 1-19. Note that wave fronts from the spherical waves interfere with the wave fronts of the plane waves. Thus the two different wave fronts vary in their phases, causing dramatic differences in pressure until the effect of the transducer edges and thus the spherical wave front becomes less pronounced farther along the z axis. This allows the sound emitted from the edges to be more or less parallel with the plane wave front, causing little interference. For sake of simplicity the area of little interference is known as the transitional zone. In the actual physical problem, however, this does not occur abruptly.

The area between the transducer and the transitional zone is termed the near field, or Fresnel zone, and the area beyond the transitional zone is termed the far field, or Fraunhofer zone.

Near field

The extent of the near field (N) is calculated by squaring the radius of the crystal (R^2) and dividing it by the wavelength, as depicted in Fig. 1-20.

$$N = \frac{R^2}{\lambda}$$

The near field is referred to as the confusion zone because of the dramatic differences in pressure that occur there. Interference of pressure is caused by superimposition of two or more wave trains with the same frequency, amplitude, and velocity but different in phase.

The pressure of a sound source with wave interference problems as shown in Fig. 1-21 can be plotted at certain points x_1 and x_2 along the z axis of propagation. Imagine that both spherical and plane waves are emitted from the transducer with the same frequency and amplitude (pressure) but with a phase difference between them. (This is not absolute but will help in the explanation of the physical problem.) As the spherical waves meet the plane waves at point x_1, the total wave will be a result of the superimposition of the two. This new wave will have the same frequency but will differ in amplitude from the original.

With the superimposition occurring at point x_1, if the phase difference is very small (compared to 180°), the resultant amplitude will be approximately twice that of either component wave. The two components (S and W) are said to be in phase with each other, causing constructive interference with a resulting increase of twice that of the initial components. This creates an increase in pressure; thus an area of maxima has been produced (Fig. 1-22).

If point x is moved a finite distance away from the transducer to point x_2 along the z axis, a new situation is evident. If the resultant waves of S and W now have a large phase difference (near 180°), the resultant amplitude will be near zero (Fig. 1-23). The resultant superimposition of the waves at point x_2 causes them to be out of phase with each other and produces de-

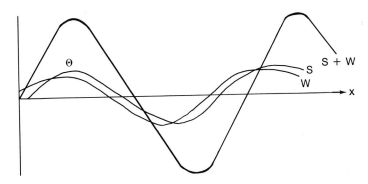

Fig. 1-22. Wave amplitude (heavy line) resulting from the constructive interferences of waves *S* and *W*.

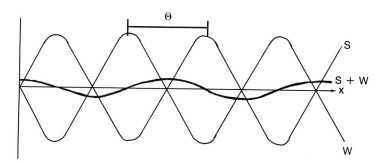

Fig. 1-23. Wave amplitude (heavy line) resulting from destructive interference of waves *S* and *W*.

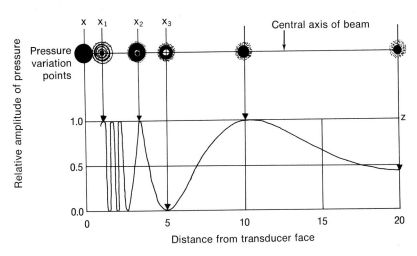

Fig. 1-24. Variation of intensity plotted in the near field.

structive interference that results in a decrease in pressure—an area of minima.

The number of points, e.g., x_1, x_2, x_3, are infinite along the z axis. The resulting maxima and minima occur rapidly near the transducer face and decrease in their pressure variations farther from the transducer until the distance ($N = R^2/\lambda$) has been reached where interference of spherical waves and plane waves no longer occurs. They transform again into planar waves at a constant pressure Pi.

The pressure on the z axis at distance $N = R^2/\lambda$ is made up of contributions of an infinite number of point sources. Each of these points varies in its pressure profile (Pi) a distance *x* from the transducer face. Each of the pressure variations can be calculated by the following equation:

$$Pi = P_0 \sin\left[2\pi\left(\frac{x - \Theta i}{\lambda}\right)\right]$$

where

P_0 is the initial pressure
x   is the distance from the transducer face
Θi is the initial phase due to different paths from the transducer to point *x*
λ is the wavelength

The individual pressure can be summed up to calculate the total pressure. Thus $\Sigma Pi = P_T$.

Far field

The far field, or Fraunhofer zone, is characterized by uniform pressure across the sound field. As the far field occurs, the amplitude of the peak acoustic pressure diminishes at increasing distances from the transitional zone. Note also (Fig. 1-20) that the beam begins to diverge from this point with an increase in its size as it progresses away from the transitional zone.

The divergence of the far field (sin Θ) is calculated as 1.22 times the wavelength divided by the diameter of the transducer.

Thus $\sin \Theta = \dfrac{1.22\lambda}{D}$.

The graph in Fig. 1-24 illustrates the concept of near and far fields, with resulting pressure variations. Again, remember that the calculations are not absolute where an actual physical problem is concerned. The true problem is quite complex, but the previous explanation should provide a basic understanding.

INTENSITY

It has been shown that the oscillating particle corresponds to the amount of displacement about the resting position, and the pressure corresponds to the displacement.

At maximum displacement (A_0), maximum pressure will be attained and is related to the intensity of the ultrasonic irradiation. Thus the greater the amplitude (a_0), the greater the pressure (P_0) and intensity (I).

The energy (e) of a particle oscillating with simple harmonic motion is the sum of its kinetic energy and potential energy. That is, the energy is related to the particle's instantaneous velocity and its displacement from its resting position and can be described by the following equation:

$$e = \tfrac{1}{2}mv^2 + \tfrac{1}{2}kx^2$$

where

> v = instantaneous velocity of the particle
> x = instantaneous displacement of the particle

The total number of particles per unit volume, as related to the mean density (P), can also help in calculating the corresponding total energy (T_E) of all the particles in that unit volume ($\Sigma e = T_E$). This energy (T_E) has both kinetic and potential terms, as noted in the previous equation. The kinetic term is related to the mean density (P) and mean particle velocity (v), whereas the potential term is related to the pressure (P) and wave velocity (c). Remember that the pressure is related to the mean displacement of the particle within the value (P). The total energy for a given volume becomes:

$$T_E = \tfrac{1}{2}\,\rho v^2 + \tfrac{1}{2}\,\frac{P^2}{P_0 c^2} \text{ in joules/cc}$$

The energy traveling through the medium, with the wave velocity and the total energy that passes through a unit volume in unit time, is defined as intensity of the wave.

Assuming that energy travels through the medium with a wave velocity, intensity can be regarded as $I = c\,(T_E)$ or W/cm². (A watt [W] equals a joule/sec.) Intensity can then be defined in the following manner:

$$I = \frac{cm}{sec} \times \frac{joule}{cc}$$

$$I = \frac{joule}{sec} \times \frac{1}{cm^2}$$

(If watt $= \dfrac{joule}{sec}$, then $I = $ W/cm².)

Intensity is described as watts per square centimeter (W/cm²). This is measured by rate of flow of energy (watts) through 1 centimeter squared of material held at right angles to the beam at that point. As the intensity of a wave increases, the pressure exerted on a particle and its corresponding displacement will similarly increase.

In the metric system the watt is a mechanical unit used to describe the rate at which work is done (watt = joule/sec). This is otherwise known as power. For smaller quantities of power the milliwatt (mW), which is equal to 1/1000 of a watt, may be used.

Ultrasonic power

The terms power and intensity are often used interchangeably. This, however, is incorrect, even though they are related.

As we have seen previously, intensity is W/cm² and in ultrasound pertains to the rate of flow of energy (joule/sec) through the unit area. Power is defined as the time rate at which work is done. The average power delivered by an agent, in this case the transducer, is the total work (W) done by the agent divided by the total time (t). Thus $p = $ W/t.

Intensity is equal to the velocity, or rate of flow, times the total energy.

$$I = cT_E$$

or

$$W/cm^2$$

Power, however, is equal to the work divided by the time taken to do the work.

Ultrasonic power (W) is calculated by the rate of flow of energy (W/cm²) times the whole cross-sectional area of the beam.

Ultrasonic power (W) = Ultrasonic intensity (W/cm²) × cross-sectional area of the beam (cm²)

It is important to remember that power stays constant throughout the beam dimensions. However, the intensity will vary depending on the cross-sectional area. To change the intensity, the cross-sectional area of the beam must be changed, for example, focusing the sound beam or changing the power. Thus intensity is equal to the power over the cross-sectional area.

$$I = \frac{Power}{Area} = \frac{W}{cm^2}$$

Decibel (dB) notation

In a comparison of two intensity levels the ratio can vary over a wide range, and the logarithm of this ratio is a convenient way to express the comparison.

Logarithms are commonly used in engineering to simplify mathematical computations. There are numerous systems (or bases) of logarithms that can be used. The common logarithm, that is, the logarithm to the base 10, is used most frequently.

The common logarithm of a number is the exponent (or power) to which 10 (the base) must be raised to produce the original number. For example, the logarithm of 100 is equal to 2, since 10^2 (or 10×10) is equal to 100. The logarithm of 1000 is equal to 3, since 10^3 (or

$10 \times 10 \times 10$) is equal to 1000. These two logarithms are expressed in the following manner:

$$\log 100 = 2$$
$$\log 1000 = 3$$

In ultrasound the ratio of two intensities is expressed in a unit called the decibel (dB). The number of decibels equals ten times the logarithm of the ratio of the two intensity levels.

$$dB = 10 \log (I_1/I_2)$$

I_1 could be the maximum intensity of the ultrasonic beam relative to the intensity of the returning echo (I_2). Since decibel indicates the ratio between two quantities, it does not express any definite amount of intensity. To associate a decibel value with a specific amount of intensity, it is necessary to establish a reference.

When it is necessary to compare the strength of an echo (reflected wave) to that of the incident wave, it is usually more convenient to measure their amplitudes or pressures rather than their intensities. In this case the number of decibels equals twenty times the logarithm of the ratio of the two amplitude levels. Since the intensity ratio is the pressure ratio squared,

$$dB = 20 \log \left(\frac{A_1}{A_2} \right)$$

ATTENUATION (ENERGY DIMINUTION THROUGH TISSUE)

The intensity of a wave of ultrasound traveling through a medium may be decreased by a number of different mechanisms. The reduction in pressure and/or intensity through tissue is known as attenuation and is affected by phenomena such as scattering, absorption, reflection, refraction, and beam divergence.

An echo returning to the transducer in the pulse-echo technique must undergo the same attenuation properties that its primary incident wave, emitted by the transducer, underwent to reach the reflective interface to produce the echo. This returning echo is, however, under far less pressure intensity.

Reflections close to the receiver or transducer will be detected far better than those arising from interfaces deep within the body. To compensate for this attenuation in depth of tissue, a time-varied gain control is placed in the ultrasonic system and aids in detection of minute intensity echoes arising from deep structures. This time-varied gain mechanism will be discussed later in the chapter.

Scattering

For reflection to occur, as in the case of Huygens' principle, in reflected and refracted waveforms, the reflecting surface must be larger than several wavelengths of the incident energy. If the ultrasonic sound energy were to strike surface dimensions smaller than the incident wavelength, the incident wave would be scattered in all directions.

This is known as Rayleigh scattering. Rayleigh scattering occurs when an ultrasonic beam strikes biologic materials such as blood cells, protein compounds, and various collagens. These and many other body tissues and organs create scattering of ultrasonic energy and cause attenuation of the ultrasonic beam.

The intensity of Rayleigh scattering has been found to be dependent on (1) the acoustic impedance change at the target or particle itself, (2) the size of the particle, and (3) the wavelength of the incident energy. The intensity of the scattered wave increases rapidly with frequency and is proportional to the square of the frequency. Therefore high-frequency sounds are scattered more readily than are low-frequency sounds.

Absorption

As the ultrasonic wave propagates through tissue, it transfers to the particles of the tissue increased energy in the form of orderly vibrations. Absorption of the ultrasonic beam traversing through tissue takes place by some orderly vibrational energy being transferred into random molecular motions, which creates an internal transfer of molecular energy to heat.

As the ultrasonic wave passes through an absorbing medium, its intensity and amplitude decrease exponentially. The graph in Fig. 1-25 represents an expo-

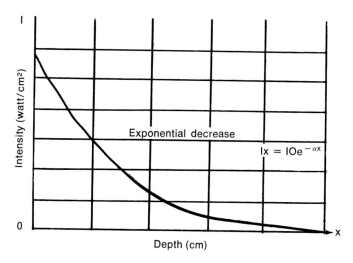

Fig. 1-25. Exponential decrease in intensity per unit depth (x).

nential decrease in beam intensity (plotted along the y axis) to an increase depth in specific tissue (plotted along the x axis). The amount of intensity per unit depth (I_x) is determined by the equation

$$I_x = I_0 e^{-\alpha x}$$

where

I_0 = original intensity
e = 2.71828 (mathematically derived number)
$-\alpha$ = absorption coefficient
x = distance in depth (cm)

The rate of fall of intensity is determined by the total absorption coefficient α. The larger the absorption coefficient of a particular tissue, the faster the decrease in intensity. The amount of absorption of α is determined by the number and the strength of the absorbent particles and is dependent on the frequency of the ultrasonic energy.

One of the mechanisms for determining absorption is the relaxation mechanism. The relaxation mechanism refers to the transfer of energy from one source to another, causing a fluctuation of kinetic energy ultimately reducing particle velocity. This causes a decrease in wave intensity.

Various types of relaxation processes occur, including the following:

1. The process of transfer of energy to internal molecular energy and back is known as thermal relaxation.

2. The transfer of energy in the form of heat going from one area to another and back is termed conductional relaxation.

3. The transfer of energy and back between two different physical structures is known as structural relaxation.

All these various forms will ultimately cause a decrease in intensity of the initial energy.

Another means of absorption is friction between moving particles. The medium tends to oppose the vibrational motion of the particles due to a resistance offered by a fluid (in this case soft tissue) and changes in form or position because of the attraction of molecules to each other. Energy is thus dissipated in driving the molecules through each wave cycle. This is known as viscosity. Because the medium tends to oppose the vibrational motion of the particles, some of this energy is converted to heat.

The relaxation mechanism, viscosity, and heat are called true absorbers and are frequency dependent. Absorption, then, is frequency dependent. The higher the frequency of the ultrasound, the higher the fluctuation in the transfer of energy. This creates a larger decrease in particle velocity and thus an increase in the absorption taking place. This is why any frequency above 20 MHz cannot be used normally for clinical practice in ultrasonic imaging.

Reflection and refraction

Nonabsorbers related to attenuation of the beam are reflection and refraction, which cause a decrease in intensity of the incident ultrasound. Beam divergence related to the Fraunhofer zone causes a decrease in intensity due to an increase in the cross-sectional area of the beam.

GENERATION OF ULTRASONIC WAVES
Piezoelectric effect

An application of a deformation force or strain to an asymmetric crystal such as quartz, tourmaline, or Rochelle salt will create an electric voltage (Fig. 1-26). This phenomenon is called the piezoelectric effect.

In ultrasound a more standardized piezoelectric effect can be obtained by the use of man-made ceramics. Some of the materials used include lead zirconate, lead metaniobate, and barium titanate.

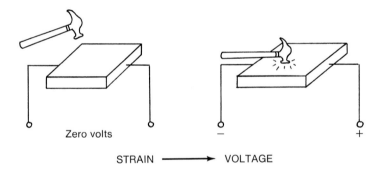

Fig. 1-26. Strain by the hammer (mechanical deformation) on the crystal creates a voltage. (From Goldberg, B. B., Kotler, M. N., Ziskin, M., and Waxham, R. D.: Diagnostic uses of ultrasound, New York, 1975, Grune & Stratton, Inc. Used by permission.)

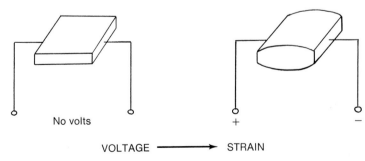

Fig. 1-27. Effect of an applied voltage on the crystal creates a mechanical deformation, thus producing sound. (From Goldberg, B. B., Kotler, M. N., Ziskin, M., and Waxham, R. D.: Diagnostic uses of ultrasound, New York, 1975, Grune & Stratton, Inc. Used by permission.)

In clinical practice the piezoelectric effect takes place as the echo returning from the reflective interface strikes the crystal and creates an electric voltage that is processed by the ultrasound equipment.

Reverse piezoelectric effect

Reverse piezoelectric effect simply means that if a voltage is applied to the crystal, a deformation or strain will take place (Fig. 1-27). This deformation creates sound at a certain frequency, and the frequency is dependent on the thickness of the crystal when manufactured.

Transducer construction

A device capable of converting energy from one form to another is called a transducer. In ultrasound the transducer, when used as a transmitting device, converts electrical energy to mechanical energy (reverse piezoelectric effect). When it is used as a receiving device, mechanical energy is converted to electrical energy (piezoelectric effect). Fig. 1-28 is a basic diagram of an ultrasound transducer. The diagram shows the piezoelectric material with electrodes on both sides. The electrodes are connected to the electrical source by means of wires and a connector. The backing material absorbs sound energy that is directed backward and also helps to provide focusing of the forward energy. Without a backing the crystal would ring for a long period of time. This is undesirable because the transducer must be prepared to accept returning echoes. Fig. 1-29 shows actual medical ultrasonic transducers.

The ultrasonic beam

With every increasing clinical application of ultrasound, sound waves of different characteristics are required to optimize the display for different types of studies. Major parameters of primary concern are frequency, diameter of transducer face, and focusing.

The amount of diffraction or divergence of the beam is related to (1) the diameter of the crystal and (2) the frequency of the sound beam. The diameter of the sound source governs the diameter of the sound beam and resulting divergence (Fig. 1-30). The larger the diameter the greater will be the depth that the sound beam will go before diverging. Since divergence is a factor in attenuation, this will allow greater concentrations of sound to deeper depths into the patient.

As the frequency increases, the ultrasound beam becomes more directional; however, the penetrating ability is decreased. Commonly used ultrasound frequencies are 1.0, 1.6, 2.25, 3.5, 5.0, and 10.0 MHz.

For each frequency there is a minimum diameter below which good beam properties are difficult to obtain. Typical transducer face diameters are 3, 6, 13, and 19 mm. The small diameters are normally found in the higher-frequency transducers and the larger diameters in lower-frequency transducers.

Resolution

Resolution is the ability to define two objects as distinct entities, that is, the greater the resolution, the closer the two objects can be seen together.

In ultrasound there are two types of resolving qualities that must be considered: lateral and axial.

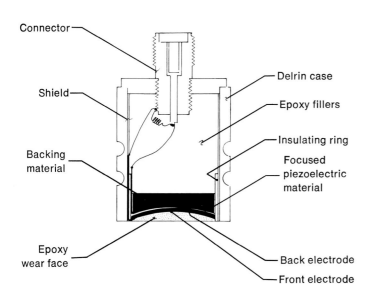

Fig. 1-28. "A" cross section of a medical transducer. (Courtesy KB-Aerotech, Lewistown, Pa.)

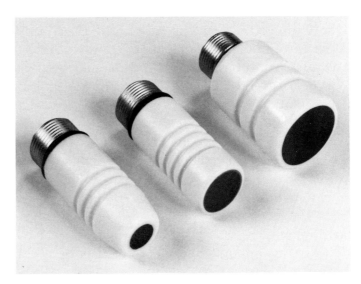

Fig. 1-29. Types of medical ultrasound transducers. (Courtesy KB-Aerotech, Lewistown, Pa.)

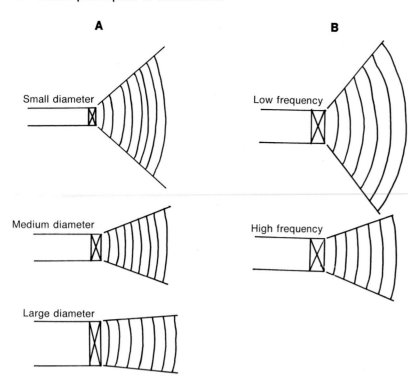

Fig. 1-30. A, Note change in divergence of the ultrasound beam with a change in the diameter of the crystal. **B,** Beam divergence with different frequency transducers. Note, however, that the diameter of the crystal has stayed the same.

Lateral resolution. Lateral, or azimuthal, resolution is the ability to distinguish objects in a line perpendicular to the axis of the sound beam. It is a measure of two objects when they are barely distinguishable by the sound beam (Fig. 1-31).

Lateral resolution is inversely proportional to the beam width, which will depend on (1) the diameter of the crystal, (2) the frequency of sound emitted by the crystal, and (3) the distance from the source at which the beam intersects the two objects. If the beam is too wide and the transducer is passed across a small echo-producing interface, the resulting echo will be as wide as the beam rather than the actual size of the structure to be sounded (Fig. 1-32). Lateral resolution can be improved with the use of focused transducers.

Axial resolution. Axial resolution is the ability to distinguish two objects on a line parallel with the sound beam axis (Fig. 1-33). The theoretical limit for axial resolution is the wavelength of the ultrasound emitted by the crystal. However, there are many factors that affect axial resolution capabilities.

In the pulse-echo technique not only the sound wavelength emitted from the crystal but also the duration of the emission or pulse must be considered. The longer the pulse, the smaller the axial resolving capabilities.

Thus the wavelength and the emitted pulse width, which is equal to and usually greater than the wavelength, determine the theoretical limit for axial resolution. The returning echo must be considered,

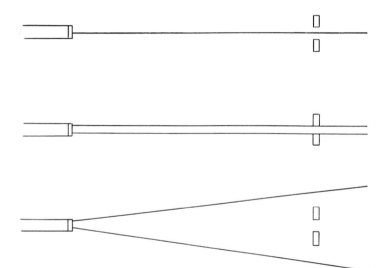

Fig. 1-31. Beam divergence and its effect on lateral resolution. (From Goldberg, B. B., Kotler, M. N., Ziskin, M., and Waxham, R. D.: Diagnostic uses of ultrasound, New York, 1975, Grune & Stratton, Inc. Used by permission.)

however, when discussing actual resolving capabilities of the machine. The pulsed wave striking the interface will reflect having a different wavelength, depending on the acoustic impedance and the angle of incidence. This returning wave pocket will then be processed by the receiver. Crystal and receiver characteristics typically limit the axial resolution to between three and five times the wavelength. Thus, if we consider the theoretical axial resolution of a 1 MHz transducer to be 1 mm, the actual resolutions will typically be 3 to 5 mm.

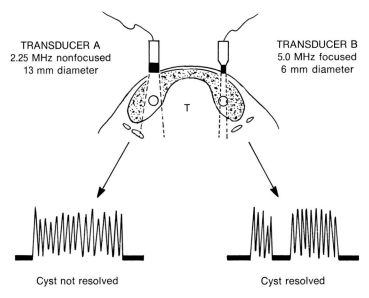

TRANSDUCER A
2.25 MHz nonfocused
13 mm diameter

TRANSDUCER B
5.0 MHz focused
6 mm diameter

Cyst not resolved

Cyst resolved

Fig. 1-32. Demonstration of the effects of beam focusing and smaller diameter transducer on lateral resolution. (From Goldberg, B. B., Kotler, M. N., Ziskin, M., and Waxham, R. D.: Diagnostic uses of ultrasound, New York, 1975, Grune & Stratton, Inc. Used by permission.)

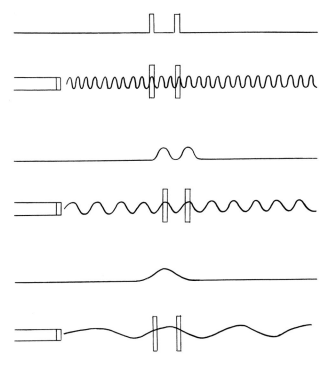

Fig. 1-33. Demonstration of wavelength and its effect on theoretical axial resolution. (From Goldberg, B. B., Kotler, M. N., Ziskin, M., and Waxham, R. D.: Diagnostic uses of ultrasound, New York, 1975, Grune & Stratton, Inc. Used by permission.)

The design of the crystal will affect axial resolution. The ability of the transducer to emit a specific pulse and to be quickly damped will determine the pulse width and thus affect axial resolution. The type of epoxy used for the manufacturing of the crystal, the housing, the damping material, and the construction of the crystal will then affect the pulse width and thus

axial resolution. The ability of the receiver to process the information coming back and the way the information is processed will also affect axial resolution. Thus the receiver-crystal combination is important when considering axial resolution and sensitivity of the machine.

Focusing

By the use of either an internal or external acoustic lens or by shaping the piezoelectric material, it is possible to shape the ultrasound beam pattern. This is called focusing.

The physics of focused ultrasound beams are similar to the physics of optical focusing, for example, a simple magnifying glass.

Through focusing the ultrasonic beam is narrowed to a "waist" at a specific point along the propagating path. This allows for maximum lateral resolution at the "waist spot" and for a focal zone about this spot of focus.

One important result of focusing the ultrasonic beam is the increase in ultrasonic intensity. At any given transverse section along the ultrasonic beam the power will be the same, regardless of attenuation; however, because of the reduced area at the focal spot, the intensity will be greatly increased. This is important when considering dosage levels.

One of the benefits of focusing the sound beam is a reduction in the length of the near field intensity variation. This allows for improvement of the image below the transducer face. For example, a transducer with a diameter of 20 mm uses a frequency of 2.25 MHz with a corresponding wavelength of approximately 0.75 mm. These figures correspond to the average abdominal transducer used in contact B scanning today.

By calculating the near zone of the sound beam with the equation $N = R^2/\lambda$, it can be seen that the confusion zone is approximately 14 cm in length. Thus the length of the near zone for the typical abdominal transducer is the thickness for an average patient. One can see from this example that the sonographer, with an unfocused transducer, will operate in the near field continually.

If the sound beam of this particular transducer is focused, the length of the near field intensity variation will be reduced and create a clearer image due to a decrease in the effects of the near zone.

Therefore focusing the beam does three things: (1) most importantly, it increases the ability to distinguish structures perpendicular to the sound beam, thus increasing lateral resolution; (2) it increases intensity to

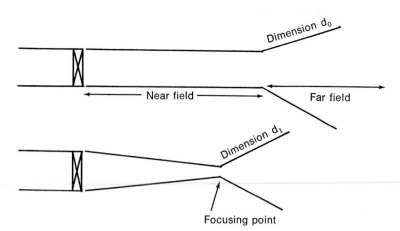

Fig. 1-34. Comparison of the beam parameter of the focused beam with the nonfocused beam.

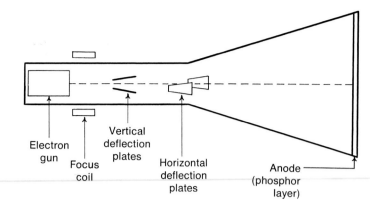

Fig. 1-35. Basic design of the cathode ray tube (CRT). (From Goldberg, B. B., Kotler, M. N., Ziskin, M., and Waxham, R. D.: Diagnostic uses of ultrasound, New York, 1975, Grune & Stratton, Inc. Used by permission.)

a specific point; and (3) it shortens the effects of intensity variations in the near field. Fig. 1-34 illustrates the difference in beam dimensions between a focused and a nonfocused ultrasonic beam.

The focal length, or the distance from the transducer face to the focal spot, is dependent on the shape of the lens used and the size of the crystal. The ability to choose different focal lengths permits optimization of the transducer to specific depths to ensure less beam divergence and greater lateral resolution.

Typical contact scanner focal lengths follow:

Short—3 to 6 cm
Medium—6 to 8 cm
Long—8 to 12 cm

To determine the lateral resolution capabilities we can determine the diameter of the spot (d) by the equation

$$d = 2.44 \left(\frac{fl \times \lambda}{A} \right)$$

where fl is the focal length, A is the diameter of the crystal, and λ is the wavelength. Note, however, that this does not show the length of the focal zone (the length of the beam affected by focusing).

NOTE: With the use of a water-delay system one typically focuses in the far field. This allows for the advantages of large diameter crystals, which give a better beam pattern or focal zone for a given focal diameter.

BASIC ULTRASOUND DISPLAY METHODS
Cathode ray tube

A cathode ray tube (CRT) is one of the most common means of displaying ultrasound information. An understanding of CRT operating principles is helpful in studying the basic modes of ultrasound.

The cathode ray tube has three basic parts—the electron gun that produces and focuses an electron beam, a system to deflect the electron beam, and a

phosphor-coated screen that changes the beam energy into visible light energy. The CRT is evacuated to prevent any gases from interfering with the movement of the electron beam. Fig. 1-35 illustrates a basic CRT.

The electron gun provides a source of free electrons as a result of heating of the cathode by passing an electric current through a filament. The control grid within the electron gun permits control of the amount and velocity of the electrons in the beam. The focusing lens causes the beam to become very narrow. Deflection occurs as the beam travels through an electrostatic field created by the deflection plates. One pair of plates serves for deflection in a horizontal (x) direction, and the other pair serves for deflection in a vertical (y) direction. The beam is deflected from its normal axis by an amount dependent on voltages that are applied to each pair of plates.

Some cathode ray tubes have external deflection coils rather than internal plates. These coils cause deflection of the electron beam by creating a magnetic field that interacts with the beam within the CRT. The amount and direction of beam deflection is determined by the electric current that is applied to the deflection coils.

When the electron beam strikes the inner surface of the phosphor-coated glass screen, the energy in the beam is converted into light energy at the point of impact. This allows the position of the beam to be observed. High voltages in the range of 3000 to 10,000 V are applied to the various elements of the CRT to ensure that the beam has sufficient energy at the time of impact on the phosphor screen. This permits a bright display on the CRT.

A mode

Fig. 1-36 illustrates a block diagram of a basic ultrasound system. The system consists of a timing unit, pulser, transmitting transducer, receiving transducer,

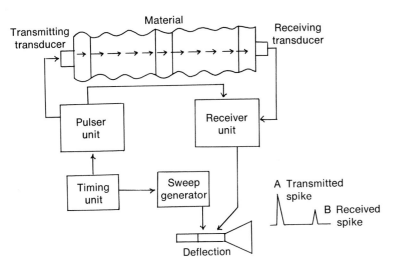

Fig. 1-36. Through-transmission system using separate transmitting and receiving crystals.

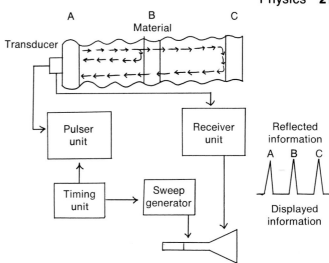

Fig. 1-37. Pulse echo system using one crystal as both transmitter and receiver. Note that reflection from material (*B* and *C*) returns to the original transmitting crystal.

receiver, sweep generator, and CRT. The pulser unit supplies the excitation to the transducer. The timing unit causes the pulser to shock the piezoelectric material at definite intervals so that it vibrates at its characteristic frequency. The pulser output is a voltage that could range from 100 to 2000 V. Typical pulse rates range from 500 to 1000 pulses per second. If the pulsed transducer is coupled to some material and directed toward a similar transducer on the opposite side, bursts of energy from the pulsed transducer will travel through the material, and the receiving transducer will respond to the impact of each burst by generating a small pulse of electric voltage. This electric voltage is amplified in the receiver unit, and, when applied to the vertical (y) deflection plates of the CRT, a spike will appear on the screen. So that the spike may be effectively displayed, the sweep generator, by applying a voltage to the horizontal (x) deflection plates, causes the electron beam to travel at a fast uniform speed across the screen of the CRT. The beam starts its horizontal movement when the sweep generator receives a starting signal from the timing unit. This starting signal is made to occur simultaneously with the start of transmission of the ultrasonic burst. The CRT will display spikes representing both the transmitted pulse and the received pulse. Because the electron beam in the CRT moves horizontally while the transmitted pulse travels through the material, the spike representing the received pulse will occur at some distance away from the spike representing the transmitted pulse. If the velocity of sound through the material and the CRT horizontal sweep speed are known, the CRT can then be used to measure the distance between the two transducers. This is possible, since the distance between transmitted and

received spikes on the CRT is a measure of the time elapsed between sending and receiving a pulse of ultrasound. Each time the electron beam completes a horizontal sweep, it quickly returns to its original position and starts again. The baseline displayed on the CRT appears to be stationary, but it is made up of many sweeps each second, the actual number being equal to the pulse rate. The two-transducer method is a simple way of measuring distances and is commonly referred to as through-transmission.

Fig. 1-37 shows how a single transducer could be used to measure distances. Assume that the transducer is being pulsed at a 1000 Hz rate. This means that a burst of energy from the transducer is occurring every 1/1000 of a second (1 msec). If each burst had a duration of 1/1,000,000 of a second (1 μsec), there would be an interval of about 999 μsec between bursts. If, during this interval, echoes return from interfaces within the material, they will be displayed on the CRT as noted. In this instance the location of the spikes will depend on the time it takes for the sound to travel from the transducer to the interface and back to the transducer. This is termed the pulse-echo method. Both methods are a form of A mode (amplitude). This is a method of data presentation in which the coordinate along the trace (horizontal) of the CRT represents time on which the amplitude of the echo is displayed as a deflection (vertical) of this coordinate. A photograph of the A-mode display is usually taken from the CRT face if a permanent record is desired.

B mode

Another method of data presentation on the CRT is B mode (brightness). In this case the coordinate along the trace represents time (distance), whereas the am-

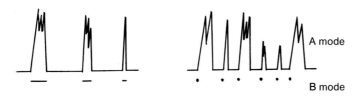

Fig. 1-38. Amplitude modulation with corresponding brightness modulation shown below.

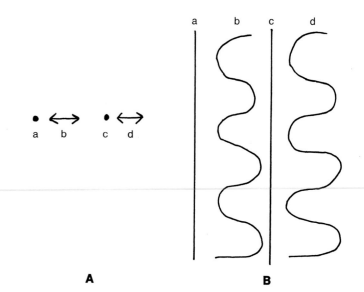

Fig. 1-39. A, Particle movement of both b and d with particles a and c stationary. B, corresponding B mode per unit time. Note horizontal motion of b and c, indicating motion of certain structures.

plitude of the echo is represented by a change of brightness or intensity of the electron beam as displayed on the CRT. Fig. 1-38 illustrates a comparison of an A-mode and a B-mode display.

M mode

In some applications distances between the transducer and reflecting interfaces are constantly changing. This occurs when studying moving tissues such as valves or other structures in the heart. To effectively record this information, a form of B mode can be used. As in A mode, time or distance is represented along the horizontal axis of the CRT. The returning echoes, however, are represented as dots of varying intensities. These dots are observed moving along the horizontal axis, constantly altering their distance from the dot on the screen representing the transducer pulse. A storage type CRT could be used to record the movement of these echoes. This type of CRT has characteristics that permit retention of an image after the signal that created the image is removed. If the moving dots on the storage CRT were permitted to drift slowly upward, the motions of the dots would be recorded as wavy lines indicating the behavior of the interfaces that produced the echoes. Fig. 1-39, A, shows motion of the brightness dots before they are caused to drift vertically on the storage CRT. Fig. 1-39, B, demonstrates the effect of vertical movement on the storage CRT. The resulting stored image can now be photographed in a manner similar to that used for A-mode recording. In the absence of a storage CRT an open-shutter technique could be used to obtain a permanent recording. This is done by placing the dot trace at the bottom of the CRT, opening the shutter of a camera with film exposed to the CRT face. The CRT trace is now permitted to drift vertically. When the trace reaches the top of the CRT, the camera shutter is closed. The storage of the dot motion actually takes place on the photographic film.

A more common method of recording the motion of the dots is to keep the trace stationary while a strip of paper with special light-sensitive characteristics is passed over the CRT. This paper when developed will

display the motion of the dots. M mode (motion) and T-M mode (time-motion) are terms commonly used to define the technique of recording the motion of echoes while the transducer remains stationary.

B scan

A-mode and M-mode presentations are only graphic representations of various structures. Actual images of cross sections of tissue can be produced by moving a transducer across the surface of the body so that the ultrasound beam slices through the tissues below it (Fig. 1-40, A). The constantly changing echo patterns are integrated on the screen of the CRT to form a picture. This is a form of B mode termed B-mode scanning, or B scan. The transducer is mounted on a scanning assembly consisting of three arms (Fig. 1-40, B). These arms are joined together by hinge assemblies. As the transducer is moved across the body, various angles are encountered between the three arms. By knowing the lengths of each arm and the angles produced, the position and direction of the scanning transducer can be plotted. Electronic means are used to transmit angular information from the arms to a computing system.

The computing system applies the necessary voltages to the deflection plates of a storage CRT so that the direction of the baseline represents the path of the ultrasound through the tissue, and the starting point of the baseline represents the position of the transducer on the surface of the body. As with A mode and stored M mode, a permanent record of the stored

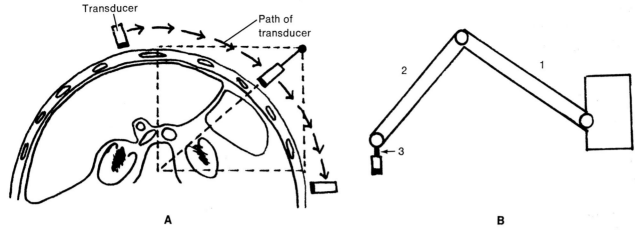

Fig. 1-40. A, Lines of movement of the transducer across the abdomen for two-dimensional imaging. **B,** Model of the three arms used in conventional contact B scanners, which give proper orientation of the transducer to the computing system for two-dimensional imaging.

B-scan image may be obtained by photographing the face of the CRT.

Operating controls

All ultrasound systems contain various operating controls that permit the operators to adjust for factors such as image size, selection, trace positioning, and scale marking. Certain operator controls deserve special attention here. These are the controls that affect the input and output levels of ultrasonic energy. It is known that sound energy encounters attenuation as it travels through tissue. Therefore echoes produced by interfaces close to the transducer will return at higher levels than echoes produced by interfaces farther away from the transducer. Compensation must be provided for those echoes which must travel greater distances and longer periods of time. Time compensated gain (TCG), or time gain compensation (TGC), is a method used to control the systems gain with respect to time to compensate for the decrease in echo amplitudes from greater depths. In addition to TGC there are other means available to the operator to control or alter the strength of received echoes, including near gain, delay, sensitivity, gain dB, reject, coarse gain, and far gain. The names of these various controls differ among ultrasound equipment manufacturers, but their primary purpose is the same—to control the amplification of received echoes (Fig. 1-41).

Some ultrasound systems include a method to control the output power available at the transducer. The controls used might be labeled output, damping, or power. The most common method of controlling the transducer output is by resistive damping. This highly effective method of damping uses a system that

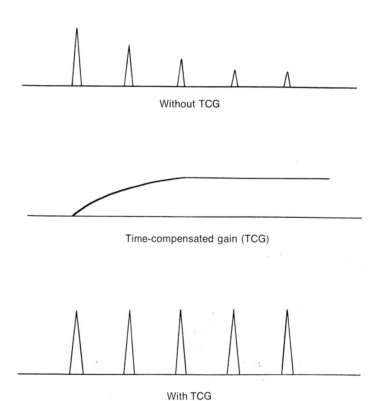

Fig. 1-41. Demonstration of the affects of amplitude corresponding to the amount of time gain compensation used. (From Goldberg, B. B., Kotler, M. N., Ziskin, M., and Waxham, R. D.: Diagnostic uses of ultrasound, New York, 1975, Grune & Stratton, Inc. Used by permission.)

switches selected resistors across the transducer output. This has the effect of controlling the width of the pulse applied to the transducer and therefore controls the average power of sound applied to the patient.

There is one important point concerning the relationship between the use of this control and the selection of high-frequency transducers. In practice it is best to use the highest-frequency transducer possible while still maintaining adequate resolution. Normally, this would ensure the best possible resolution. As higher-frequency transducers are selected for use, less damping is desirable for proper penetration. Since the type of damping regulator under consideration controls the width of the pulse applied to the transducer, a point could be reached when the width of the pulse would be so great that the resolution normally associated with the higher-frequency transducer would not be obtained. Thus a combination of proper receiver and output controls, along with the proper and optimal frequency for the task at hand, must be thoroughly understood and used.

IMAGE PROCESSING AND DISPLAY
Signal processing

The incoming signal produced by the returning echo has the characteristic of a radiofrequency wave (Fig. 1-42). This signal is further amplified and then encounters rectification, which removes one half of the radiofrequency wave. This rectified wave then encounters a process where it becomes enveloped and creates a simple wave packet. The normal A-mode display is a representation of this enveloped wave.

Other types of signal processing are often used for B-mode applications. One of these is the leading edge. Fig. 1-43 illustrates leading edge processing. Note that B-mode dots produced in the leading edge configuration do not represent the entire echo complex but only that portion of each echo as it leaves the baseline.

Display devices

Although the echoes displayed in Fig. 1-43 have different amplitudes, the B-mode dots are displayed with equal intensity. One reason for this is that the standard storage cathode ray tube is a bistable device, causing all echoes above a given threshold to store with equal intensity. Because of this limitation, this display method did not utilize the amplitude information present in the reflected signal. The bistable CRT produces black and white images with no grey shades present.

A possible method of producing grey-scale imaging involves the photography of a nonstorage CRT image, with the camera shutter open. With the shutter open it is necessary to scan with a constant velocity motion to produce artifact-free images. If, as the transducer is being moved across the body, the velocity is not kept constant, the image will be brighter in areas where the transducer is moved slower than the initial speed. One way to attack this problem is with the use of complex, constant velocity, mechanical scanners in a water bath. Since a nonstorage CRT is used, the resulting image cannot be viewed as the scan is being made; one must audit film development to determine the quality of results.

Scan convertor display systems

Scan convertors have the ability to write in one mode (x-y in this case) and display in another, such as TV Raster scanning. The x-y and intensity information is stored on a target surface and is then displayed in a TV format.

The standard method of TV scanning is the 2:1 interlace method. If the scanning beam is started at the top left of the image, the horizontal sweep system causes the beam to rapidly move to the right. When the beam is at the right edge of the image, retrace occurs and the beam is very rapidly returned to the left edge of the image, where it will again start moving to the right. During this horizontal movement the beam is gradually being pulled down by a slower vertical sweep system. The vertical sweep rate is 60 Hz. This was

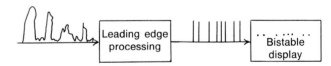

Fig. 1-43. Leading edge processing using a CRT as opposed to quantification using a scan convertor.

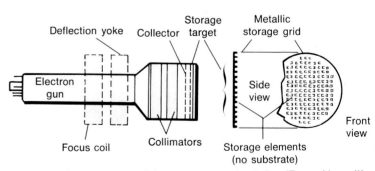

Fig. 1-44. Components of the scan convertor tube. (From Alvarelli, J., Hagen, S., McKay, L., and Schorzman, L.: Body scanning, Cleveland, 1976, Picker Corp.)

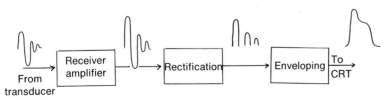

Fig. 1-42. Various phases of the receiver affecting the returning echo information.

chosen because it is rapid enough to eliminate the illusion of flicker to the human eye and it corresponds to the power line frequency in the United States, thus providing an easy method of synchronization. Every 1/60 second vertical retrace occurs, and the beam that had reached the bottom of the image is returned to the top to start a new sequence. This sequence is repeated continuously even in the absence of intensity information. The TV system beam reflection will continue, but the intensity of the scanning beam varies in accordance with the incoming signal.

The key component of the system is the scan convertor tube (Fig. 1-44). This tube is an electromagnetically focused and deflected cathode ray tube that functions in a manner analogous to that of the familiar TV picture tube, except that the electron beam is directed toward a small charged storage target rather than a phosphor viewing screen. The target of the scan convertor tube cannot be viewed directly but is simply used to store information.

The storage target basically contains a dielectric substrate with a large number of microscopic elements. Each element is a discrete storage bit. A matrix of 1000×1000 storage elements is formed, producing a storage system with high-resolution capability.

The scan convertor operating mode may be changed at will to read the charge-stored image, and a television type signal can then be transmitted to display monitors in full grey scale. This is a well-established technology that has been used for years both commercially and in aerospace. Displaying the grey-scale image while it is being written involves time-sharing for the scan convertor's electron beam.

During a certain period of time the beam is used to read the image stored on the target. A block of time, a few television lines wide, is then used to write the information obtained from the target. The result is a slight flicker corresponding to the read and write time of the convertor.

Recent developments in technology have produced a scan convertor with a solid-state image memory, as compared to the storage tube memory previously discussed. The solid-state memory resembles the memory in a digital computer. One major advantage of this type of storage would be increased stability of the system.

2 □ Instrumentation and techniques

EQUIPMENT

There are numerous commercially available ultrasound systems, which makes it difficult for the novice to evaluate equipment objectively. Important considerations to be seriously evaluated when purchasing equipment follow:

1. Resolution quality of the image (before and after magnification)
2. Ease of operation (minimum of gain-control knobs)
3. Movement of mechanical arm from transverse to longitudinal position with ease
4. Lightness of scanning arm with counterbalance feature
5. Reproducibility
6. Reliability
7. Serviceability
8. Educational opportunities

The equipment discussed in this chapter will be represented throughout this book by examples of various ultrasonic scans. Comparative knobology among the systems will be discussed to present an objective evaluation of equipment relative to specific needs of the laboratory.

A mode. A-mode equipment has multiple uses in echoencephalography, ophthalmology, localizing masses for biopsy, aspiration, or internal consistency, and localizing pleural effusion. Thus A-mode equipment is portable and generally compact with a minimum of gain controls to adjust. It should have the internal capability of visualizing small superficial structures, as well as the adaptability of penetrating the dense skull for internal cranial detail. Therefore it should be capable of handling a selection range from a high-frequency 10 MHz transducer to a low-frequency 1 MHz transducer. An electronic through-transmission is optional to produce an electronic midline for encephalography examinations. (See Fig. 2-1.)

Doppler technique. Continuous-wave Doppler technique is used in the detection of peripheral vascular disease, fetal heart viability, and placental localization. Most systems produce an audible flow sound but provide no means for recording such pat-

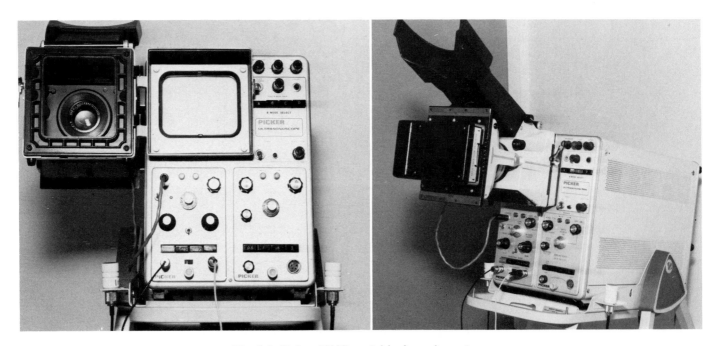

Fig. 2-1. Picker EV VI portable A-mode system.

terns. A tape recorder may be used to permanently record the sounds, or some type of strip-chart recorder can be attached for a more permanent recording. Various frequency Doppler capabilities will be required if the Doppler technique is to be used for multiple examinations. Most systems are quite compact. Some have earphone attachments, and others are battery charged for ease of operation. (See Fig. 2-2.)

M mode. Used mainly for echocardiography, M-mode equipment should have electrocardiography capabilities with an option for phonocardiography and carotid pulse tracings. The unit should be small and compact and have large wheels to aid in its portability

(for emergency procedures and examining critically ill patients). Gain controls should allow independent adjustment of near gain, far gain, slope, delay, and ramp. The coarse gain should have flexibility for rapid adjustment to separate the posterior wall from the pericardium. Some equipment has an enhance, or grey-scale, capability to distinguish low-level echoes from stronger reflections. The variable-gain pod may

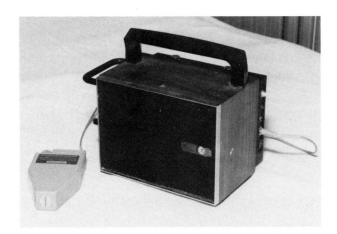

Fig. 2-2. Medsonics Doppler system for peripheral vascular disease.

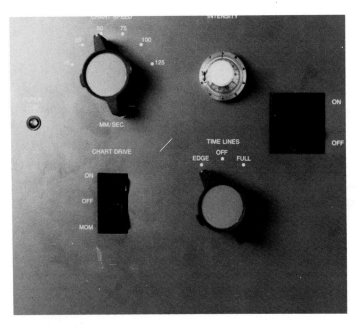

Fig. 2-3. Picker 80C echocardiology strip-chart system.

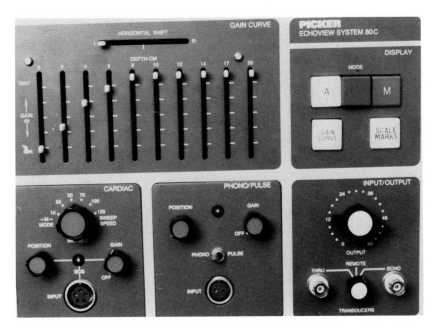

Fig. 2-4. Picker 80C echocardiography variable depth control.

allow more flexibility in adult cardiac examinations but may be limiting in the pediatric age group. The time lines should be legible through the vertical echo trace, with millisecond time lines across the horizontal tracing.

There are several strip-chart recorders available to interface with the M-mode equipment. The recorder may process the tracing on light- or heat-sensitive paper. Light-sensitive paper presents with pink and grey tones and, if further exposed to excessive sunlight, will fade. The heat-sensitive paper provides greater contrast, although processing is more cumbersome. The strip-chart recorders have variable-speed and intensity knobs for optimum control. (See Figs. 2-3 and 2-4.)

M mode with pulsed Doppler. This combined unit allows separate M-mode echo recording or Doppler and M-mode recording simultaneously. The unit is compact and portable. The Doppler provides an additional diagnostic tool in the evaluation of regurgitation and ventricular or atrial septal defects. (See Fig. 2-5.)

B-mode grey scale. Most commercial systems are very close in resolution capabilities if they are working at their maximum capacity. Their differences lie within ease of operation, scanning arm maneuverability, and reliability. Some units employ a variable-gain pod control, and others offer independent near-gain, far-gain, and slope controls. Most all units offer coarse-gain, attenuation, or output controls. Some equipment allows individual transducer frequency selection range to specifically tune in on the frequency bandwidth for better resolution. All systems have enhance controls to balance the echo image. Some units have too many variables for routine scans to be performed effectively. The routine scan converter allows the image to be magnified with a slight loss of resolution and focus as the image is enlarged. Some equipment will electronically allow for magnification without significant loss of resolution.

Each unit has specific writing speed characteristics that influence the speed of performing scans. Centimeter markers or scale factors are included in some way on all equipment. Permanent markers are preferable to manual markers.

The scanning arm ideally should move from transverse to longitudinal positions without occupying excess space in the room. The transducer should be

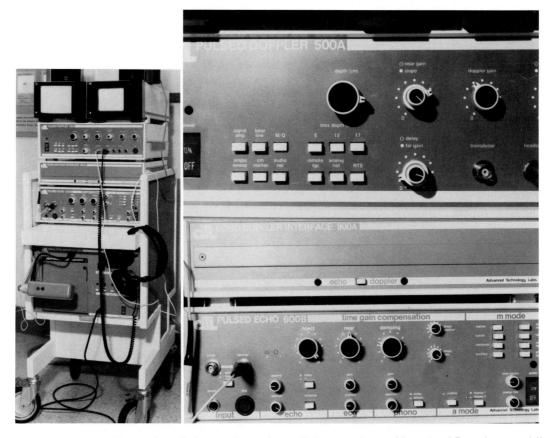

Fig. 2-5. Advanced Technology Laboratories echocardiology system with pulsed Doppler capabilities.

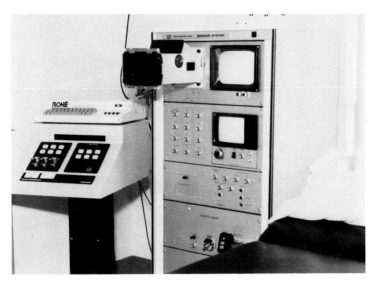

Fig. 2-6. Rohe grey-scale system.

small, flexible along the lateral abdominal walls, and easily interchangeable.

The A-mode scope should be representative of a quality reflection for diagnostic interpretation of mass consistency and size. (See Figs. 2-6 to 2-9.) Table 2-1 contains pertinent characteristics of selected scanners.

REAL TIME

The Bronson unit is a high-frequency real-time unit used for superficial areas such as the *eye, thyroid,* and *breast.* The small transducer is manually held over the area of interest with the image projected on a large TV monitor. (See Fig. 2-10.)

There are several real-time units commercially available for *abdominal* and *obstetric* use. One type offers a linear array transducer with variable fre-

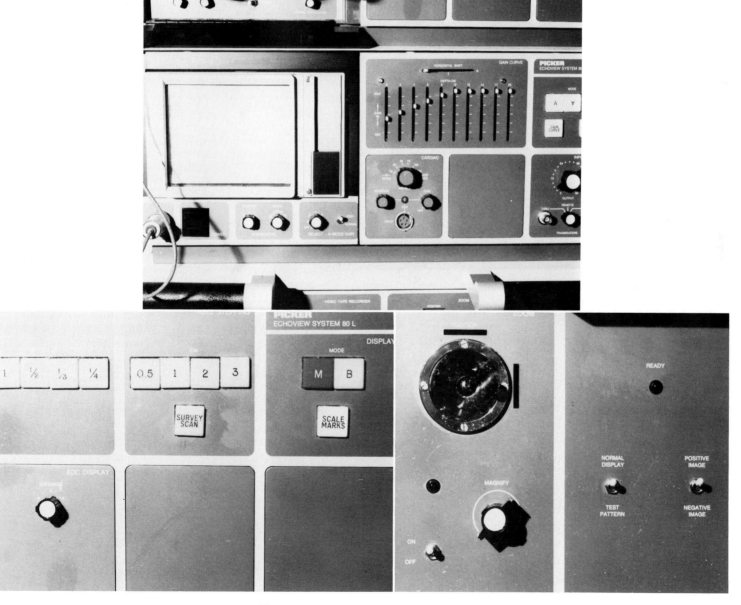

Fig. 2-7. Picker 80L grey-scale system.

Table 2-1. Features of selected commercially available scanners

Characteristic	Picker 80L	Rohe 5550	Unirad Sonograph III	Characteristic	Picker 80L	Rohe 5550	Unirad Sonograph III
Varies receiver amplification of received echoes from specific depths of tissue	10 sliding potentiometers controlling amplification every 2 cm	System gain, near gain, slope start, slope, far gain, pedestal (position, width, height)	Initial dB, slope, gain, delay	Sets magnification factor of image before scan is performed by varying sweep amplitude prior to application to scan convertor	B-scan scale (magnification factor: 1, ½, ⅓, ¼)	B-scan: 1, 2, 3, 4 cm	Field of view: 0.5, 1, 2, 3, 4, 5 cm/div
Varies transducer output by controlling width of pulse applied to transducer	20-step input/output control	3-position acoustic power switch	Not available	Controls degree of magnification of stored scan convertor image being displayed on TV monitors	Magnify	Zoom magnification	Zoom
Varies frequency response of receiver to match transducer being used	Uses wideband receiver	6-position frequency selector	Uses wideband receiver	Erases image stored on scan convertor tube	Erase	Erase	Erase
Selects level of echo suppression after amplification by receiver; used to eliminate electrical noise from display	Reject	Reject	Not available	Places spaced marker dots on scanned image; each dot represents 1 cm of tissue	B-scan mark (automatic)	Cm marks (used with *write* pedal depressed)	Markers (automatic)
				Inverts A-mode trace on oscilloscope for echoencephalography	A, ∀	Function (R, L)	Not available
Selects method of processing amplified echoes from receiver to provide bistable or grey-scale display	Signal-processing selector (EDC-video, leading edge, peak)	Fixed grey scale only	Image control (outline, video, gretone)	Changes polarity of video signal displayed on TV monitors by altering signal taken from scan convertor tube	Positive image/ negative image (controls both TV monitors)	Image polarity, white/ black (controls both TV monitors)	Video invert; separate switch for each TV monitor
Shifts *read* and *write* levels on scan convertor storage tube to emphasize or de-emphasize lower or higher shades of grey	Enhance	Enhance	Post–data processing				

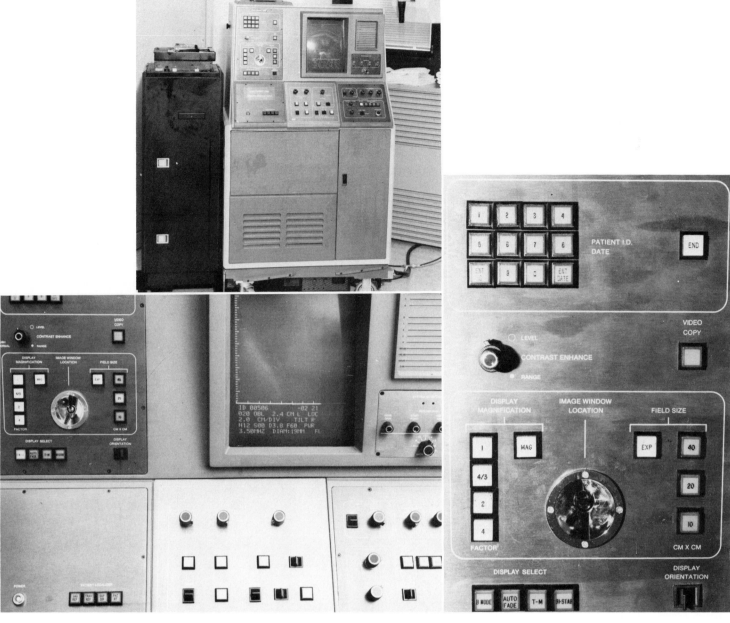

Fig. 2-8. Searle grey-scale system.

quencies. The transducer is manually manipulated over the area of interest. Longitudinal scans offer the best contact for this type of transducer, since its rigid framework prohibits good contact along the lateral abdominal wall. Portability is offered with linear array systems, with a reduction in resolution quality compared with more elaborate systems.

The other real-time system is the water bath system, with a single transducer mounted within its water bath. Several crystals are mounted on this transducer, which rotates a certain number of times each second to produce the real-time image. The pliable water bath allows excellent contact over the heart, upper abdomen, and pregnant uterus.

Gain controls on both types of equipment are simple, with controls for near gain, far gain, and balance or reject. All use Polaroid photography, which has its limitations in a real-time system. (See Figs. 2-11 and 2-12.)

There are also several commercially available real-time *cardiology* units. Most systems offer a "pie" sweep variable-degree arc to visualize intracardiac structures. The smaller the arc, the better the resolution; the smaller the transducer face, the better the angulation beneath the sternum. Some transducers have water bath couplers for better near-field resolution in pediatric patients. Combined real-time and M-mode capabilities allow qualitative and quantita-

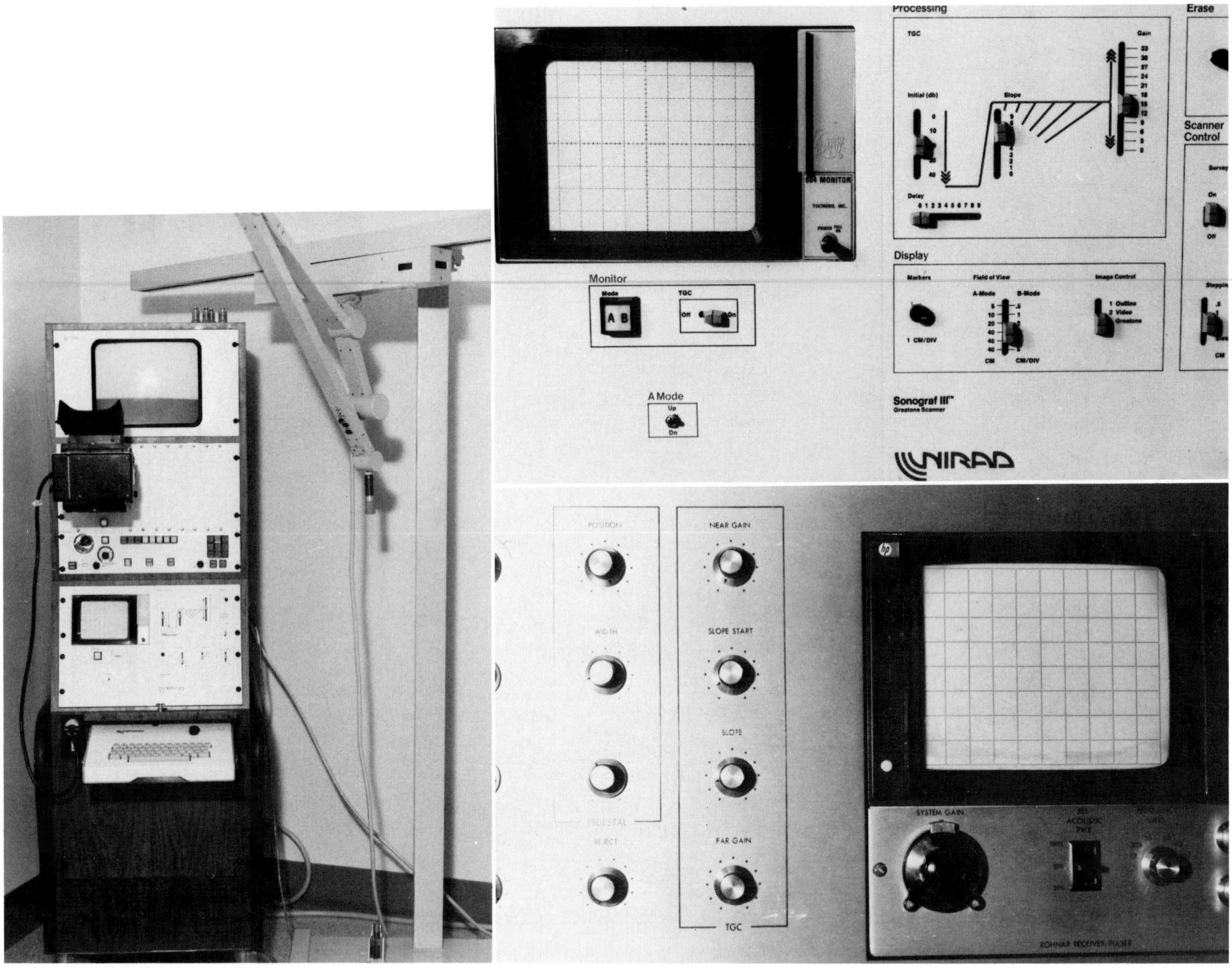

Fig. 2-9. Unirad Sonograf III grey-scale system.

tive information to be recorded. Videotape, scan convertors, and computer systems allow data to be processed for future reference.

Gain controls are either independent (far gain, near gain, slope) or step-decibel pod controls with overall gain sensitivity. Most have interchangeable frequency transducers for all ages. Selected systems are available for suprasternal notch evaluation.

AUTOMATED EQUIPMENT

The U. I. Octoson was developed by Kossoff and colleagues in Australia as the first automated system with eight transducers mounted completely in a water bath. Transducer movement is controlled from a

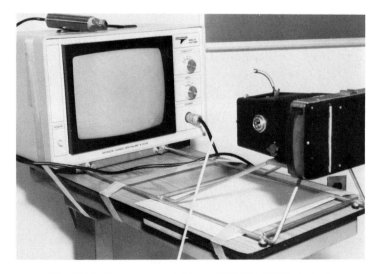

Fig. 2-10. Bronson real-time ophthalmology system.

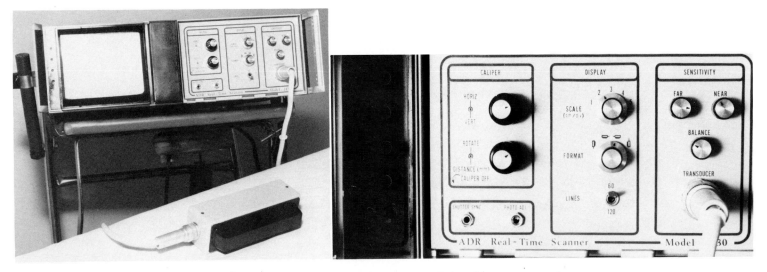

Fig. 2-11. Advanced Diagnostic Research real-time linear array system.

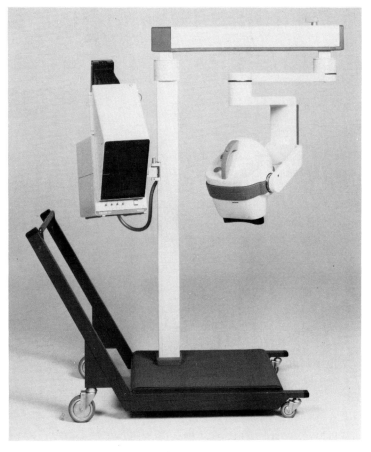

Fig. 2-12. Seimens water bath real-time system.

streamlined panel. This panel allows the operator to control the angle of sweep, the scan center angulation, and the increment movement of the transducers. It can perform transverse, longitudinal, or oblique scans with or without angulation. The transducer arm may be moved closer or farther from the patient's skin surface to control the quality of penetration. It has the capability of utilizing all eight transducers, or a single transducer, or a combination of transducers. It also has manual capabilities if the area of interest needs to be specifically outlined. The manual control may also be used with the M-mode sweep to further outline motion (e.g., fetal heart, pulsatile aortic movement, or delineation of cardiac structures). (See Fig. 2-13.)

The gain controls are interprogramed with one another, with flexibility to control near gain, far gain, and overall attenuation. The transducer arm may be controlled automatically or manually. Increment movement can be implemented from 1 mm to 2 cm intervals. The camera can be controlled manually or integrated with the automatic scan sweep movement so that once the direction of movement is established with correct gain settings, a series of scans can be made and recorded in minutes. Protocol is established for each ultrasound examination, further expediting each study.

The concept of automation versus contact scanning is an intriguing one. The question that arises in regard to the operation of the equipment is "Will this replace the intensified sonography training put forth in ultrasound laboratories throughout the United States?" It is a well-known fact that contact scan equipment demands a high degree of manual dexterity and hand-eye coordination. The Octoson eliminates this facet of

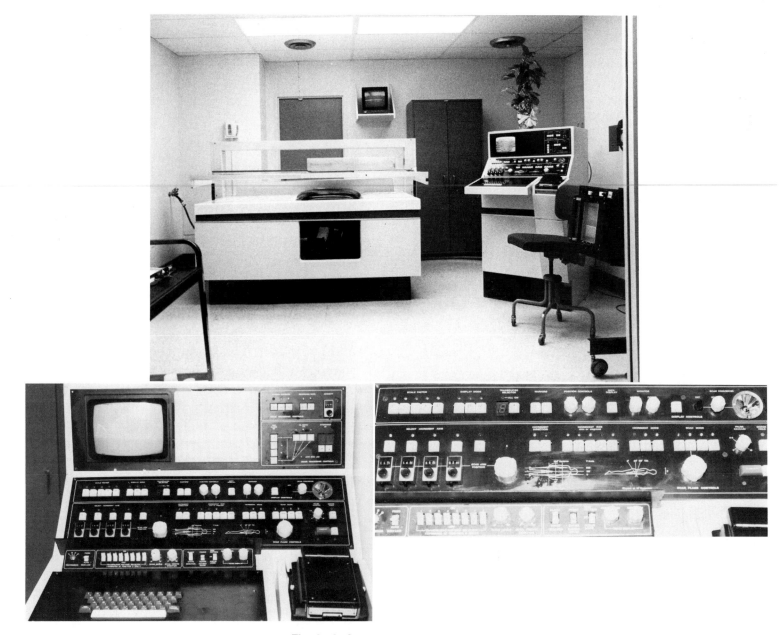

Fig. 2-13. Octoson automated system.

operation by automatically producing quality scans. However, from our experience in training ultrasound students, we have found those students who took command of the contact scanner early in their training consistently produced quality scans as their knowledge of anatomy and pathology improved. Although it is extremely important in contact scanning to know how to produce a diagnostic scan, I think the real secret lies within one's knowledge of cross-sectional and sagittal anatomy.

The Octoson provides no sonographer contact with the transducers, and thus initially it may be difficult to understand anatomic presentation without constantly looking through the plastic-covered window in the side of the system. However, once digital incre-

ments and anatomic relationships are understood, the sonographer no longer needs to check for transducer location in relation to the patient's skin surface.

The role of the sonographer will be just as vital with the automated ultrasonic systems as it has been with the contact ultrasonic systems. The difference will be in the recognition of anatomic structures and relationships and the time involved to demonstrate such anatomy. Scans should consistently be of better quality with the automated water bath system. Patients who were difficult to scan with conventional contact equipment because of chest configuration, unusual abdominal contour, or postsurgical incisions are not affected by this water bath system.

PART TWO ECHOCARDIOGRAPHY

3 □ Anatomic and physiologic relationships

Before a discussion of the heart, the thoracic cavity and its organs will be briefly considered.

THORAX

The thorax constitutes the upper part of the trunk. Within the thorax lies the thoracic cavity. This is separated from the abdominal cavity by the dome-shaped diaphragm, which reaches upward as high as the midaxillary level of the seventh rib. Superiorly the upper thoracic cavity gives access to the root of the neck. It is bounded by the upper part of the sternum, the first ribs, and the body of the first thoracic vertebra. Anteriorly the sternum consists of three parts: the manubrium, the corpus sterni (body), and the xiphoid. The junction between the manubrium and the body of the sternum forms a prominent ridge. Together they form the angle of Louis. This palpable landmark is important in locating the superior mediastinum or the second rib cartilages, which articulate with the sternum at this point.

The greater part of the thoracic cavity is occupied by the two lungs, which are enclosed by the pleura. To understand the pleural sac, imagine a deflated plastic bag covering your fist. Both sides of the bag should be reflected onto your fist to simulate the pleural sac. The internal layer (visceral pleura) is adherent to each individual lobe of the lung. The external layer (parietal pleura) is adherent to the inner surface of the chest wall (costal pleura), the diaphragm (diaphragmatic pleura), and the mediastinum (mediastinal pleura). The costophrenic sinus is the pleural reflection between the costal and diaphragmatic portions of the parietal pleura. This space lies lower than the edge of the lung and in most cases is never occupied by the lung. When pleural fluid accumulates, its most common location is in the costophrenic sinus. On radiographic examination this costophrenic angle is blunted by pleural effusion.

The space between the two pleural cavities is the mediastinum. It extends superiorly to the root of the neck and inferiorly to the diaphragm. Anteriorly it extends to the sternum and posteriorly to the twelfth thoracic vertebra, the thymus, the heart and great blood vessels, the trachea and esophagus, the thoracic duct and lymph nodes, the vagus and phrenic nerves, and the sympathetic trunks.

An imaginary plane from the sternal angle to the lower body of the fourth thoracic vertebra divides the mediastinum into superior and inferior mediastina. The inferior mediastinum is subdivided into three parts: (1) middle, which contains the pericardium and heart; (2) anterior, which is a space between the pericardium and sternum; and (3) posterior, which lies between the pericardium and vertebral column.

It is helpful to remember the anteroposterior locations of the following major mediastinal structures:

1. Superior mediastinum
   a. Thymus
   b. Large veins
   c. Large arteries
   d. Trachea
   e. Esophagus and thoracic duct
   f. Sympathetic trunks
2. Inferior mediastinum
   a. Thymus
   b. Heart within the pericardium, with the phrenic nerves on each side
   c. Esophagus and thoracic duct
   d. Descending aorta
   e. Sympathetic trunks

HEART

Contrary to the usual illustrated anatomic position, the heart is not situated with the right chambers lying to the right and the left chambers to the left. It may be better considered as an anteroposterior structure with the right chambers more anterior than its posterior left chambers. During embryologic development the heart forms as a right-to-left structure. However, with further embryologic development the right side becomes more ventral although the left side remains dorsal. In addition, another change in axis causes the apex, or inferior surface of the heart, to tilt anteriorly.

Thus the final development of the heart presents the right atrium anteriorly to the right of the sternum and the right ventricle anterior and beneath the sternum or slightly to the left; the left atrium then becomes the most posterior chamber to the left of the sternum, and the left ventricle swings its posterior apex slightly toward the anterior chest wall.

The heart and the roots of the great vessels lie within the pericardial sac. Like the pleura of the lungs, the pericardium is a double sac. The fibrous pericardium limits the movement of the heart by attaching to the central tendon of the diaphragm below and the outer coats of the great blood vessels above. The sternopericardial ligaments attach it in front.

The serous pericardium is divided into the parietal and visceral layers. The parietal layer lines the fibrous pericardium and becomes continuous with the visceral layer of serous pericardium. The visceral layer is very closely applied to the heart and is often called the epicardium. The small slit between the parietal and visceral layers is the pericardial cavity. This cavity normally contains a small amount of fluid that lubricates the heart as it moves.

The pericardium, of course, does not totally encompass the heart. On the posterior left atrial surface of the heart the reflection of serous pericardium around the pulmonary veins forms the recess of the oblique sinus. This is an important landmark in the separation of pericardial effusion from pleural effusion in echocardiography. The transverse sinus lies between the reflection of serous pericardium around the aorta and pulmonary arteries and the reflection around the large veins.

The heart has three surfaces—sternocostal (anterior), diaphragmatic (inferior), and base (posterior). It also has an apex (Fig. 3-1).

The right atrium and right ventricle (separated by the vertical atrioventricular groove) form the sternocostal surface. The right atrium forms the right border of the heart to the right of the sternum. The left border is formed to the left of the sternum by the left ventricle and left auricle. The right and left ventricles are separated by the anterior interventricular groove.

The diaphragmatic surface of the heart is formed principally by the right and left ventricles separated by the posterior interventricular groove. A small part

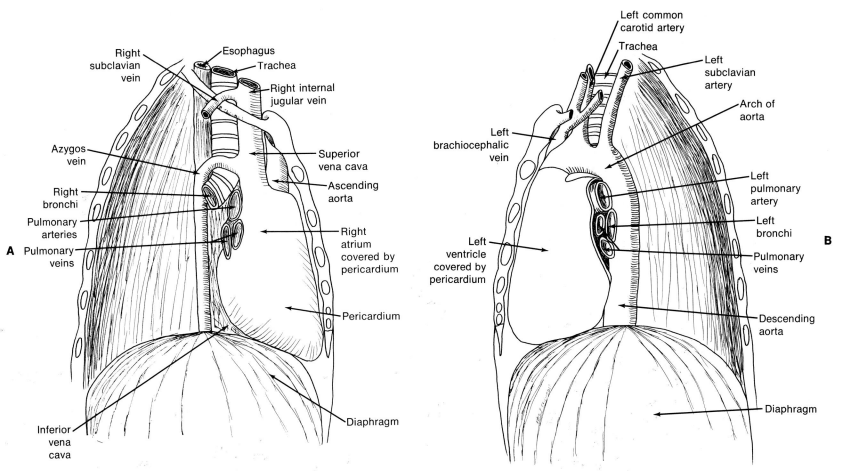

Fig. 3-1. A, Right side of mediastinum. **B,** Left side of mediastinum.

of the inferior surface of the right atrium also forms this surface.

The base of the heart is formed by the left atrium, into which open four pulmonary veins. The right atrium contributes a small part to this posterior surface. The left ventricle forms the apex of the heart, which can be palpated at the level of the fifth intercostal space, 9 cm from the midline.

The chambers of the heart are lined by an endothelial layer, the endocardium. The myocardium is part of the cardiac muscle in the contractile walls of the chambers. The epicardium is sometimes referred to as the third layer of muscle but is actually part of the visceral layer of the pericardium.

Right atrium. The right atrium has a posterior, smooth-walled portion into which enter the superior and inferior venae cavae, the coronary sinus, and a thin-walled trabeculated part. They are separated by the crista terminalis. Lateral to the crista terminalis run a large number of pectinate muscles along the free wall of the atrium. The ear-shaped right auricle also contains pectinate muscles.

Medial to the inferior caval valve the coronary sinus enters the right atrium. The interatrial septum forms the posteromedial wall of the right atrium. The thin, shallow depression in the septum is the fossa ovalis. The atrioventricular part of the membranous septum separates the right atrium and left ventricle. (Atrial defects can occur in this area, causing blood to flow from the high-pressured left ventricle into the right atrium.) The bundle of His arises from the atrioventricular node and serves as an important structure in the conduction pathway of the heart. The limbus fossa ovalis is the remainder of the atrial septum and forms a ridge around the fossa ovalis.

The tricuspid valve gives access to the right ventricle. Its three cusps, septal, inferior, and anterior, are attached by their bases to the fibrous atrioventricular ring. The chordae tendineae attach the cusps to the papillary muscles. These muscles contract, as the ventricle contracts, to pull the cusps together and prevent them from being pulled into the atrium. To help in this process, the septal and anterior cusps are connected to the same papillary muscle.

The pulmonary orifice is guarded by the semilunar pulmonary valve. The curved lower border of each of its cusps is attached to the arterial wall. The open mouths of the cusps are directed upward. The sinuses are dilatations external to each cusp.

The walls of the right ventricle are thicker than those of the right atrium and display ridges formed by irregular muscle bundles. Some of these bundles form

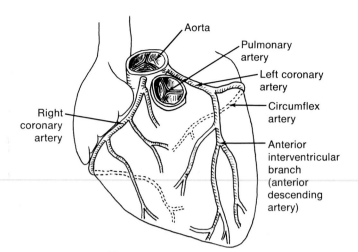

Fig. 3-2. Coronary arteries.

papillary muscles. The moderator band conveys the right branch of the atrioventricular bundle. It is a muscular bundle that crosses the ventricular cavity from the septal to the anterior wall.

Left atrium. The most posterior structure of the left atrium is situated behind the right atrium. Four pulmonary veins open into the left atrial wall.

Left ventricle. The bicuspid mitral valve guards the atrioventricular orifice. The anterior cusp is the larger cusp and is contiguous with the posterior aortic root. Chordae tendineae attach the cusps to the anterior and posterior papillary muscles of the left ventricular wall.

The tricuspid aortic valve is similar in structure to the pulmonary valve. The anterior cusp is often referred to as the noncoronary cusp, since there is no coronary artery originating from this cusp. The other cusps are termed right and left, with respective coronary arteries arising from the posterior bulging of each cusp (coronary sinus). (See Fig. 3-2.)

The upper posterior part of the left ventricle below the aortic orifice is relatively smooth and is known as the aortic vestibule.

Physiology

The heart is a muscular pump. The cardiac cycle is the series of changes the heart undergoes as it fills with blood and empties. The normal adult cardiac cycle is about 70 beats a minute, whereas in children that rate is almost double.

Rhythmic contraction of the heart causes blood to be pumped through the chambers of the heart and out through the great vessels (Fig. 3-3). Systole is the forceful contraction of the heart chambers; diastole is the relaxed phase of the cardiac cycle.

The cardiac cycle consists of the following stages:
1. *Atrial systole.* As the atria contract, the blood is

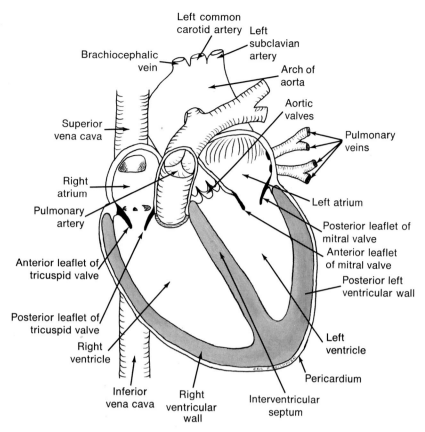

Left common
carotid artery   Left
subclavian
artery

Brachiocephalic
vein

Arch of
aorta

Aortic
valves

Superior
vena cava

Pulmonary
veins

Right
atrium

Left atrium

Pulmonary
artery

Posterior leaflet of
mitral valve

Anterior leaflet
of mitral valve

Anterior leaflet of
tricuspid valve

Posterior left
ventricular wall

Posterior leaflet of
tricuspid valve

Right
ventricle

Left
ventricle

Pericardium

Inferior
vena cava

Right
ventricular
wall

Interventricular
septum

Fig. 3-3. Anatomy of cardiac structures.

forced into the pulmonary artery and aorta. (The atrioventricular valves are closed.)

2. *Ventricular systole.* As the ventricles contract, the blood is forced into the pulmonary artery and aorta. (The atrioventricular valves are open.)

3. *Atrial diastole.* During ventricular systole, as the atria refill with blood from the great veins, atrial diastole begins.

4. *Ventricular diastole.* During atrial systole, as blood from the atria fills the ventricles, ventricular diastole begins.

The blood enters the right atrium through two large veins, the inferior and superior venae cavae. The tricuspid valve prevents the blood from entering the right ventricle during ventricular systole. As ventricular diastole occurs, the tricuspid valve opens to allow blood flow into the ventricular chamber. The blood is then forced through the pulmonary artery into the lungs for filtration.

Oxygenated blood then enters the left atrium through the four large pulmonary veins. The mitral valve prevents blood from flowing into the left ventricle during ventricular systole. As with the right side of the heart, ventricular diastole causes increased pressure in the left atrium to force the mitral leaflets open, allowing blood to flow into the left ventricle. (See Fig. 3-4.)

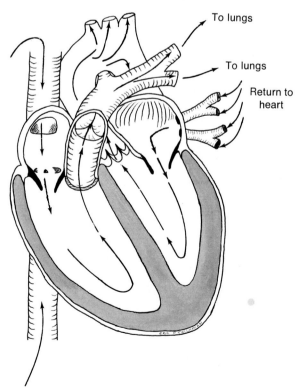

To lungs

To lungs

Return to
heart

Fig. 3-4. Arrows show blood circulation through the heart.

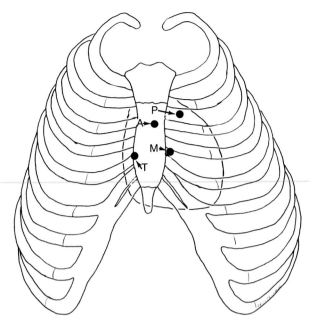

Fig. 3-5. Position of the heart valves. *P*, Pulmonary; *A*, aortic; *M*, mitral; *T*, tricuspid.

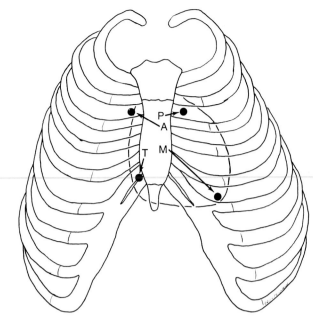

Fig. 3-6. Position of heart valves (valve sounds may be best heard with the least interference at the location of the arrows). *P*, Pulmonary; *A*, aortic; *M*, mitral; *T*, tricuspid.

The left ventricle maintains the highest pressures in the heart. As a result its walls are much thicker than those on the right side of the heart.

Heart valves

Surface anatomy (Fig. 3-5). The tricuspid valve lies behind the right half of the sternum, opposite the fourth intercostal space. The mitral valve lies behind the left half of the sternum, opposite the fourth costal cartilage. The pulmonary valve lies behind the medial end of the third left costal cartilage and the adjoining part of the sternum. The aortic valve lies behind the left half of the sternum, opposite the third intercostal space.

Auscultation (Fig. 3-6). The first heart sound is produced by ventricular contraction and closure of the tricuspid and mitral valves. The second sound is produced by sharp closure of the aortic and pulmonary valves.

Sound from the tricuspid valve is best heard over the right half of the lower end of the body of the sternum; from the mitral valve over the apex beat. Sound from the pulmonary valve is heard with the least interference over the medial end of the second left intercostal space and from aortic valve over the medial end of the second right intercostal space.

Electrocardiographic timing

To study electric timing of the cardiac chambers, an ECG lead is attached to the patient (right arm, left arm,

and a ground on the abdomen or leg). The ECG has three components—P, QRS, and T waves.

The P wave characterizes depolarization from the sinoatrial node tangentially along the atrial walls to the left atrium and the atrioventricular node. (Absence of the P wave may indicate atrial fibrillation.) The P wave indicates onset of atrial contraction.

Electric depolarization of the ventricle produces the QRS wave. It indicates the onset of ventricular contraction (ventricular systole) and is the point of maximal end diastole.

The T wave indicates electric repolarization of the atrium.

In diastole the ventricle relaxes and the mitral valve opens to allow blood to flow from the left atrium into the left ventricle. In systole the mitral valve closes as the ventricle contracts to send blood through the aortic cusps to the body (Fig. 3-7).

Apexcardiogram

Apexcardiography is used to describe a method for graphic recording of precordial movements. Most echocardiographic equipment may be used in conjunction with the apexcardiogram. Thus this combined technique permits observation of valve movements and chamber dimensions to provide information regarding the pathogenesis of auscultatory and palpable phenomena.

When the heart begins to contract, pressure in the ventricle is very low. The increasing pressure first

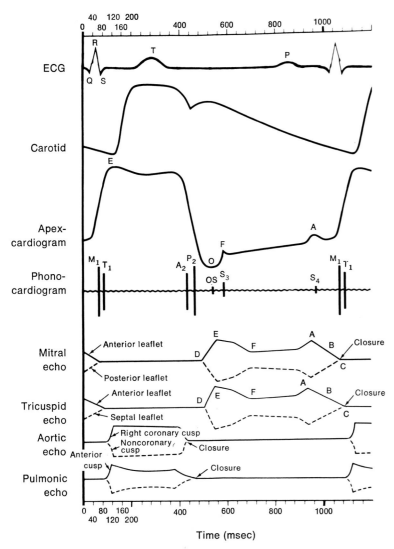

Fig. 3-7. Correlation of heart sounds, pulse tracings, and electric timing with the four heart valves.

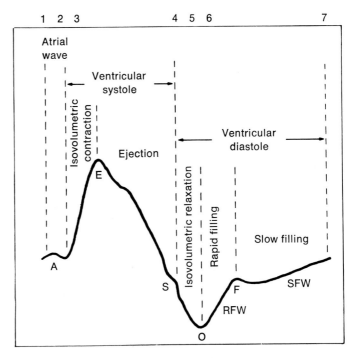

Fig. 3-8. Apexcardiogram.

closes the mitral valve. It does not open the aortic valve until pressure in the ventricle begins to *exceed* pressure in the aorta. The time between mitral closure and aortic valve opening is called *isovolumic contraction* (the shape of the ventricle changes but not the volume). After the P wave the lag period is 0.08 to 0.10 second. The ECG indicates electric phenomena; the mechanical events follow after a delay (in about 0.08

second). Therefore mechanical ventricular systole does not actually begin until about 0.06 to 0.08 second after the QRS wave.

Fig. 3-8 describes the apexcardiogram as follows:

1. Ventricle contracts; mitral valve closes; no blood goes out.

2. Ventricular pressure exceeds aortic pressure; aortic valve opens.

3. Ventricle gets smaller in volume and begins to relax.

4. Mitral leaflets open; first sharp opening of mitral leaflets.

5. Blood from atrium begins to fill ventricle (atrium has been filling with blood from lungs); during ventricular systole, atrium enlarges.

6. Early rapid ventricular filling occurs, followed by a slower filling phase.

7. Electric atrial depolarization takes place (A wave on echocardiogram); atrial contraction causes active ventricular filling, or *a* kick.

4 □ Ultrasonic detection techniques

TRANSDUCERS

Several types of transducers are available for echocardiography. Ideally, one should use as high a frequency as possible to improve the resolution of returning echoes. Remember, the higher the frequency, the less the penetration; therefore compromises will have to be made.

Many echocardiographers use a 3.5 MHz transducer with a medium focus. A larger patient may require a 2.25 MHz transducer and a barrel-chested, emphysematous patient a 1.6 MHz transducer. The pediatric patient generally requires a 5.0 or a 7.5 MHz transducer for good resolution and near-field definition.

Most transducers are now internally focused to improve resolution by shaping the beam and reducing distortion. Most cardiac transducers are of medium focus to concentrate the maximum resolution in the area of the mitral valve (Fig. 4-1).

A smaller crystal or diameter of the transducer allows better skin contact between rib interspaces and also gives more freedom to "sweep" the beam. Thus the transducer remains in one interspace, but the beam angle is changed to record cardiac structures in an oblique path.

Special transducers may be advantageous, depending on the specific patient population and the type of examination offered. An aspiration transducer may be useful in the location of pericardial effusion for pericardicentesis. The small suprasternal transducer may be employed for the detection of a dissecting aortic aneurysm, right atrial myxomas, or left atrial thrombi, and in measuring the left atrium, ascending aorta, or left brachial cephalic vein.

DISPLAY OF NORMAL HEART PATTERNS

The conventional M-mode display of echocardiographic techniques reveals the cardiac structures from anterior to posterior, just to the left of the sternal border. The patient is generally examined in the supine or left lateral semidecubitus position. Early literature described the "cardiac window" at the fourth intercostal space to the left of the sternal border. The cardiac window is the area on the anterior chest where the heart is just beneath the skin surface, free of lung interference (Fig. 4-2). With high gain we have found it more advantageous to cover a larger area along the left sternal border in the initial search for typical echocardiographic patterns to determine which inter-

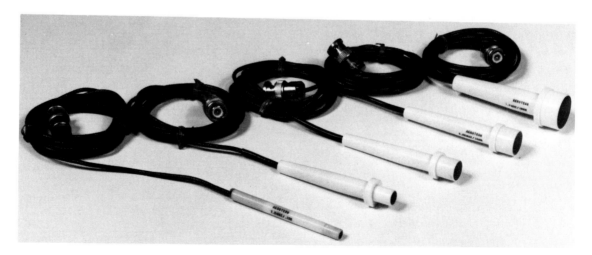

Fig. 4-1. Transducers should be used with the highest frequency and smallest diameter to improve resolution of the cardiac structures. Pediatric transducers vary in diameter from 3 to 6 mm with varying frequencies of 3.5, 5.0, and 7.5 MHz. Adult transducers also vary in diameter, including those of 6, 13, and 19 mm and frequency of 3.5, 2.25, and 1.6 MHz. (Courtesy KB-Aerotech, Lewistown, Pa.)

42

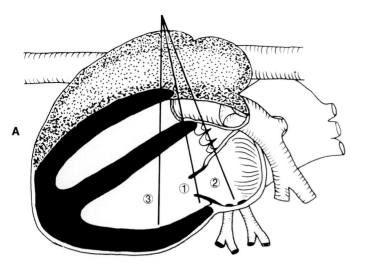

A

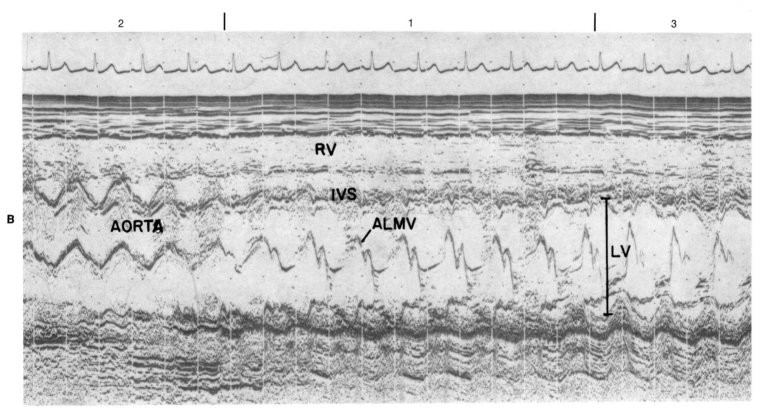

B

RV

IVS

AORTA

ALMV

LV

Fig. 4-2. A, Transducer positions. *1,* Perpendicular angulation with the anterior chest wall to record the right ventricular cavity, interventricular septum, anterior and posterior leaflets of the mitral valve, and left ventricular cavity. *2,* Medial cephalic angulation to record the aortic root, cusps, and left atrium. *3,* Lateral inferior angulation from the anterior leaflet of the mitral valve to record the right ventricle, interventricular septum, left ventricular cavity, and posterior heart wall. **B,** M-mode sweep from aorta (position 2), to mitral valve (position 1), to left ventricular cavity (position 3).

space is best. Once the transducer is placed along the left sternal border, the examiner should run up and down the chest wall to define the pericardial echo, which has the strongest, or "loudest," echo reflection. After the pericardium is defined, one can search for the mitral and aortic valve patterns and determine which interspace is best for demonstrating the continuity of cardiac structures (Fig. 4-3).

The echocardiographer must keep in mind that different body shapes will require variations in transducer position. These positions are guidelines for the average patient. An obese patient may have a trans-

verse heart and thus require lateral movement from the sternal border to record all cardiac structures. A tall thin patient may have a long and slender heart, requiring a lower, more medial transducer position. Barrel-chested patients may present echographic difficulties because of the lung absorption interference. One may have to turn these patients completely on the left side or even prone to eliminate this lung interference. Sometimes the upright or slightly bent forward position is useful to force the heart close to the anterior chest wall (Fig. 4-4).

Moving the transducer freely along the left sternal

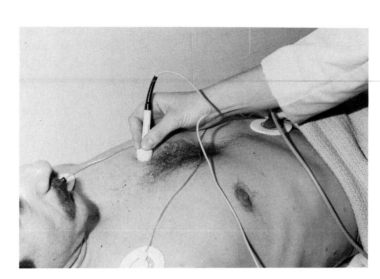

Fig. 4-3. Transducer position for aortic valve localization.

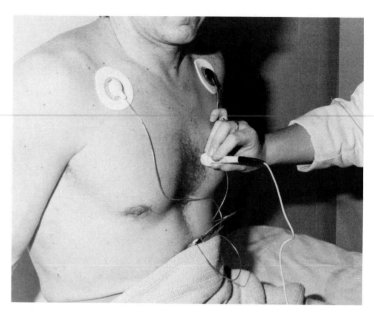

Fig. 4-4. Transducer position for mitral valve localization with patient in the upright position.

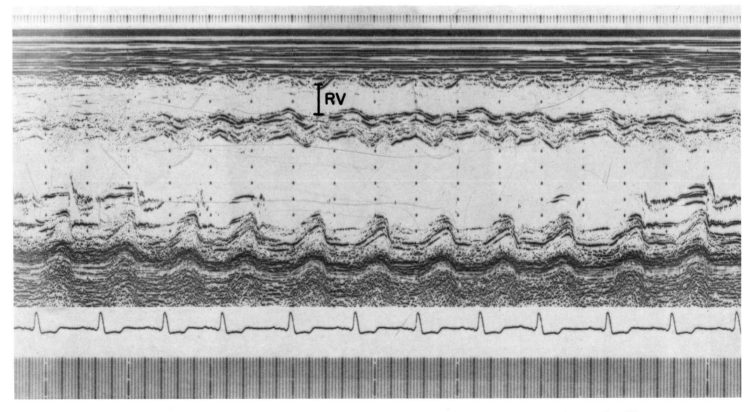

RV

Fig. 4-5. Right ventricular cavity is shown as the first echo-free space in the cardiac cavity. The anterior wall of the right ventricle is identified as the first moving echo as seen on A mode and M mode.

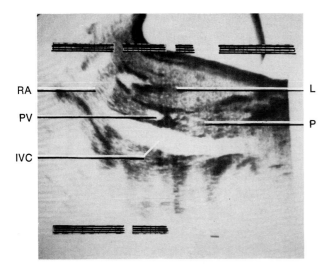

Fig. 4-6. Right atrium is best seen on the longitudinal B scan of the abdomen. The inferior vena cava can best be seen with the patient in deep inspiration. The cava pierces the diaphragm and empties into the right atrial cavity.

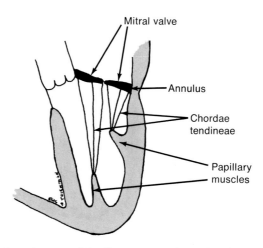

Fig. 4-7. Attachment of leaflets to annulus, chordae tendineae, and papillary muscles.

border until all the cardiac structures are easily identified is better practice than restriction to one interspace in the initial echocardiographic study. This saves time and gives the examiner a better understanding of cardiac relationships. If there is difficulty examining the patient in the supine position, a semidecubitus position should be used. Sometimes the best study is performed with the patient completely on the left side if the heart is actually medial. If too much lung interference clouds the study, the patient should exhale for as long as possible. This will usually give the examiner enough time to record a valid study.

The gain is usually increased for the initial searching period and decreased to obtain a clear tracing. The highest gain will be in the left ventricle and mitral valve area, but the aorta and tricuspid and pulmonary valves require less gain.

Table 4-1 contains locations and characteristics of intracardiac structures.

The right ventricle lies anterior to the left heart and is consistently shown on the echocardiogram as an anterior echo-free space between the first moving echo and the anterior interventricular septum. Near-field adjustments should be made to record the initial movement of the right side of the heart and the anterior side of the interventricular septum (Fig. 4-5).

The right atrium is best seen on the longitudinal real-time or B-mode display as the inferior vena cava empties into it. Suprasternal approach directed toward the right hip also allows visualization of this chamber (Fig. 4-6).

The mitral and tricuspid valves are thin saillike formations attached by chordae tendineae to the papillary muscles. The chordae tendineae are thin fibrous strands much like the guide ropes that hold up a tent. They prevent the valves from "swinging in the breeze." The ring, or annulus, surrounds the orifice of the valves. The leaflet is attached on one end to the annulus, and the "free" end is attached to the chordae tendineae and papillary muscle (Fig. 4-7).

The tricuspid valve is easily seen in patients with right ventricular enlargement. Its appearance is similar to the mitral leaflet, although only the anterior leaflet is usually shown (Fig. 4-8). With medial transducer angulation from the mitral leaflet the normal tricuspid valve may be partially demonstrated (Fig. 4-9). The systolic upswing is commonly seen.

Several differences are apparent between the anterior and posterior mitral leaflets. The anterior leaflet is much larger than the posterior, accounting for markedly greater excursion. In echocardiography the anterior leaflet moves 2 to 4 cm; this is one of its distinguishing features. The other is its amplitude echo strength with a biphasic motion (M movement), caused by the initial rapid opening and closing of the leaflet in early diastole and reopening in late diastole, secondary to atrial contraction, just before the final closure of the valve with ventricular systole. The chordae tendineae of the posterior leaflet are more closely allied to the papillary muscles, thus reducing the amount of excursion. Characteristically, the posterior leaflet moves opposite the anterior leaflet as in a mirror image, or W movement, with both anterior and posterior leaflets coming together during systole and moving anteriorly together until diastole.

Echographically the mitral valve should be re-

Table 4-1. Approximate locations of intracardiac structures

Structure	Distance from transducer	Transducer position	Characteristics
Posterior heart wall (PW)	9 to 12 cm	Usually found in third, fourth, and fifth interspace with transducer directed perpendicular to chest wall	1. Strong, pulsating echo complex 2. Pericardium strongest reflection in cardiac cavity 3. Three layers of posterior heart wall, endocardium, myocardium, epicardium, are seen anterior to pericardium
Anterior leaflet of mitral valve (ALMV)	6 to 9 cm	Transducer perpendicular to chest wall; may need slight medial or lateral angulation	1. Biphasic kick (M pattern seen on M mode) 2. Moves at least 2 to 3 cm in A or M mode 3. Strong reflector
Posterior leaflet of mitral valve (PLMV)	9 to 10 cm	From ALMV, angle *slightly* inferior and lateral (must maintain part of ALMV and watch for "clapping hands" movement of ALMV and PLMV moving opposite one another)	1. W pattern on M mode 2. Weak echo (be careful reject is not turned up to wipe out this echo)
Aortic root	4 to 6 cm	From MV, angle transducer superior and medial toward right shoulder	1. Parallel echo movement on A mode 2. Anterior part of aorta comes off IVS 3. Posterior part of aorta comes off ALMV 4. Normal aortic valve size: 1.2 to 1.9 cm
Cusps		Slight angulations to record cusp movement (may be medial, lateral inferior, or superior); if there is trouble recording noncoronary cusp, move slightly down and lateral or have patient stop breathing; may have to move up an interspace or roll patient to left side to see cusps	1. Internal echo seen within parallel echo complex on A mode 2. When both noncoronary and right coronary cusps recorded, "box" pattern is seen on M mode 3. Third cusp (left coronary) moves throughout center of "box"
Tricuspid valve (TV)	2 to 4 cm	From aortic root, angle inferior and slightly medial, or from MV, angle medial	1. Similar in appearance to MV (biphasic kick, wide excursion) 2. Because of location under sternal border, difficult to record completely; usually initial opening recorded
Right ventricle (RV)	1 to 3 cm	Right ventricle seen anterior to IVS and MV, aortic root with transducer on left sternal border	1. Anterior side of RV can be identified as first moving structure beyond crystal artifact and chest wall 2. Posterior surface anterior side of IVS 3. Normal size less than 2-3 cm
Interventricular septum (IVS)	2 to 4 cm	Usually seen with transducer perpendicular to chest wall or angled inferior and lateral to MV	1. Should be able to identify both sides of septum well by using near gain (suppression) and delay; if too many echoes in RV, turn near gain up; If not enough, turn near gain down (counterclockwise) (delay should be increased until it breaks off at anterior edge of septum) 2. Should equal posterior wall thickness (ratio 1.3:1.0 cm)
Left ventricular wall (LVW) (endocardium, myocardium, epicardium, pericardium)	9 to 12 cm	Inferior and lateral to ALMV	1. Extremely important to "sweep" from ALMV to left ventricle 2. Chordae tendineae may be demonstrated anterior to LVW (appears as denser echo than endocardium and has less excursion); endocardium has characteristic "notch" ⟵Chordae tendineae ⟵Endocardium 3. By decreasing gain, three layers of LVW may be demonstrated, with pericardial echo remaining as strongest moving reflection (demonstration of pericardial effusion is done by this method if fluid layer would dampen movement of pericardium)
LV and IVS		Transducer inferior and lateral to ALMV, but may angle slightly superior to this position to record IVS (use care to record IVS movement in correct position; when transducer is angled toward aorta, paradoxical motion may be seen)	1. For LV dimensions important to record IVS and LVW together (in systole they contract, in diastole they relax, and normal movement requires IVS and LVW to move toward one another); conversely, paradoxical septal motion means IVS moving opposite LV in systole
Pulmonary valve (PV)	1 to 3 cm	From aortic root, angle superior and lateral toward left shoulder; may have to move up one interspace	1. Parallel movement on A mode 2. Cusp echo may be seen within echo complex 3. Usually only posterior cusp seen, which moves posteriorly with systole

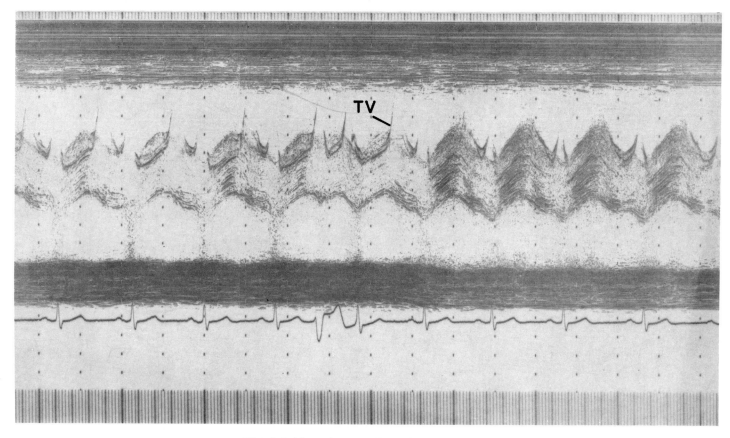

Fig. 4-8. M-mode recording of tricuspid valve.

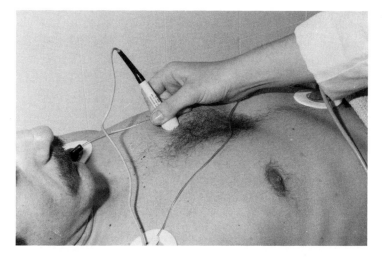

Fig. 4-9. Medial, slight caudal angulation of the transducer to demonstrate the tricuspid valve.

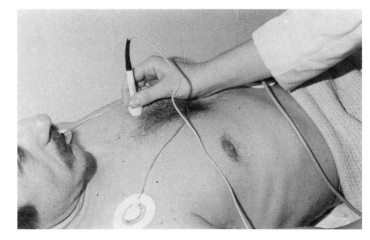

Fig. 4-10. Perpendicular angulation of the transducer to record mitral valve apparatus.

corded with the transducer perpendicular to the chest wall (Fig. 4-10). Good excursion of the valve is shown when the beam is directed toward the tip of the leaflet. If the beam is directed slightly superior toward the base of the valve or annulus, a sine wave will take the place of the valve or will run posterior to the anterior leaflet. The posterior leaflet is best recorded as the beam is directed slightly inferior and lateral toward the left ventricle (Fig. 4-11).

The aortic valve can be recorded by a sweep superior and medial toward the right shoulder (Fig. 4-12). The posterior aortic root is continuous with the anterior mitral leaflet, and the anterior aortic wall is continuous with the interventricular septum. With slight medial angulation or change in patient position to a more decubitus lie, the cusps of the aorta may be recorded (Fig. 4-13). Usually, the right coronary (anterior) and noncoronary (posterior) cusps are best shown

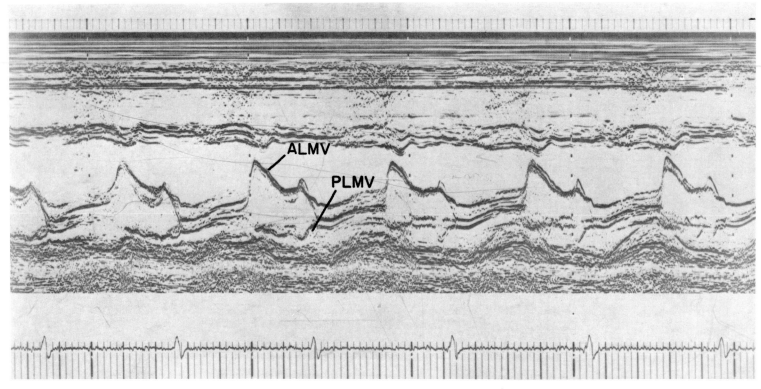

Fig. 4-11. M-mode recording of anterior and posterior leaflets of the mitral valve.

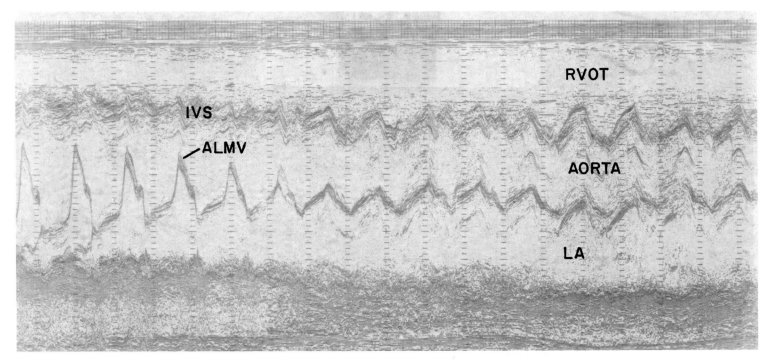

Fig. 4-12. M-mode sweep from the anterior leaflet of the mitral valve to the aortic root.

echographically. The left coronary cusp is sometimes shown in the middle of these two cusps (Fig. 4-14). Careful angulation will enable the examiner to record clear aortic root and cusp structures. Often both walls of the anterior and posterior aortic roots are shown, enabling the examiner to measure the lumen and the outer width of the vessel.

The pulmonary valve may be shown lateral and slightly superior to the aortic valve (Fig. 4-15).

Generally, as one sweeps from the aorta to the left shoulder, a large 2 to 4 cm space is shown anteriorly, with the left atrium posterior. It is within this space that part of the pulmonary valve is best shown (Fig. 4-16).

The left atrium is shown posterior to the aortic root. The size ratio of aorta to left atrium should be 1:1, thus making it easy to assess left atrial enlargement. The left atrial wall is immobile, since it is a filling chamber; thus no movement should be recorded on the tracing. As the examiner moves slightly inferior, the atrioventricular junction may be seen as a shallow boxlike movement along the left atrial wall. Often the left pulmonary vein can be faintly seen within the left atrial chamber and should not be confused with the left atrial wall (Fig. 4-17). Sweeps from the left atrium into the left ventricle can help determine the left atrial wall from the pulmonary vein if there is confusion.

The most obvious difference between cardiac chambers is wall thickness. The atria have thin walls because they are filling chambers, whereas the ventricles have thick walls for pumping activity. The pressures on the right side of the heart are not as great as those on the left side. The left ventricle is the real powerhouse and has the thickest walls of all the chambers.

Echographically the left ventricle is best shown by sweeping from the mitral valve inferiorly and laterally

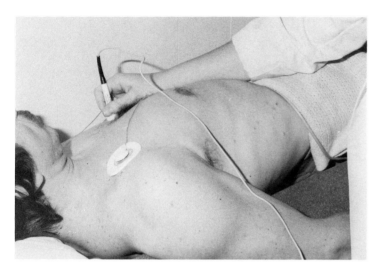

Fig. 4-13. Medial transducer angulation with patient in semidecubitus position to record the aortic root and cusps.

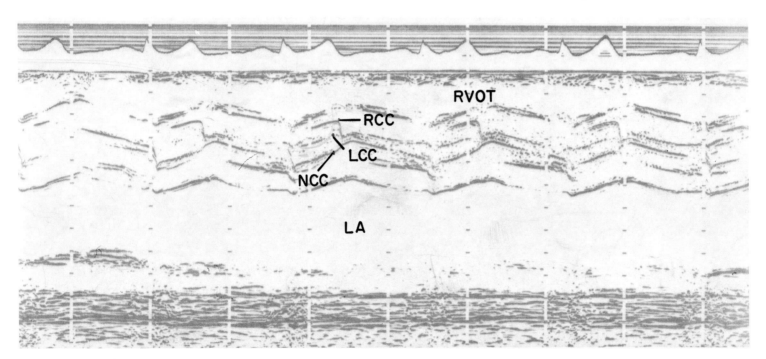

Fig. 4-14. M-mode demonstration of the aortic root with three cusp patterns. *RVOT,* Right ventricular outflow tract; *RCC,* right coronary cusp; *LCC,* left coronary cusp; *NCC,* noncoronary cusp; *LA,* left atrium.

toward the left hip (Fig. 4-18). At this point, just inferior to the mitral leaflets, the widest diameter of the left ventricle is seen. The examiner should be able to separate the right ventricle and the interventricular septum from chordae tendineae and the posterior heart wall (Fig. 4-19). Good motion of the interventricular septum and posterior heart wall is the best indicator of correct transducer position. This is probably the hardest cardiac structure to record because several sweeps are usually made before the best tracing is completed. The septum is best shown medially, and the posterior wall is best shown more laterally; thus, with slight patient obliquity in the left lateral decubitus position, careful

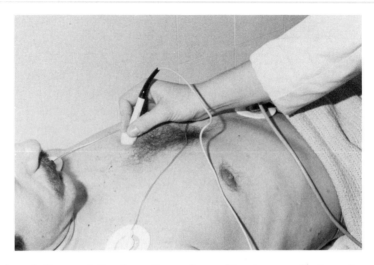

Fig. 4-15. Lateral cephalic angulation from the aortic position to record echoes from the pulmonary valve.

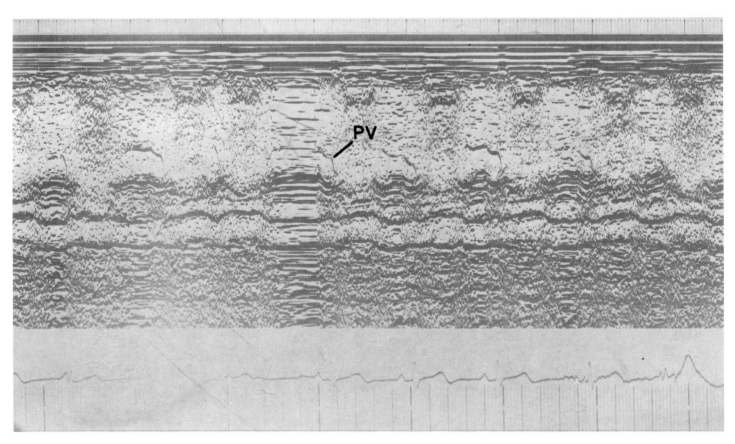

Fig. 4-16. M-mode demonstration of the pulmonary valve.

sweeps may be made to record both the septum and the posterior wall together. Gain adjustments should be lowered to further define the chordae, endocardium, myocardium, epicardium, and pericardium (Fig. 4-20). Chordae tendineae are usually more dense than the endocardium echo pattern, whereas the endocardium has a much greater velocity than the chordae. Endocardium is generally a continuous pattern; chordae may be more sporadic in the cardiac cycle. As the gain is decreased, the myocardium, or middle posterior wall layer, may be separated from the epi pericardium. The gain should be reduced dramatically to separate endocardium from pericardium to define posterior wall thickness.

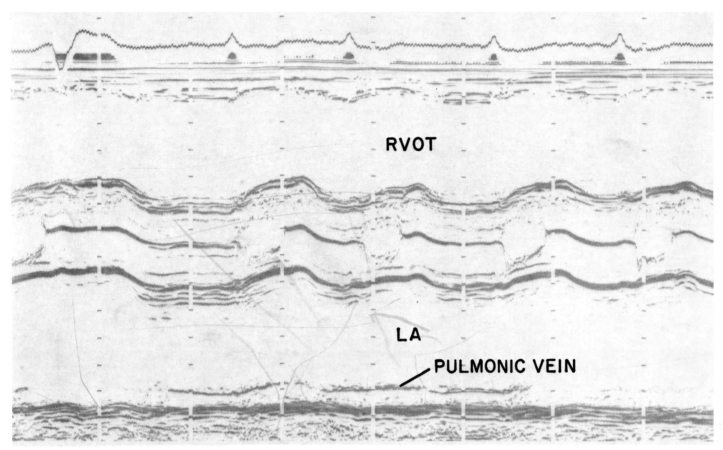

Fig. 4-17. Left atrium is recorded posterior to the aortic root. The left pulmonary vein can often be seen as a fine echo within the left atrial cavity.

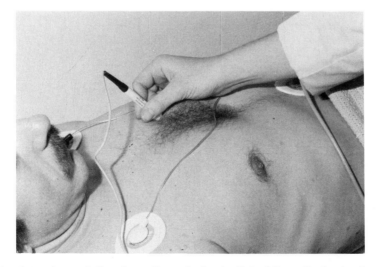

Fig. 4-18. Inferior lateral angulation from the anterior leaflet of the mitral valve to record left ventricular dimensions.

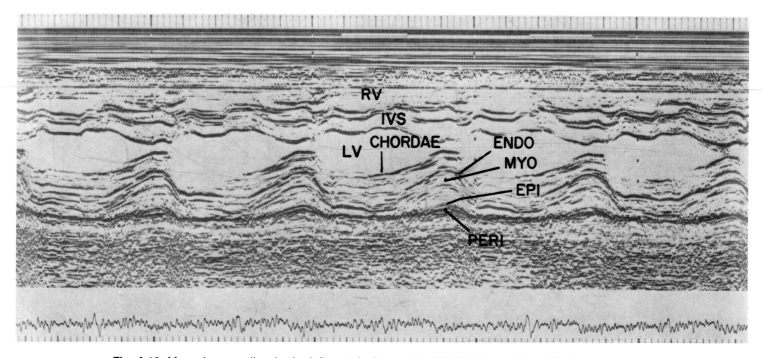

Fig. 4-19. M-mode recording in the left ventricular cavity. *RV,* Right ventricle; *IVS,* interventricular septum; *LV,* left ventricle; *ENDO,* endocardium; *MYO,* myocardium; *EPI,* epicardium; *PERI,* pericardium.

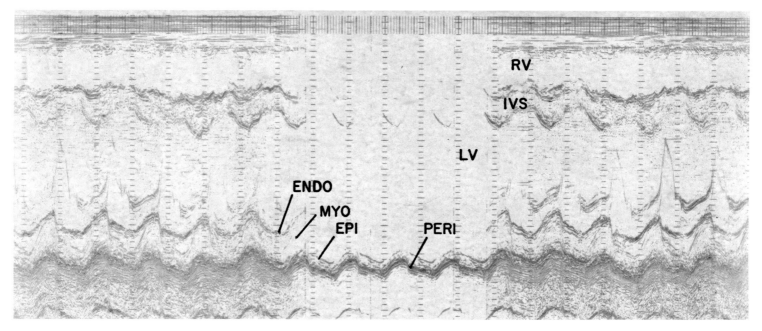

Fig. 4-20. Sweep into the left ventricular cavity to demonstrate reduced gain settings to separate the posterior heart wall from the pericardium.

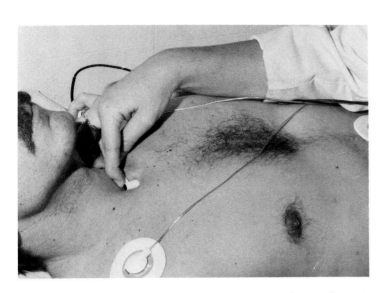

Fig. 4-21. Suprasternal approach to demonstrate the aortic arch, right pulmonary artery, and left atrium.

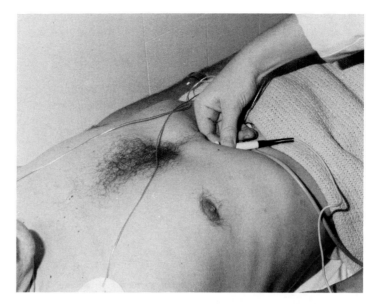

Fig. 4-22. Subxyphoid technique used for patients with too much lung interference in the conventional ultrasonic approach.

OTHER METHODS OF ULTRASONIC EXAMINATION

In a small percentage of the patients scanned, the examiner will not be able to record adequate information from the conventional left sternal approach. This may be a function of lung interference, an unusual angulation of the cardiac structures, or pathophysiology. Therefore other useful approaches should be employed to obtain the echographic information.

Suprasternal approach. The suprasternal technique was first described by Goldberg (1972). A special flattened transducer is placed in the suprasternal notch with the beam directed caudad. The transducer beam passes through the left brachiocephalic artery, aortic arch, right pulmonary artery, and left atrium. This technique has proved useful in the further detection of aneurysmal growth, tumor invasion, and arterial size in the pediatric and neonatal groups (Allen et al., 1977) (Fig. 4-21).

Subxyphoid approach. Chang first described the subxyphoid approach as an alternative method in the evaluation of cardiac structures obscured by lung tissue. The transducer is directed in a cephalic angulation from the subxyphoid approach. Recordings can then be made of the left ventricular wall, the mitral valve, and the aortic valve. Although accurate measurements cannot be obtained from this tangential approach, it has proved a useful technique in ruling out certain cardiac problems such as valvular disease, pericardial effusion, and tumor formation (Fig. 4-22).

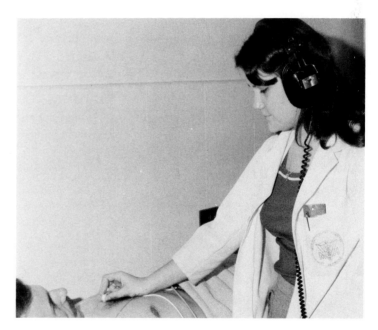

Fig. 4-23. Pulsed Doppler technique with earphones to hear forward and reverse flow within the heart.

Pulsed Doppler approach. The pulsed Doppler apparatus has been especially useful in the detection of regurgitation flows, septal defects, and certain kinds of arrhythmias. The transducer is directed over the area of interest while audible and direct printouts are recorded to demonstrate forward and reverse flow (Fig. 4-23).

5 □ Echocardiographic measurements

with assistance of
LINDA MEIXELL, R.T., *and* **PAT HETRICK, B.S.**

The ability to evaluate echographic data has been of great interest to the clinicians and investigators involved in ultrasonic techniques. The early pioneers in ultrasound (Feigenbaum, Popp, Gramiak, and Joyner) were able to consistently correlate their ultrasonic data with other diagnostic studies to confirm the validity of ultrasonic measurements in echocardiography. The data must be evaluated along with the patient's clinical history and symptoms to have meaning (pp. 55 to 60). Although many laboratories have discontinued certain echocardiographic measurements, we have found the echocardiogram a very useful teaching tool. Instructing the students how to evaluate the echocardiogram by the use of measurements improves their technique and sharpens their echo tracings for interpretation. We have also found that eyeballing can mislead an inexperienced sonographer to overread or underread a particular study. Therefore this chapter is devoted to echocardiographic measurements and their explanation. These data have accumulated from the various investigators in the field with specific references to normal values. In addition, an outline of specific diseases and their echographic significance is provided in Table 5-1.

To fully evaluate the cardiac patient, we have found it useful to perform the conventional M-mode and real-time applications of ultrasound (Fig. 5-1). Thus, when we calculate our measurements, the added dimension of the real-time image adds to our understanding of the total picture of cardiac function and contractility.

Calipers facilitate the measurement process and should be used for uniformity and accuracy in data accumulation. The scans and data sheets are then reviewed by the sonographer and physician for final interpretation.

Text continued on p. 62.

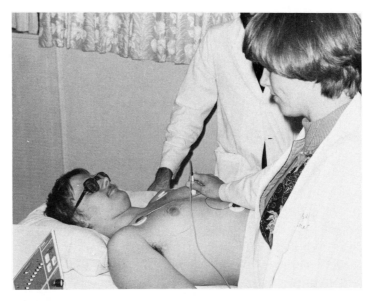

Fig. 5-1. Conventional M-mode technique to record the intracardiac structures from the aortic root, mitral valve, tricuspid valve, pulmonary valve, and ventricular cavities.

DIVISIONS OF ULTRASOUND AND CARDIOLOGY
Echocardiographic Data Research Form

Patient identification

Adult 25 years or over	_____
25 years or under	_____
Adolescent 2 to 12 years	_____
Infant under 2 years	_____
Neonate	_____
Age	_____
Previous echocardiographic examination	Yes____ No____
Blood pressure	_____/_____
Height	_____
Weight	_____
Body surface area	_____

Mitral valve

C-E amplitude	_____ cm
↑ _____	
↓ _____	
C-D amplitude	_____ cm
↑ _____	
↓ _____	
LVO at *c* point	_____ cm
↑ _____	
↓ _____	
LVO at *d* point	_____ cm
↑ _____	
↓ _____	
E-F slope	_____ mm/sec
↑ _____	
↓ _____	

Characteristics

Flutter	Yes____ No____
Arrythmias	Yes____ No____
Calcification	Yes____ No____
Thickening	Yes____ No____
SAM	Yes____ No____
Pseudo-SAM	Yes____ No____
Separation of ALMV/PLMV	_____ cm
Prolapse PLMV	Yes____ No____
Midsystolic	_____
Late systolic	_____
Holosystolic	_____
Prolapse ALMV	Yes____ No____
Midsystolic	_____

Late systolic	_____
Holosystolic	_____
Prolapse ALMV/PLMV	_____
PLMV moves	
Posterior	_____
Anterior	_____
Myxoma shown	Yes____ No____
Vegetations on MV	_____
PR-AC interval	_____
↑ _____	
↓ _____	
Premature closure of MV	Yes____ No____
Amputated *e*; prominent *a*	Yes____ No____
Calcified mitral annulus	Yes____ No____

Aorta

Dimension aortic root	_____ cm
↑ _____	
↓ _____	
Multiple or increased echoes	Yes____ No____
Dissection	Yes____ No____

Aortic valve

Cusps shown

RCC ____	
NCC ____	
LCC ____	
Systolic opening rate _____ mm/sec	
Systolic time interval	_____ _____
	_____ msec
Systolic separation	_____ cm
↑ _____	
↓ _____	
Thickening	Yes____ No____
Midsystolic closure	Yes____ No____
Eccentric	Yes____ No____
Coapt	Yes____ No____

Left atrium

Dimension	_____ cm
↑ _____	
↓ _____	
Left atrial wall motion	
Normal _____	
Exaggerated _____	

Continued.

DIVISIONS OF ULTRASOUND AND CARDIOLOGY—cont'd
Echocardiographic Data Research Form—cont'd

Left atrial index	_____	
↑ _____		
↓ _____		
Tumor echoes	Yes____ No____	
Pericardial effusion behind LA wall	Yes____ No____	
Tricuspid valve		
Normal	Yes____ No____	
Flutter	Yes____ No____	
Flattened	Yes____ No____	
Amplitude	_____ cm	
Pulmonary valve		
Normal	Yes____ No____	
Flutter	Yes____ No____	
a dip	Yes____ No____	
Amplitude	_____	
Prosthetic valve		
Type _____ (ball, disk, homograft)		
Model _____		
Aorta _____		
Mitral _____		
Tricuspid _____		
Excursion _____		
Opening slope _____		
Closing slope _____		
Unusual echoes _____		
Right ventricle		
Dimension	_____ cm	
↑ _____		
↓ _____		
Interventricular septum		
Thickness	_____ cm	
↑ _____		
↓ _____		
Septal wall amplitude	_____ cm	
↑ _____		
↓ _____		
Septal wall motion		
Normal _____		
Paradoxical _____		
Flat _____		

Left ventricle

LVIDd	_____ cm
↑ _____	
↓ _____	
LVIDs	_____ cm
↑ _____	
↓ _____	
PLVW	_____ cm
IVS/PLVW	_____/_____
↑ _____	
↓ _____	
Normal _____	
LVDV (Dd^3)	_____ cm
LVDV (Ds^3)	_____ cm
SV = LVDV − LVSV	_____
↑ _____	
↓ _____	
Normal _____	
CO = HR × SV/1000 =	_____
HR	_____
↑ _____	
↓ _____	
Normal _____	
E. F. = 1 − (Ds^3/Dd^3) =	_____
↑ _____	
↓ _____	
Normal _____	
LV mass	_____
↑ _____	
↓ _____	
Normal _____	
Pericardial effusion	
Anterior _____	
Posterior _____	
Separation epicardium to pericardium	_____ cm
PLVW amplitude	_____ mm
↑ _____	
↓ _____	
Normal _____	

DIVISIONS OF ULTRASOUND AND CARDIOLOGY—cont'd
Echocardiographic Data Research Form—cont'd

Endocardial velocity	_____ mm/sec	Ebstein's anomaly	_____
↑ _____		Atresia	_____
↓ _____		Discontinuity—aorta	_____
Diagnosis		**Pulmonary valve**	
Mitral valve		Stenosis	_____
Stenosis	_____	Insufficiency	_____
Regurgitation	_____	**Right ventricle**	
Prolapse	_____	Enlargement	_____
Myxoma	_____	Paradoxical septal motion	_____
Vegetations	_____	Diminution	_____
Calcified mitral annulus	_____	**Interventricular septum**	
Atresia	_____	Thin	_____
Other	_____	Concentric thickening with PLVW	_____
Aorta		Eccentric thickening with PLVW	_____
Stenosis	_____	Atrial septal defect	_____
Subaortic stenosis	_____	Akinesis	_____
Regurgitation	_____	Hyperdynamia	_____
Vegetations	_____	LBBB movement	_____
Bicuspid valve	_____	ASH without obstruction	_____
Dissection	_____	ASH with obstruction (IHSS)	_____
Truncus arteriosus	_____	Enlargement	_____
Patent ductus	_____	Diminution	_____
Coarctation	_____	**Left ventricle**	
Atresia	_____	Enlargement	_____
Other	_____	Thin PLVW	_____
Left atrium		Thick PLVW	_____
Enlargement	_____	Akinesis	_____
Tumor	_____	Hyperdynamia	_____
Tricuspid valve		Aneurysm of LVW	_____
Stenosis	_____	Cardiomyopathy	_____
Insufficiency	_____	Pericardial effusion	_____
Vegetations	_____	Other	_____

ECHOCARDIOLOGY DATA SHEET
Preliminary report
Physician ______________________________
Sonographer ______________________________

Patient ______________________________
Age ________ Ht. ________ Wt. ________ BSA ________ m²
Location ______________________________
Date ______________________________
Clinical diagnosis ______________________________

C-E ampl.	E-F	LVOc	LVOd	Cusp	Width	LA	RV	IVS	PLVW	LVIDd	LVIDs	SV	E.F.	LV mass
	220 mm													
	215													
	210													
	205													
	200													
	195													
	190													
	185													
	180													
	175													
	170													
	165													
	160													
	155													300
	150													290
	145													280
	140													270
	135													260
	130	48 mm	48 mm											250
	125	46	46											240
	120	44	44											230
	115	42	42											220
40 mm	110	40	40					4.0 cm						200
38	105	38	38					3.8	3.8 cm					190
36	100	36	36			9.0 cm		3.6	3.6				0.95	180
34	90	34	34			8.5		3.4	3.4	9.0 cm			0.90	170
32	85	32	32			8.0		3.2	3.2	8.5	8.5 cm	160	0.85	160
30	80	30	30			7.5		3.0	3.0	8.0	8.0	150	0.80	150
28	75	28	28		7.0 cm	7.0		2.8	2.8	7.5	7.5	140	0.75	140
26	70	26	26		6.5	6.5		2.6	2.6	7.0	7.0	130	0.70	130
24	65	24	24		6.0	6.0	6.0 cm	2.4	2.4	6.5	6.5	120	0.65	120
22	60	22	22		5.5	5.5	5.5	2.2	2.2	6.0	6.0	110	0.60	110
20	55	20	20		5.0	5.0	5.0	2.0	2.0	5.5	5.5	100	0.55	100
18	50	18	18		4.5	4.5	4.5	1.8	1.8	5.0	5.0	90	0.50	90
16	45	16	16		4.0	4.0	4.0	1.6	1.6	4.5	4.5	80	0.45	80
14	40	14	14	3.5 cm	3.5	3.5	3.5	1.4	1.4	4.0	4.0	70	0.40	70
12	35	12	12	3.0	3.0	3.0	3.0	1.2	1.2	3.5	3.5	60	0.35	60
10	30	10	10	2.5	2.5	2.5	2.5	1.0	1.0	3.0	3.0	50	0.30	50
8	25	8	8	2.0	2.0	2.0	2.0	0.8	0.8	2.5	2.5	40	0.25	40
6	20	6	6	1.5	1.5	1.5	1.5	0.6	0.6	2.0	2.0	30	0.20	30
4	15	4	4	1.0	1.0	1.0	1.0	0.4	0.4	1.5	1.5	20	0.15	20
2	10	2	2	0.5	0.5	0.5	0.5	0.2	0.2	1.0	1.0	10	0.10	10
Mitral valve				Aorta		LA	RV	IVS	Left ventricle					

DIVISIONS OF ULTRASOUND AND CARDIOLOGY
Echocardiography Consultation Form

Case number _____

Interpretation

Height _____ Weight _____

Clinical findings _____

_____

_____

_____

Indicated measurements

Interventricular septum	_____ cm	Ejection time	_____
LV posterior wall	_____ cm	Septal-aortic continuity	_____
Aortic root dimension	_____ cm	Septal motion	_____
Intra-aortic cusp spacing	_____ cm	Pericardial effusion	_____
RV cavity	_____ cm	Stroke volume	_____
LV internal dimension(ed)	_____ cm	Ejection fraction	_____ (above
LV internal dimension(es)	_____ cm		65%)
Left atrial dimension	_____ cm	Cardiac output	_____
Mitral valve amplitude	_____ cm		
Mitral valve velocity	_____ cm		

$$Vcf = \frac{LVID(ed) - LVID(es)}{LVID(ed) \times LVET} = \underline{\qquad}$$

Prolapse ALMV _____

PLMV _____

Holosystolic, midsystolic,

typical _____

Suggestive _____

Possible _____

Suprasternal notch

Aorta (arch) _____ cm

Right pulmonary artery _____ cm

Left atrium (y axis) _____ cm

LV mass _____

Endocardial velocity _____

Sonographer _____

Physician _____, M.D.

DIVISIONS OF ULTRASOUND AND CARDIOLOGY
Echocardiography Report

Case number _____

Height _____ Weight _____

Interpretation

Clinical findings _____
_____
_____
_____

Indicated measurements

Interventricular septum	_____ cm (0.7-1.1 cm)	Ejection time _____
LV posterior wall	_____ cm (0.7-1.1 cm)	Septal-aortic continuity _____
Aortic root dimension	_____ cm (2.0-3.7 cm)	Septal motion _____
Intra-aortic cusp spacing	_____ cm (1.3-1.9 cm)	Pericardial effusion _____
RV cavity	_____ cm (0.7-2.6 cm)	Stroke volume _____
LV internal dimension(ed)	_____ cm (4.0-5.5 cm)	Ejection fraction _____ (above
LV internal dimension(es)	_____ cm (2.5-4.0 cm)	65%)
Left atrial dimension	_____ cm (1.9-4.0 cm)	Cardiac output _____
Mitral valve amplitude	_____ cm (20-35 mm)	
Mitral valve velocity	_____ cm (70-150 mm/sec)	

$$\text{Vcf} = \frac{\text{LVID(ed)} - \text{LVID(es)}}{\text{LVID(ed)} \times \text{LVET}} = \underline{\qquad}$$

Prolapse ALMV _____

LV mass _____

    PLMV _____

Endocardial velocity _____

    Holosystolic,

      midsystolic,

      typical _____

    Suggestive _____

    Possible _____

Suprasternal notch

    Aorta (arch) _____ cm

    Right pulmonary artery _____ cm

Sonographer _____

    Left atrium (y axis) _____ cm

Physician _____, M.D.

Table 5-1. Echocardiographic structures

Disease	LA	LV	LVO	RV	Mitral valve (anterior and posterior)	Aortic valve	IVS	Posterior heart wall	Other
MV stenosis	↑				↓ E-F slope (<35 mm/sec) ↓ C-E amplitude (severe) No *a* kick (usually) PLMV moves anterior (usually)				Calcification (thickening)
MV regurgitation	↑	↑	↑		*e* point touches IVS ↑ C-E amplitude E-F slope >180 mm/sec Flutter ALMV				Prolapse?
MV prolapse	↑ (MR)	↑ (MR)	↑ (MR)		Posterior motion in systole (3 to 5 mm)				"Hump" in pericardial effusion (pseudoprolapse)
Aortic insufficiency		↑	↑		↓ E-F slope Flutter of ALMV		↑ Amplitude (may have) ? Flutter IVS		
Aortic stenosis					↓ E-F slope ? Calcified mitral annulus	Calcified walls ↓ Systolic septal wall motion	↑ Thickness	Concentric hypertrophy	Bicuspid (eccentric cusps)
CCM (congestive cardiomyopathy)	↑	↑	↑	↑	↓ Amplitudes PLMV clearly recorded ALMV/PLMV clearly recorded		Thin Poor contractility	Thin	Cardiomegaly; pericardial effusion
IHSS or HOCM	? ↑ MR	↑	↓		*e* point touches IVS ↓ E-F slope SAM (obstructive)	Midsystolic closure	>1.8 to 2.0 cm IVS/PHW > 1.3 cm		Pseudo-SAM in hypertension
Vegetations	↑ MR	↑ AI	↑ AI	↑ TR	Multilayered thickening Coarse diastolic flutter	Coarse diastolic flutter			Vegetations 2 to 3 mm thick
Normal heart	1.9 to 4.0 cm; 1:1 LA/Ao	4.0 to 5.5 cm	20 to 35 cm	0.7 to 2.6 cm	M shape of ALMV PLMV moves posterior E-F slope 80 to 150 mm/sec C-E amplitude = 20 to 35 mm	Box shape Systolic separation 1.5 to 2.6 cm LA index † <2.2	0.6 to 1.2 cm IVS/PHW = 1.3	1.1 cm	

*SAM = Systolic anterior motion.

†LA index = LA/BSA (body surface area).

Mitral valve

C-D amplitude   From c point to d point (Fig. 5-2). This is the closed systolic position during which the valve leaflets move with the annulus. This measurement has nothing to do with the valve itself but concerns the heart movement.

C-D slope   Slope, is measured over a period of time. The line must be extended through a 1-second interval, which is three time lines. The line will be drawn through points c and d.

C-E amplitude   From c point to e point. This measures the amplitude at which the mitral valve is opening; e point is the most anterior excursion.

LVO at c point   Left ventricular outflow tract. Measure from the left side of the septum to the c point on the mitral valve echo.

LVO at d point   Left ventricular outflow tract. Measure from the posterior wall of the septum to the d point on the mitral valve echo.

D-E slope   Opening movement of the mitral valve in early diastole (Fig. 5-3).

D-E amplitude   Maximum mobility or excursion of the valve.

E-F slope   Measures the rate of motion of the cusp in early diastole and expresses the rate of left atrial emptying. Since a slope is being measured, extend the line connecting e and f through three time lines.

A-C slope   The systolic closing slope is measured from points a to c through three time lines.

Fluttering   You may see fine flutter of the anterior leaflet in diastole. This could be due to aortic insufficiency, mitral regurgitation, or, if the flutter is coarse, atrial fibrillation.

SAM   Systolic anterior motion. The valve moves anteriorly in systole. SAM occurs in idiopathic hypertrophic subaortic stenosis (IHSS). (See Fig. 5-4.)

Multiple echoes   In the absence of calcification, the mitral valve echo is thin, single, or double; more echoes are compatible with calcification.

Thickening   If the echoes are thick and confluent, heavy calcification is present.

PLMV   Designate whether the posterior leaflet moves posteriorly in diastole or anteriorly.

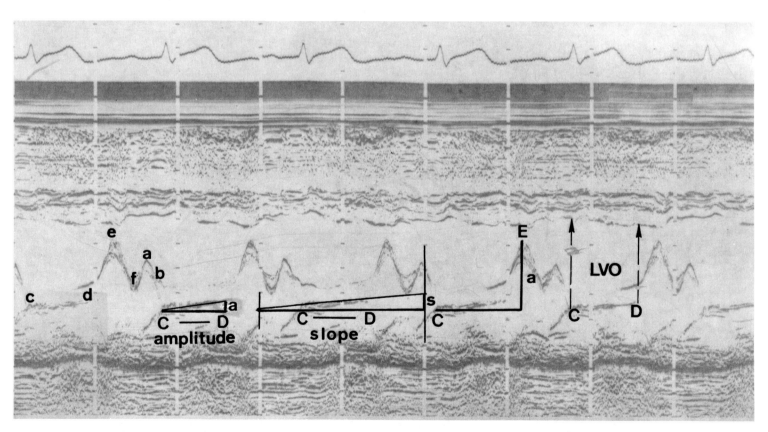

Fig. 5-2. Mitral valve has been given letters to represent systolic components (c-d) and diastolic components (d, e, f, a, b, c). For an explanation of C-D amplitude (a) and slope (s) C-E amplitude (a) and left ventricular outflow tract at c and d see text.

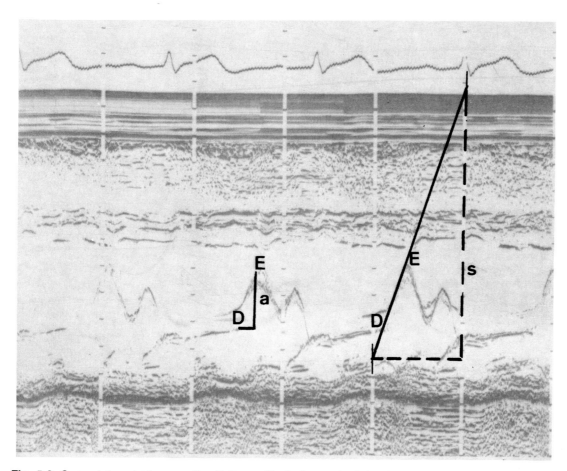

Fig. 5-3. Some laboratories use the D-E amplitude instead of the C-E amplitude for mitral valve excursion. See text for explanation.

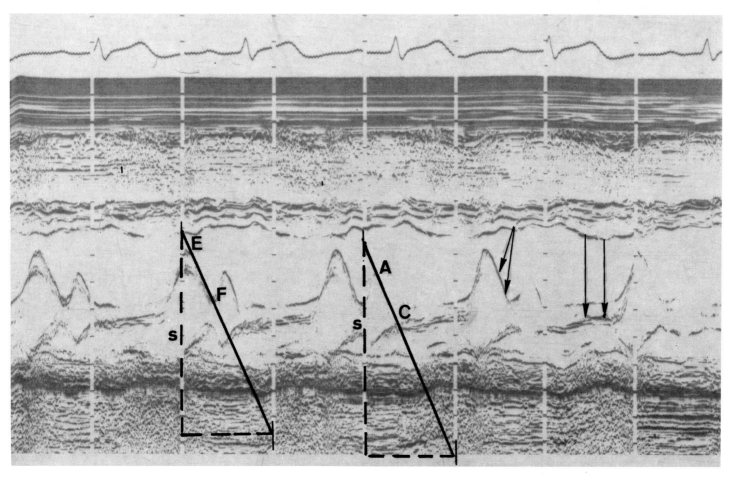

Fig. 5-4. Mitral leaflet should be measured at its greatest excursion. The best excursion is normally below the aorta near the tip of the leaflet (the posterior leaflet may also be seen at this point). In figuring the E-F slope the steepest slope should be measured. See text for explanation of A-C slope, flutter, and SAM.

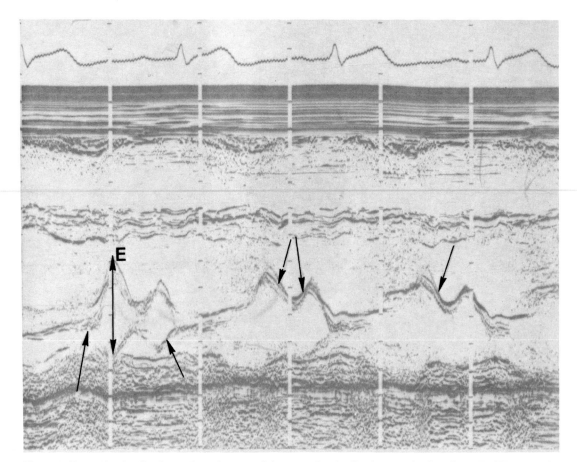

Fig. 5-5. Posterior leaflet is a mirror image of the anterior leaflet in ventricular diastole. The anterior and posterior leaflets should meet in systole at points C-D. See text for explanation of mitral valve separation, thickening, and multiple echoes (as seen in mitral stenosis).

MV separation	Measures the separation from the ALMV to the PLMV in diastole. Measure the *e* point of the anterior leaflet to the posterior leaflet at the same point. (See Fig. 5-5.)
Posterior bulging	The posterior leaflet will be displaced posteriorly in systole. The normal anterior systolic movement is interrupted by a posterior steplike motion, usually 3 to 5 mm in magnitude but sometimes as large as 10 mm. This motion occurs in prolapse.
Space beneath MV clear	Echoes behind the mitral value in diastole that do not disappear as the gain is decreased slightly. If there is an echo-free space behind the mitral valve in early diastole followed by an increase of echoes, this could represent a myxoma (Fig. 5-6).
Vegetations	Bacterial endocarditis can be visualized as ragged echoes on the anterior leaflet (may simulate flutter).
PR-AC interval	Measure from the beginning of the P wave to the beginning of the QRS complex, and from the *a* point to the *c* point on the mitral valve. Measure both on the 40 msec time line. Subtract the AC from the PR interval to obtain the PR-AC interval.
Premature closure	The *c* point of the mitral valve occurs before the QRS complex.

Amputated *e*, prominent *a*	Occurs with elevated left ventricular end-diastolic pressure. The *e* point is diminished, and the *a* point is accentuated.

Normal measurements

E-F slope	80 to 150 mm/sec
E-F slope in mitral stenosis	Under 35 mm/sec (Gramiak, Feigenbaum) Under 70 mm/sec (Popp)
C-E amplitude	23 to 32 mm
D-E amplitude	20 to 30 mm (Popp)
PR-AC interval	More than 0.06 second (Feigenbaum)

Aortic root

Dimension	Measure at end diastole, leading edge of anterior aortic root to leading edge of posterior aortic root (Fig. 5-7).
Multiple or increased echoes	Heavy lines appearing in the aorta are calcification.
Dissection	Dilatation of the aortic root, plus a continuous echo appearing at least 1 cm from the walls of the aorta (maybe along both walls or along only one wall).

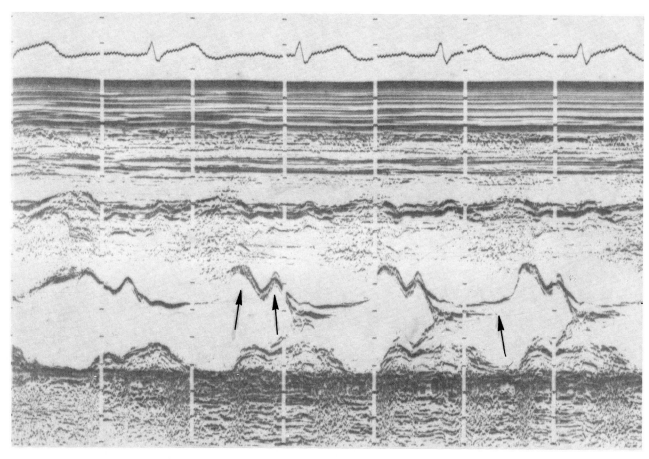

Fig. 5-6. Space beneath the mitral valve's anterior leaflet should be clear of echoes. The systolic segment of the valve should move in an anterior direction.

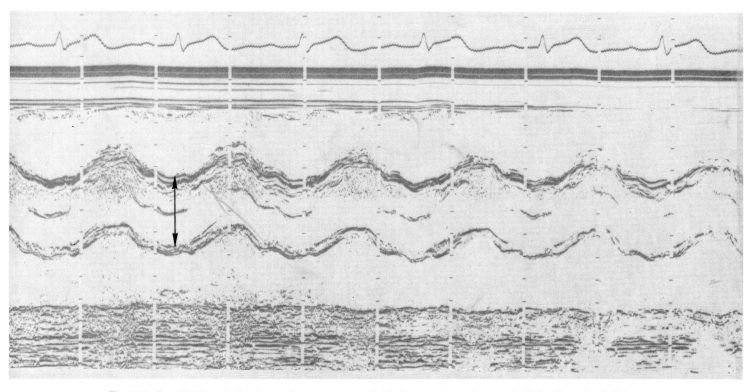

Fig. 5-7. Parallel band of echoes that move anteriorly in systole and posteriorly in diastole delineate the walls of the aorta. The leading edge to leading edge is measured because it is a finite and initial point (according to Popp), and there should be little difficulty separating the walls from the lumen of the aorta.

Aortic valve

Cusps shown	Right coronary (anterior), left coronary (middle), and noncoronary (posterior).
Systolic opening rate	Rate at which the cusps open in systole (Fig. 5-8).
Systolic closing rate	Rate at which the cusps close in systole.
Systolic separation	The cusps' separation is measured in systole. Draw a perpendicular line from the right coronary cusp to the noncoronary cusp at the opening movement
Flutter	Fine flutter may occur in the cusps.
Thickening	This indicates calcification of the aortic cusps.
Interrupted opening	There would be an indentation in the box-type figure in midsystole (as seen in IHSS).
Eccentric	Positioning of the cusps during diastole to one side of the aortic wall rather then in the middle of the aorta.
Coapt	The cusps normally come together in diastole. (See Fig. 5-9.)

Normal measurements

Aortic width (EDD—end-diastolic diameter)	2.1 to 4.4 cm (Popp)
Aortic value opening	16 to 26 mm (Feigenbaum)

Left atrium (Fig. 5-10)

Dimension	The left atrium is measured at the end of systole. Measure from the anterior portion of the posterior aortic wall to the anterior edge of the posterior atrial wall.
Wall motion	Draw a straight line horizontally from the posterior atrial wall in systole to above the point where the posterior atrial wall is in diastole. Measure this distance for atrial wall motion.
Left atrial index	Divide the body surface area into the left atrial size. This equals the left atrial index.

Normal measurements

End-systolic diameter, uncorrected	1.9 to 4.0 cm (Feigenbaum) 2.3 to 4.0 cm (Popp)
End-systolic diameter, corrected to body surface area (BSA)	1.2-2.1 cm/m² (Feigenbaum)
End-systolic diameter, corrected to left atrial size/aortic size	0.87 to 1.2 cm (Popp)

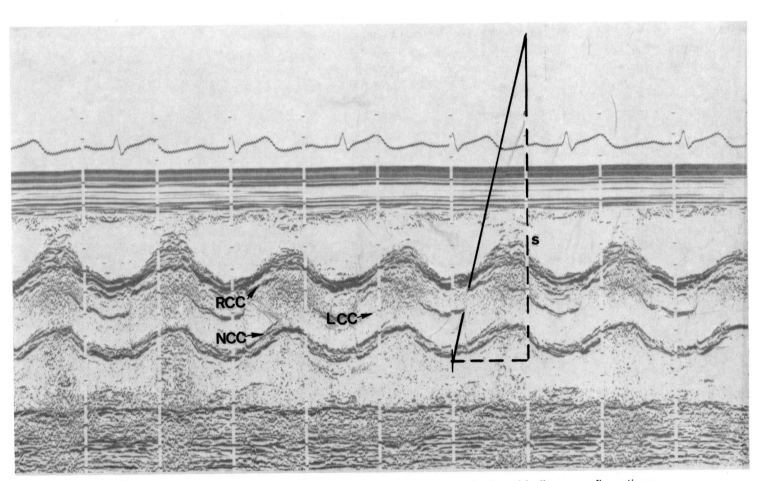

Fig. 5-8. Gramiak (1970) states that the valvular cusps are recognized as thin linear configurations moving to the periphery of the aorta in systole and occupying a midaortic position. The right and noncoronary cusps show significant systolic movement in the opposite direction and produce a boxlike configuration. The left coronary cusp is normally not visualized, since it lies at right angles to the sonic beam. See text for systolic opening rate.

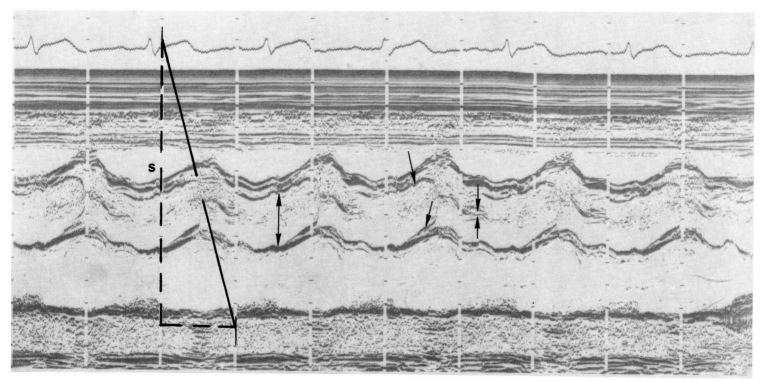

Fig. 5-9. See text for explanation of systolic closing rate, systolic separation, flutter, thickening, interrupted opening, eccentricity, and coapt signs.

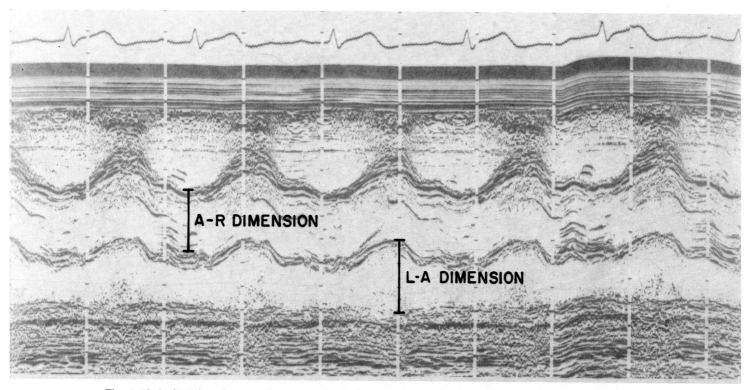

Fig. 5-10. Left atrium is recorded posterior to the aortic root and usually presents a 1:1 ratio to the aortic root dimension. The measurement of the left atrium includes the anterior edge of the posterior aortic wall. This is a source of error, but if all left atrial dimensions are measured in this fashion, the error will be consistent and constant.

Right ventricle (Fig. 5-11)

Dimension   The right ventricle is measured in end diastole. The measurement is taken from the anterior wall of the right ventricle to the anterior wall of the septum.

Normal measurements

End-diastolic diameter (values greater than these suggest right ventricular dilatation)

Supine   7 to 23 cm (Feigenbaum)

Lateral decubitus   11 to 26 cm (Feigenbaum)

5 to 21 cm (Popp)

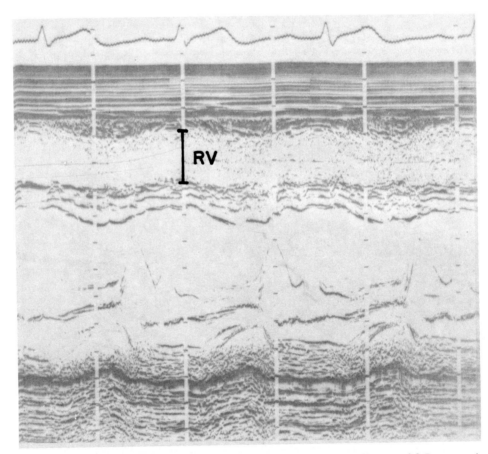

Fig. 5-11. If the right ventricular wall echo cannot be visualized, an estimate of 0.5 cm posterior to the last nonmoving chest wall echo as the location of the right ventricular wall can be made. The right ventricle will appear slightly enlarged as the patient assumes the semidecubitus position because of the tangential angulation of the transducer. Generally, it does not exceed 2.6 cm in either direction in normal subjects.

Interventricular septum (Fig. 5-12)

Thickness — The septum is measured in ventricular diastole (R wave on the ECG). Measure from leading edge to leading edge.

Amplitude — Measure from the most posterior to the most anterior movement of the posterior wall of the septum.

Motion — Normal—the septum moves posteriorly as the posterior heart wall moves anteriorly.

Type A—both septum and PLVW move anteriorly (paradoxical motion).

Type B—the left side of the septum moves poorly or not at all.

Normal measurements

Normal values at end diastole

	IVS	*PLVW*
Thickness	8 to 11 mm	8 to 11 mm
Excursion	3 to 8 mm	9 to 14 mm
Movement in systole	Posterior	Anterior

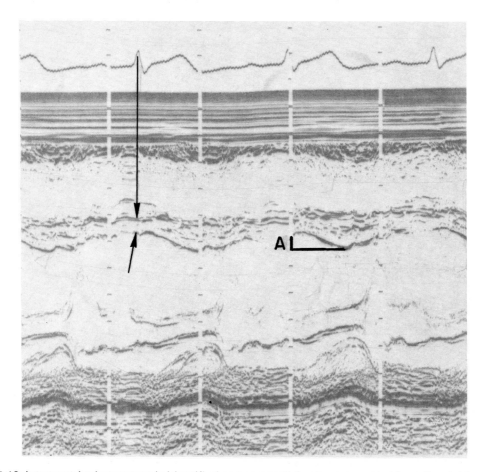

Fig. 5-12. Interventricular septum is identified as two parallel echoes recorded from the right and left sides of the septum. The membranous portion of the interventricular septum is continuous with the anterior wall of the aorta. Therefore the basal portion of the interventricular septum moves anteriorly in systole and posteriorly in diastole. This is paradoxical motion because the septum moves like the left ventricle (this is normal in the basal portion of the septum). The septal motion and measurements are not made at this basal portion. Instead, the measurements are made from the muscular septum, which is much thicker than the membranous septum and moves anteriorly in diastole and posteriorly in systole. See text for discussion of septal wall thickness, septal wall amplitude, and motion.

Left ventricle (Fig. 5-13)

LVIDd	Left ventricular internal dimension in diastole. Draw a verticle line from the left side of the IVS to the endocardium at the R wave on the ECG.
LVIDs	Left ventricular internal dimension in systole. This is the ventricle's minimal dimension. It should be measured around the T wave of the ECG or when the endocardium is most anterior. Measure from the left side of the septum to the endocardium.
Posterior LVW amplitude	Measure from the anterior wall of the endo-cardium in diastole to the same point in systole.
Endocardial velocity	Draw a line from the endocardium in systole to the endocardium in diastole. Extend the line through three time lines. (See Fig. 5-14.)

Normal measurements

Normal end-diastolic diameter	35 to 56 mm (Feigenbaum) 35 to 53 mm (Popp)
Endocardial velocity	20 to 35 mm/sec
Ejection fraction	Over 0.67

PLVW	Posterior left ventricular wall. Measure from endocardium to epicardium/pericardium at the R wave on the ECG.

Septum/PLVW	Septal wall thickness/posterior left ventricular wall. This should be a 1:1 ratio (Fig. 5-15).
LVDV (Dd^3)	Left ventricle dimension in diastole cubed.
LVSV (Ds^3)	Left ventricle dimension in systole cubed.
SV = LVDV − LVSV	Stroke volume—this is the amount of blood ejected per beat.
$CO = \dfrac{HR \times SV}{1000}$	Cardiac output—the heart rate multiplied by the the stroke volume divided by 1000 cc/liter. This is the amount of blood ejected in liters per minute.
E.F. = 1 − (Ds^3/Dd^3)	Ejection fraction—this figure supplies the percentage of blood filling the ventricle in diastole that is ejected in systole.
LV mass = $\dfrac{(Dd + 2W)^3 - (Dd^3) \times 1.050}{BSA}$	This is the weight of the ventricle.
Pericardial effusion	Pericardial effusion will appear as a clear space between the pericardium and the epicardium. It could be anterior *and* posterior or just posterior.

To obtain mean blood pressure
EXAMPLE: systolic pressure/diastolic pressure = 120/80

$$\frac{(SP \times 2) + (DP \times 3)}{5} = \frac{(120 \times 2) + (80 \times 3)}{5} = \frac{240 + 240}{5} = \frac{480}{5} = 96$$

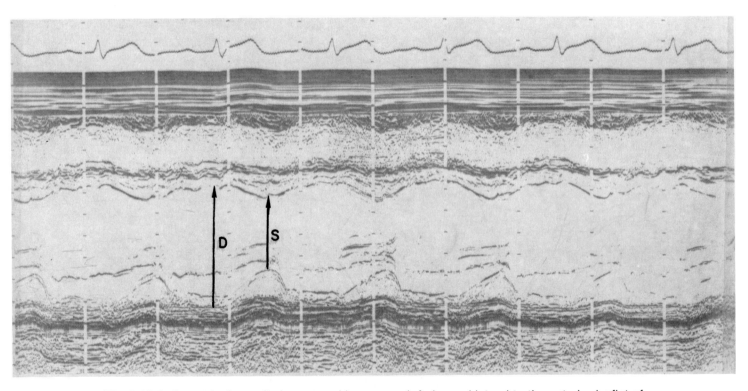

Fig. 5-13. Left ventricular cavity is assessed in a sweep inferior and lateral to the anterior leaflet of the mitral valve. It is important to identify the dense chordae structures from the endocardial surface of the posterior heart wall for measurement purposes. There seems to be a small twisting motion of the heart at the end of systole and at the onset of diastole. The two heart walls apparently move anterior together for a few milliseconds as a result of this twisting motion. The systolic measurement is essentially the same, whether taken at the peak downward movement of the septal motion or at the peak upward motion of the posterior endocardium. The only precaution is that this measurement be taken perpendicular. The diagonal connection of the peak downward motion of the septum with the peak upward motion of the posterior endocardium would result in a measurement error (Feigenbaum, Popp, 1976).

To obtain stroke output

$$\frac{CO}{Heart\ rate} = \frac{7200\ ml/min}{72\ beats/min} = \frac{100\ ml}{beat}\ (Normal = 77 \pm 25)$$

To obtain stroke index
Divide stroke output by BSA

$$\frac{100\ ml/beat}{2\ m^2} = 50\ ml/beat/m^2\ (Normal = 45 \pm 12)$$

To obtain stroke work index
Multiply stroke index by mean pressure and conversion factor

$$50 \times 96 \times 0.0136 = 4800 \times 0.0136 = 65\ g\text{-}m/beat/m^2\ (Normal = 56 \pm 12)$$

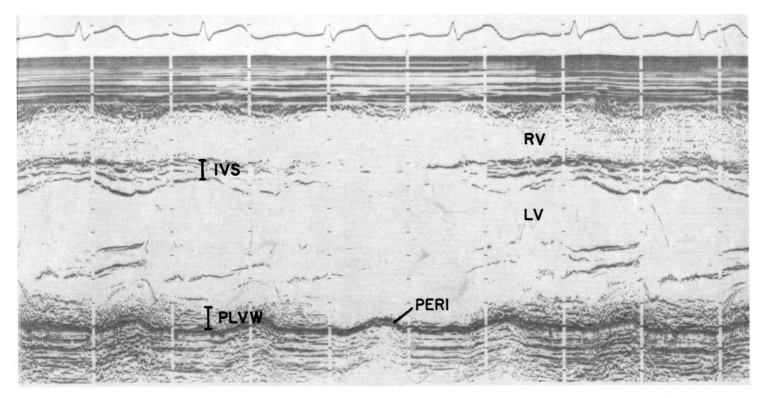

Fig. 5-14. Posterior left ventricular wall should be considered with the septal thickness to evaluate for hypertrophy or thinning of these structures.

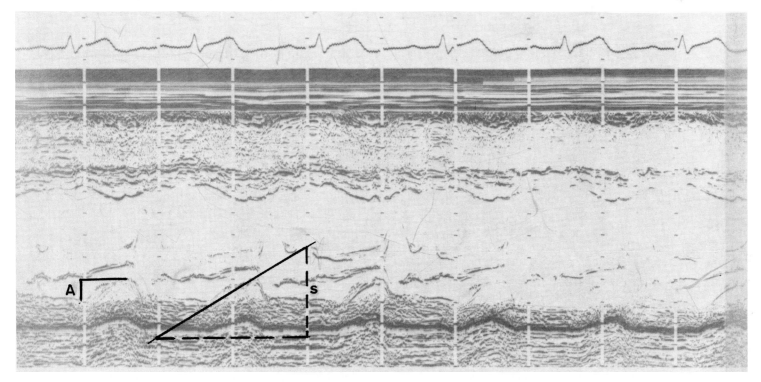

Fig. 5-15. See text for discussion of posterior left ventricular amplitude and endocardial velocity.

6 □ Mitral valve

NORMAL MITRAL VALVE

The bicuspid atrioventricular valve located between the left atrium and left ventricle is the mitral valve (Fig. 6-1). It consists of the extension of the endocardial layer of the left atrial wall and the lateral posterior wall of the aortic root. The mitral ring, or annulus, is the superior border of the valve structure, and the multiple saillike chordae tendineae serve to attach the anterior and posterior leaflets to the papillary muscle of the left ventricular heart wall (Fig. 6-2).

Echographically the mitral valve is one of the easiest cardiac structures to recognize. The transducer should be directed perpendicular to the patient's chest wall, slightly to the left sternal border, in approximately the fourth intercostal space. With proper gain settings the A-mode tracing is often the most sensitive recorder of initial mitral valve motion. The sonographer can recognize the initial echo of the right ventricular wall, the echo-free cavity of the right ventricular cavity, the anterior and posterior walls of the interventricular septum, and, finally, the mitral valve area as shown in the left atrial cavity or left ventricular cavity (depending on transducer angulation). The mitral valve pattern is usually seen 6 to 9 cm from the patient's skin surface. It has the greatest amplitude and excursion and can be unquestionably recognized by its "double," or biphasic, kick. This is caused by the initial

opening of the valve in ventricular diastole and the atrial contraction at end diastole. Thus the valve opens with its maximum excursion in early diastole, the ventricle relaxes, and the valve starts to close. The atrium then contracts, forcing the valve open with reduced amplitude. The ventricle is then fully relaxed, the mitral valve closes, and the onset of ventricular systole occurs. (See Fig. 6-3.)

It is critical to find the maximum excursion of the leaflet for recording purposes. The scanner should glide along the left sternal border to ensure maximum amplitude. The transducer should be perpendicular to the mitral valve for an adequate scan. (See Fig. 6-4.)

When diastole begins, the anterior mitral leaflet executes a rapid anterior motion, coming to a peak at point *e*. As the ventricle fills rapidly with blood from the left atrium, the valve drifts closed—point *f*. The rate at which this movement takes place represents the rate of left atrial emptying and serves as an important indicator of altered mitral function.

As the left atrium contracts, the mitral valve opens in a shorter anterior excursion and terminates at *a*, which occurs just after the P wave of the ECG. This is followed by a rapid posterior movement from point *b* to point *c*, which coincides with the QRS systolic component on the ECG produced by left ventricular contraction closing the valve. (See Figs. 6-5 to 6-12.)

Text continued on p. 79.

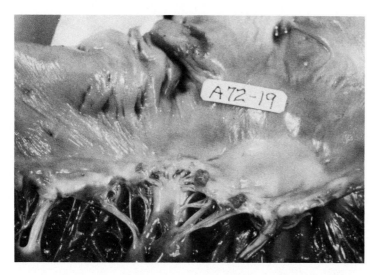

Fig. 6-1. Gross specimen of the mitral leaflet, mitral annulus, and chordae tendineae of the anterior and posterior leaflets.

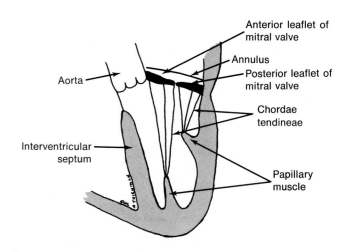

Fig. 6-2. Mitral apparatus as shown in the systolic segment.

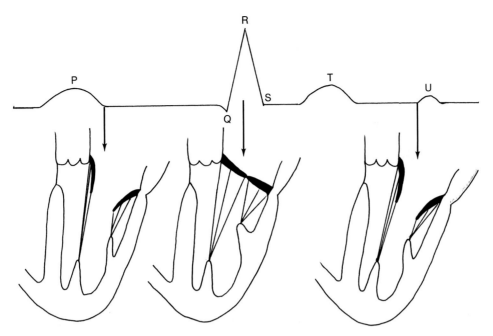

Fig. 6-3. Correlation of the electrocardiogram with the mitral apparatus. The P wave triggers the onset of atrial contraction, which gently forces the mitral leaflet open—A wave. The QRS complex is the onset of systole, at which point the mitral valve closes completely to allow blood to flow through the aortic root. The T wave on the ECG signifies the end of systole, and at that point the mitral valve opens to its full extent in early diastole.

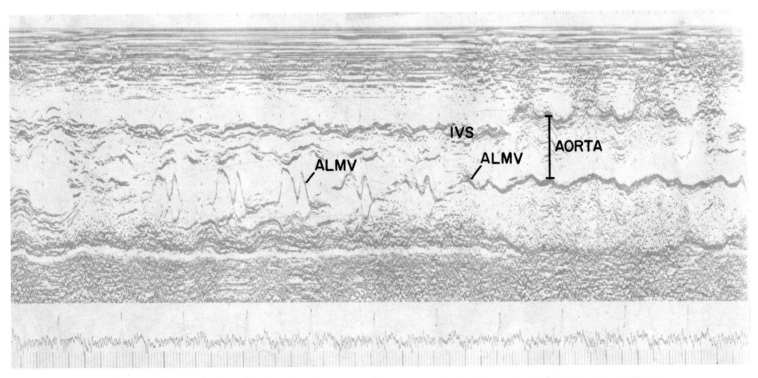

Fig. 6-4. Generally, it is best to localize to maximum excursion of the mitral leaflet by the cardiac sweep from the left ventricle to the aortic leaflet area. The tip of the anterior leaflet is seen just before the area of the left ventricle is seen.

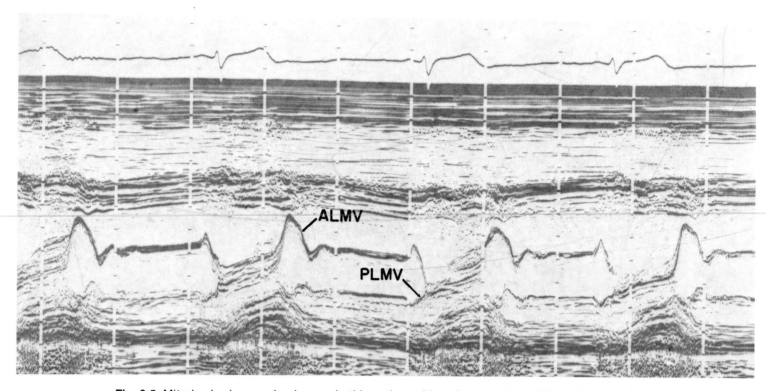

Fig. 6-5. Mitral valve is very clearly seen in this patient with a slow heart rate. The systolic segment moves anterior slightly until diastole begins, which causes the anterior leaflet to sweep anterior while the posterior leaflet dips posterior. The atrial contraction gives rise to the smaller *a* kick until the valve closes at end diastole.

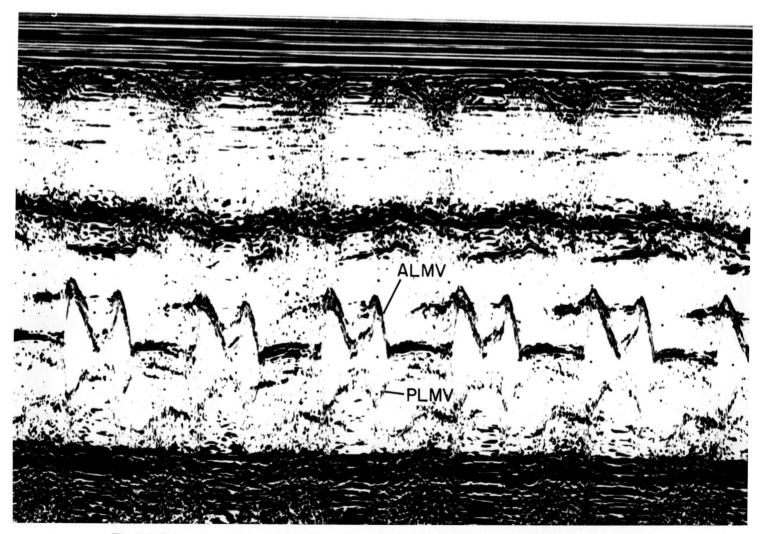

Fig. 6-6. Extra echo shown near the tip of the anterior leaflet of the mitral valve represents part of the mitral annulus, or ring, and signifies that the transducer is directed toward the base of the valve.

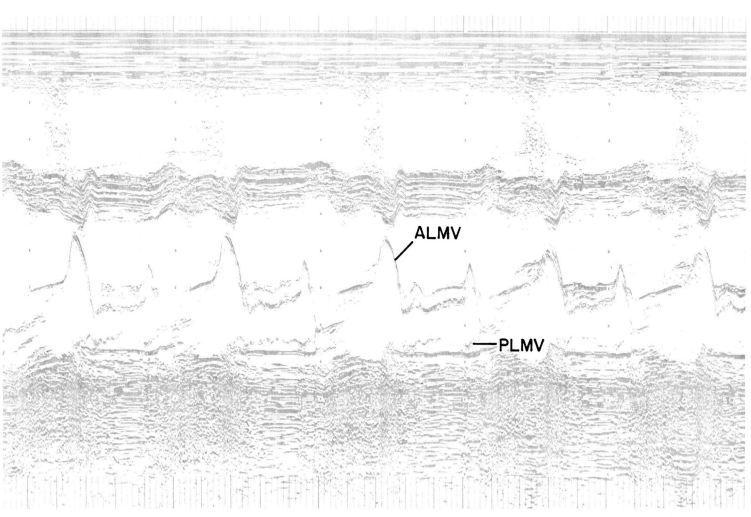

Fig. 6-7. Posterior leaflet is usually best shown as the transducer is swept slightly inferior and lateral from the tip of the anterior leaflet.

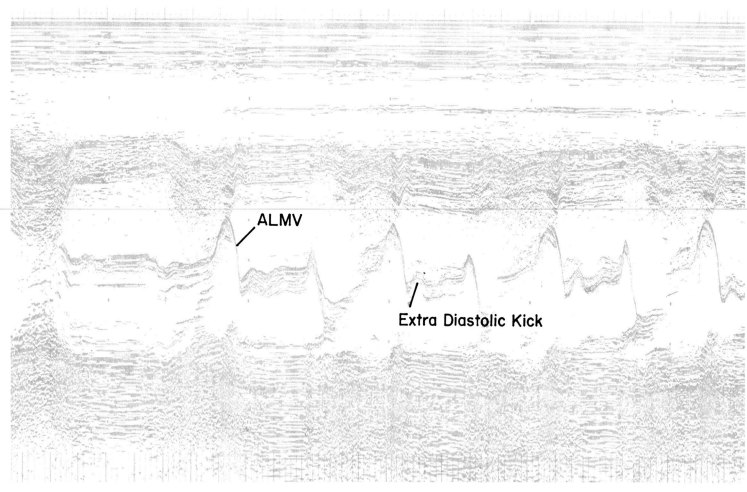

Fig. 6-8. Extradiastolic kick is a normal variant in patients with slow heartbeat and should not be mistaken for an abnormality.

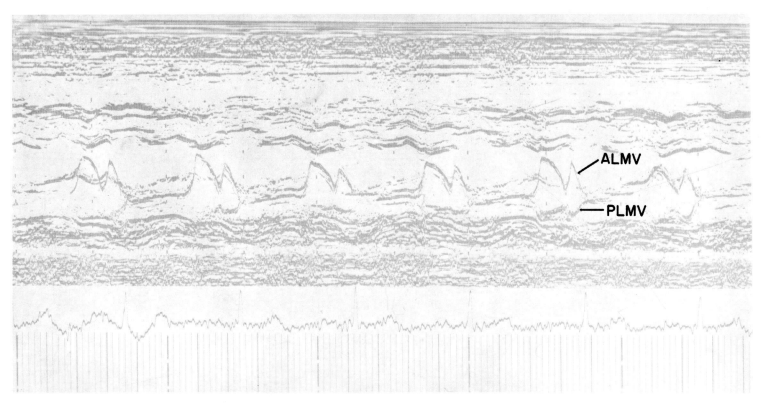

Fig. 6-9. Various angulations of the transducer demonstrate how recordings of the mitral valve and annulus, the tip of the leaflet, and reduced excursion of the leaflet are seen on continuous trace.

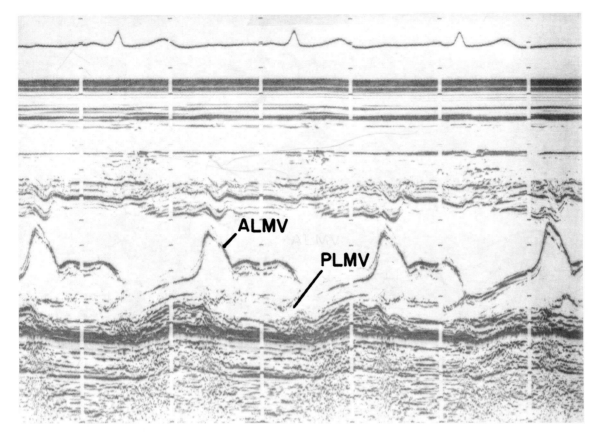

Fig. 6-10. Anterior leaflet of the mitral valve generally has at least three times the amplitude of the posterior leaflet.

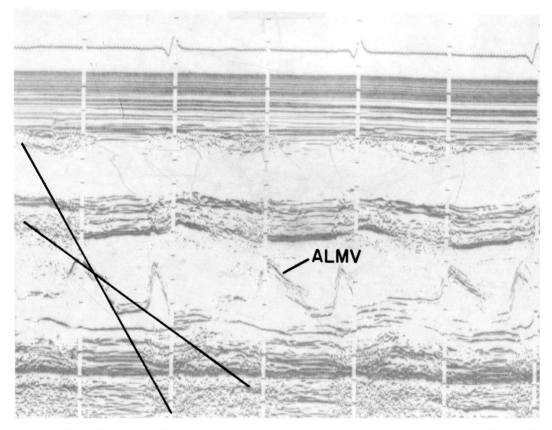

Fig. 6-11. Diastolic slope (E-F) measurement of the anterior leaflet should be made at the first initial closure of the mitral valve.

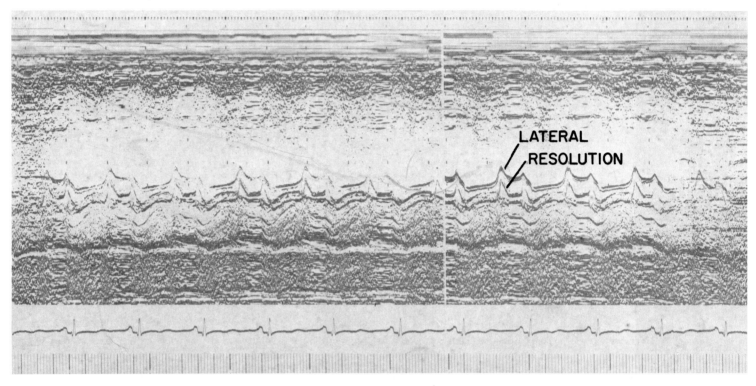

Fig. 6-12. Because of the diameter and focus of each transducer, the lateral beam width resolution may cause reverberation artifacts to simulate more than one mitral leaflet. Usually, slight angulation of the transducer allows a definitive recording.

On the phonocardiogram, point c for the mitral valve coincides with the first heart sound, representing the position of maximum closure of the mitral valve. During systole the closed valves move slightly anterior in a smooth, continuous manner. This is most likely caused by the emptying of the left ventricular cavity and the drawing of the whole valve and its ring toward the base of the heart. The second heart sound can then be heard because it indicates the closure of the aortic valve. (See Figs. 6-13 to 6-19.)

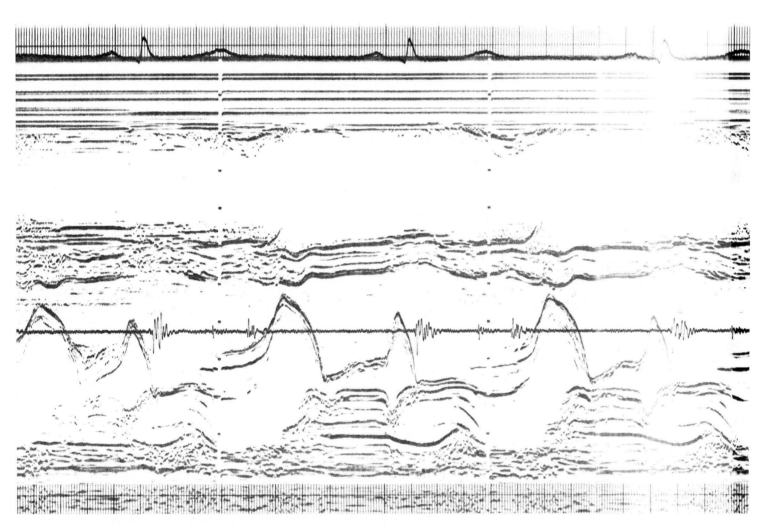

Fig. 6-13. The phonocardiogram may be added to the echogram simultaneously to record the first and second heart sounds in relation to the valve motion (midsystolic click is noted on phonocardiogram). (Courtesy Paul Walinsky, M.D., Philadelphia.)

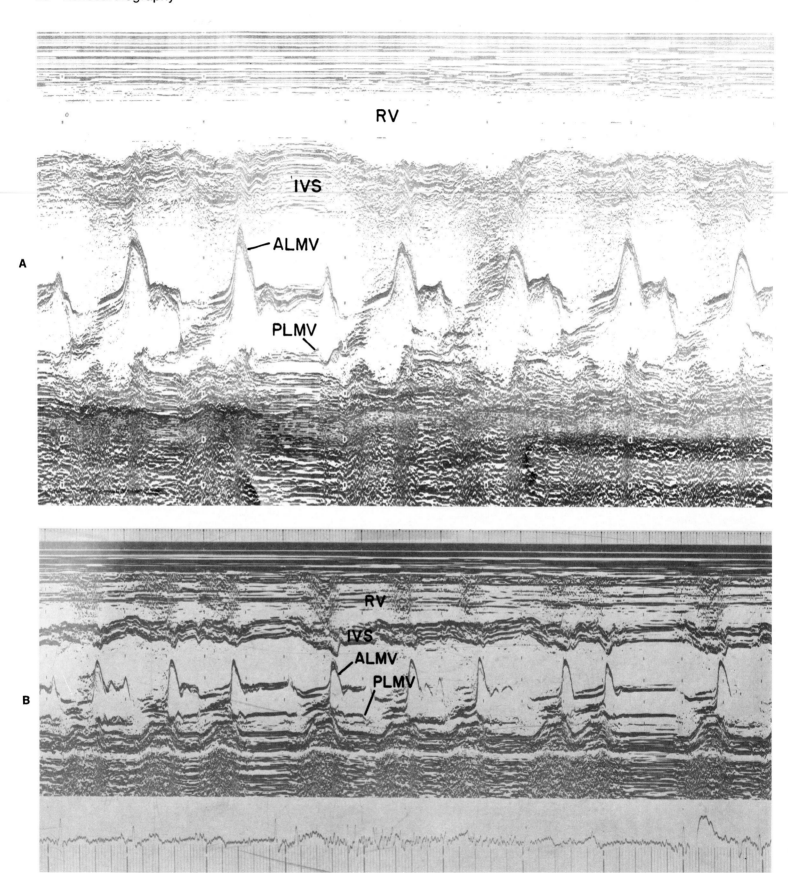

Fig. 6-14. A, Intermittent prolonged diastolic intervals may be noted occasionally during an echo-cardiogram. The extradiastolic kick should be disregarded when routine cardiac measurements are being taken. **B,** If multiple arrhythmias occur during an echocardiogram, it may be difficult to measure the mitral apparatus accurately. In this case multiple measurements should be made on several mitral complexes to determine the average measurement. Complexes without an *a* kick should be disregarded.

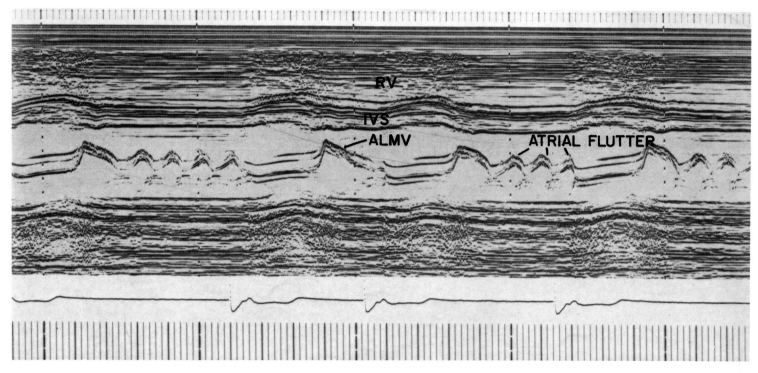

Fig. 6-15. Coarse flutter of the *a* kick indicates atrial flutter. It may be difficult to obtain measurements when this occurs.

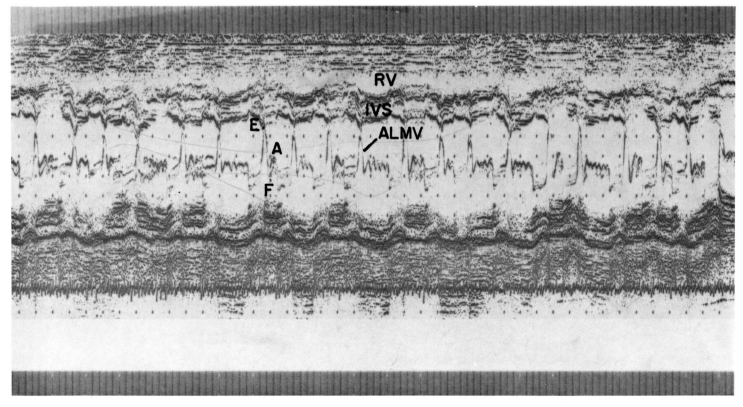

Fig. 6-16. Coarseness of atrial flutter should not be mistaken for the coarse flutter of ruptured chordae. In atrial fibrillation the C-E amplitude and E-F slope remain normal, whereas the *a* kick fibrillates as shown with the ECG.

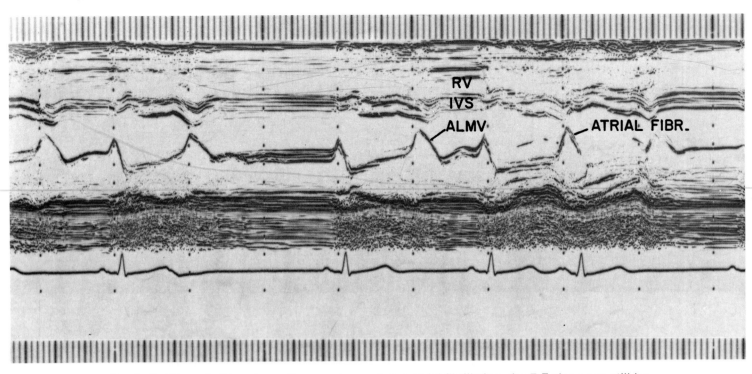

Fig. 6-17. Although this echocardiogram demonstrates atrial fibrillation, the E-F slope can still be calculated on the normal complexes.

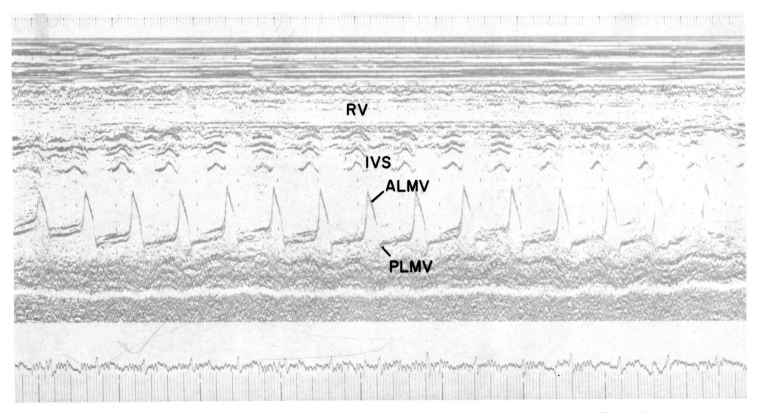

Fig. 6-18. Tachycardia makes it extremely difficult to assess mitral valve parameters. The only evaluation that could be made would be that of mitral stenosis. The patient should be reexamined when in normal sinus rhythm.

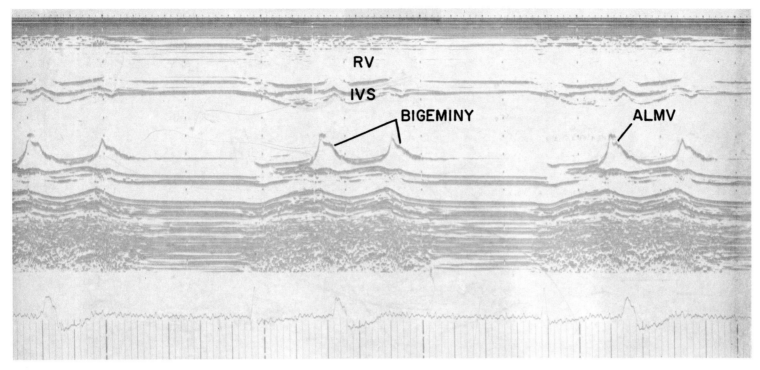

Fig. 6-19. Echocardiogram demonstrates a bigeminy arrhythmia. No measurements would be made on this patient.

PATHOLOGIC CONDITIONS

Specific echographic patterns of a diseased leaflet are demonstrated in pathologic states. Since the mitral valve is the most common site of origin for many of these lesions to develop, echography has been a diagnostic aid in demonstrating the complexity or severity of such lesions.

Rheumatic fever

Rheumatic fever is probably the primary cause of most valvular stenosis and regurgitation cases. The fever follows an infection with a particular *Streptococcus* bacterium. Rheumatic fever is actually secondary to the infection. The patient with rheumatic fever becomes hypersensitive to antibodies made by his own system. A continuing reaction goes on in all tissues between the *Streptococcus* organism, its poisons, and the antibodies. This is the beginning of rheumatic fever. The interaction between antigens and antibodies keeps the inflammation of rheumatic fever going in many tissues of the body. The inflammation is found in the joints, tissues, brain, heart, and under the skin. Masses of these inflamed areas form and heal, but the most dangerous characteristic of the disease is its tendency to leave scar tissue as it heals. Whereas one out of a hundred individuals contracts rheumatic fever, only one half of these develop heart disease.

Mitral stenosis

Obstruction at the mitral orifice can be acquired or congenital or caused by interposition of a nonleaflet. Even though rheumatic heart disease may be viewed as a disease of the mitral valve, other valves may also be involved. The mitral leaflets may be diffusely thickened by fibrous tissue and/or calcium deposits, or the commissures may be fused together. The chordae tendineae may be shortened and fused. Sometimes, in rheumatic disease, the chordae are so retracted that the leaflets appear to insert directly into the posterior papillary muscle. When this does occur, the stenosis is always severe because the interchordal spaces are obliterated. Sometimes the chordae inserting into one papillary muscle are well preserved, whereas those inserting into the other are completely fused. A commissurotomy on such a valve usually must include a splitting of the papillary muscle as well as the leaflet commissure.

The amount of calcium in the heart varies considerably with age and sex. There appears to be more in men than in women and, of course, more in older patients than in younger. Rheumatic fever accounts for 99% of all cases of mitral stenosis, which occurs four times as frequently in women as in men.

The congenital obstruction to left atrial flow may be caused by (1) congenital mitral stenosis, (2) the parachute mitral valve, (3) a supravalvular stenosing ring,

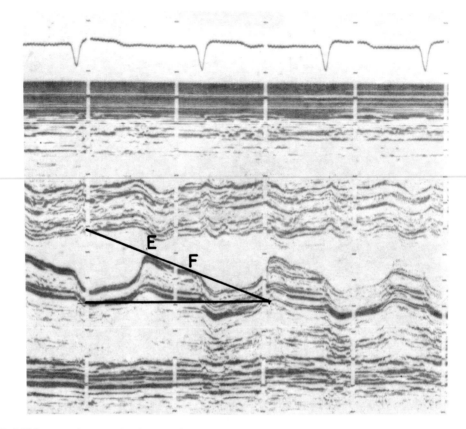

Fig. 6-20. Mild to moderate mitral stenosis with a decreased E-F slope and reduced C-E amplitude. The posterior leaflet moves anteriorly with the anterior leaflet.

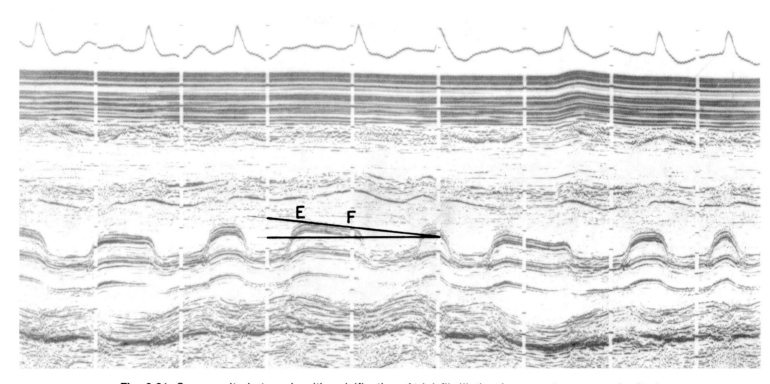

Fig. 6-21. Severe mitral stenosis with calcification. Atrial fibrillation is present, so several mitral complexes should be measured before determining the E-F slope.

where the obstruction is at the orifice itself, (4) cor triatriatum, which is caused by a partition within the left atrial cavity, with a normal mitral valve and chordae tendineae, or (5) congenital pulmonary vein stenosis. The most common cause of congenital mitral stenosis is the parachute mitral valve or single papillary muscle syndrome. This is usually accompanied by other cardiovascular anomalies as well.

Echographically the most consistent finding in mitral stenosis is the reduction of the E-F slope of the anterior leaflet of the mitral valve, that is, velocity is less than 35 mm/sec. Since the E-F slope is an indicator of the rate of left atrial emptying, in mitral stenosis the decreased slope signifies an obstruction caused by the stenosed mitral orifice. (See Figs. 6-20 and 6-21.)

In addition to the decreased E-F slope, the posterior leaflet moves in the same direction as the anterior leaflet, as a result of commissural fusion. In very mild cases of mitral stenosis the posterior leaflet may move in its normal posterior position if there is little thickening or calcification (Figs. 6-22 to 6-24). The amplitude, or C-E excursion of the valve, assesses the degree of mobility or restriction of the leaflet. In a heavily calcified valve this amplitude is reduced.

Careful angulation must be used to assess the maximum mobility of the valve. Once the leaflet is demonstrated, the examiner should search for the greatest excursion of the leaflet by slight angulations of the transducer or by moving the beam up or down an interspace. (See Figs. 6-25 and 6-26.)

Increased echoes indicate the amount of calcification present. Gramiak (1975) states that one echo indicates mild calcification, two indicate moderate, and three, severe calcification. The gain settings must be carefully adjusted properly to distinguish calcification from reverberation. Once the posterior leaflet is well shown, the sensitivity should be gradually reduced to assess the degree of calcification from the remaining echoes (Fig. 6-27). Real-time evaluation in the horizontal plane allows the anterior and posterior leaflets to be visualized with a "fishmouth" appearance. A planimeter can be used to measure the area of the leaflets and thus more precisely assess the degree of mitral stenosis.

Approximately 40% of mitral stenosis patients develop atrial fibrillation (Fig. 6-28). This condition is related to the patient's age and the size of the left atrium. The older patient with a large left atrium is more likely to develop atrial fibrillation. On the

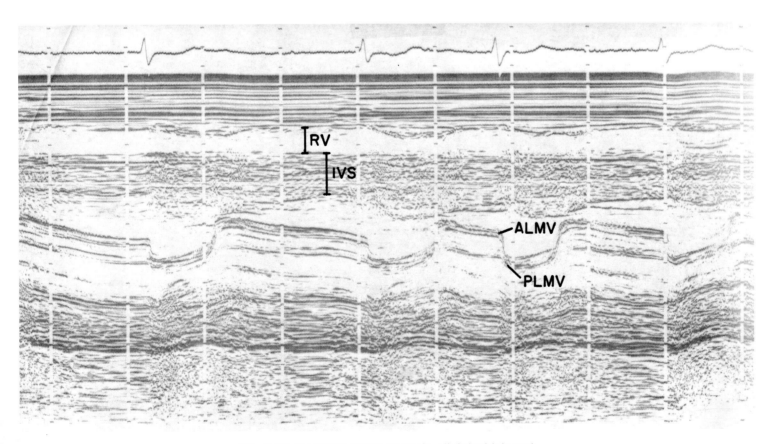

Fig. 6-22. Moderate mitral stenosis, slightly thickened.

echocardiogram the *a* point is lost on the mitral leaflet with atrial fibrillation, and a beat-to-beat variation occurs. It has been reported that in mitral stenosis the *a* point disappears with or without atrial fibrillation. This may be the result of fibrosis and thickening of the leaflet.

In the evaluation of our own laboratory data we found that 62% of our patients with mitral stenosis also had atrial fibrillation. Of the remaining patients 53% demonstrated no *a* point in cases of moderate to severe stenosis, whereas those with increased left atrial dimensions and moderate to mild stenosis demonstrated a small *a* point. The *a* point in these cases was not as relevant to the atrial fibrillation as it seemed to be to the degree of stenosis. Following is a breakdown of our data.

Mitral stenosis

With atrial fibrillation	23	(62%)
Without atrial fibrillation	13	(35%)
With arrhythmia	1	(2%)
TOTAL	37	

Mitral stenosis without atrial fibrillation

No *a* point		7 (53%)
Small *a* point		6 (46%)
Enlarged left atrium	5	
Normal left atrium	1	

Patient data for mitral stenosis without atrial fibrillation

No *a*, severe	1
No *a*, moderate	1
No *a*, mild, with mitral regurgitation	1
No *a*, good; C-E, severe	1
No *a*, severe	2
No *a*, moderate, enlarged left atrium	1
Small *a*, enlarged left atrium, mitral regurgitation	4
Small *a*, enlarged left atrium, moderate	1
Small *a*, normal left atrium, mild	1

Other echographic findings can also be seen with mitral stenosis. The size of the left atrial cavity can be evaluated to help assess the degree of stenosis. In the case of an extremely large atrial cavity, mitral regurgitation must also be considered as part of the diagnosis. Thus the left atrium is quite a sensitive indicator of valvular disease. (See Figs. 6-29 and 6-30.)

Text continued on p. 93.

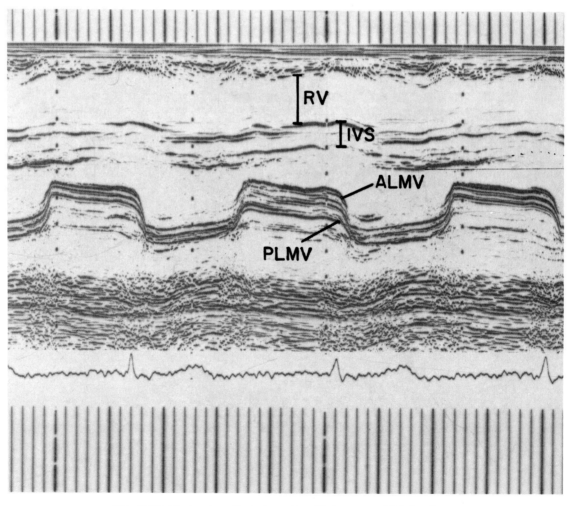

Fig. 6-23. Moderate mitral stenosis with increased thickening.

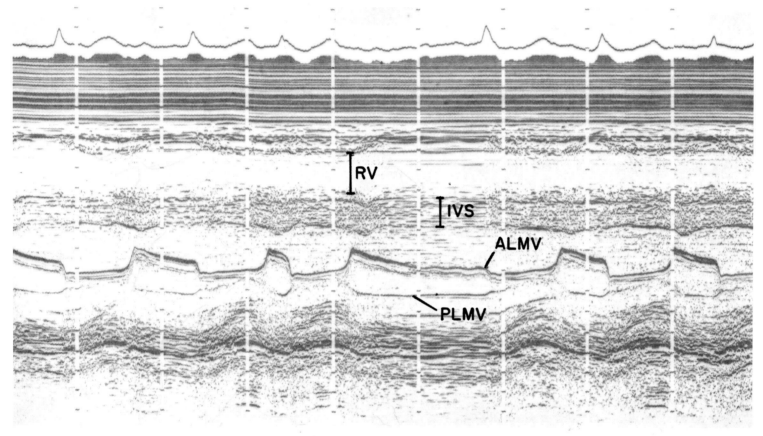

Fig. 6-24. Mild mitral stenosis with little thickening or calcification. The posterior leaflet is shown to move in its normal posterior direction.

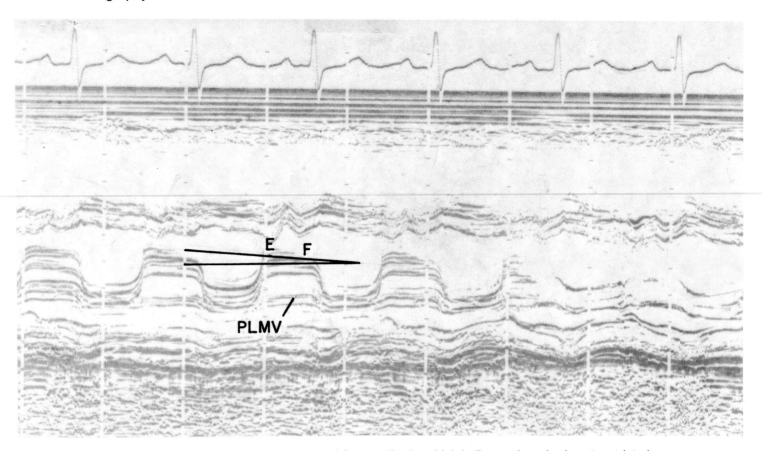

Fig. 6-25. Severe mitral stenosis with good C-E amplitude, which indicates the valve is not restricted by fibrous tissue formation.

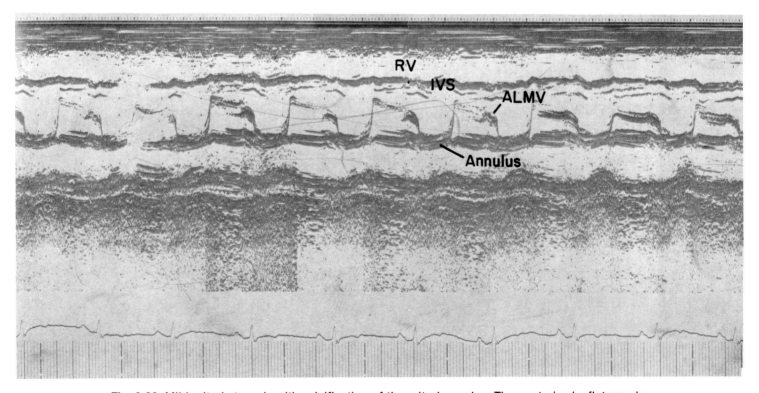

Fig. 6-26. Mild mitral stenosis with calcification of the mitral annulus. The posterior leaflet may be seen to flow anterior just above the annulus.

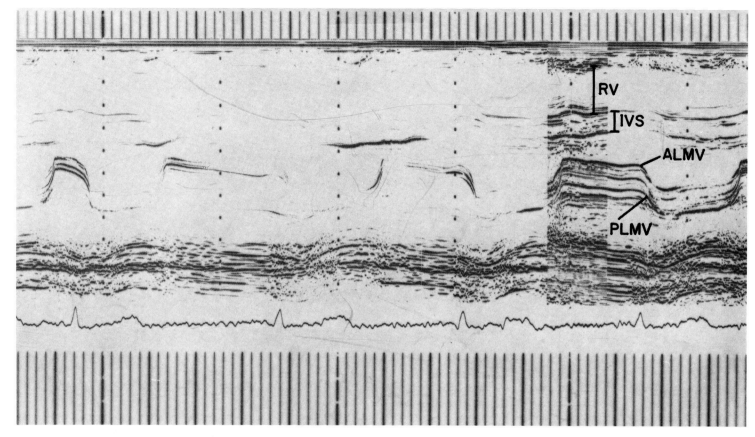

Fig. 6-27. Increased sensitivity is important to assess the degree of calcification and thickening a rheumatic valve may have.

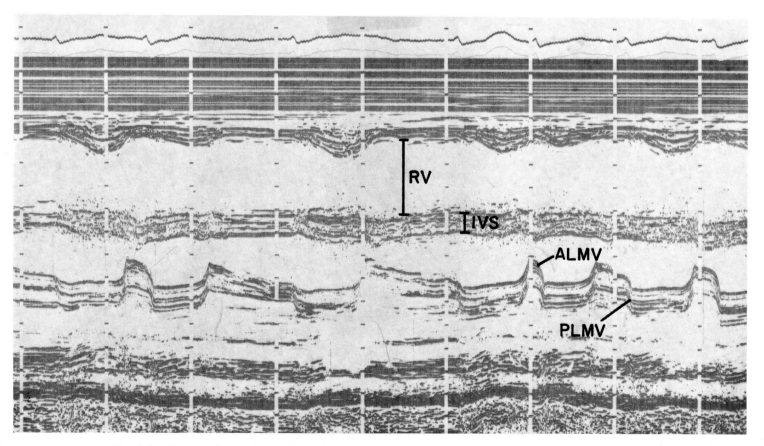

Fig. 6-28. Frequently, patients with mitral stenosis will display atrial fibrillation. See text for discussion.

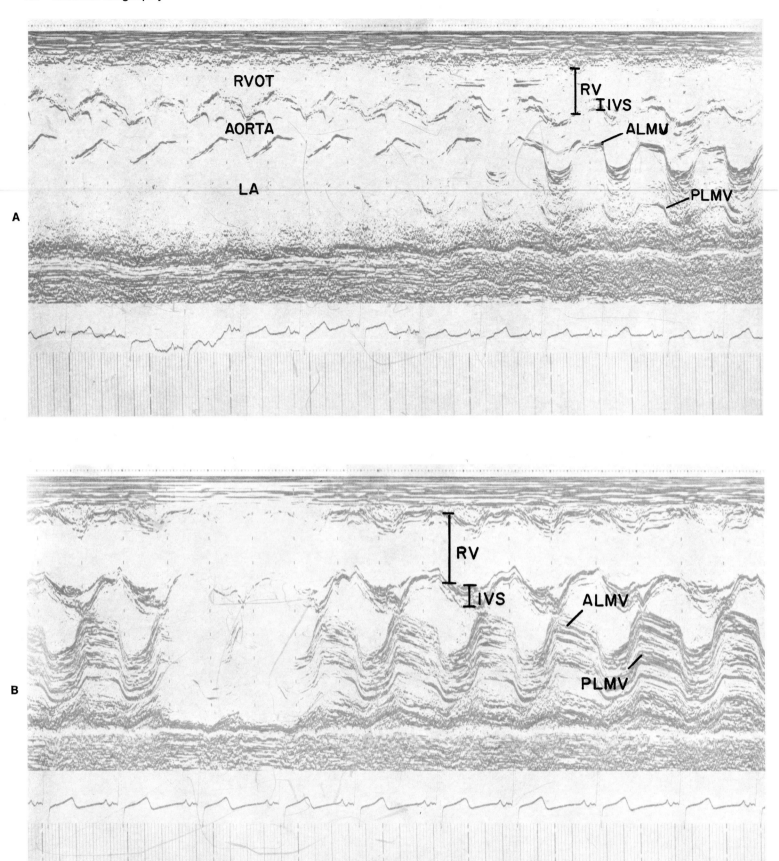

Fig. 6-29. A, Young patient with history of rheumatic fever in adolescence. Sweep from the aorta to the mitral valve demonstrates an enlarged left atrium with decreased slope of the anterior leaflet of the mitral valve. The excursion is good, and the posterior leaflet moves anteriorly to indicate mitral stenosis. **B,** As the gain is increased, intense echoes can be seen within the mitral apparatus indicating scarring of the leaflets. With good excursion the valve does not appear to be restrictive.

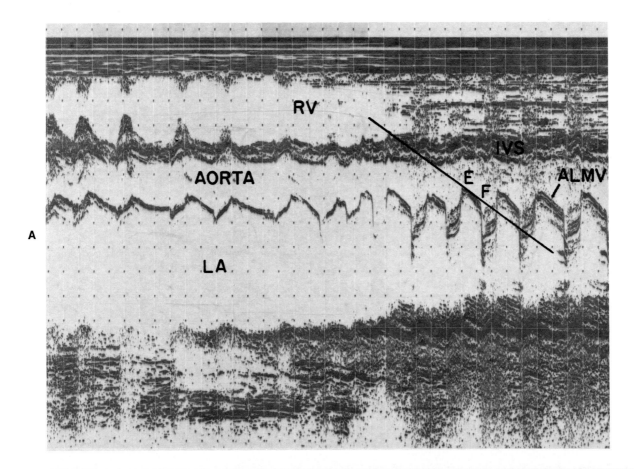

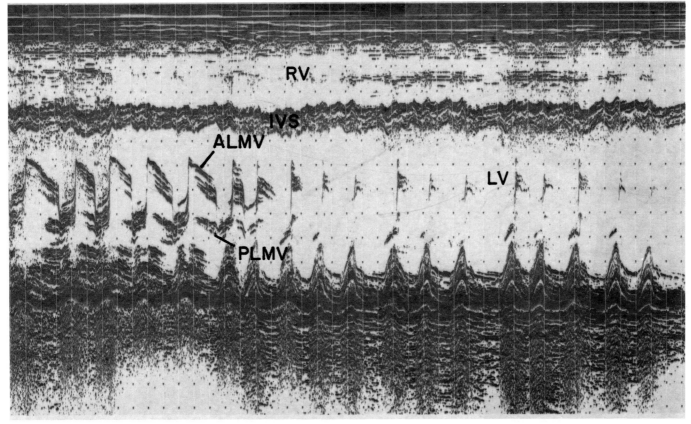

Fig. 6-30. A, Sweep from the aorta to the mitral valve demonstrates an enlarged left atrium, 6.0 cm, with mitral stenosis. **B,** The sweep into the left ventricle demonstrates an enlarged cavity, 6.0 cm, indicating that the mitral regurgitation is chronic.

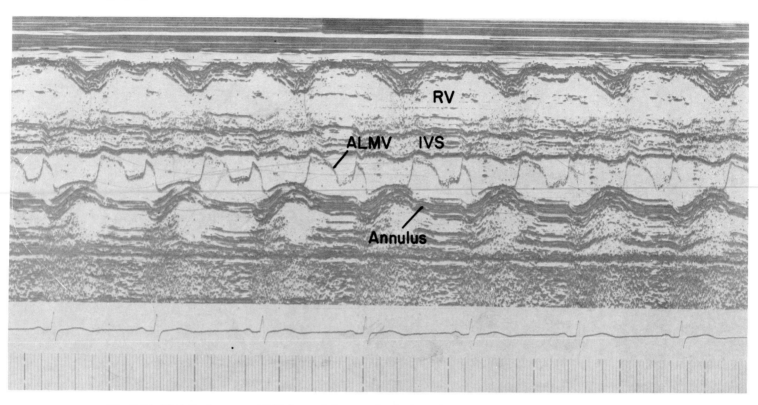

Fig. 6-31. Slightly decreased E-F slope of the anterior leaflet without mitral stenosis and calcification of the mitral annulus extending from aortic wall calcification.

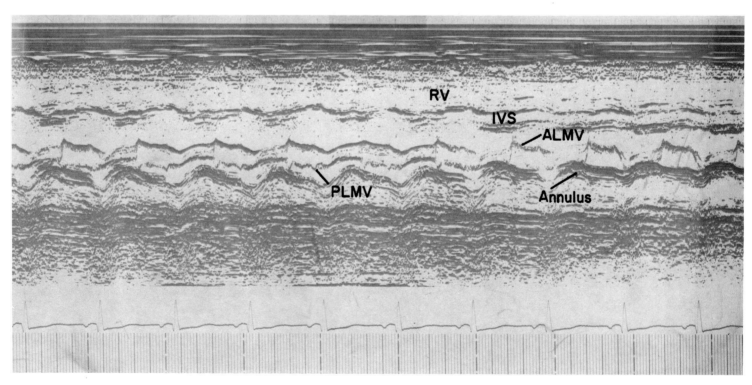

Fig. 6-32. Aortic stenosis and insufficiency can cause the E-F slope of the mitral valve to be reduced. Calcification of the mitral annulus is also shown. Fine flutter of the anterior leaflet is secondary to aortic insufficiency.

Decreased mitral valve slope without mitral stenosis

Decreased contractility of the left ventricle can cause a pseudo mitral stenosis, with a decreased amplitude and reduced E-F slope of the anterior leaflet. Generally, the E-F slope does not fall below 35 mm/sec as it does in mitral stenosis. The posterior leaflet moves in its posterior direction during diastole.

Aortic stenosis may also cause a reduced mitral slope and amplitude due to the pressures within the left ventricle. Calcification of the mitral annulus may make it difficult to visualize the posterior leaflet. (See Figs. 6-31 to 6-34.)

Tumor from the left atrium may flop posterior to the mitral valve in diastole, causing a decreased mitral valve slope. Idiopathic subaortic stenosis may give rise to a flattened E-F slope of the anterior leaflet with systolic anterior motion. The posterior leaflet would be unaffected. (See Fig. 6-35.)

A left atrial myxoma is another form of obstruction to the left atrial flow. It may be small or may completely obstruct the left atrial outflow tract. The myxoma is attached to the atrial wall by a pedicle and prolapses into the ventricular chamber after the onset of diastole (Fig. 6-36). It can be distinguished from thrombosis by its characteristic appearance on angiography—a myxoma floats in the left atrial cavity with smooth and shiny surface, whereas a thrombus may appear in the body or appendage of the atrium with ill-defined borders and a ragged surface. The left atrium enlarges with thrombus but may not enlarge with a myxoma.

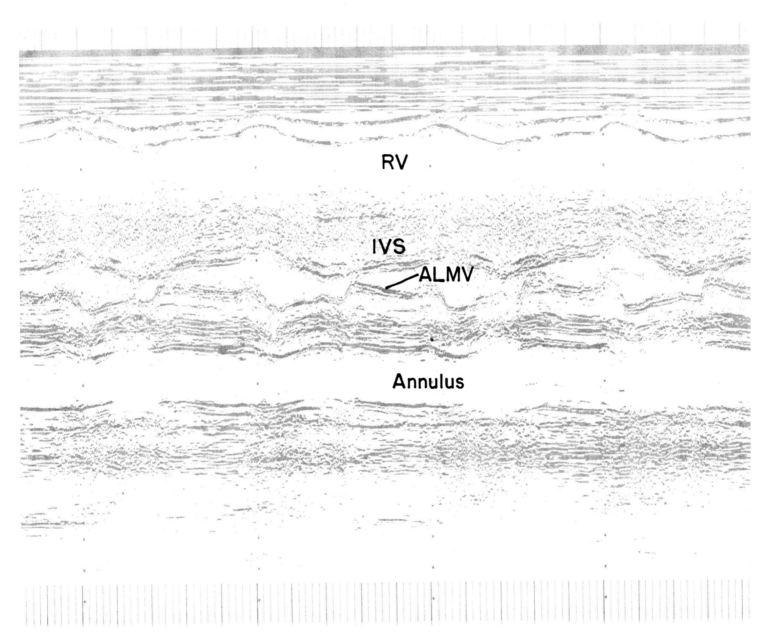

Fig. 6-33. Decreased E-F slope with good *a* kick secondary to aortic stenosis. Patients with mitral stenosis usually lose the *a* kick. Calcification of the annulus is also noted.

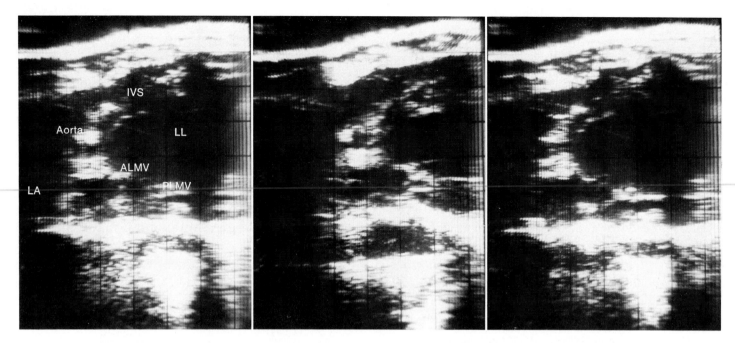

Fig. 6-34. Restriction of the mitral apparatus may sometimes be difficult to assess with conventional M-mode equipment. Real-time studies allow the investigator to observe the movement of the valve and to evaluate thickness or calcification on the leaflet. This patient shows a heavily calcified posterior leaflet that moved anteriorly, as in mitral stenosis. However, the anterior leaflet moves normally. Real-time evaluation demonstrated a pliable anterior leaflet with a calcified, restricted posterior leaflet.

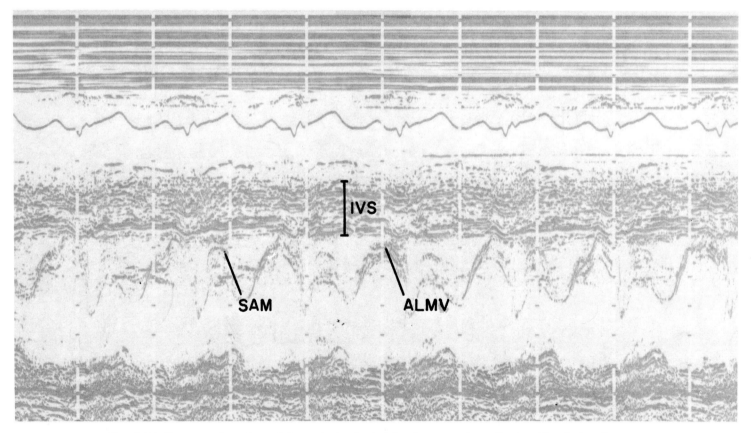

Fig. 6-35. Decreased motion of the anterior leaflet is also seen in patients with obstructive cardiomyopathy. The anterior leaflet is shown to hit the left side of the hypertrophied septum, restricting its normal motion.

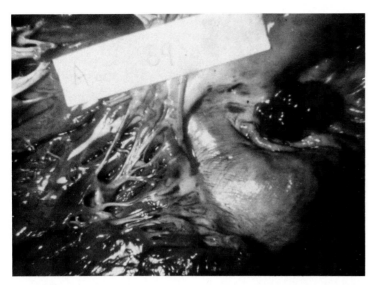

Fig. 6-36. Gross specimen of a left atrial myxoma attached to the left atrial wall.

Mitral regurgitation

The inability of the mitral leaflets to close completely or to appose precisely may be caused by a wide variety of lesions. The valve leaflets may be damaged by rheumatic fever, the effects of which could cause regurgitation due to leaflet thickening, distortion and calcification of valve cusps allowing insufficient tissue for opposition, shortening of the chordae tendineae pulling the cusps into the ventricle, ruptured papillary muscle, or mitral valve prolapse. Idiopathic hypertrophic subaortic stenosis may also give rise to mitral valve dysfunction and cause minor regurgitation. Other effects of regurgitation are infective endocarditis, congenital regurgitation, increased diameter of the valve ring, and ruptured chordae tendineae.

Regurgitation is the failure of the valve to achieve complete closure in systole. This permits the high-pressured flow of the ventricle to regurgitate, or jet back, into the low-pressured left atrial cavity. This in turn results in an added load on the left ventricle. As a result the left ventricle may hypertrophy or fail.

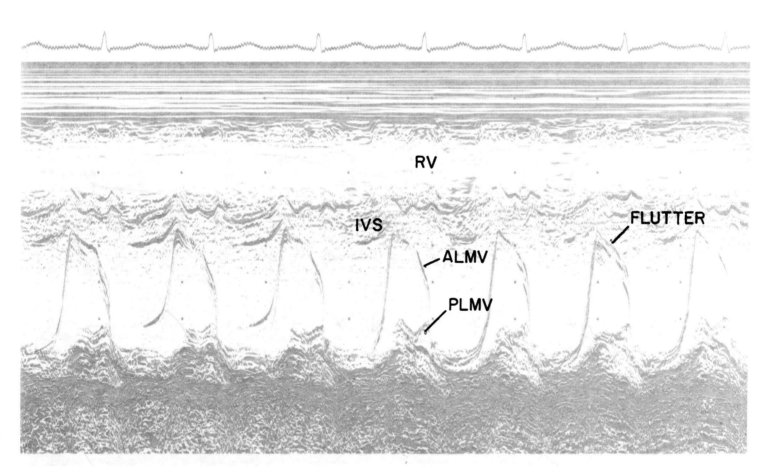

Fig. 6-37. The *e* point is shown to touch the septum in patients with mitral regurgitation. The C-E amplitude is increased (over 35 mm), and there is holosystolic sagging of the leaflets to indicate prolapse.

Likewise, left atrial enlargement is common with regurgitation of long duration.

Echographically the C-E amplitude, or excursion of the mitral valve, is greater than normal, often touching the left side of the interventricular septum and covering the entire left ventricular outflow tract (Fig. 6-37). This is probably the most dramatic assessment of the degree of mitral regurgitation. The E-F slope is very rapid, usually with velocities over 180 mm/sec (Figs. 6-38 and 6-39). Often very fine flutter can be seen in the early closure of this diastolic slope because of the extreme overload in the left atrium (Fig. 6-40).

The leaflets may demonstrate systolic sagging into the left atrium, indicative of prolapse (Fig. 6-41). The left atrium is always enlarged, whereas the left ventricle enlarges with the duration and severity of the disease (Fig. 6-42). In rheumatic regurgitation the leaflets appear somewhat thicker than do normal echo patterns. Again, this should be assessed by the variance of the sensitivity control. Recent studies have demonstrated that nonrheumatic forms of mitral regurgitation, that is, papillary or chordae rupture and prolapse, occur more frequently than was previously believed.

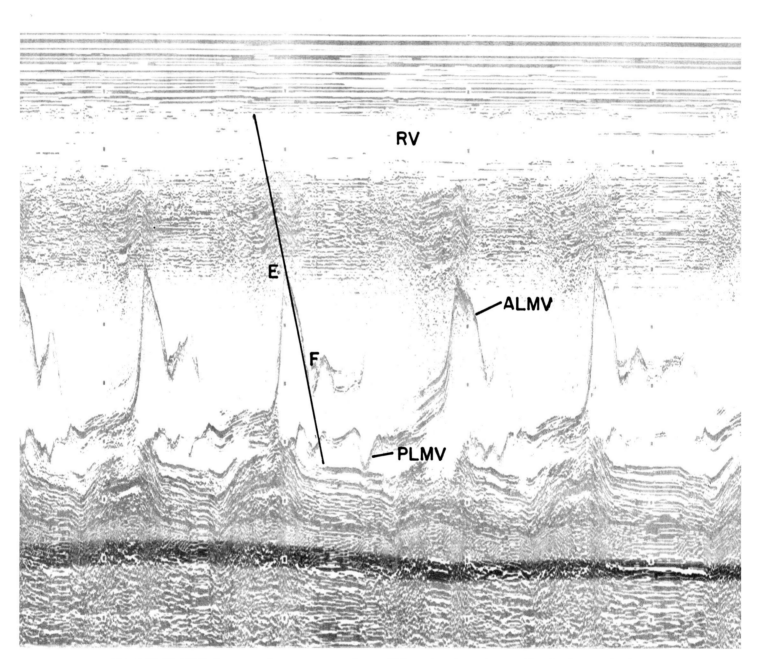

Fig. 6-38. The E-F slope usually measures well over 180 mm/sec in patients with mitral regurgitation, reflecting the incompetence of the leaflet.

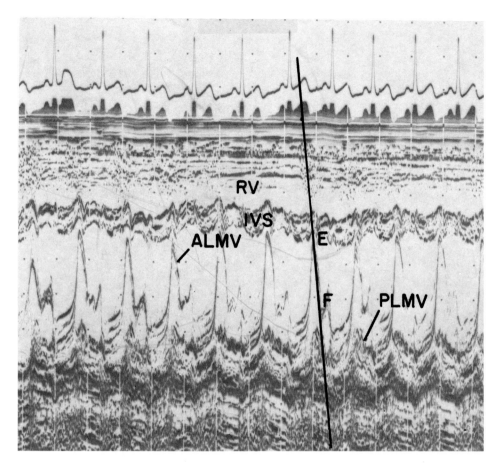

Fig. 6-39. Patient with mitral regurgitation. E-F slope measures 180 mm/sec.

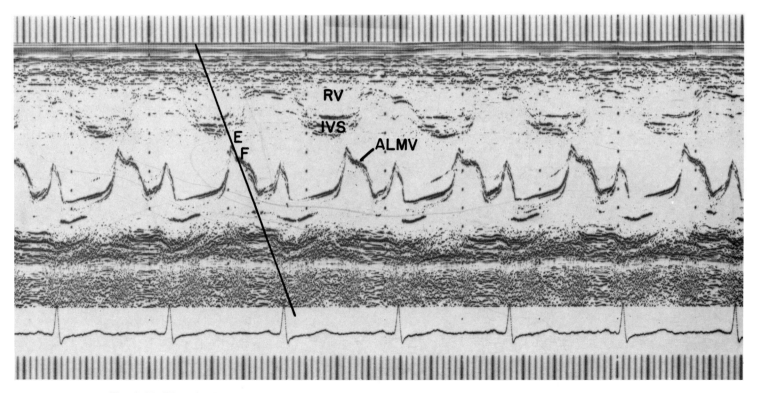

Fig. 6-40. Rheumatic origin of mitral regurgitation without thickening of the leaflets. The rapid E-F slope and fine flutter are shown in early diastole.

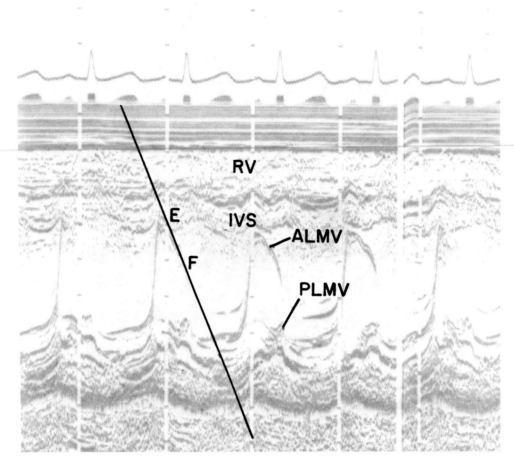

Fig. 6-41. Slight sagging of the systolic segment is shown on the anterior leaflet. As the beam is angled toward the left atrial cavity, this systolic segment dips more posterior.

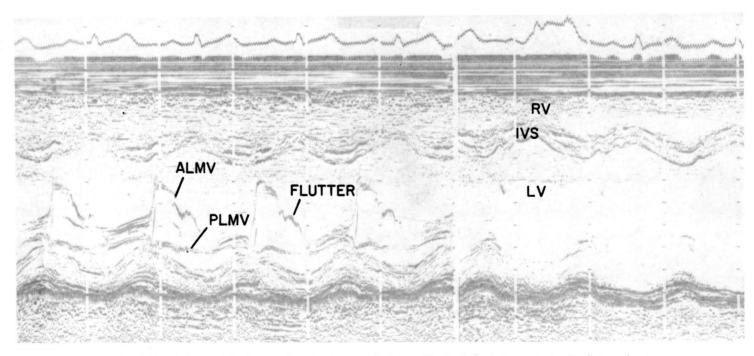

Fig. 6-42. Patient with rheumatic mitral regurgitation with flutter of the anterior leaflet and an enlarged left ventricular cavity.

Ruptured chordae

In most cases of mitral regurgitation the posterior leaflet moves posteriorly with no increased excursion. With ruptured chordae tendineae the posterior leaflet becomes a mirror image of the anterior leaflet (Figs. 6-43 and 6-44). Its excursion is tremendous, almost equaling that of the anterior leaflet. Fine or coarse flutter during diastole may be demonstrated in accordance with the respective ruptured chordae. There may be an increased amplitude of systolic excursion of the left atrial wall caused by the hyperdynamic movement of the heart. The left atrial dimension may or may not be enlarged, depending on the longevity of the rupture. Usually, the anterior and posterior leaflets do not coapt, or come together, during systole. The interventricular septum and posterior left ventricular wall may demonstrate hyperdynamic motion.

Prolapse

The exact cause of prolapse is a topic of controversy, and numerous studies have been conducted in an effort to relate information about prolapse with other clinical data. One acknowledged condition is a change in the consistency of the leaflet, or papillary muscle. Roberts and Henry (1973) reports that a myxomatous degeneration of the mitral apparatus can lead to prolapse of the leaflet. Elongation of the anterior leaflet is common in prolapse and causes the valve to close deep near the posterior heart wall.

Barlow and associates (1963) demonstrated that the relationship between a midsystolic click and late systolic murmur did in fact result from a billowing or prolapsed mitral leaflet, earlier referred to as Barlow's syndrome. Other researchers have noted similar findings and have described the disease as such at different time intervals. Barlow noted that these particular patients did have mitral regurgitation during the latter part of systole. Some of these patients had unusual anatomic deformities of the mitral valve apparatus, which were characterized by prolapsing in middle to late systole. Other associated conditions include Marfan's syndrome, in which the echo demonstrates an enlarged aortic root, flutter of the anterior leaflet of the mitral valve caused by aortic regurgitation, and holosystolic prolapsing of the mitral apparatus. The cause of such a "floppy" valve could not be

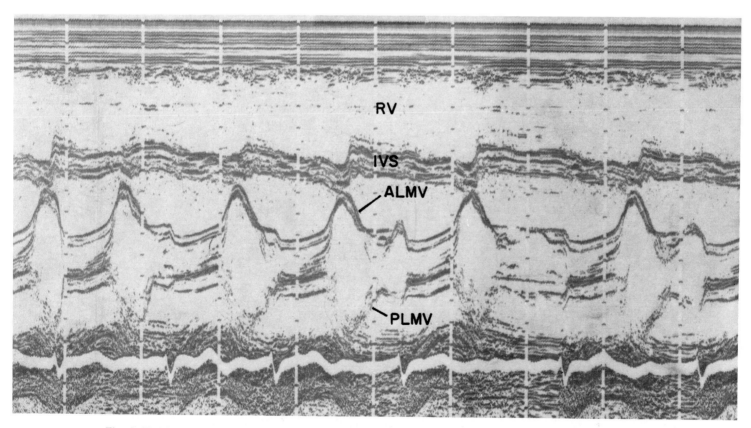

Fig. 6-43. Elderly man with a history of mitral regurgitation. The posterior leaflet is shown to move with the same amplitude as the anterior leaflet. Flutter is shown on the diastolic segment of the posterior leaflet to indicate a ruptured chorda tendineae.

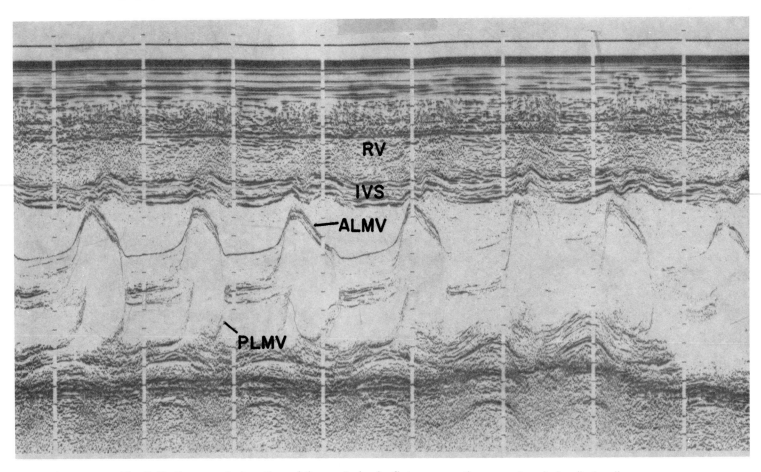

Fig. 6-44. Exaggerated motion of the posterior leaflet representing a ruptured chorda tendineae.

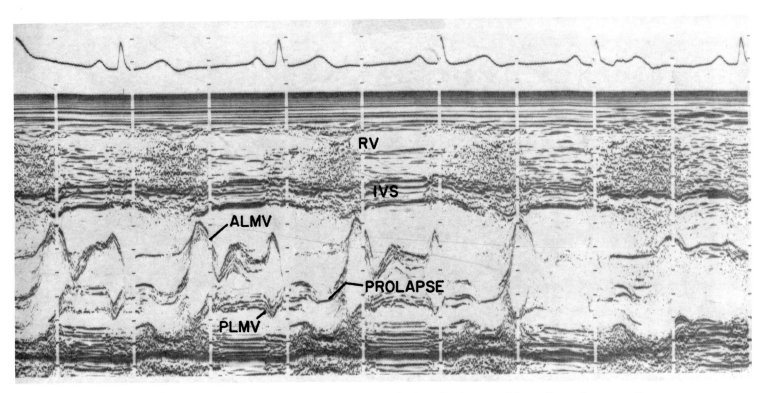

Fig. 6-45. Patient with a midsystolic click on auscultation displays a midsystolic prolapse on the echocardiogram.

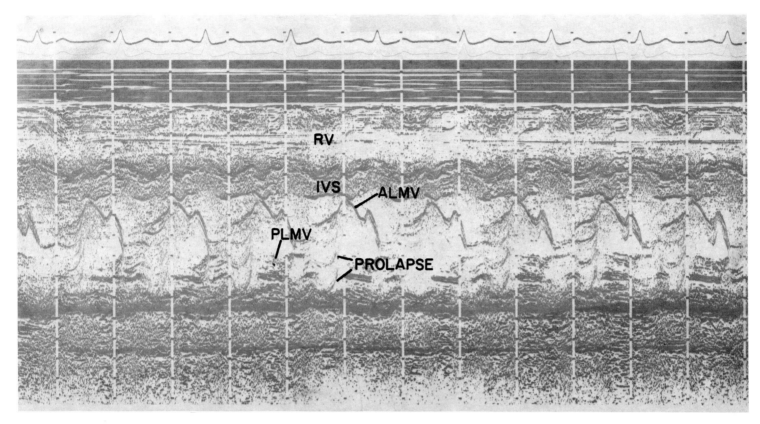

Fig. 6-46. Increased gain and careful angulation into the left atrial cavity are necessary to demonstrate the systolic prolapse of the mitral apparatus.

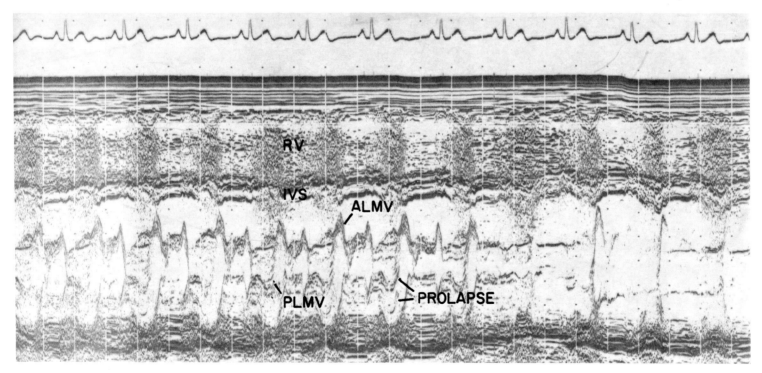

Fig. 6-47. Echocardiogram demonstrating a midsystolic prolapse and ruptured chordae tendineae.

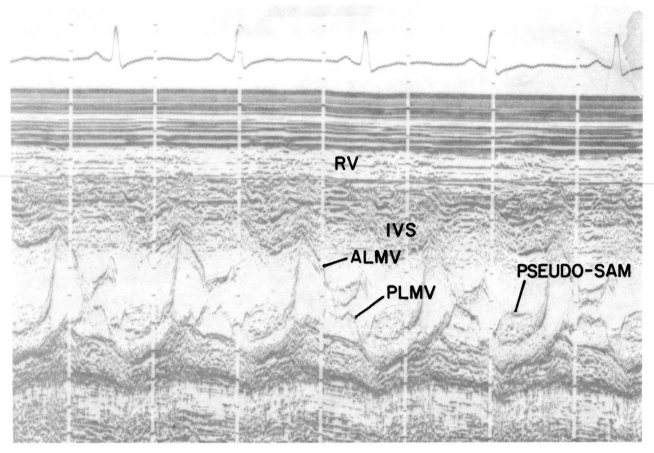

Fig. 6-48. We have noted the anterior motion of the posterior chordae tendineae in several patients who have a midsystolic murmur. This anterior prolapse of the posterior leaflet was first described by Gramiak (1975) and was thought to represent redundant chordae prolapsing anterior to represent a pseudo-SAM.

explained, but several studies suggest a genetic factor. A high percentage of patients with valve prolapse have chest pain, significant ECG changes, and ventricular arrhythmias at some point in their clinical course, which support the belief that the syndrome of a prolapsed mitral leaflet is a significant component of left ventricular disease.

Echography of the mitral valve apparatus is specific for prolapse. The systolic segment is the important factor to evaluate. Prolapse can occur throughout systole (holosystolic), in midsystole, or in late systole. In all cases the *d* point must fall below 2 mm of the *c* point in systole to be considered a prolapse (Fig. 6-45). The examiner must be extremely careful of transducer angulation to avoid artifactitious prolapses into the left ventricle. The transducer should be held perpendicular to the mitral apparatus and directed toward the left atrial cavity to record the maximum prolapse (Figs. 6-46 to 6-48). Often ventricular arrhythmias can be noted throughout the trace. Mitral regurgitation may be present and should be evaluated. The patient may be provoked with amyl nitrite to better demonstrate

the prolapse. In our laboratory we have found that patients who presented with a click and murmur demonstrated positive echo findings of prolapse. If they had only one of these findings, no prolapse was shown.

The other interesting feature of mitral prolapse is that the patient may demonstrate a prolapse only during the time arrhythmias are occurring. If the click-murmur is intermittent, we cannot demonstrate the prolapse on echo. We try to examine the patient in the same manner in which auscultation is performed—supine, semidecubitus, upright, standing, and squatting. We have found some patients who presented with a prolapse in the upright and squatting positions but appeared normal at rest.

Two-dimensional real-time scanning allows a more precise evaluation of mitral prolapse. The long axis view of the heart provides the opportunity to visualize the mitral apparatus as it prolapses into the left atrial cavity. A more precise evaluation of the posterior leaflet may be made with real time. The amplitude of the leaflets and the structure of the chordae tendineae can be evaluated in the long axis and horizontal views.

7 □ Aortic valve and left atrium

NORMAL AORTIC VALVE AND LEFT ATRIUM

The aorta has many subdivisions as it leaves the left ventricle. The base of this vessel is the aortic root, which has three cusps to prohibit a free flow of blood to the body (Fig. 7-1). The ascending aorta rises from the aortic root and begins its posterior descent at the arch of the aorta. The descending aorta then proceeds posteriorly to pierce the diaphragm and the abdominal aorta (Fig. 7-2).

Our particular interest is with the aortic root, the semilunar cusps, and the left atrial cavity. The transducer should be directed from the area of the mitral valve cephalad and medial to the patient's right shoulder. The sonographer should be able to identify the anterior leaflet of the mitral valve flowing with the posterior aortic wall at the same time the interventricular septum flows into the anterior aortic wall (Fig. 7-3). Often we note a double parallel echo appearance

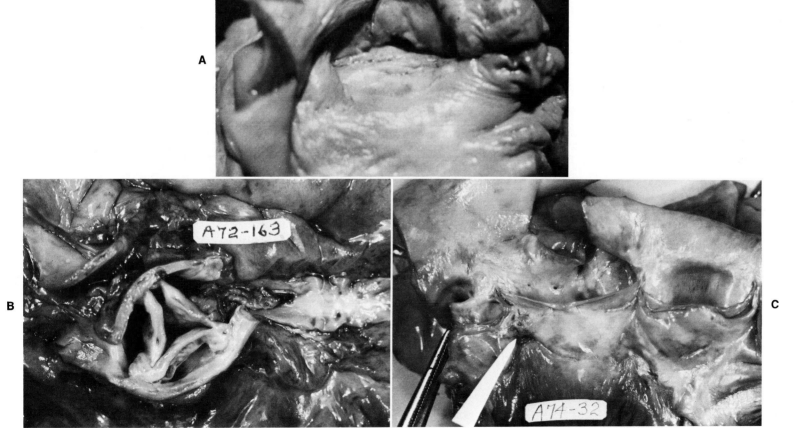

Fig. 7-1. A, Gross specimen of the aortic valve as seen from the inferior to superior angle and looking up the barrel of the aorta. **B,** Gross specimen of the aorta looking down into the ventricular cavity. The aortic sinus is seen to lie between each cusp and wall of the aorta. **C,** A direct view of the aortic root split open for visualization of the right coronary cusp and artery, left coronary cusp, and noncoronary cusp.

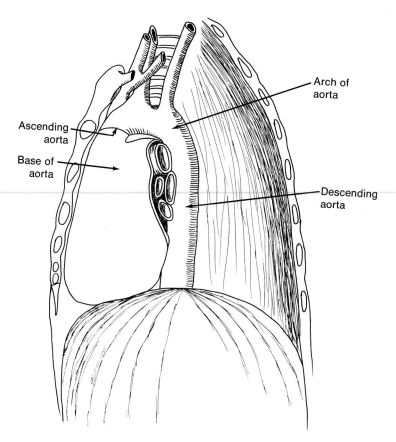

Fig. 7-2. Left side of the mediastinum.

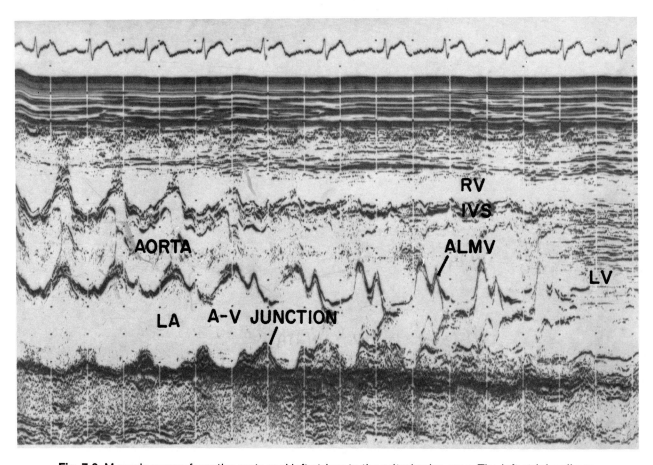

Fig. 7-3. M-mode sweep from the aorta and left atrium to the mitral valve area. The left atrial wall can be seen to flow into the atrioventricular junction behind the mitral valve area.

along the anterior and posterior aortic walls that indicates wall thickness (Fig. 7-4). Care should be taken to record both wall echoes to ensure proper measurement of the aortic root dimension. Adjustment of the near-gain control allows excellent visualization of the anterior wall. The echoes recorded from the aortic root should move in parallel, anterior in systole and posterior in diastole. The chamber posterior to the aortic root is the left atrium, which can be recognized by its immobile wall (Fig. 7-5). As one sweeps from the mitral apparatus medially and superiorly, the left ventricular wall flows into the atrioventricular groove and finally into the left atrial wall (Fig. 7-6). Thus the sweep demonstrates good movement in the left ventricle with anterior wall motion in systole to the atrioventricular area, where the posterior wall starts to move posterior in systole, to the left atrium, where there is no movement. Sometimes it is possible to record the left pulmonary vein within the left atrial cavity. This appears as a thin double-walled vessel and can be a problem in determining left atrial measure-

ments. Care should be taken to sweep from the mitral valve to the aortic root and back to the mitral apparatus several times to note the continuity of the posterior ventricular wall to the left atrial wall and to avoid confusion. The pulmonary vein will never appear continuous.

As the transducer is angled slightly medial, two of the three semilunar cusps can be visualized (Fig. 7-7). Gramiak (1968) has proved that the right coronary cusp is shown anterior and the noncoronary cusp posterior (Fig. 7-8). When seen, the left coronary cusp is in the midline of these two cusps. The onset of systole causes the cusps to open the full extent of the aortic root (Fig. 7-9). The extreme force of blood through this opening causes fine flutter to occur during systole (Fig. 7-10). As the pressure relaxes in the ventricle, the cusps begin to drift to a closed position, until they are fully closed in diastole.

Chang (1977) states that the anterior "humping" of the aortic valve following its closure is a common occurrence in patients with efficient cardiac outputs. It

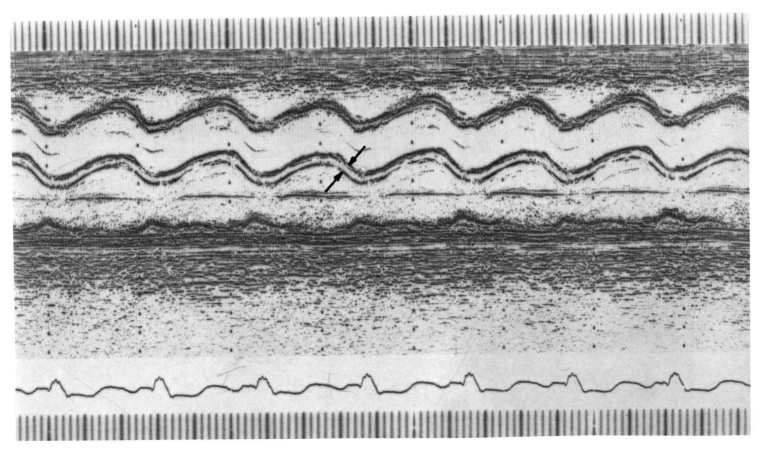

Fig. 7-4. Parallel double lines on the posterior aortic wall demonstrate that the transducer was not exactly perpendicular to the aortic wall. Sometimes it is possible to record the inner and outer dimensions of both anterior and posterior walls of the aorta with good resolution. A dissecting aneurysm would display a widened distance in the aortic wall (more than 1 to 1.6 cm) if the dissection occurred at the root of the aorta.

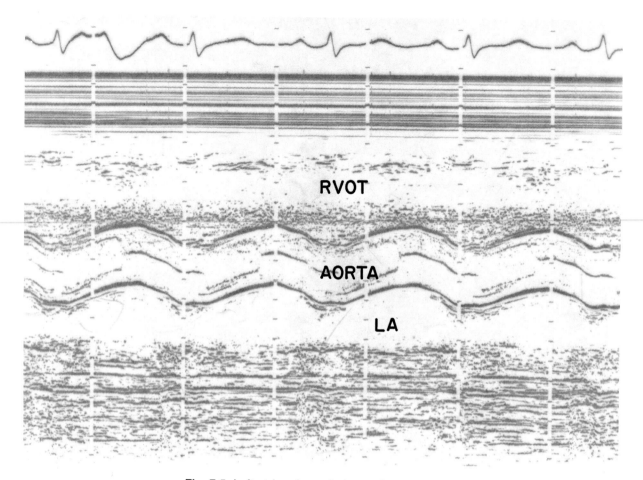

Fig. 7-5. Left atrium is posterior to the aortic root.

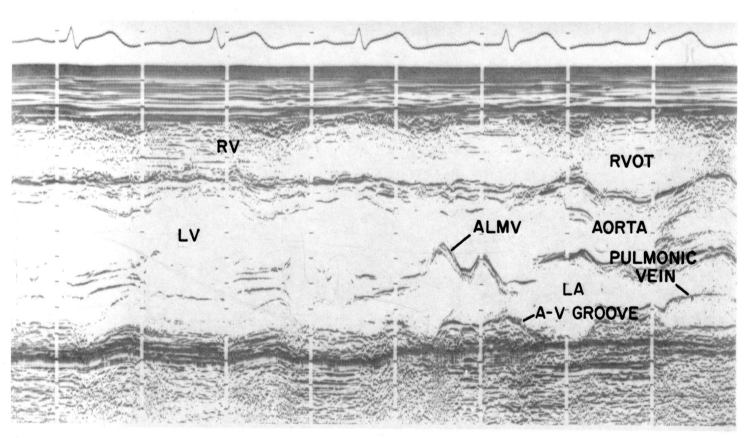

Fig. 7-6. Sweep from the left ventricle to the mitral area and medial to the aortic root demonstrates good posterior wall motion in the left ventricle, a box-type motion in the atrioventricular groove, and no motion in the left atrial cavity.

may be a total displacement of the aortic root anteriorly following systolic completion and does not seem to indicate abnormality (Fig. 7-11). In our experience we found at least one cusp, usually the right coronary, in 86% of the cases. In 70% of the patients two cusps were demonstrated, and 14% demonstrated all three cusps.

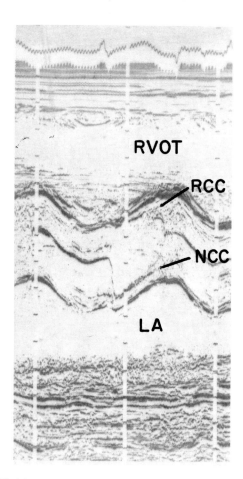

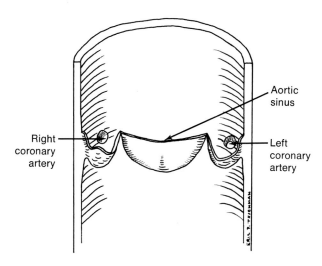

Fig. 7-7. Semilunar cusps with their respective coronary arteries.

Fig. 7-8. Right coronary cusp is the most anterior cusp seen in the aortic sweep, and the noncoronary cusp is the most posterior.

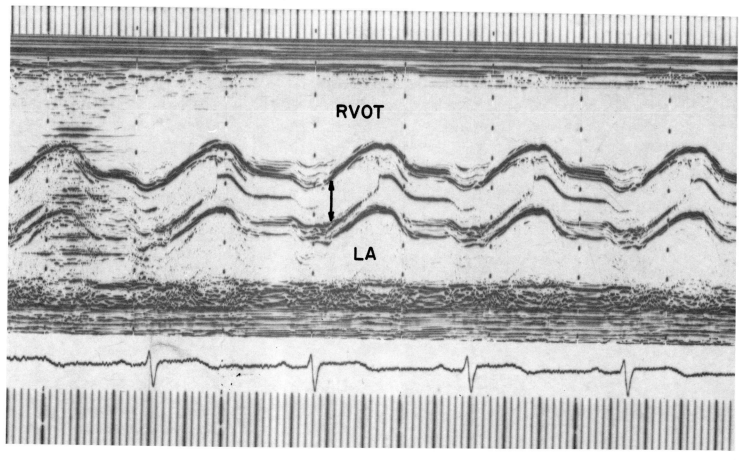

Fig. 7-9. Systolic opening of the aortic cusps.

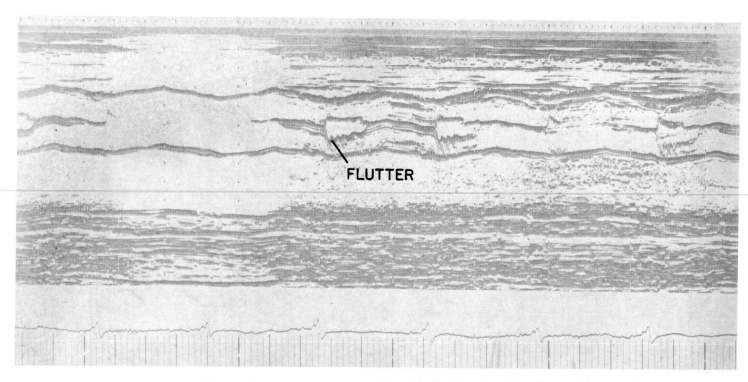

Fig. 7-10. Flutter of the aortic cusps was once considered indicative of cardiac disease. However, it is now recognized as a normal occurrence in the aorta from the high-pressure blood flow through its orifice. These cusps do not open to their full extent, but flutter is still demonstrated in their systolic component.

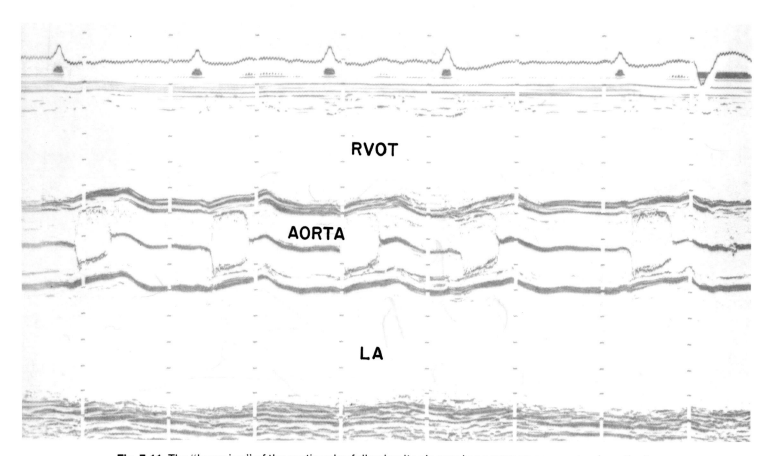

Fig. 7-11. The "humping" of the aortic valve following its closure is a common occurrence in patients with efficient cardiac output, according to Chang (1977).

PATHOLOGIC CONDITIONS
Aortic stenosis

Aortic stenosis will be discussed in relation to isolated aortic stenosis, acquired aortic stenosis, and congenital lesions.

The most common cause of fatal valvular dysfunction in patients past late adolescence is isolated valvular aortic stenosis. This is nearly always nonrheumatic in origin and commonly represents a congenital malformation. The mitral apparatus is normal anatomically in the majority of patients with isolated aortic stenosis. In patients under 15 years of age the aortic valve is either unicuspid or bicuspid in cases of isolated aortic stenosis. In patients from 15 to 65 years the aortic valve is congenitally malformed in 60% of these cases. The valve is usually tricuspid, with a small percentage of bicuspid valves, in patients over 65.

Acquired aortic stenosis, the result of calcification and fibrosis, is generally of two types: that involving a congenitally malformed but initially normally functioning valve and that involving a previously normal valve. Congenitally malformed valves are determined by the number of cusps and commissures. (A commissure is a small bump on the end of each cusp. It helps the cusps close completely so that no blood can leak through.) Two types of unicuspid aortic valves are (1) a cusp devoid of lateral attachments to the wall of the aorta with a centrally located orifice (this is usually the type underlying valvular pulmonary stenosis) and (2) a unicommissural cusp, in which the valve orifice is eccentrically located with one lateral attachment to the aortic wall, and that at the level of the orifice. (This is frequently fatal aortic stenosis found in children less than 1 year of age.)

The most frequent malformation of the aortic valve is the presence of only two cusps—bicuspid valve. There are two types of bicuspid valves, with equal distribution among patient populations. In the first type the cusps are located in the right and left and the commissures anteriorly and posteriorly. If a raphe false commissure is present, it is always in the right cusp. A coronary artery arises from behind each cusp. In the second type the cusps are located anterior and posterior, and the commissures are right and left. A raphe, if present, is always in the anterior cusp, and both coronary arteries arise in front of the anterior cusp. Possibly as many as 2% of infants have bicuspid valves at birth. Aortic stenosis is the most common complication of this congenital malformation.

Occasionally, a tricuspid aortic valve is malformed in such a way that the cusps are of unequal size. Some

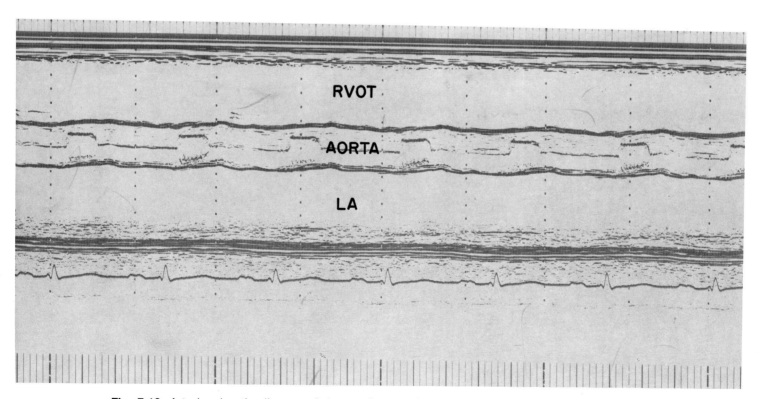

Fig. 7-12. Arteriosclerotic disease of the aortic root demonstrates little anterior motion during systole.

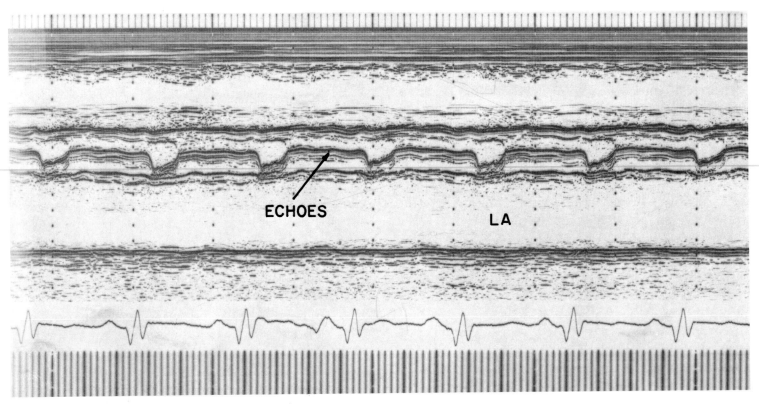

Fig. 7-13. Arteriosclerotic disease and calcification result in decreased motion of the aortic root.

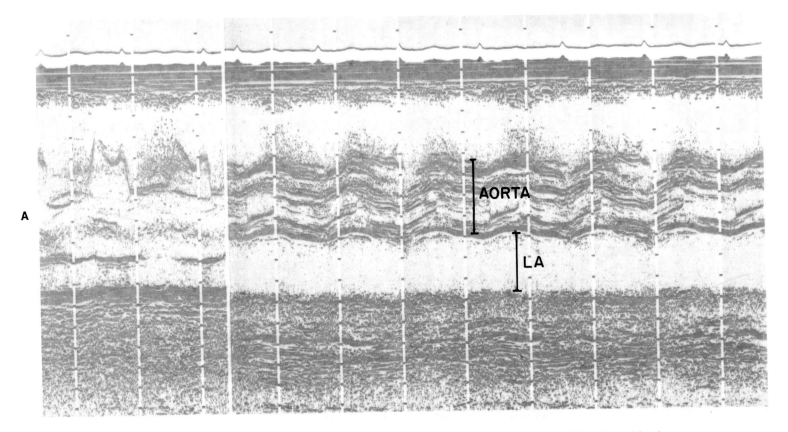

Fig. 7-14. A, Heavily calcified aortic valve as shown with moderate gain settings. The tricuspid valve is seen to the left of the tracing.

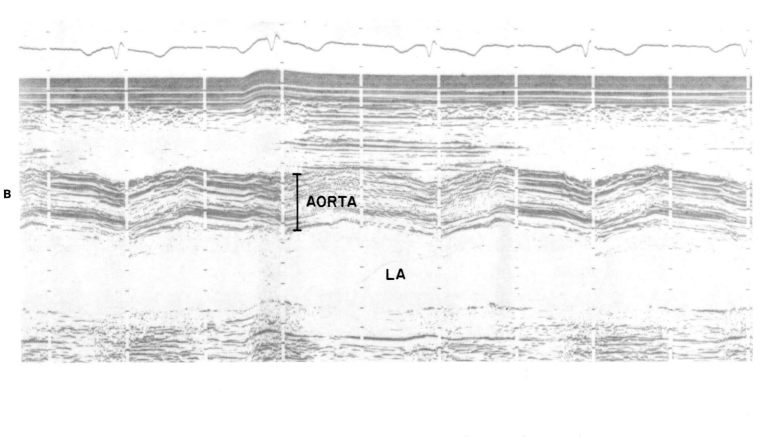

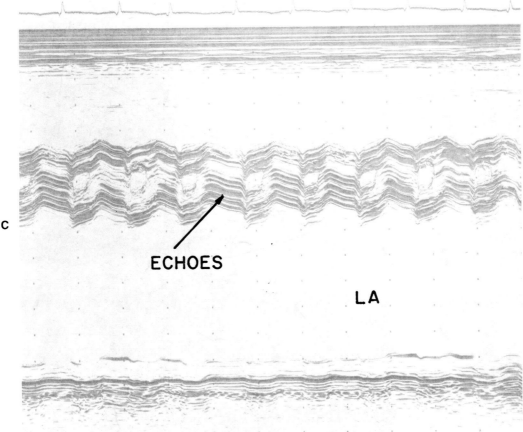

Fig. 7-14, cont'd. B, Reduced gain settings demonstrate the calcification to remain as the left atrial wall begins to fade. **C,** Moderately calcified root with good motion of the systolic component. Enlarged left atrium indicates associated mitral disease.

professionals believe that the contact of unequal sized cusps can lead to focal cuspal fibrosis with eventual calcification and stenosis.

Acquired aortic stenosis in a normal aortic valve is commonly associated with rheumatic fever. The aortic obstruction results from calcium deposits that prevent the cusp from retracting adequately during ventricular systole. The cause of aortic stenosis in elderly individuals has not been ascertained. The wear and tear on the aortic valve is the probable cause of calcium deposits. It is not uncommon to find calcification in the aortic wall extending into the mitral annulus.

Echographically it is possible to assess calcification and thickness of the aortic wall and cusps. As the aortic root is demonstrated on the sweep, the motion of the aortic root itself can be observed as it swings forward anterior in systole and moves posterior in diastole. Lack of motion indicates some calcification and arteriosclerotic heart disease (Figs. 7-12 and 7-13). The fine echoes on the anterior and posterior aortic walls should have intensities equal to or less than the left atrial wall. As the gain is decreased, these wall echoes will disappear. In calcification of the aortic wall these echoes appear very dense and will not disappear as readily when the gain is reduced (Fig. 7-14). Also, as

the transducer beam sweeps from the calcified aortic root to the area of the mitral valve, calcification of the mitral annulus will probably be noted as a thick continuous echo arising from the posterior aortic wall and extending throughout the mitral apparatus (Fig. 7-15).

Calcification and thickening of the aortic cusps can also be demonstrated by echography. Normally, the anterior and posterior cusps are thin fluttering echoes within the aortic root. With thickening and fibrosis these echoes increase in intensity and lose their characteristic flutter (Fig. 7-16). The wide systolic opening of the cusps diminishes with the degree of calcification (Fig. 7-17). If the valve is severely calcified, it is difficult to separate the systolic component of the aortic cusp from the diastolic, since there are so many increased echoes within the aortic root (Fig. 7-18). Although the mitral valve is often pathologically unaffected by aortic stenosis, changes can be shown on the echo. The increased pressure in the left ventricle, secondary to aortic stenosis, causes echographic changes on the mitral valve. The amplitude becomes reduced, and the E-F slope flattens according to the severity of the aortic stenosis (Fig. 7-19). The posterior leaflet of the mitral valve remains in its normal posterior motion, and the *a* kick of the anterior leaflet is generally

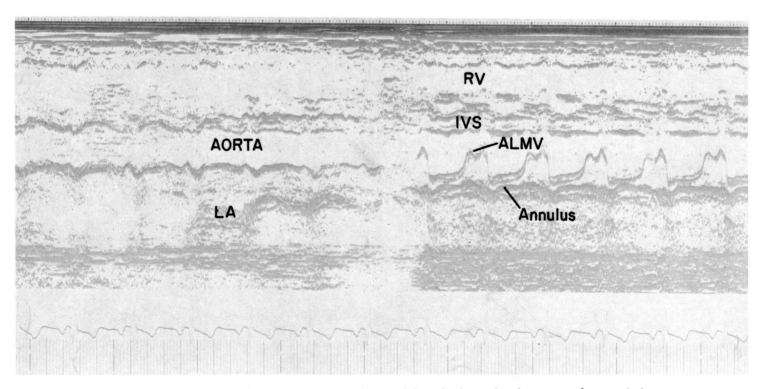

Fig. 7-15. Calcification of the aorta can extend around the mitral annulus. In a sweep from aorta to mitral apparatus a very heavy echo can be seen toward the posterior part of the mitral valve that represents the mitral annulus. Depending on transducer angulation, this echo may weave through the upper part of the valve or toward the posterior leaflet of the mitral valve.

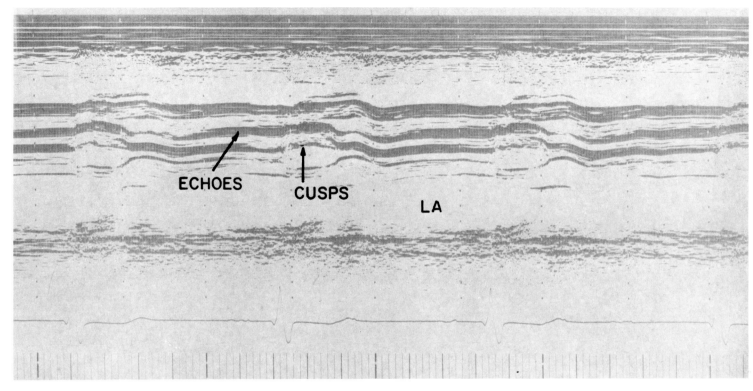

Fig. 7-16. Heavily calcified cusps lose their flutter capability with fibrosis.

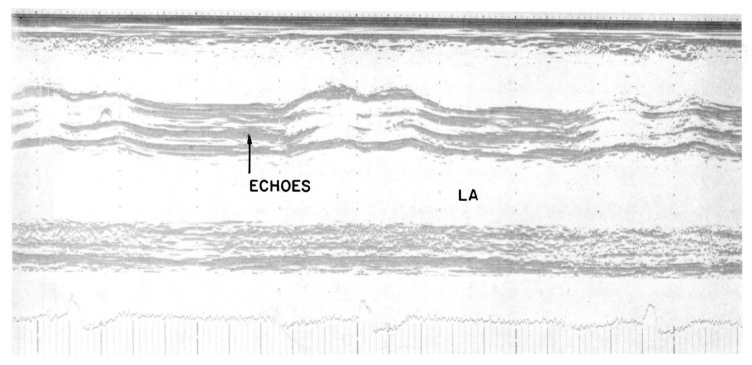

Fig. 7-17. Systolic cusp separation can be measured and, if reduced, indicates aortic restriction. However, this is not a strong indicator of the severity of aortic valve disease.

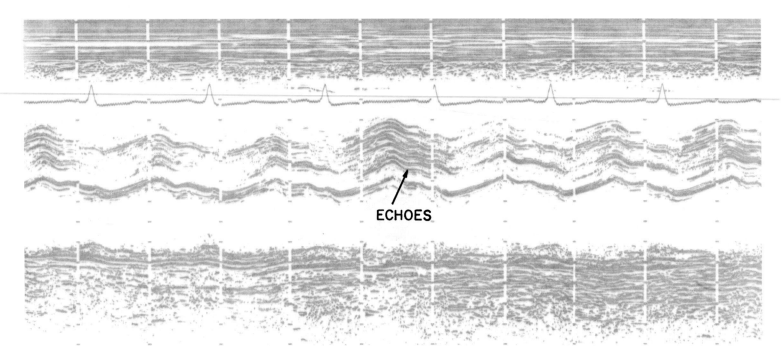

Fig. 7-18. Often, with severely calcified cusps and root, it becomes difficult to assess the cusp separation.

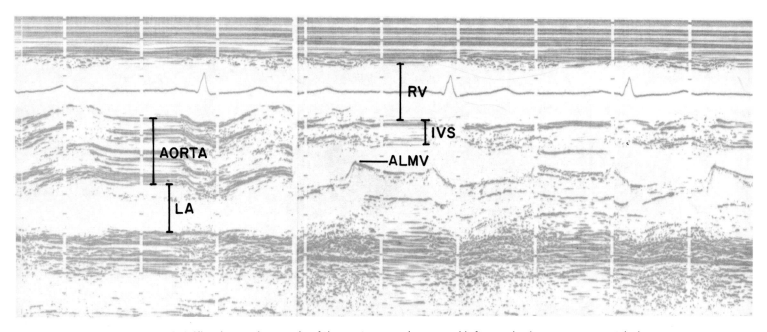

Fig. 7-19. Calcification and stenosis of the aorta cause increased left ventricular pressure, restricting the opening of the anterior leaflet of the mitral valve and giving it a stenotic appearance.

still apparent, so the examiner should not confuse the mitral valve's decreased E-F slope in aortic stenosis with that of mitral stenosis. We have also seen concentric hypertrophic changes of the left ventricle and septum with severe aortic stenosis.

Bicuspid valve

The normal cusps of the aorta close concentrically in diastole, whereas the bicuspid valve closes eccentrically. It is important to record the aortic cusps in various positions to ascertain whether this eccentricity shown in bicuspid valves is present. It is well known that transducer beam angulation can cause the normal cusps to appear to close eccentrically. We always evaluate the cusps with the patient supine and in a slight left decubitus position, carefully searching the aortic root area to determine the accurate appearance of the aortic cusps. In our studies we found that normal valves

could be made to look bicuspid in some sweeps but not consistently. In bicuspid valves the cusps usually closed quite eccentrically. In most cases one cusp barely appeared to move to the midline for closure. Generally, the posterior cusp appeared to have the reduced diastolic closure (Fig. 7-20). As the bicuspid valve became calcified, it was difficult to ascertain whether the valve was normal or bicuspid because of the increased echoes within the aortic root. A bicuspid valve cannot be ruled out completely by echo, but if the eccentricity is demonstrated, the valve is bicuspid.

Real-time evaluation provides an additional method of evaluating aortic cusp closure. The short-axis view of the aorta demonstrates normal aortic cusp motion to simulate a "Mercedes-Benz" sign. The bicuspid valve would clearly demonstrate the cusp closure eccentrically located to one of the valves.

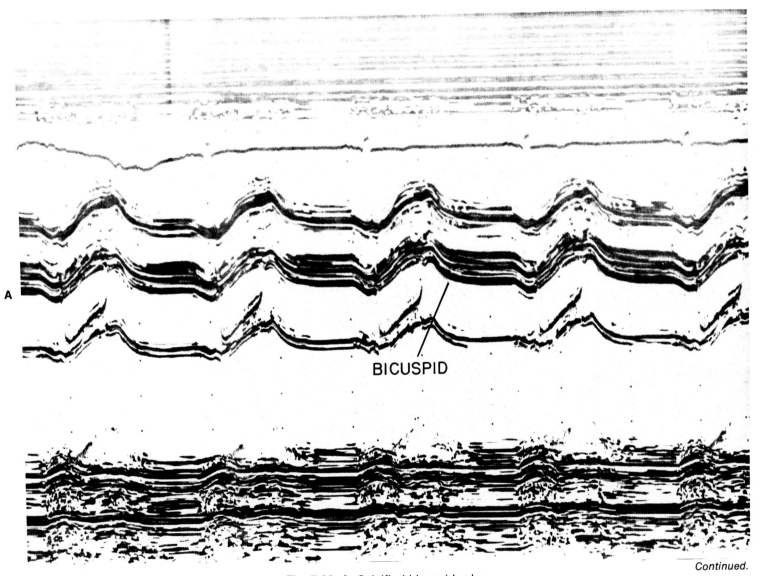

A

BICUSPID

Continued.

Fig. 7-20. A, Calcified bicuspid valve.

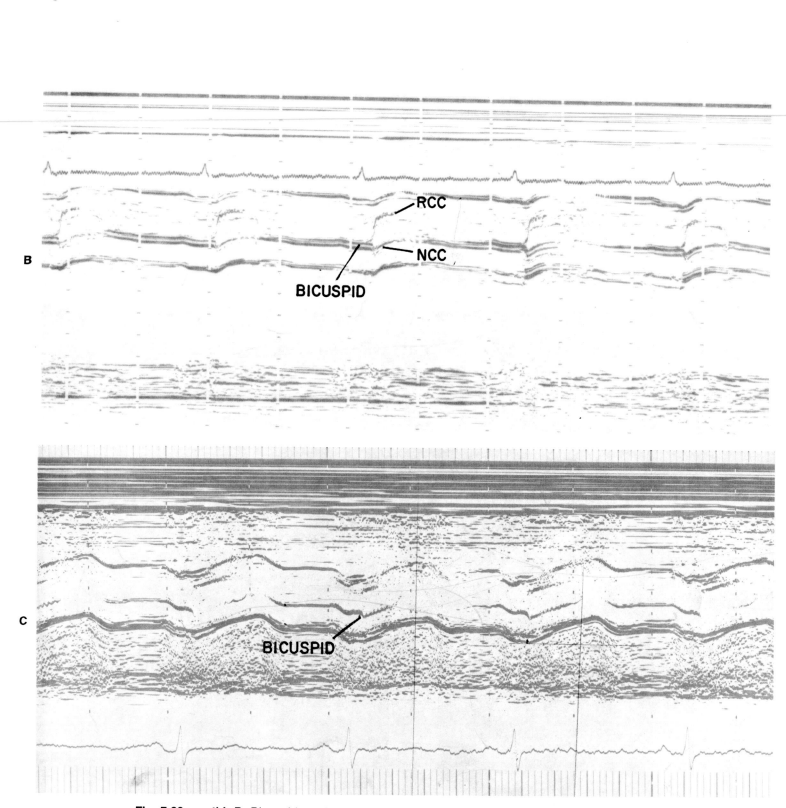

Fig. 7-20, cont'd. B, Bicuspid aortic valve. **C,** The aortic cusps close eccentrically in diastole to represent a bicuspid valve.

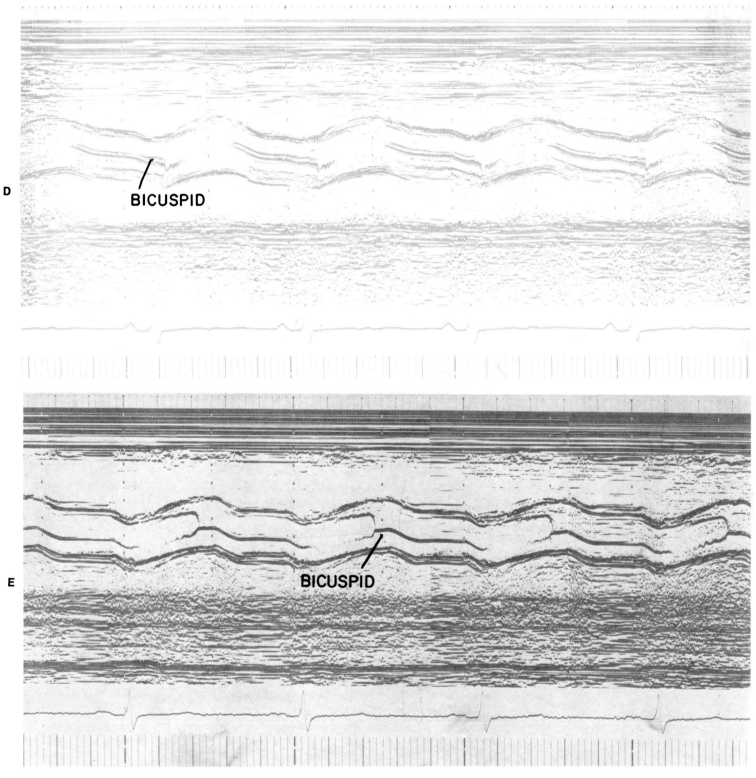

D

BICUSPID

E

BICUSPID

Fig. 7-20, cont'd. D, Slightly calcified bicuspid valve. **E,** Biscuspid valve.

Supravalvular aortic stenosis

Stenosis above the aortic valve may be a narrow ring, a longer hourglass deformity, or a hypoplastic ascending aorta. In a continuous sweep from the aortic root and cusp area to the area above the valve, until no aorta can be visualized, the dimension of the valve should become wider, since the beam is transecting the aorta in a tangential plane. However, if this area narrows consistently, supravalvular aortic stenosis is probably present.

Subvalvular aortic stenosis

The midsystolic closure of the aortic cusps is generally seen in cases of idiopathic hypertrophic subaortic stenosis (IHSS) or discrete subvalvular aortic stenosis. In cases of IHSS there is a hypertrophied septum with a systolic bulging of the anterior leaflet of the mitral valve. As the left ventricle contracts to eject blood through the outflow tract, this thickened septum and systolic bulge cause the aortic leaflets to close in midsystole (Fig. 7-21). (We have never seen the cusps remain closed throughout systole.) As the obstruction on the anterior leaflet moves away from the septum, the pressure relaxes in the left ventricle and the blood continues through the aortic cusps. This causes the cusps to reopen in late systole, although not as fully as in early systole. In discrete subaortic stenosis there is no septal hypertrophy or midsystolic obstruction, as seen in IHSS. A piece of tissue shaped like a diaphragm sits below the aortic valve and obstructs the flow from the left ventricle. This causes the aortic cusp to close in midsystole and reopen in late systole (Fig. 7-22).

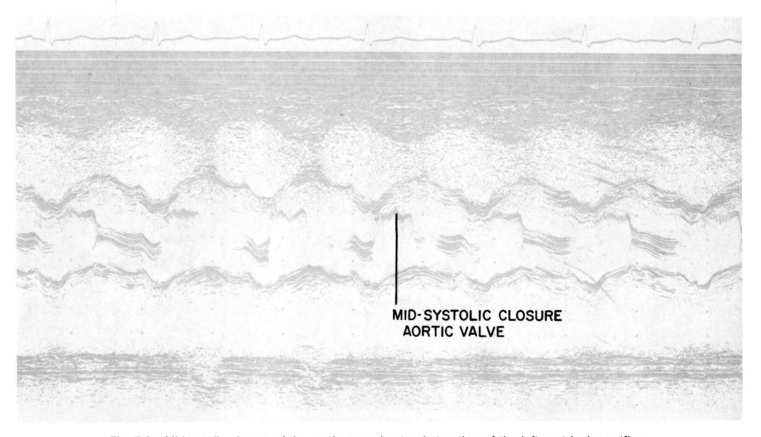

MID-SYSTOLIC CLOSURE
AORTIC VALVE

Fig. 7-21. Midsystolic closure of the aortic cusp due to obstruction of the left ventricular outflow tract, a result of idiopathic hypertrophic subaortic stenosis.

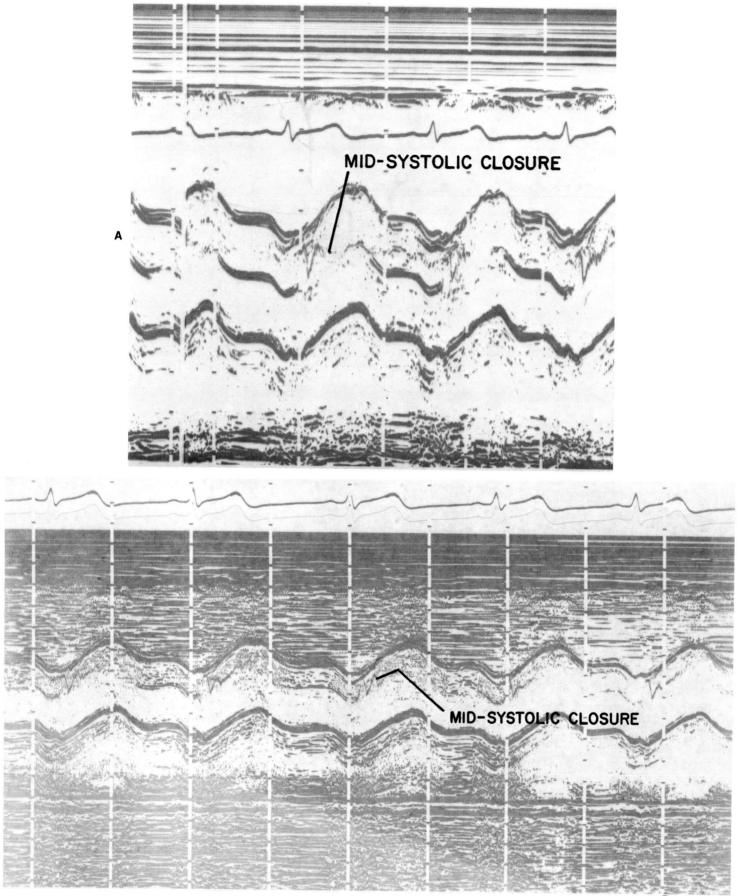

Continued.

Fig. 7-22. A, Subvalvular aortic stenosis can also cause a midsystolic closure of the aortic valve.
B, Midsystolic closure of the aortic valve.

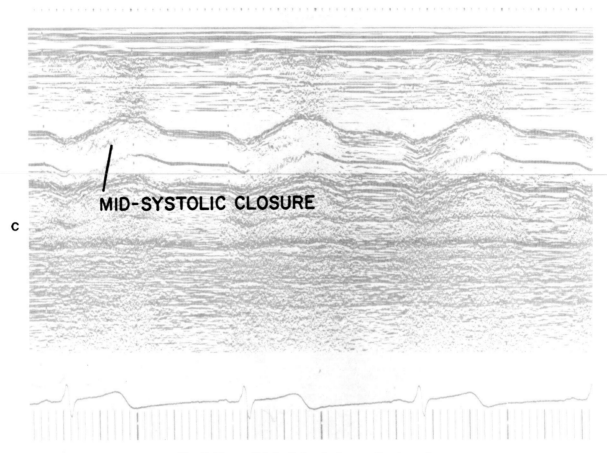

MID-SYSTOLIC CLOSURE

C

Fig. 7-22, cont'd. C, Subvalvular aortic stenosis.

Aortic regurgitation

Causes of aortic regurgitation include rheumatic fever, bacterial endocarditis, syphilis, aneurysm of the ascending aorta, ruptured aortic cusp, myxomatous degeneration of aortic valve cusps, and hypertensive dilatation of the aortic root.

Rheumatic fever may involve the aortic cusps, leaving them shrunken and fibrotic. Often aortic stenosis and insufficiency are the resulting diseases. Echographically the combined diseases cause the aortic root to display increased echoes representing calcification (Fig. 7-23). The aortic insufficiency appears on the anterior leaflet of the mitral valve as fine flutter during diastole (Fig. 7-24). The amplitude of the mitral valve decreases, as does the E-F slope, because of the increased pressures in the left ventricle.

Bacterial endocarditis may be spread to the aortic valve from other infected areas of the heart. Any lesion of the aortic valve can be the site for bacterial invasion, whether it is congenital, rheumatic, or syphilitic. The most dramatic echographic changes are demonstrated in diastole. As the cusps of the aortic valve close, the vegetations appear as fuzzy coarse echoes (Fig. 7-25, A). The amount of vegetation damage may determine the degree of associated aortic insufficiency. Acute aortic insufficiency can be recognized with early mitral valve closure by measuring the PR-AC interval (Fig. 7-25, B).

Syphilis infection may affect the aorta, the aortic valve ring, and the coronary artery ostia. As the aortic ring dilates, progressive regurgitation results (Fig. 7-26). The echo demonstrates dilatation of the aortic root and fine flutter of the anterior leaflet of the mitral valve. Every patient in the tertiary stage of this disease whom we examined had these features.

Text continued on p. 127.

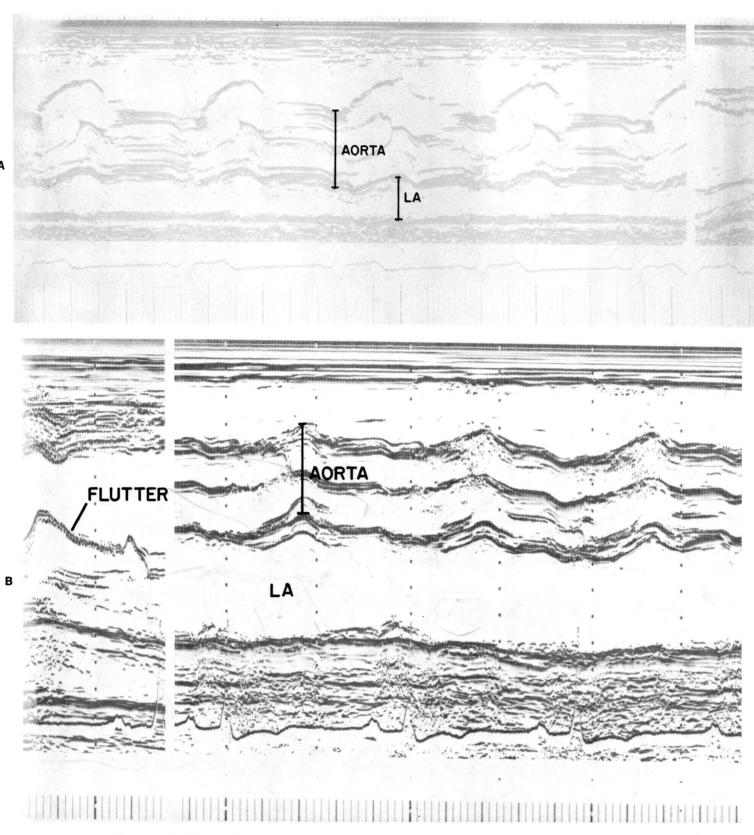

Fig. 7-23. A, Rheumatic disease with slight calcification of the aorta. The aorta appears dilated compared with the left atrial size. **B,** Rheumatic disease involving the aorta and mitral valves. Fine flutter is shown on the anterior leaflet of the mitral valve due to aortic insufficiency. The left atrium is enlarged due to mitral disease.

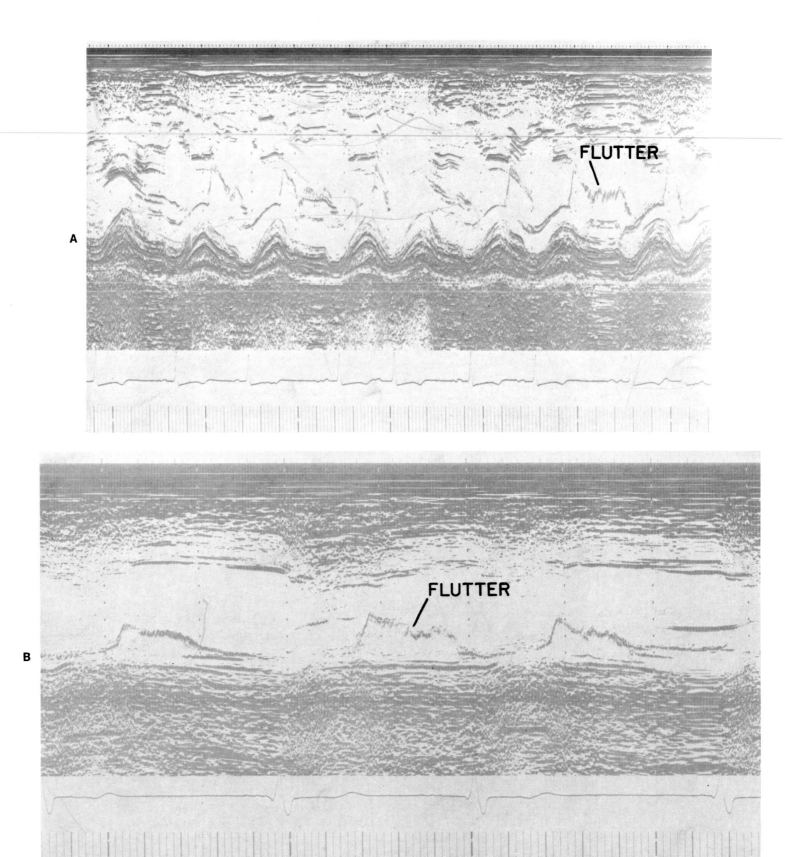

Fig. 7-24. A, Fine flutter on the anterior leaflet of the mitral valve due to aortic insufficiency. **B,** Flutter on the anterior leaflet of the mitral valve due to aortic insufficiency.

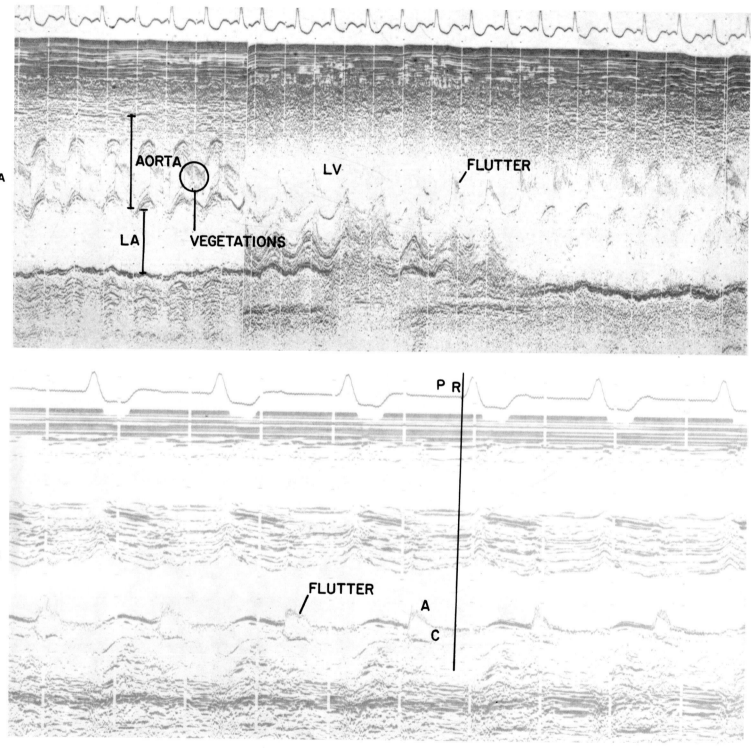

Fig. 7-25. A, Increased echoes in diastole represent vegetations on the aortic valve. Aortic insufficiency is shown on the anterior leaflet of the mitral valve and is caused by the destruction of the
cusps. **B,** Premature closure of the mitral apparatus (PR-AC interval less than 0.06 sec) represents
acute aortic insufficiency.

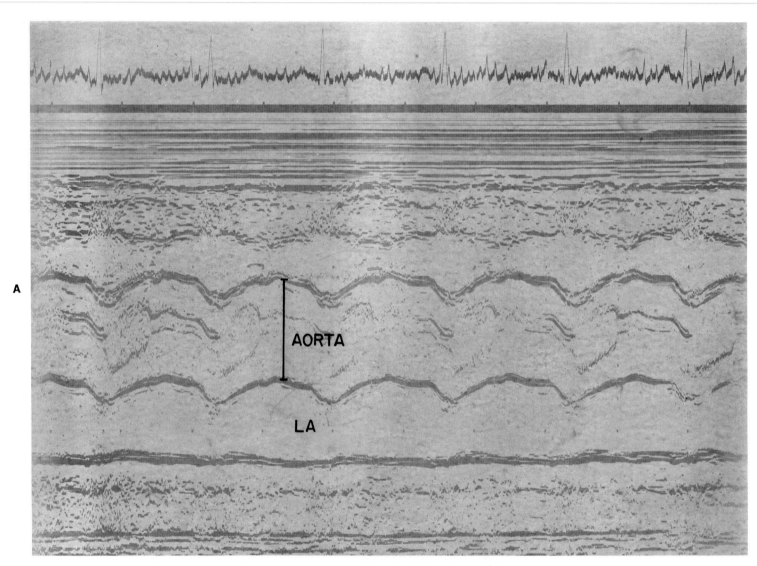

Fig. 7-26. Aortic insufficiency **(A)** can result from the later stages of syphilis and demonstrates an enlarged aortic dimension with fine flutter **(B)** on the mitral valve.

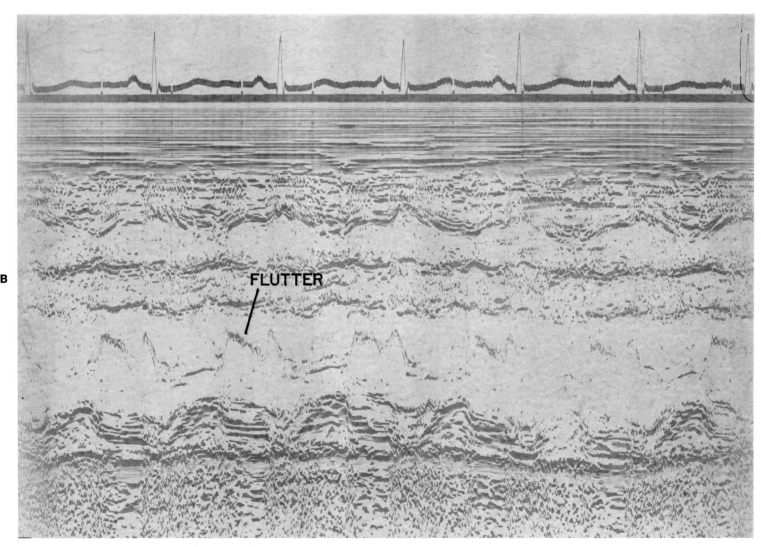

Fig. 7-26, cont'd. For legend see opposite page.

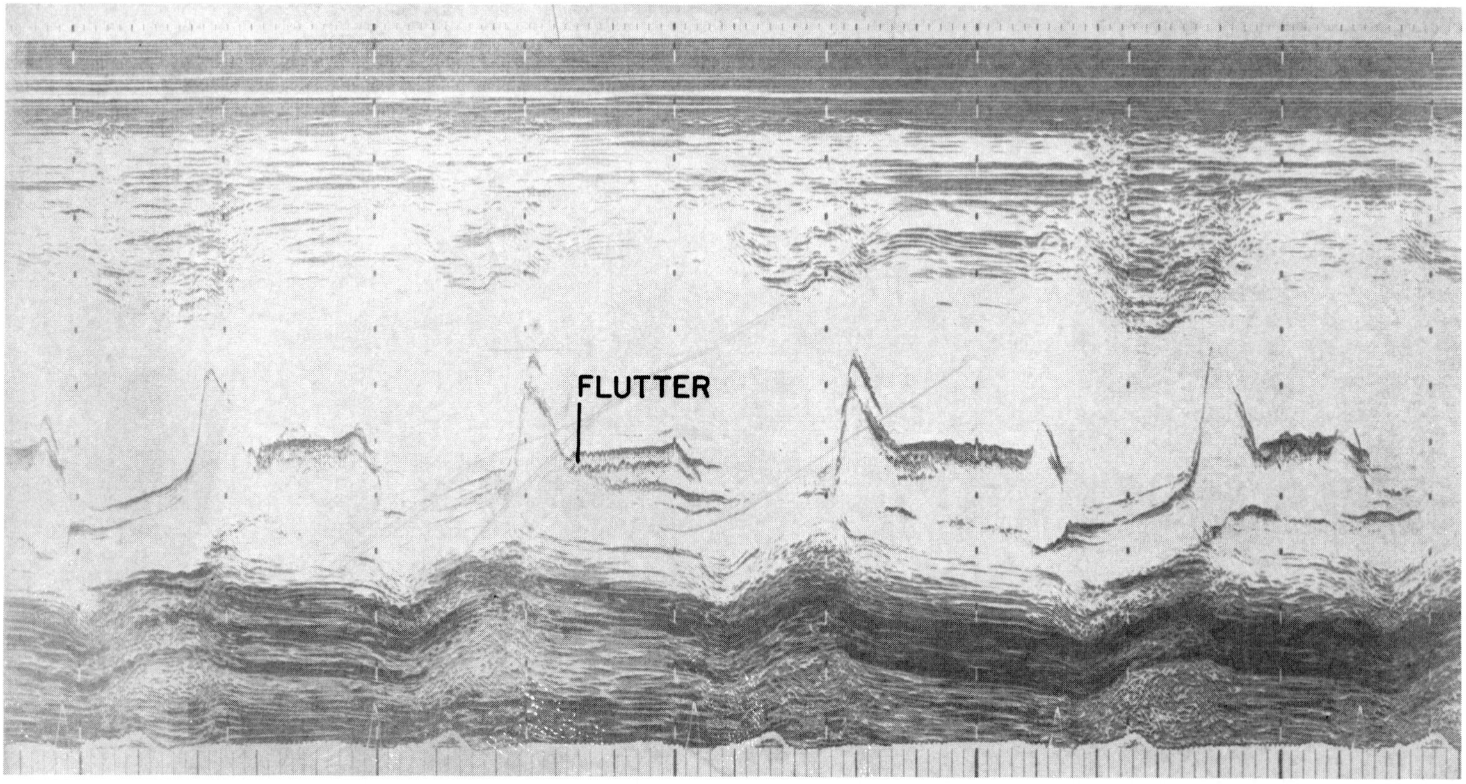

Fig. 7-27. A, Young man with Marfan-type syndrome. Echo demonstrates an enlarged aortic root. **B,** Flutter of the anterior leaflet of the mitral valve from the aortic insufficiency, with positive regurgitant sounds from the pulsed Doppler.

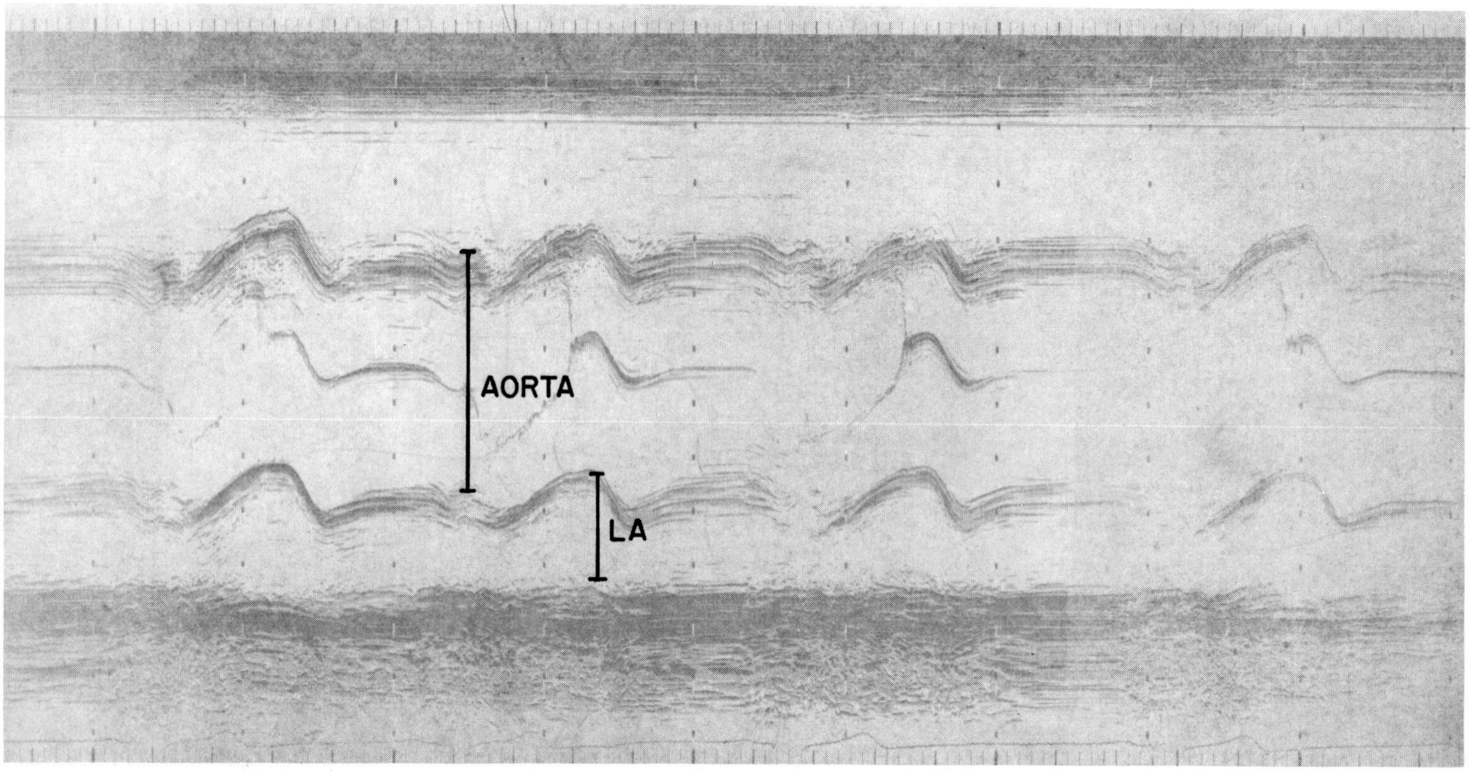

Marfan's syndrome

Marfan's syndrome is considered a stretch lesion of the valve. The aortic and mitral leaflets stretch and overshoot their normal closing, with resulting mitral or aortic regurgitation. The ascending aorta is also subject to dilatation and weakness, which may lead to dissection. Marfan's syndrome patients have the following other physical symptoms: long thin fingers, tall stature, double-jointedness, and an abnormal metacarpal index.

Patients with Marfan's syndrome display several echographic features. They usually have a huge aortic root with associated aortic insufficiency, shown on the mitral valve as fine flutter (Fig. 7-27). Usually, associated mitral regurgitation is shown with increased amplitude of the anterior leaflet and "spooning" or holosystolic prolapse of both leaflets in systole.

LEFT ATRIAL CAVITY

The left atrium is located posterior to the aortic root. Normally, a 1:1 ratio exists between the left atrial cavity and the aortic root. The left atrial dimension should be calculated at the end-systolic dimension from the leading edge of the posterior aortic wall to the leading edge of the left atrial wall. Enlargement of the left atrium most likely reflects mitral valve disease, cardiomyopathy, or congestive heart failure. (See Fig. 7-28.)

Tumors

Determination of tumor echoes vs. reverberation echoes is important to assess in the left atrial cavity. In a sweep into the left atrial cavity, intense echoes from tumor formation should appear in systole. As the sweep is made into the mitral valve area, these tumor echoes should flop behind the anterior leaflet of the mitral valve in diastole. There should be a small space just after the opening of the mitral valve before the tumor flops from the left atrium. (In some cases the tumor will be firmly adhered to the left atrial wall and will not flop posterior to the mitral apparatus.) The echoes appear much like a calcified mitral valve, occurring in diastole and flopping into the left atrium in systole. On the other hand, reverberation echoes can be seen in the left atrium because of patient respiration. As the sweep is performed, these echoes will appear in the systolic segment but will not flop into the mitral area. If the patient holds respiration, these echoes will disappear. (See Fig. 7-29.)

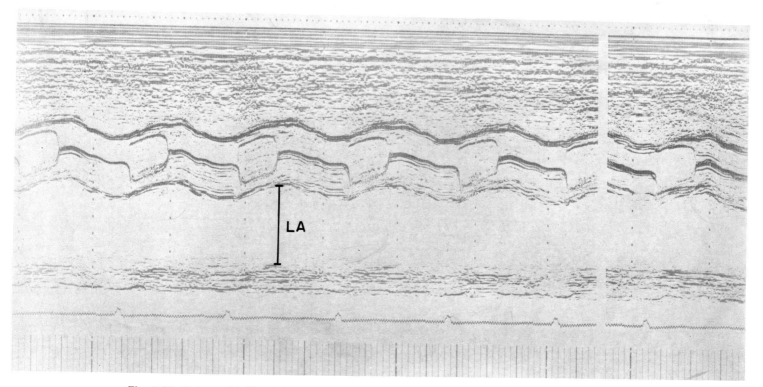

Fig. 7-28. Enlarged left atrial cavity secondary to rheumatic involvement of the mitral valve.

We have noted a bizarre movement of the left atrial wall extending into the left ventricular cavity in several patients. Two of those patients developed bronchogenic carcinoma and Hodgkin's disease. Both had hyperdynamic cardiac movement, which may account for the increased activity of the left atrial wall.

Real time demonstrated increased echoes just superior to the atrioventricular groove in the left atrial cavity. Some patients with moderate-to-large pericardial effusions have also shown this peculiar movement. (See Fig. 7-30.)

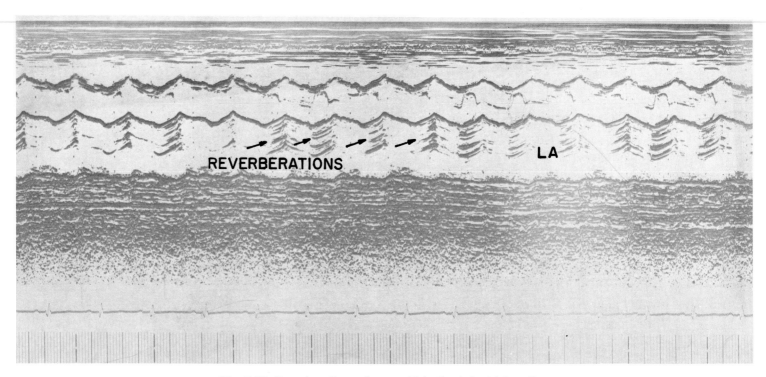

Fig. 7-29. Reverberations shown within the left atrial cavity.

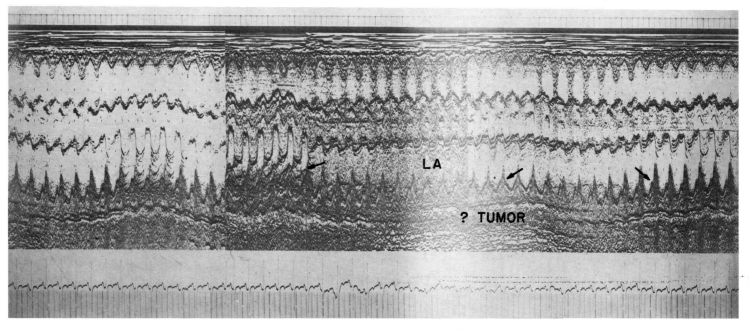

Fig. 7-30. Hyperdynamic left atrial wall motion could be secondary to tumor formation or a large pericardial effusion.

8 □ Tricuspid valve

NORMAL TRICUSPID VALVE

The tricuspid valve is not as easily identified as the mitral valve because of its substernal location in most patients (Fig. 8-1). Recordings are easily made if the right ventricle is slightly enlarged or if the heart is rotated to the left of the sternum. Once the transducer has recorded the mitral apparatus, the beam should be directed slightly medial to record the tricuspid valve (Fig. 8-2). It is fairly easy to identify the "whipping" motion of the anterior valve in systole and early diastole. However, the diastolic period reveals the pathologic changes of stenosis and regurgitation, and careful angulation may allow this phase to be recorded. An alternate method of recording is to locate the aortic root. The transducer beam should sweep inferiorly and medially toward the patient's right foot to record the tricuspid valve (Fig. 8-3).

Sometimes it is confusing to differentiate the tricuspid from the pulmonary valve. In the normal patient the tricuspid valve is always inferior and medial to the aortic root, whereas the pulmonary is superior and lateral. The other difference is that the tricuspid valve moves anterior with atrial contraction, and the pulmonary *a* valve dips posteriorly (Fig. 8-4).

It is very easy to record the tricuspid valve in children with the transducer directly on the sternum. There is virtually no lung interference, as is often found in adults (Fig. 8-5). In our experience the tricuspid valve has been displayed in over 60% of patients (Figs. 8-6 and 8-7).

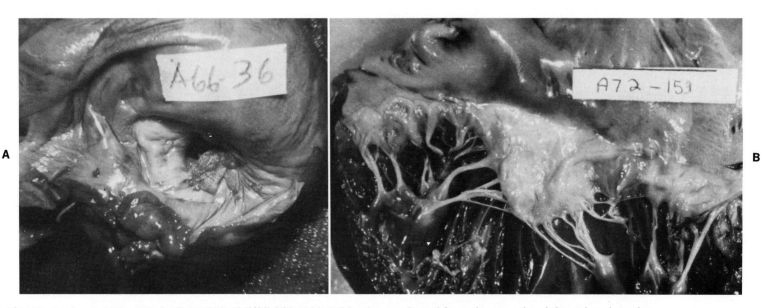

Fig. 8-1. A, Gross specimen of the tricuspid valve as viewed from the superior right atrium into the barrel of the valve leaflets. **B,** The gross specimen of the tricuspid valve demonstrates the large anterior leaflet (middle) attached by chordae tendineae to both walls of the heart. The posterior leaflet (right) is much smaller and can be seen on echo posterior to the anterior leaflet. The septal leaflet (left) is not seen on echo, since it lies parallel to the transducer beam.

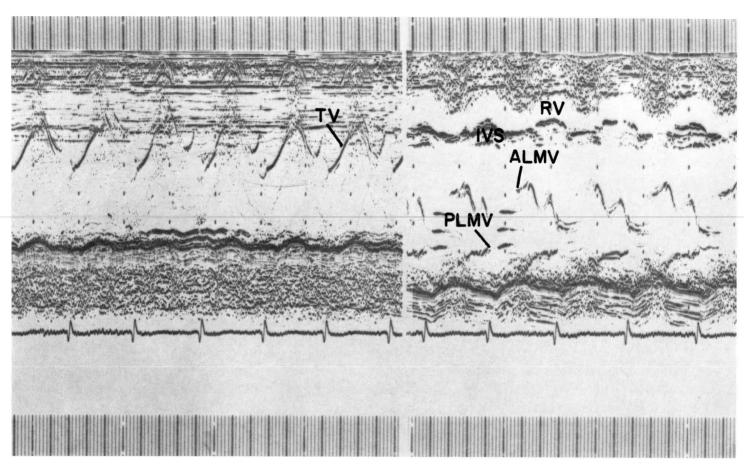

Fig. 8-2. Anterior leaflet of the tricuspid valve can be identified as a sweep is made medial and slightly inferior from the mitral valve. It should demonstrate the same motion as the mitral valve.

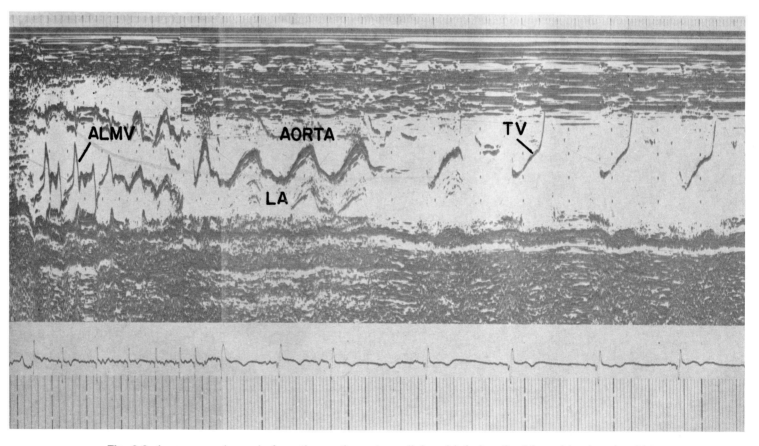

Fig. 8-3. As a sweep is made from the aortic root, medial and inferior, the tricuspid valve should appear at the level of the anterior aortic wall.

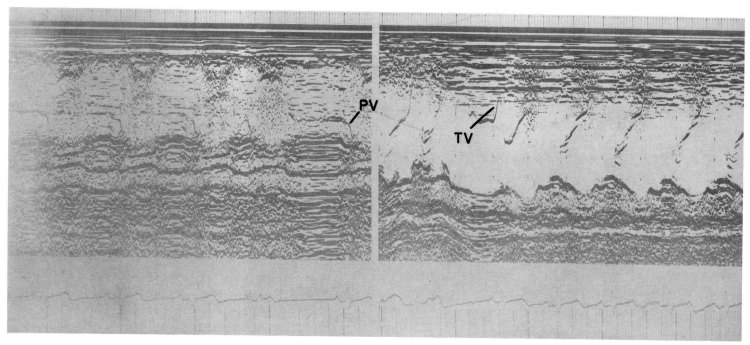

Fig. 8-4. Distinction of tricuspid valve from pulmonary valve is one of position and movement. The tricuspid valve moves anterior after atrial contraction, whereas the pulmonary valve dips posterior.

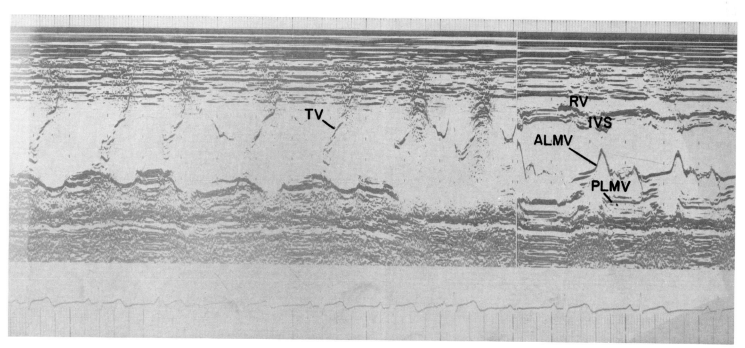

Fig. 8-5. Tricuspid valve of young children, adolescents, and slim adults is very easy to record. In most cases the transducer may be held directly over the sternum, or the patient may be rolled into a left decubitus or lateral position to allow the right side of the heart to be viewed.

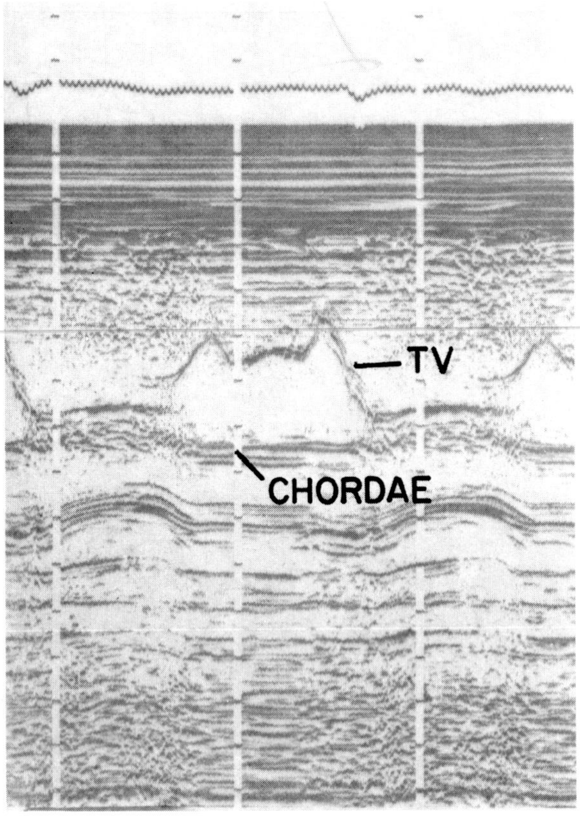

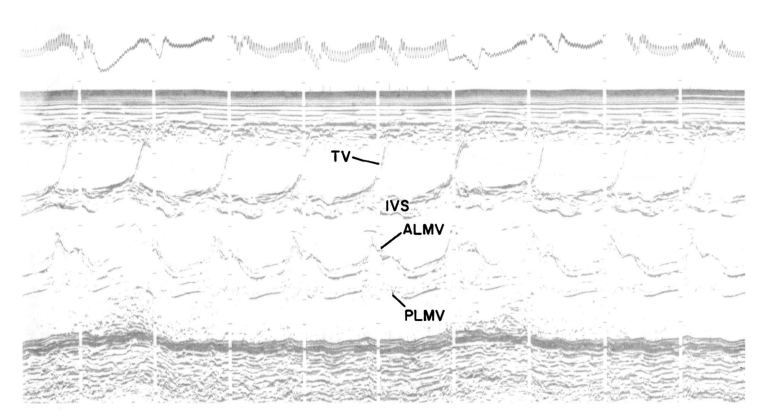

Fig. 8-6. Normal tricuspid valve with chordae tendineae posterior. These chordae may be confused as part of the right side of the septum, and careful gain settings and transducer position should allow one to separate the chordae from the right side of the septum.

Fig. 8-7. Sometimes the tricuspid valve can be seen at the same time as the mitral leaflet is recorded. This is caused either by cardiac position or disease (enlarged right ventricle, Ebstein's anomaly).

PATHOLOGIC CONDITIONS

Tricuspid stenosis

Most cases of tricuspid stenosis are rheumatic in origin, with the mitral and aortic valves being affected first. Other possible causes are congenital tricuspid stenosis, systemic lupus erythematosus, and carcinoid tumors. The stenotic leaflets usually fuse, leaving a roundish hole in the central area of the leaflets and some degree of incompetence in the valve. As in mitral stenosis, the right atrium dilates and hypertrophies in tricuspid stenosis.

Echographic evaluation of stenosis is very difficult to accomplish. Since the pressures are so low on the right side of the heart, it is possible for the valve to be badly diseased and yet produce no pressure gradient at cardiac catheterization, thus showing no decreased slope on the anterior leaflet.

Tricuspid regurgitation

There are two types of regurgitation—functional and organic. Functional tricuspid regurgitation is the result of right ventricular failure, which causes right ventricular dilatation. This dilatation causes the tricuspid ring also to dilate, producing tricuspid valve regurgitation. Organic regurgitation is caused by rheumatic disease process, congenital lesions of Ebstein's disease and endocardial cushion defects, or bacterial endocarditis.

The right atrium enlarges with regurgitant flow from the tricuspid valve. Likewise, during diastole, the right ventricle receives this blood from the right atrium in addition to that reaching the right atrium from the great veins, causing hypertrophy and dilatation. The dilated right side of the heart enables the examiner to visualize the tricuspid valve echographically with ease (Figs. 8-8 to 8-11).

Bacterial endocarditis can result as a complication of drug addiction. Vegetations may form in the right side of the heart if infection occurs. Echographically the increased echoes in diastole may represent vegetations (Fig. 8-12). Care must be used to avoid increased echoes caused by respiratory motion (Fig. 8-13). Vegetations adhere to the valve apparatus and do not disappear in continual tracings, whereas artifacts of respiration may.

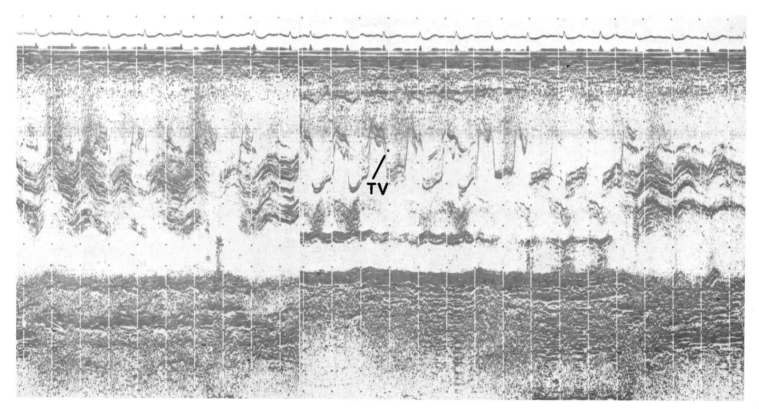

Fig. 8-8. Tricuspid valve is noted to have increased amplitude, although no flutter is seen.

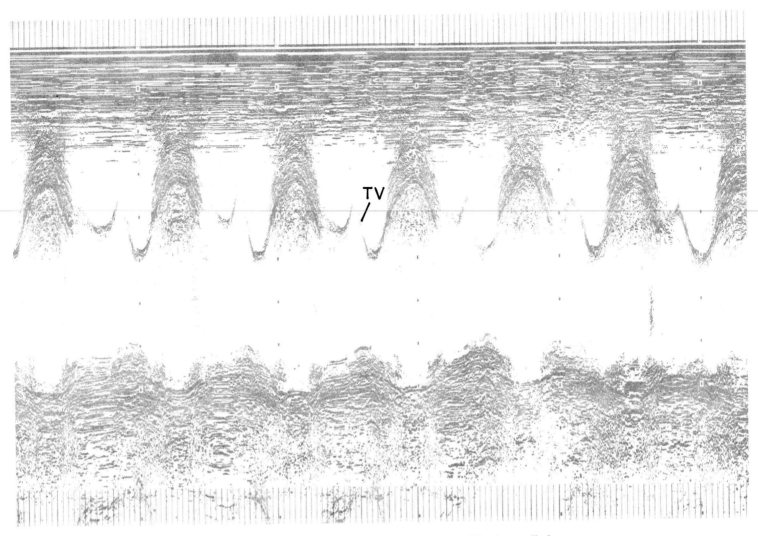

Fig. 8-9. Dilated right ventricular cavity with tricuspid valve well shown.

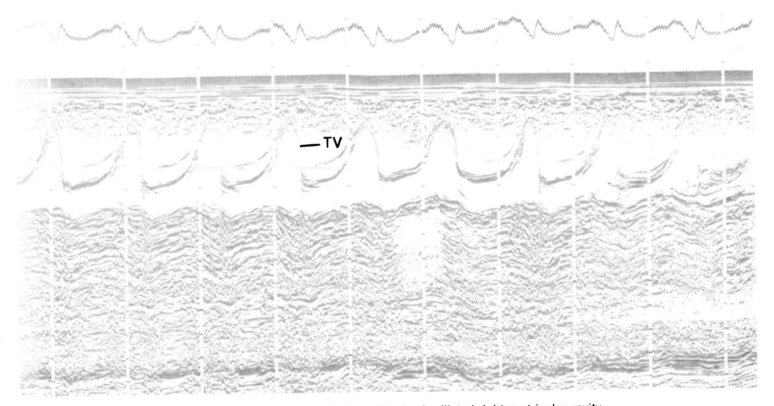

Fig. 8-10. Anterior leaflet of tricuspid valve in dilated right ventricular cavity.

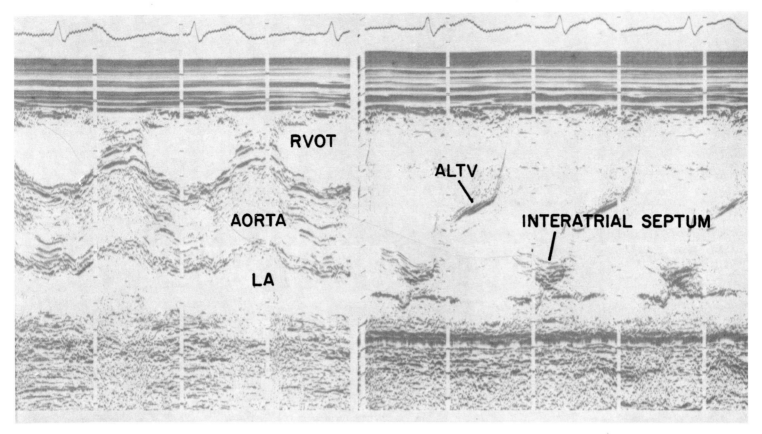

Fig. 8-11. Tricuspid valve well seen with interatrial septum posterior.

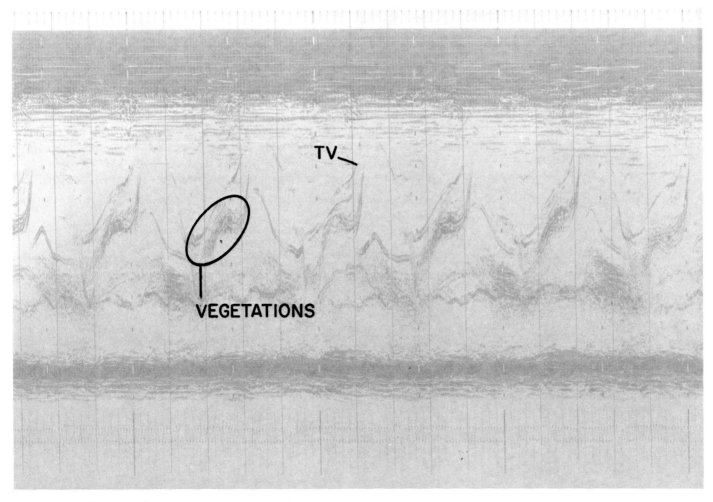

Fig. 8-12. Scan of a young heroin addict with spiking fevers and systolic murmur. The tricuspid valve demonstrates increased echoes in early diastole, which represent vegetation growth on the anterior leaflet. Tricuspid incompetence was noted on subsequent scans.

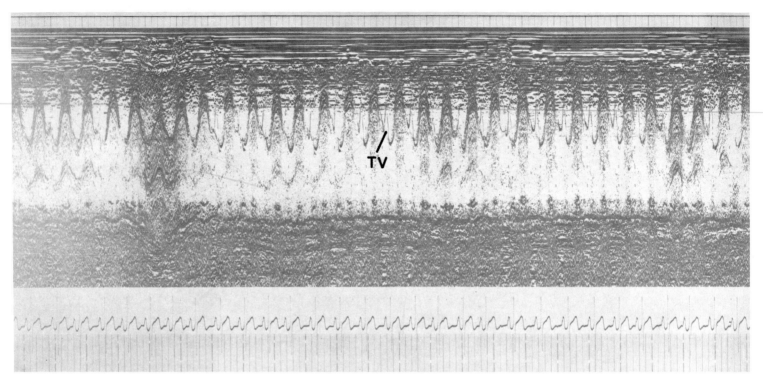

Fig. 8-13. Respiratory echoes can sometimes be confusing when seen in early diastole. They appear as equidistant lines at the time of respiration and vary with increased respiratory motion.

Fluttering

The tricuspid leaflet generally opens and closes as the mitral leaflet does, with no fine fluttering motion. If fine flutter is noted, there may be one of several causes. Pulmonary insufficiency is probably the most common cause of fine flutter. The regurgitation from the pulmonary valve acts the same as aortic insufficiency does on the mitral apparatus. The backflow of blood strikes the tricuspid leaflet, causing high-frequency flutter. Small vegetations may be difficult to analyze if there is flutter on the leaflet. Generally, however, the bacterial lesions must be 2 to 3 mm for diagnosis, causing a coarser flutter on the tricuspid leaflet. Occasionally, tricuspid regurgitation causes fine flutter on the leaflet as well as dilatation of the right chambers (Figs. 8-14 and 8-15).

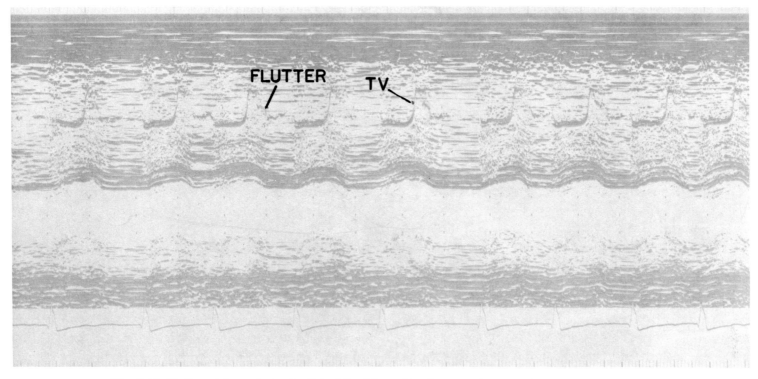

Fig. 8-14. Flutter of the anterior leaflet of the tricuspid valve may denote pulmonary insufficiency, tricuspid regurgitation, or an elongated chorda.

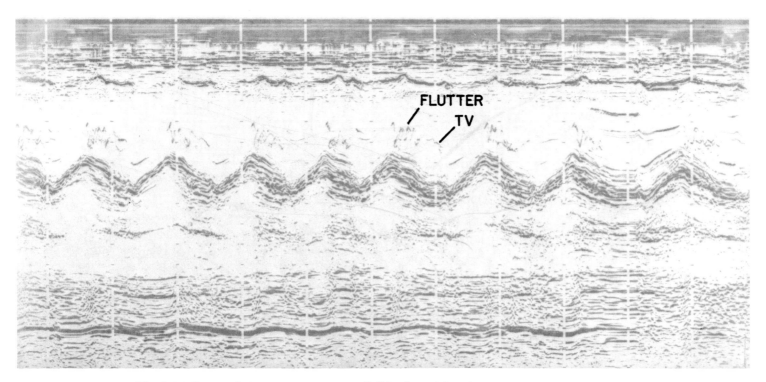

Fig. 8-15. Coarse flutter may represent a flail leaflet, giving rise to tricuspid incompetence.

9 □ Pulmonary valves

NORMAL PULMONARY VALVE

The normal pulmonary valve was the last of the four valves to be adequately visualized by ultrasound. Gramiak and Nanda (1972) were the first to document its echographic pattern through the aid of contrast studies. Although it is a tricuspid valve, only the left, or posterior cusp, can be adequately demonstrated on echographic evaluation. Prior to Walter L. Henry's (of NIH) visit to our laboratory, we had little success in demonstrating the pulmonary valve in patients without right heart dilatation. It is more difficult to visualize this valve in obese women or muscular males, but with continued practice we are able to see the pulmonary valve in approximately 85% of our patients. We generally have greater success as we slowly sweep from the aortic valve area laterally and superiorly toward the left shoulder to the pulmonary valve area. The parallel aortic echoes serve as a landmark in the sweep to the pulmonary valve. The anterior aortic root forms the posterior boundary of the pulmonary valve area. There should be a 2 to 4 cm space beneath the anterior chest wall and in front of this posterior border in which to visualize the pulmonary valve. Gramiak (1972) has identified these posterior structures as the junction of the right ventricular outflow tract and pulmonary artery and the atriopulmonary sulcus with the left atrium posterior.

When this structure-complex is identified, small adjustments in beam position and direction will usually pass the beam through the left pulmonary valve cusp, which lies in a posterior position in the right ventricular outflow space. We have found the A-mode trace very helpful in recognizing the fleeting posterior cusp motion of the pulmonary valve. Its appearance is similar to that of the aortic cusp and requires very slight angulation to demonstrate fully. We have not found it easier to locate this valve in one particular position. We usually look for the cusp with the patient in a slight left lateral decubitus position, and, if none is found, the patient lies in a supine position. Of course, patients with increased right heart dimensions enable much easier visualization of the pulmonary valve.

The other method for locating the pulmonary valve is to direct the transducer beam from the area of the mitral valve superiorly, without changing the lateral angle. We have found this to be more difficult because of lung interference, but in some cases it succeeds when the aortic sweep fails.

Gramiak (1972) describes the physiologic parameters as shown in the echocardiogram. At the beginning of diastole the pulmonary valve is displaced downward and is represented anteriorly on the ultrasound record. The low transducer position with upward beam angulation, together with the vertical inclination of the pulmonary ring, results in examination of the valve from below. All elevations of the pulmonary valve in the stream of flow are represented as posterior movements on the echo. Likewise, downward movements are represented by anterior cusp positions on the trace.

The valve begins to move posteriorly in a gradual manner as the right ventricle fills in diastole. Atrial systole elevates the valve and produces a 3 to 7 mm posterior movement—a dip. The valve moves upward with ventricular systole and thus shows a rapid posterior motion on the echo. (See Figs. 9-1 to 9-7.)

The normal measurements of the pulmonary valve follow:

a depth	2 to 7 mm (Feigenbaum)
	3 to 13 mm (Shah)
B-C opening	13.9 ± 1.8 mm (Feigenbaum)
(os)	8.7 ± 0.92 mm (Shah)
B-C slope	Under 300 mm/sec (Feigenbaum)
(os)	211 ± 12.7 mm/sec (Shah)

Text continued on p. 143.

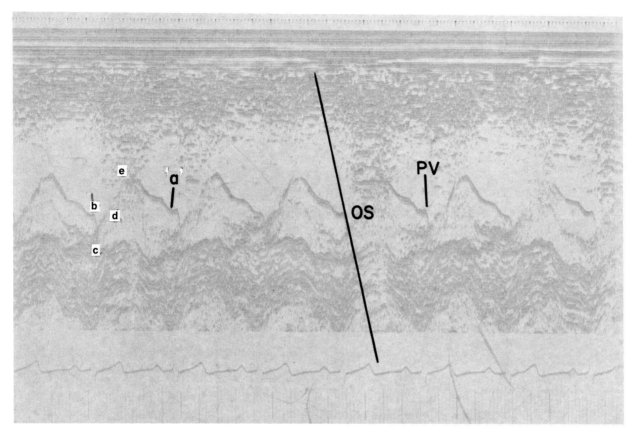

Fig. 9-1. *A* point occurs just before the pulmonary valve opening and is identified by a posterior deformity on the pulmonary valve caused by atrial systole. The amplitude of the *a* point varies with respiration, increasing on inspiration and decreasing on expiration. The opening of the pulmonary valve occurs between points *b, c, d,* and *e.*

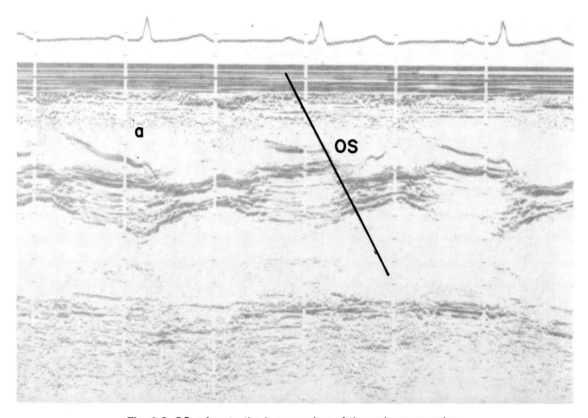

Fig. 9-2. *OS* refers to the b-c opening of the pulmonary valve.

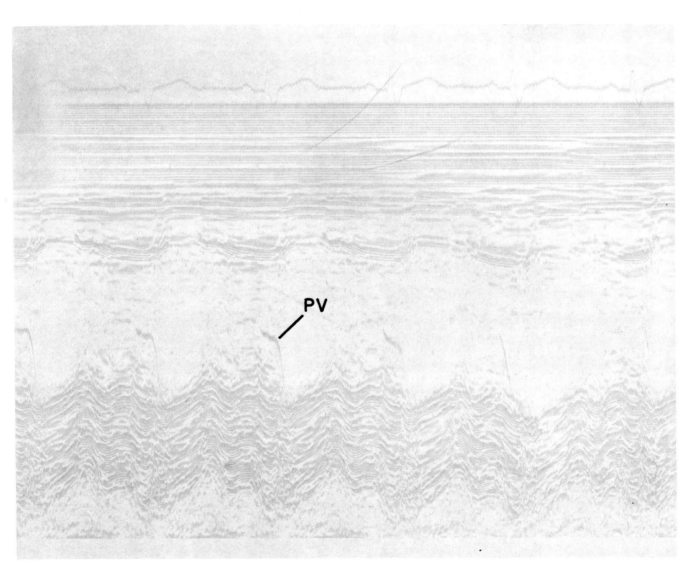

Fig. 9-3. Scale should be expanded when the pulmonary valve is recorded to allow better visualization of this anterior valve.

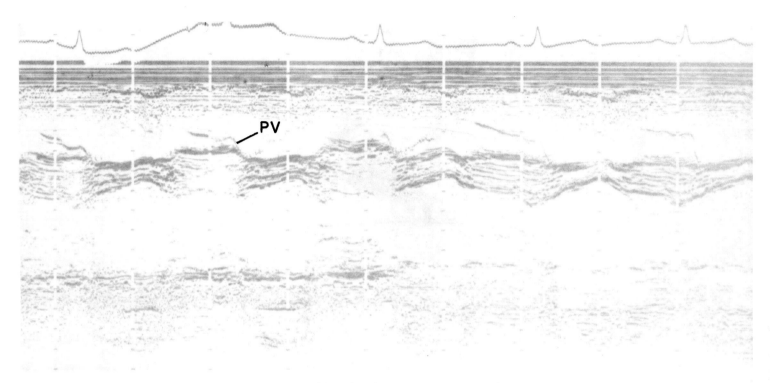

Fig. 9-4. Normal pulmonary valve with atriopulmonary sulcus posterior to valve opening. The left atrial cavity is posterior to the sulcus.

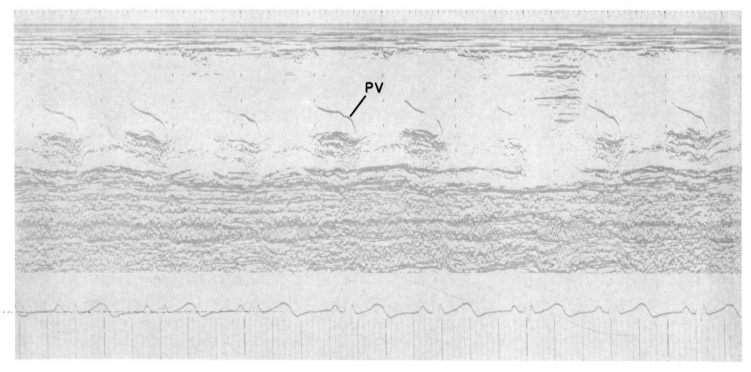

Fig. 9-5. Normal pulmonary valve.

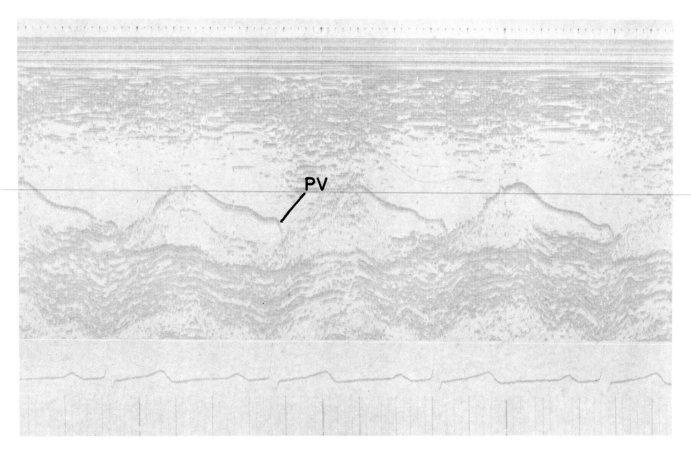

Fig. 9-6. Normal pulmonary valve.

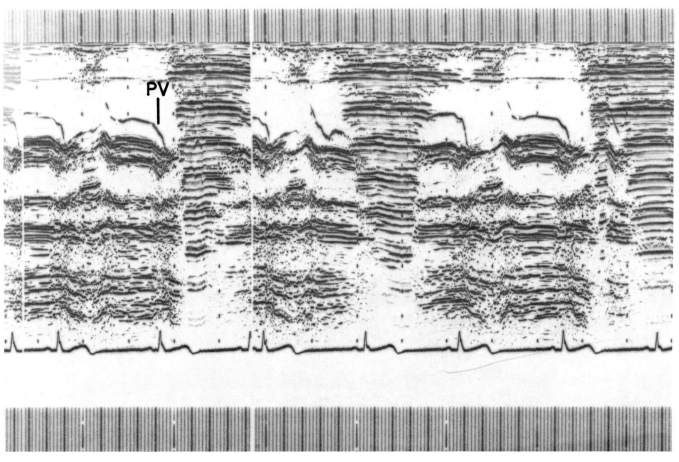

Fig. 9-7. Normal pulmonary valve.

PATHOLOGIC CONDITIONS
Pulmonary stenosis

Pulmonary valve stenosis is almost always congenital. The valve is either bicuspid or tricuspid, and thickened. Chang (1977) states that severe pulmonary stenosis will cause the pulmonary valve to open completely with the onset of systole; the *a* wave will appear to be absent echographically because it never returns toward the baseline before the onset of systole. Goldberg, Allen, and Sahn (1974) have reported increased hypertrophy of the right ventricular wall and dilatation of the right ventricular dimension. Moderate pulmonary stenosis may produce an exaggerated *a* dip, exceeding the normal 7 mm (Fig. 9-8).

Pulmonary insufficiency

The cause of pulmonary insufficiency is usually pulmonary hypertension, which causes dilatation of the main pulmonary artery and valve ring (Fig. 9-9). It can also result from bacterial endocarditis, congenital absence of the valve, or pulmonary valvotomy. Echographically the pulmonary valve is easier to demonstrate in cases of pulmonary hypertension resulting from dilatation of the vessel. The *a* dip diminishes with increased pressures, and the E-F slope flattens (Figs. 9-10 and 9-11). With increased hypertension a midsystolic notching appears; this was termed the "flying W" sign by Goldberg, Allen, and Sahn (Fig. 9-12).

Fine flutter may appear on the pulmonary cusp but not as frequently as shown in other valve lesions such as aortic and mitral insufficiency.

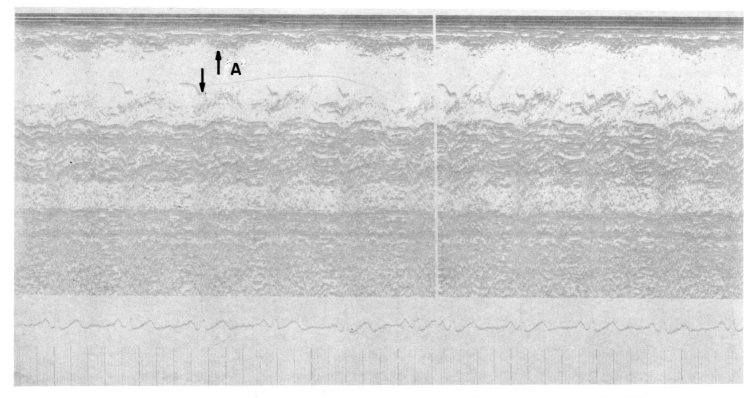

Fig. 9-8. Pulmonary stenosis may be identified by the increased *a* dip on the pulmonary valve. This *a* dip should exceed 7 mm.

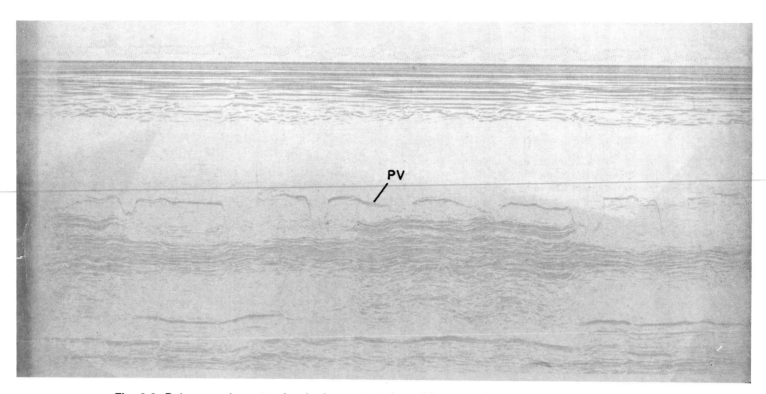

Fig. 9-9. Pulmonary hypertension is demonstrated on this scan of a patient with a dilated right ventricle and flattened E-F slope.

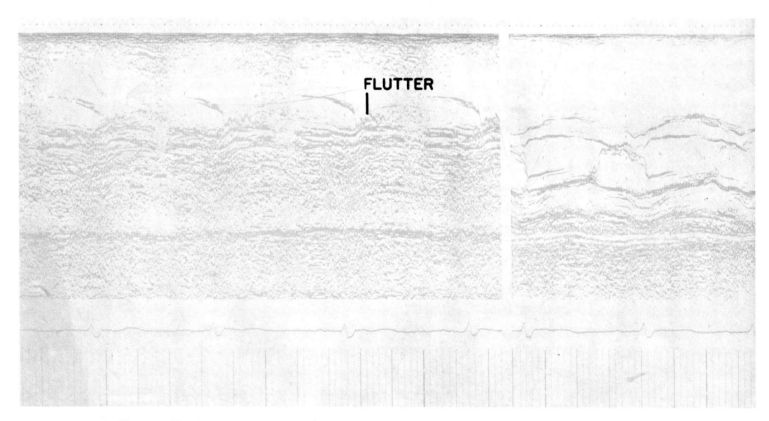

Fig. 9-10. Fine flutter of the pulmonary valve is shown in systole. The enlarged right ventricular cavity is seen anterior to the mitral valve.

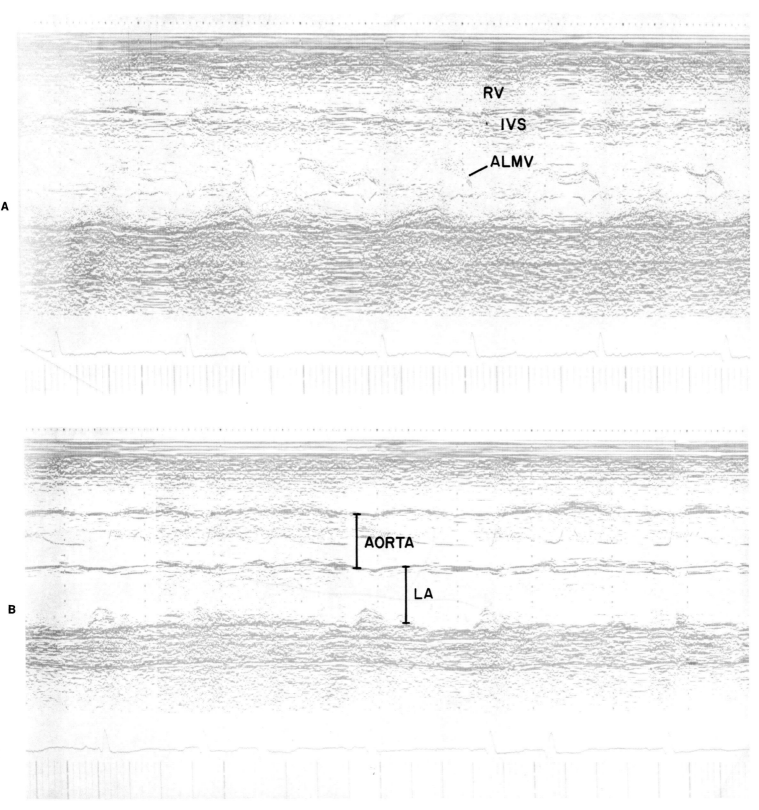

Fig. 9-11. A, Patient with cor pulmonale. Echo is difficult to obtain because of lung interference. Right ventricular cavity is generally enlarged. **B,** Normal aorta and left atrial dimension in same patient.

Continued.

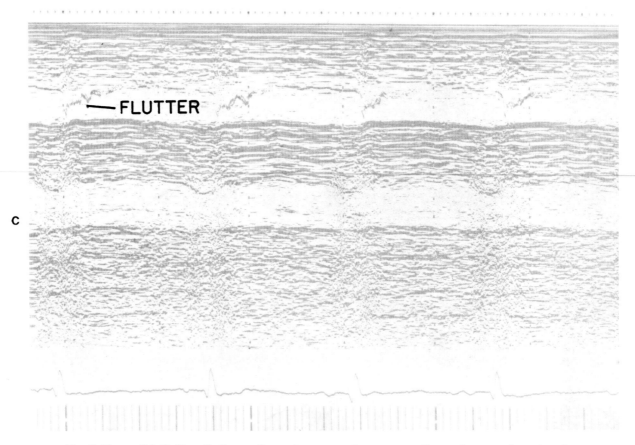

Fig. 9-11, cont'd. C, Fine flutter on the pulmonary valve representing pulmonary hypertension.

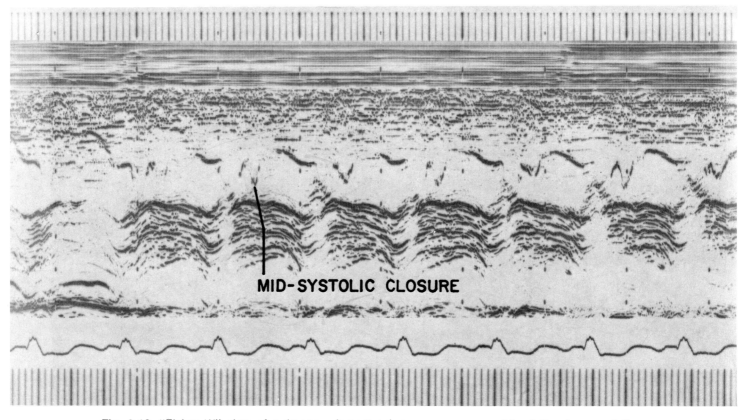

Fig. 9-12. "Flying W" sign of pulmonary hypertension appears as a midsystolic closure of the pulmonary valve.

10 □ Prosthetic valves

Our laboratory has had experience with three basic types of prosthetic valves—the cage with ball (Starr-Edwards), the cage with disk (Beall), and the tilting disk or hinge (Björk-Shiley) (Fig. 10-1). It is important for the echographer to know the type of prosthetic valve in use for adequate recording of its most perpendicular axis.

There are three basic parts to each type of valve—the disk or ball, the strut or cage, and the sewing ring or seating of the valve (the upper and lower round attachment of the valve). Any of these components is subject to changes. The Starr-Edwards ball is composed of silicon and is subject to ball variance, or a grooving irregularity. This ball variance is not seen in Teflon disk valves. Some of the valves are cloth covered and not as subject to thrombus.

The incidence of thrombus with good anticoagulation is 30%. The upper and lower seating is frequently subject to thrombosis, which in turn narrows the valve. The lower-seating thrombosis interferes with the closure of the valve and eventually can lead to regurgitation. In addition to these problems with thrombosis, the sutures around the area of the valve can come loose, causing regurgitation.

The evaluation of defects in the valve is sometimes very difficult. The majority of patients are asymptomatic. Some demonstrate signs of fatigue; some go into congestive heart failure because of a sticking poppet. Embolisms to various organs may be seen in some patients as a result of thrombosis formation on the valve. Bacterial endocarditis is one complication of prosthetic valves, since the malfunctioning valve is a seedbed for bacteria.

The disk and hinge types of valve can be used interchangeably in the aorta and the mitral valve by reversing their positions. During auscultation the valves should make two noises during one cycle. At the onset of systole the mitral valve should have a closing click, whereas the aortic valve should have an opening click. Likewise, during diastole the mitral valve should have an opening click and the aortic a closing click. With the valve in the aortic area there is normally a slight gradient. In the mitral area there is a small gradient as the blood flows from a low pressure to a high pressure, giving rise to the middiastolic murmur. The various valves have different intensities in their opening and closing clicks. For example, a Björk-Shiley prosthesis has a soft opening and loud closing.

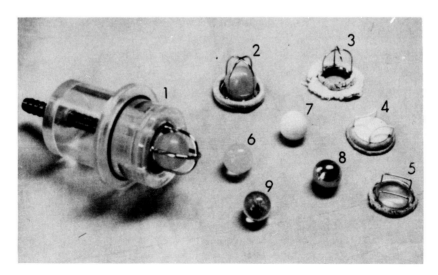

Fig. 10-1. Plastic chamber with 3M Starr-Edwards valve *(1)*. Other valves are model 6100 Starr-Edwards valve *(2)*, specially modified Starr-Edwards cage *(3)*, Beall mitral prosthesis *(4)*, Kay-Shiley mitral prosthesis *(5)*, nonradiopaque Silastic rubber *(6)*, radiopaque Silastic rubber *(7)*, Stellite metal *(8)*, and glass *(9)*. Glass is not used clinically. (From Gramiak, R., and Waag, R.: Cardiac ultrasound, St. Louis, 1975, The C. V. Mosby Co.)

The presence of a systolic murmur in the mitral valve area is abnormal and is frequently attributed to a paravalvular leak. If there is a clot inside the cage, it causes the valve to close improperly, and regurgitation results.

Phonocardiography has become an important aid in assessing prosthetic valvular function. In the aortic valve the onset of systole should give a loud S_I, and the onset of diastole should give a soft S_{II}. In the mitral valve area the soft S_I coincides with systole, whereas diastole gives a loud S_{II}. The duration of these sounds can also be measured. Usually, the S_{II} distance is fixed and does not change with diastole. In the mitral valve area, thrombus can increase the duration of the aortic and mitral valve openings. Thus phonocardiography can assess (1) the presence or absence of valve sounds, (2) muffled or attenuated click, (3) timing of the S_{II} opening click and the Q-S interval, and (4) the ratio of aortic closing to aortic opening click (this ratio may indicate ball variance caused by poppet swelling or the appearance of a clot around the ball).

Other studies helpful in assessing prosthetic function are chest x-ray examinations, fluoroscopy, angiography, and echography.

The chest x-ray examination can determine cardiac enlargment or position of the prosthesis. Fluoroscopy is helpful if there is a detachment of the valve or a paravalvular leak causing tilting of the valve in the mitral position. In the aortic valve position the movement is usually very dramatic, and, if there is a problem, side-to-side "flipping" is recorded.

Angiography can detect leakage, but, since there is a slight degree of regurgitation with the prosthesis, it may be more difficult. Diagnostic regurgitation is physiologic in the mitral valve area. In pathologic regurgitation the dye goes to the ventricle during systole.

Echography has proved to be a useful technique in the assessment of valve function because of the strong reflecting interface between the artificial valve and the surrounding structures. The exact model and size of the prosthesis is noted prior to recording the valve. If the examiner is not careful, only the supporting structures of the cage may be recorded without disk or ball movement. By angling the transducer so that the beam is more perpendicular to the prosthesis, the proper echoes may be recorded (Fig. 10-2). This transducer angle is critical in the assessment of valvular motion and excursion. The motion of the prosthesis is determined by valve characteristics and the entire cardiac structure. To provide the most accurate assessment of valve function, recordings should be made shortly after surgery (five to seven days) and followed at specified time intervals (three months, six months, etc.).

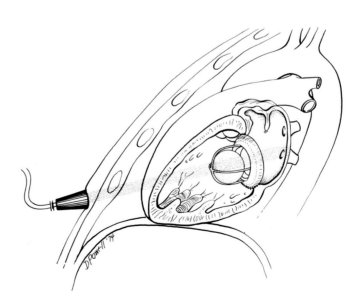

Fig. 10-2. Diagram depicting location of transducer on anterior chest wall in patient with mitral prosthetic ball valve. Beam is perpendicular to the longitudinal axis of the valve. Ball opens toward the transducer during diastole. (From Gramiak, R., and Waag, R.: Cardiac ultrasound, St. Louis, 1975, The C. V. Mosby Co.)

MITRAL VALVE

The best mitral recording is one that clearly records the valve opening and closure and most closely approximates the valve's normal excursion. Disk or hinge valves can generally be recorded in their usual mitral position. However, Starr-Edwards valves may have to be located on the chest x-ray film for proper transducer angulation. Often the examiner has to move to the apex of the heart and angle the transducer severely cephalad to record the valve at its most perpendicular angle. Simultaneous phonocardiograms can be added to most echographic equipment and will help in measuring the interval of the aortic valve closure to mitral valve opening.

The actual thrombus formation is difficult to distinguish on echo, but the alteration of the valve motion may be recorded. Sometimes there is a delay in the valve opening, or there is no opening at all during some cycles. Decreased amplitude of valve opening must be assessed with the transducer in various angles to ascertain the maximum excursion. Because of the intense echo reflection of the valve apparatus, there often appear to be large "clumps" or ring down echoes behind the open valve. This should not be confused with thrombus and usually can be eliminated by slight transducer angulations or a reduction in the sensitivity of the equipment (Fig. 10-3).

Johnson (1975) described the actual measurement of the older type of ball valve by echo and has multiple charts available for analysis of individual tracings. He also discovered that the Starr-Edwards ball was made of Silastic rubber, a slower sound-conduction material. Thus, when recordings are made from such a valve, it appears that the posterior edge of the ball is actually beyond its posterior cage (Figs. 10-4 and 10-5). A correction factor of 0.64 can be applied to the measurement of the ball diameter to adjust for this factor (Figs. 10-6 and 10-7).

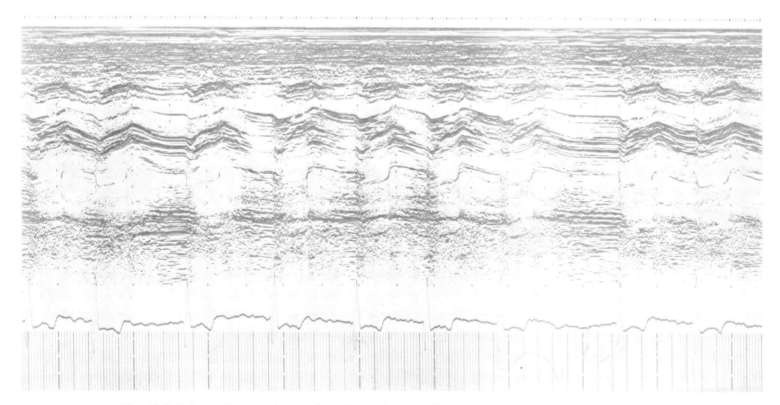

Fig. 10-3. Echocardiogram from a Starr-Edwards valve. The sweep is made from the aorta to the prosthetic area. The apex of the cage is demonstrated as one sweeps from the aorta to the mitral area. The surface of the ball closest to the transducer is then shown with the suture ring and ball surface posterior.

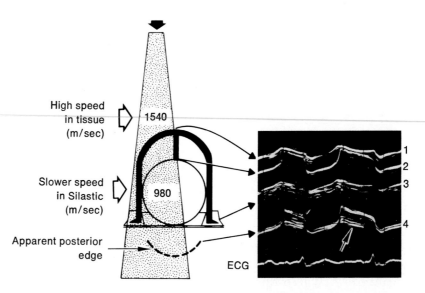

High speed
in tissue
(m/sec)

1540

Slower speed
in Silastic
(m/sec)

980

Apparent posterior
edge

ECG

1
2
3

4

Fig. 10-4. Left, schematic diagram showing sound beam traversing a Starr-Edwards ball valve. Sound travels at a slower speed through Silastic rubber than through body tissue. Because the oscilloscope is calibrated for the faster speed, the diameter of ball seems to be greater than it actually is. Right, echocardiogram from a patient with a Starr-Edwards mitral valve. Traces *1* to *4* are apex, anterior surface of the ball, suture ring, and posterior surface of the ball, respectively. Arrow points to the suture ring as seen through the ball in diastole. (From Gramiak, R., and Waag, R.: Cardiac ultrasound, St. Louis, 1975, The C. V. Mosby Co.)

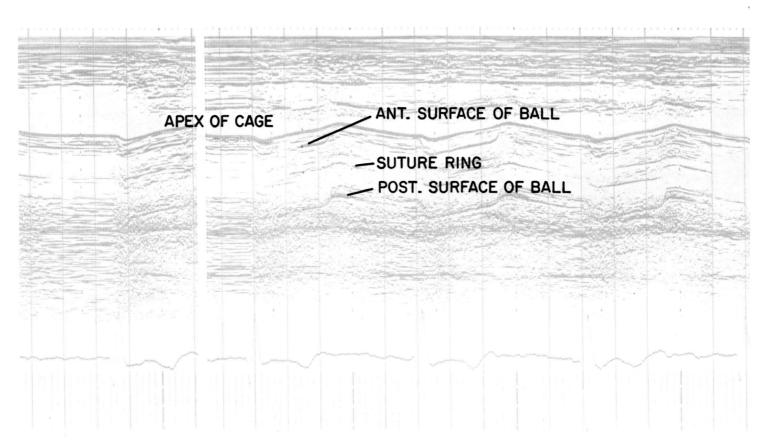

APEX OF CAGE

ANT. SURFACE OF BALL

SUTURE RING
POST. SURFACE OF BALL

Fig. 10-5. Starr-Edwards mitral prosthesis.

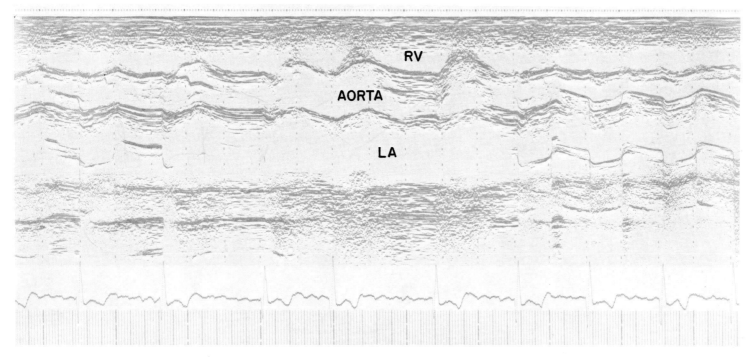

Fig. 10-6. Sweep from prosthesis to aorta to prosthesis. This sweep is not always possible because of the beam angulation. It depends on the location of the prosthetic valve to obtain such a sweep.

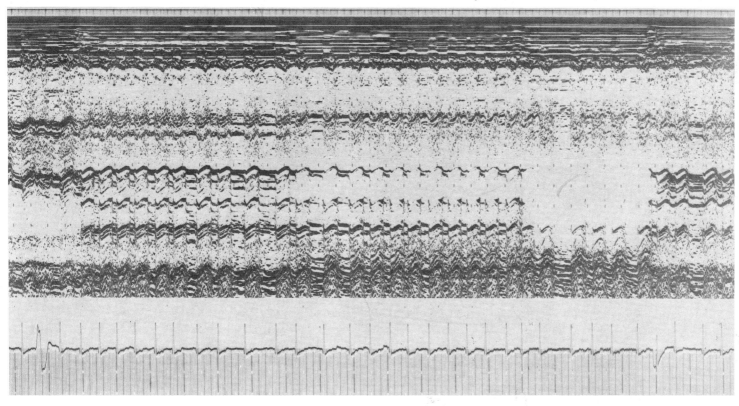

Fig. 10-7. Sometimes the prosthetic valve will appear as an aortic valve (normal), and the examiner must be certain the beam is perpendicular to obtain the opening and closing movements of the artificial valve.

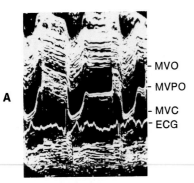

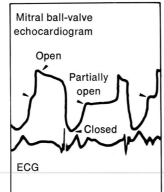

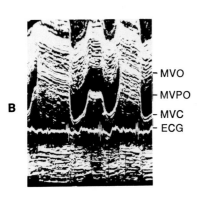

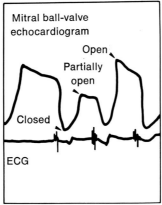

Fig. 10-8. Echocardiogram from a malfunctioning Smeloff-Cutter mitral valve. Posterior ball surface is visualized. **A,** Note the marked delay in the opening of the ball. **B,** Ball fails to open at all. (From Belenkie, I., Carr, M., Schlant, R. C., Nutter, D. O., and Symbas, P. N.: Am. Heart J. **86**:399, 1973.)

AORTIC VALVE

Usually, the aortic valve is more difficult to assess because of its surgical position. Often it is difficult to observe the poppet motion in a perpendicular path. Various angles of the transducer are used to record the greatest amplitude.

As in the mitral valve, a loss of motion may represent thrombus formation (Figs. 10-8 and 10-9). Many prostheses are associated with aortic regurgitation. In this case the echographic changes are shown on the anterior leaflet of the mitral valve as fine flutter during diastole or premature closure caused by acute aortic regurgitation.

Changes can also be noted in the interventricular septal motion. Both normal and paradoxical septal motion have been noted in postsurgical patients. It has not been ascertained whether the paradoxical motion is the result of superimposed tricuspid insufficiency, some effect of the prosthetic valve, or surgery on left ventricular dynamics (Johnson, 1975). However, it has been noted in serial evaluation of patients with a paradoxical septum that the development of normal septal motion and an inappropriately large stroke volume are highly suggestive of a mitral or possibly aortic paraprosthetic or intraprosthetic leak.

Pericardial effusion is not an uncommon finding in post–valvular surgery patients and may be serially followed by echography.

TRICUSPID VALVE

It is often confusing to evaluate patients with two or three prosthetic valves, and careful evaluation must be done to separate each. If the sonographer does routine cardiac sweeps, the transducer may record the individual valves to help the sonographer evaluate the most perpendicular axis. Then the transducer can be moved to the tricuspid area or to the apex of the heart for recording maximum amplitudes of the valves.

Fig. 10-9. Surgical specimen of Smeloff-Cutter valve from patient discussed in Fig. 10-8. The thrombus was found extending into the orifice of the suture ring, which hampered normal movement of the ball and resulted in the sticking of the ball in a partially open position. Valve is shown in partially open (**A**) and open (**B**) positions. (From Belenkie, I., Carr, M., Schlant, R. C., Nutter, D. O., and Symbas, P. N.: Am. Heart J. **86**:399, 1973.)

11 □ Endocarditis

Bacterial endocarditis presents a constantly changing pattern of disease. It is an infective lesion of the endocardial surface of the heart, usually affecting one or more valves. There are two types of infectious endocarditis, depending on the virulence of the invading organism—acute and subacute bacterial endocarditis.

Acute bacterial endocarditis can occur during an attack of acute septicemia from organisms such as *Staphylococcus aureus, Neisseria gonorrhoeae,* or *Streptococcus pyogenes.* The cardiac valves may be invaded and destroyed by these bacteria. In subacute bacterial endocarditis, organisms of a low-grade virulence invade a valve or an area of the endocardium that has been damaged by a previous acquired heart disease such as rheumatic fever or congenital heart defect (Fig. 11-1). In this case *Streptococcus viridans* is the most common invading organism. The organism can enter the bloodstream as a result of one of several circumstances—dental extraction, apical tooth abscess, diarrhea, osteomyelitis, cardiac surgery, or drug abuse.

INCIDENCE

Generally, bacterial endocarditis occurs between the third and seventh decade of life, with the peak occurrence in the fourth decade. The majority of patients (75%) with bacterial endocarditis suffer left heart valvular disease, with 45% affected in the aortic valve, 35% in the mitral valve, and 19% in both valves. A smaller percentage (12%) are afflicted with right heart disease, in which the tricuspid valve is always affected and the pulmonary valve is very rarely affected. Approximately 13% of these patients suffer bilateral infections.

PATHOPHYSIOLOGY

Previously damaged valves are more susceptible to bacterial formations than are normal valves, although 50% to 60% of patients have no preexisting valvular lesion. Prolapse, IHSS, and similar anomalies are probable risks with subacute bacterial endocarditis. The jet effect plays a significant role in the collection of bacteria, on the valves as well as on the chordae tendineae. This effect is related to the insufficiency of one valve, causing a high-pressure source with a low-pressure "sink." The infection usually occurs on the low-pressure side. Thus a patient with aortic insufficiency would have a jet stream from the aortic root into the left ventricle. The stream would flow directly into the chordae tendineae, causing satellite regions of bacterial formation to develop on the chordae.

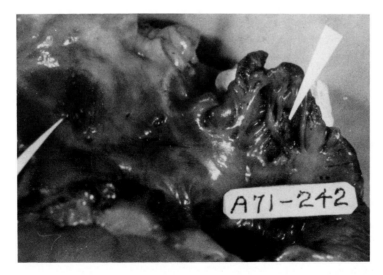

Fig. 11-1. Gross specimen of the tricuspid valve demonstrating vegetation destruction of the valve and cardiac wall (arrow).

CLINICAL MANIFESTATIONS

The patient usually develops anemia and spiking fevers. The disease then may progress with the infectious process on the valve, an embolism to the coronary arteries, spleen, kidneys, or brain, metastatic infection, or degenerative verrucous endocarditis. In the subacute variety the white count is not elevated; however, in the acute variety it is.

COMPLICATIONS

Valve incompetence results from the destruction of the endocardium and rupture of the chordae tendineae. Embolic incidents occur when a fragment of the vegetation becomes detached. Systemic embolism indicates vegetations on the left side of the heart.

Echographic evaluation of vegetation on the left side of the heart is more successful than on the right because of the difficulty in assessing the diastolic parameter of the tricuspid valve. Look for very course flutter in the diastolic phase of the valvular cycle. If associated regurgitation or insufficiency occurs, the flutter of the leaflet will have to be evaluated for its courseness to indicate vegetations. Lesions smaller than 2 or 3 mm are difficult to evaluate echographically. Careful evaluation of the mitral and tricuspid valves should be made to separate respiration artifacts from vegetations (Fig. 11-2). This can be done by angling the transducer slightly; the vegetation will adhere consistently to the valve, whereas respiration artifacts will occur intermittently. The aortic area is probably one of the easiest to evaluate in a search for course flutter in the diastolic period, since its cusps close (Fig. 11-3, A). Associated aortic insufficiency may be noted with fine flutter of the anterior mitral leaflet (Fig. 11-3, B). Premature closure of the mitral leaflet may be helpful in assessing if the insufficiency is acute, in which case the PR-AC interval should measure less than 0.06 mm/sec to qualify as premature closure.

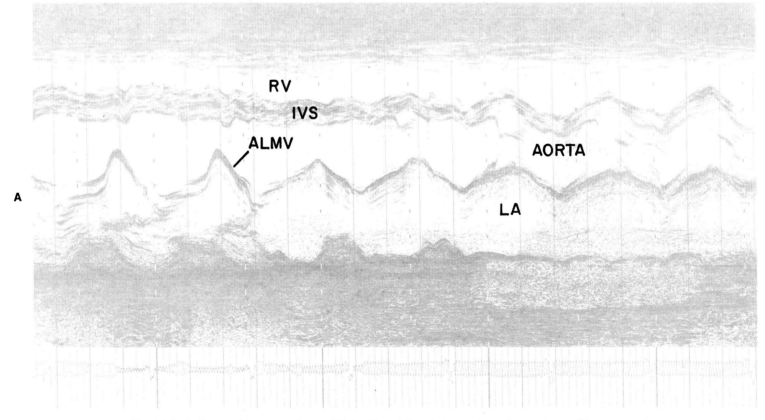

Fig. 11-2. A, Scan of a young drug addict with spiking fever and cardiac murmur. The sweep from the anterior leaflet of the mitral valve into the aortic root appears normal. There is no thickening of the leaflet or cusps during diastole.

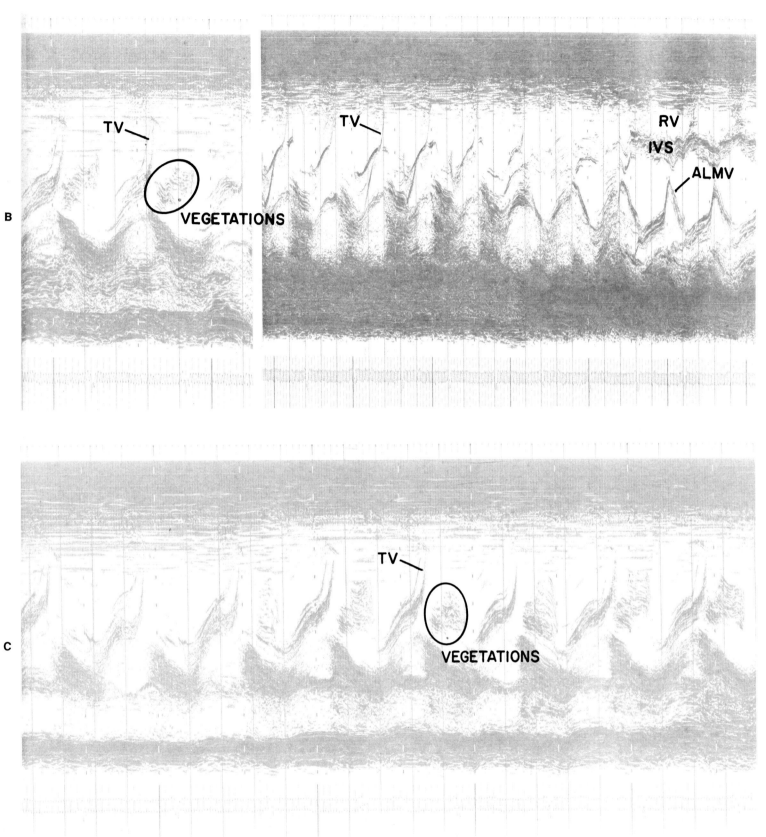

Continued.

Fig. 11-2, cont'd. B, As the sweep is made into the tricuspid area, dense echo formations are seen attached to the diastolic portion of the valve. These echoes measure approximately 10 mm and are recorded on real time as heavy-dense echoes attached to the tricuspid leaflet. Right-sided vegetations are secondary to the drug addiction. **C,** Subsequent studies performed at weekly intervals demonstrate the echo formation to decrease or increase with the patient's clinical condition.

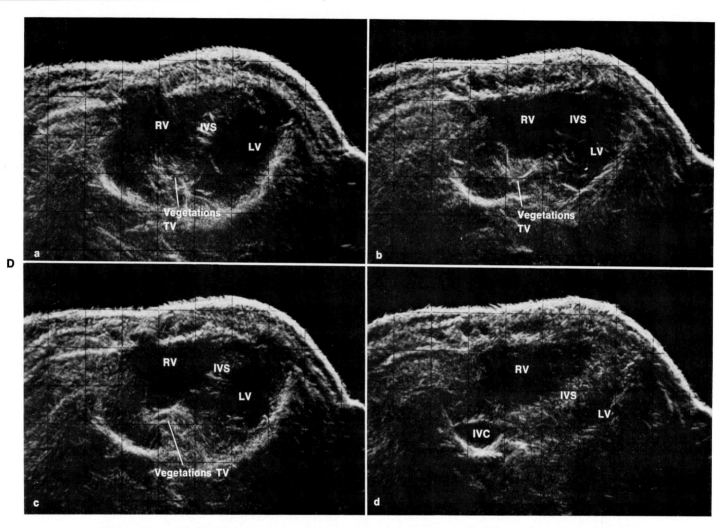

Fig. 11-2, cont'd. D, Two-dimensional scans with the Octoson are utilized to better ascertain the involvement of the lesion. The scans were performed in a horizontal plane with the right side shown on the left of the scan. **a,** An enlarged right ventricle with the tricuspid valve and vegetations shown at the lower border, medial to the septum and mitral valve. **b,** Vegetations with some tricuspid motion within. **c,** Vegetations. **d,** Inferior vena cava.

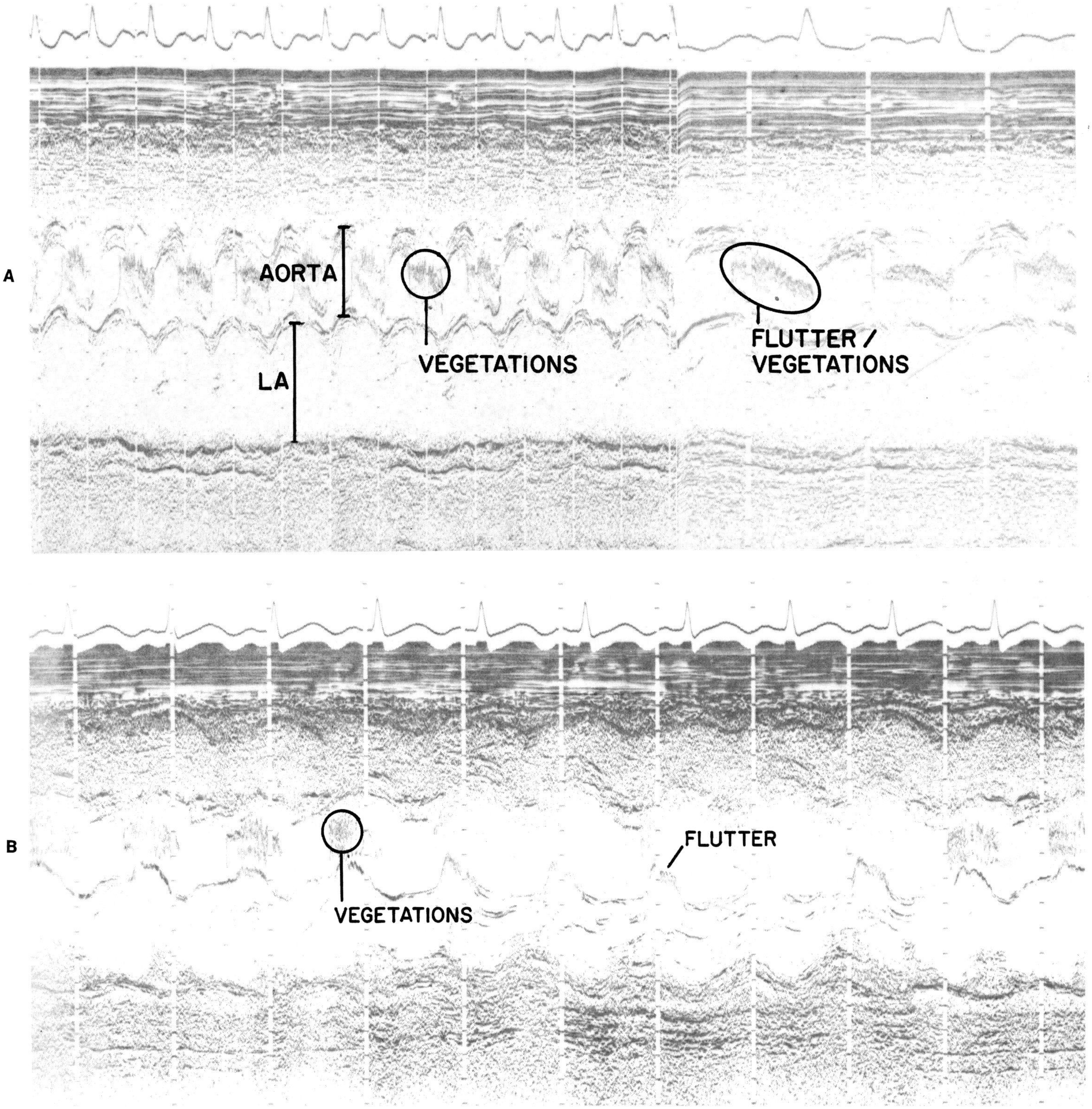

Fig. 11-3. Scan of a young man with fever of unknown origin. **A,** Initial echogram demonstrates aortic root with increased coarse echoes in diastole. **B,** As the sweep is completed to the mitral valve area, fine flutter is shown on the anterior leaflet to represent incompetence of the aortic valve.

12 □ Right ventricle

The right ventricle is the most anterior chamber of the heart. The anterior wall of this chamber may be demonstrated with proper near-gain settings adjusted so the first moving echo shown after the immobile main bang and chest wall echoes represents the right ventricular wall. If this echo is not clearly defined, Popp has suggested an arbitrary measurement of 0.5 cm from the last nonmoving echo to serve as the right ventricular wall for chamber size determination. Most ventricular measurements are made in the supine position and must be adjusted if the patient is examined in an upright or decubitus position.

Right ventricular enlargement may result from overload of the right ventricle caused by tricuspid insufficiency, pulmonary insufficiency, or septal defect. Right ventricular pressure overload may result from pulmonary stenosis obstructing the blood flow from the right ventricle. Congestive cardiomyopathy or congestive heart failure will cause right ventricular enlargement along with other chamber enlargement. (See Figs. 12-1 to 12-13.)

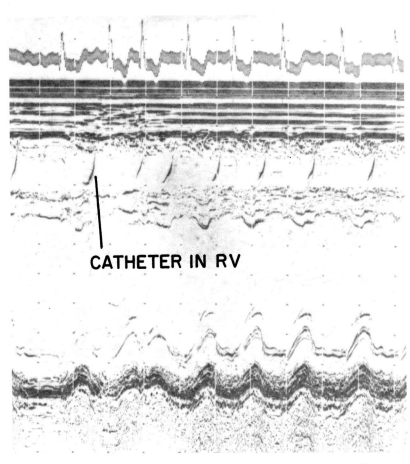

CATHETER IN RV

Fig. 12-1. Right ventricle may be identified as the anterior chamber after the first moving echo. The dense echo within the cavity represents a catheter.

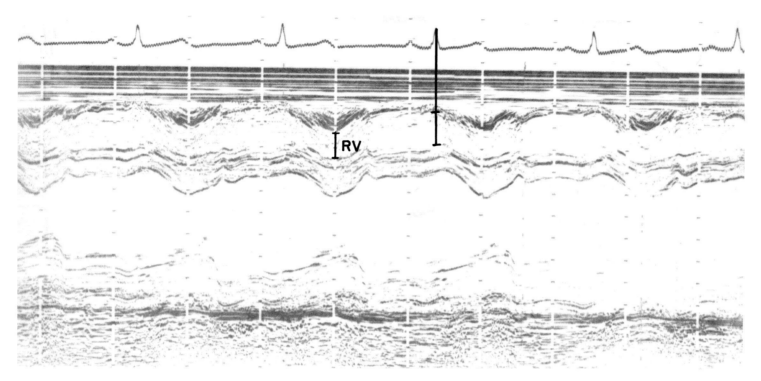

Fig. 12-2. Right ventricle should be measured at end diastole at the *r* point on the ECG.

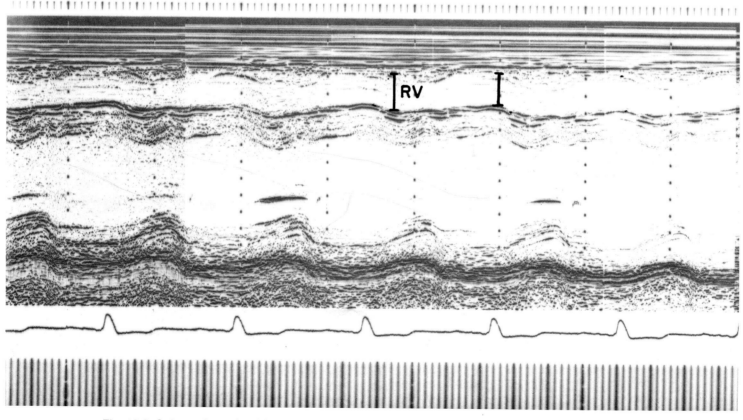

Fig. 12-3. Gain settings should be reduced to separate the right side of the septum from the chordae tendineae of the tricuspid valve.

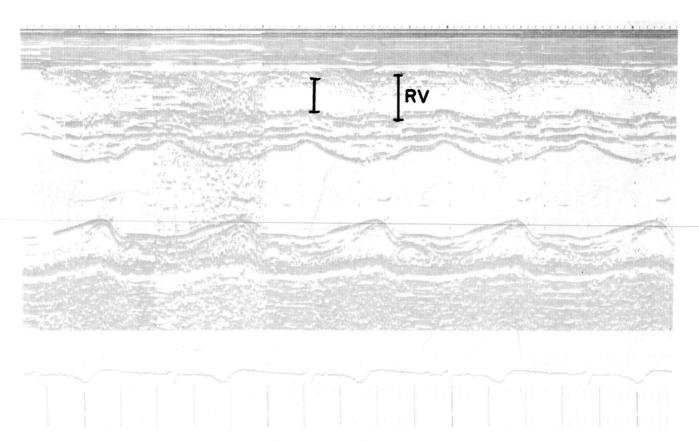

Fig. 12-4. Right side of the septum should move as the left side of the septum. If it does not, the transducer position should be altered to obtain this parallel movement. If it still remains immobile, it could represent multiple chordae along its right side or disease involving the anterior side of the septum.

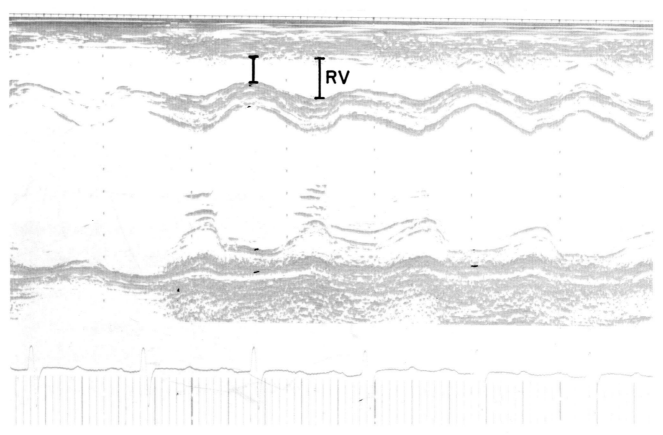

Fig. 12-5. In a sweep into the ventricular cavity the anterior right ventricular wall is identified.

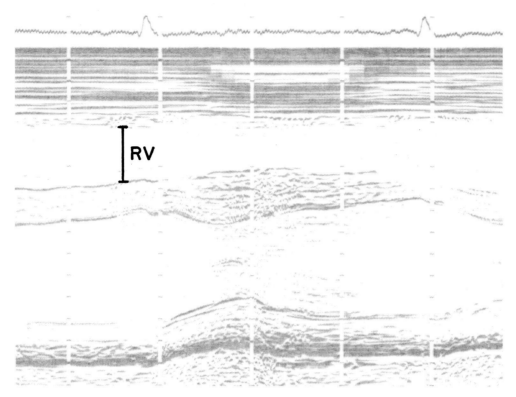

Fig. 12-6. Top normal right ventricle.

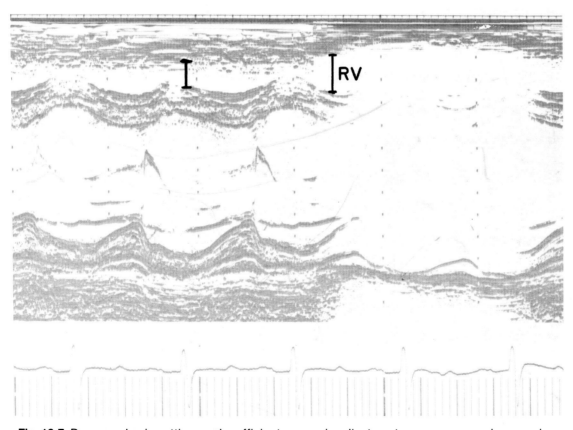

Fig. 12-7. Decreased gain settings or insufficient near-gain adjustment may cause error in assessing the right ventricular dimension.

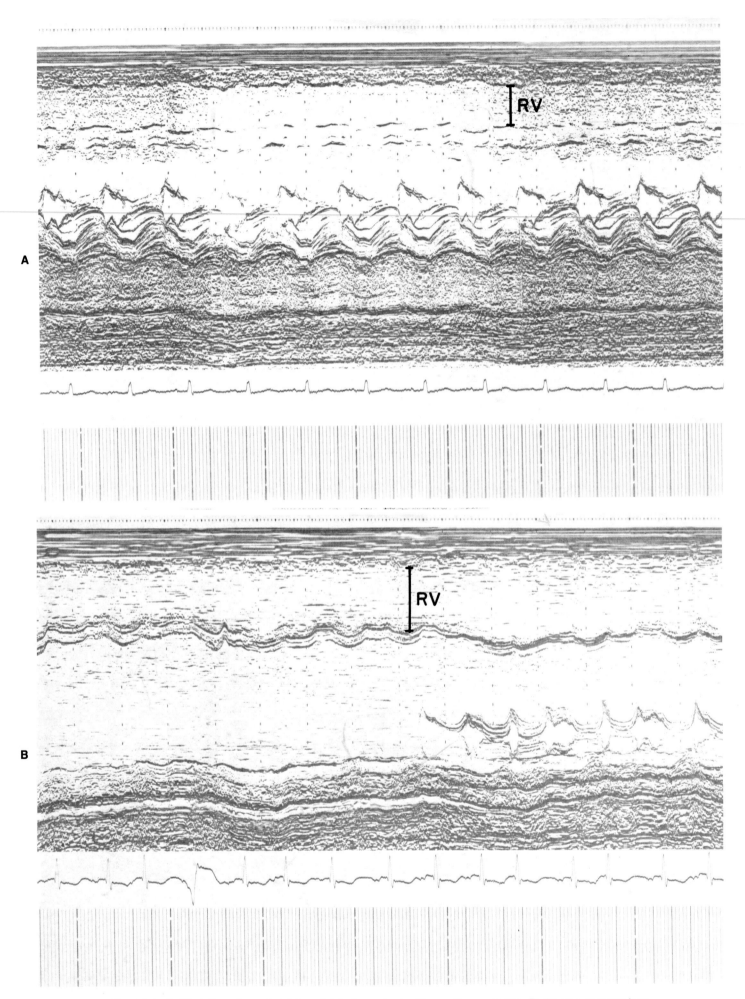

Fig. 12-8. A, Slightly enlarged right ventricle in patient with cardiomyopathy. **B,** As one sweeps into the left ventricular cavity, right ventricular dilatation is noted.

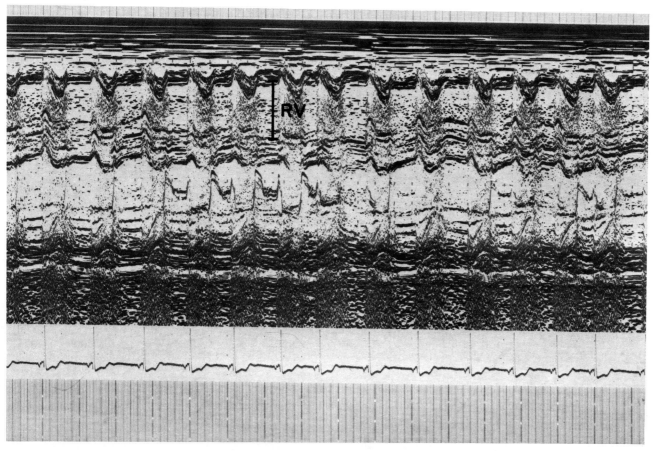

Fig. 12-9. Respiratory artifacts make it difficult to assess chamber dimensions. The scan should be repeated with the patient in full expiration.

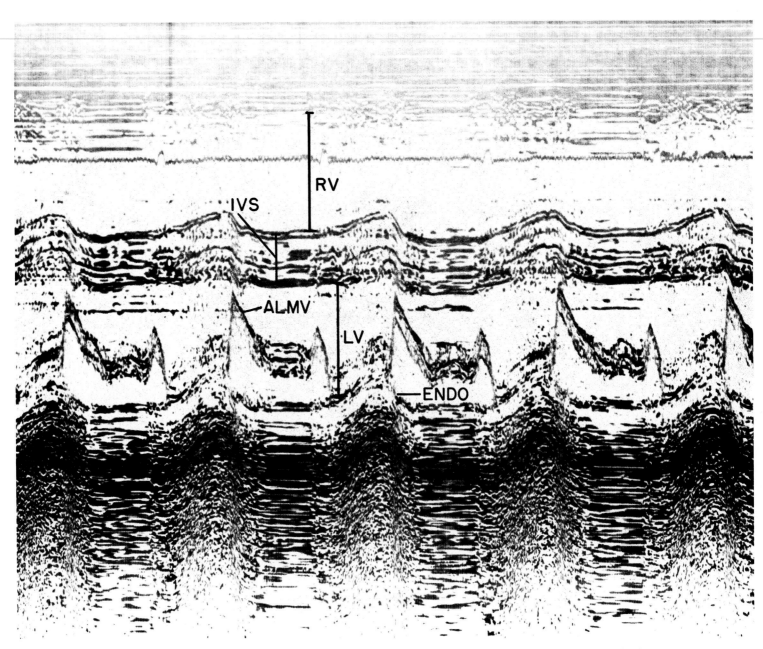

Fig. 12-10. Enlarged right ventricle and paradoxical septal motion in a patient with right ventricular volume overload due to atrial septal defect.

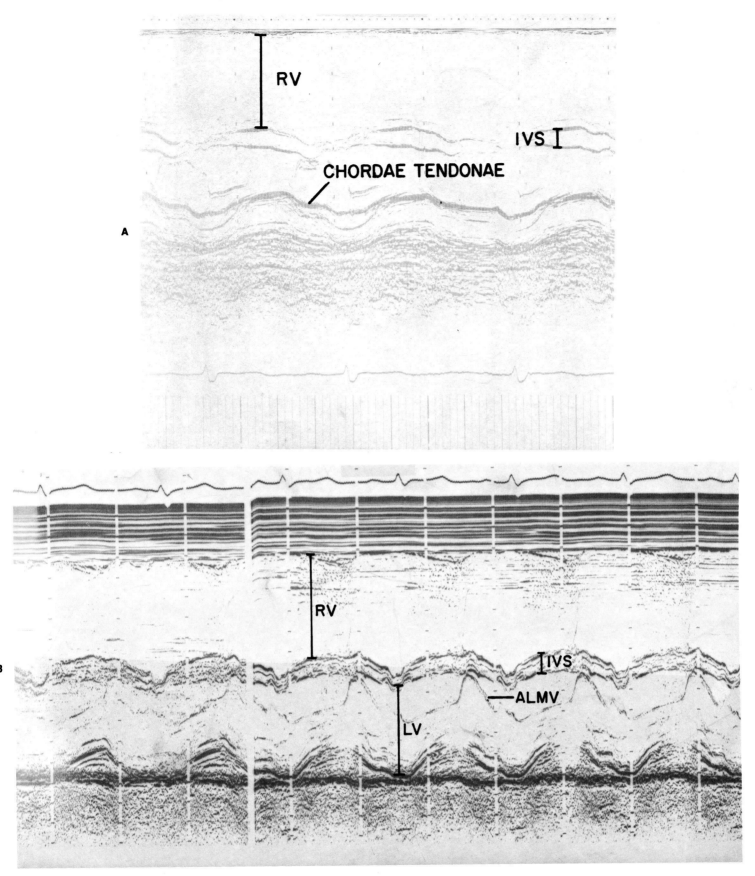

Fig. 12-11. A, Enlarged right ventricle secondary to atrial septal defect. **B,** Enlargement of the right ventricle can still be noted as the beam is swept toward the mitral area.

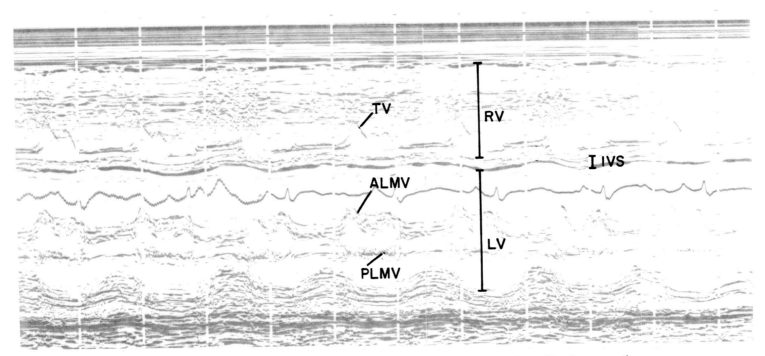

Fig. 12-12. Enlargement of the right ventricle permits visualization of the tricuspid valve, sometimes at the same time the mitral valve is seen.

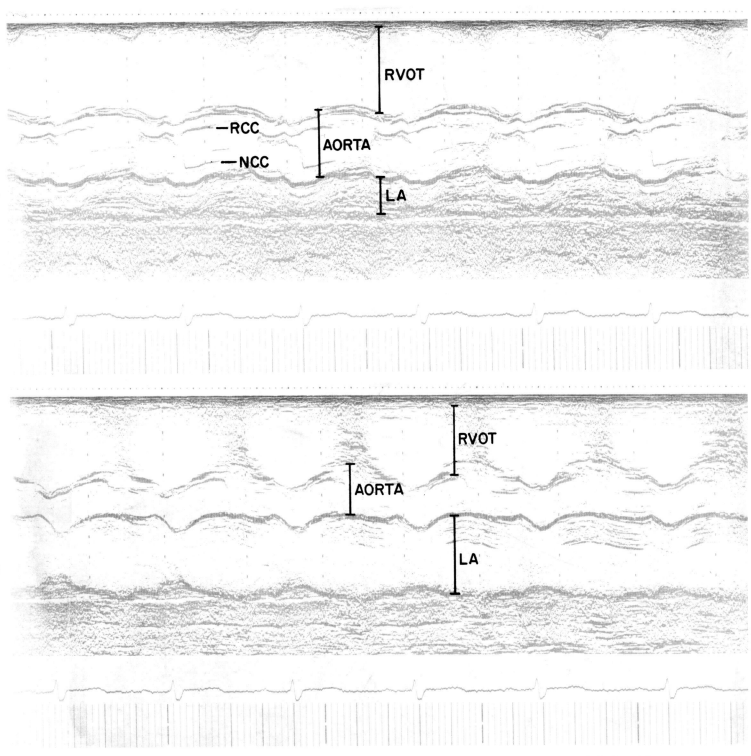

Fig. 12-13. A, Enlargement of the right ventricular outflow tract anterior to aortic root. **B,** Left atrial enlargement in the same patient, shown as the transducer is angled slightly more medial.

13 □ Interventricular septum

The interventricular septum divides the right and left ventricles. Its right side is contiguous with the anterior aortic root (Fig. 13-1). At this junction the movement of the septum is influenced by the movement of the aorta and thus may appear to move abnormally, or paradoxically, to the posterior heart wall. As the transducer is angled slightly inferior and lateral to the mitral valve, the septum moves slightly anterior in early systole and posterior at the end of systole and early diastole. Both sides of the septum should move symmetrically. If they do not, the transducer should be placed more medial on the chest wall, or the patient should roll into a more decubitus position.

The septum thickens in the midportion of the ventricular cavity. The measurement and evaluation of septal thickness and motion should be made at this point. Normal septal thickness should match that of the posterior left ventricular wall and not exceed 1.3 cm (Fig. 13-2). Congestive cardiomyopathy usually produces concentric thinning of the septum and posterior wall and reduced septal motion (Fig. 13-3).

Coronary artery disease or anterior myocardial infarction can produce reduced or flat septal motion or paradoxical movement of the septum (Fig. 13-4). Right ventricular volume overload results in paradoxical septal motion when scanned in the left ventricular plane (Fig. 13-5).

Thickening of the septum may be produced by asymmetrical septal hypertrophy or poor technique in defining the right ventricular wall (Figs. 13-6 to 13-8). Idiopathic diastolic thickening of the septum has been seen more frequently and clinically does not produce obstruction to the left ventricular outflow tract (Fig. 13-9). Concentric hypertrophy from hypertension or aortic stenosis results in symmetrical thickening of the septum and posterior wall (Fig. 13-10).

Left bundle branch block reveals an abrupt posterior movement of the septum in early systole with a ragged motion following in diastole (Fig. 13-11). Postcardiac surgery patients may reveal abnormal septal motion, but the septum may return to normal in time.

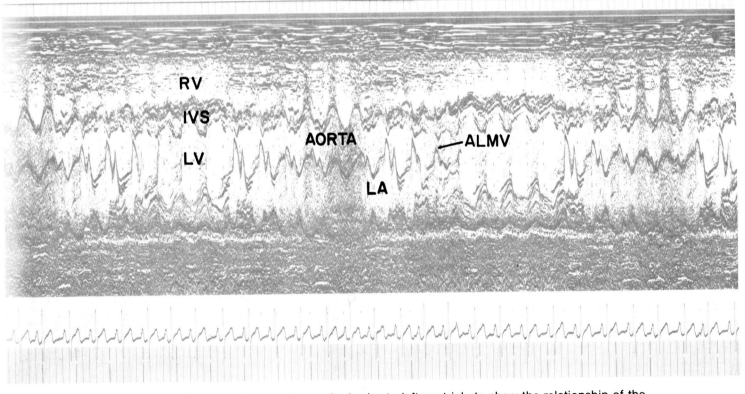

Fig. 13-1. Normal sweep from aorta to mitral valve to left ventricle to show the relationship of the interventricular septum to other cardiac structures.

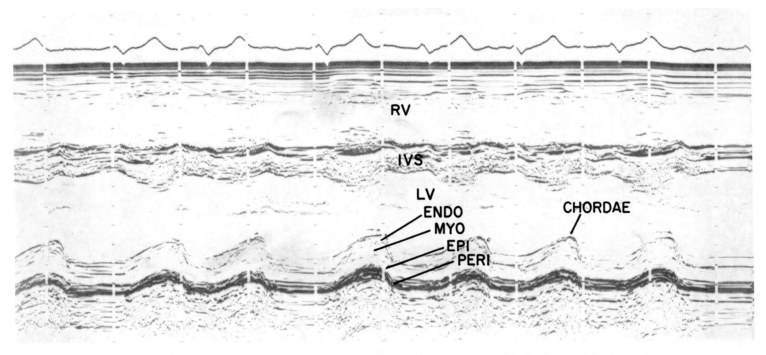

Fig. 13-2. Normal septum moves posterior at end systole to contract with the left ventricular wall.

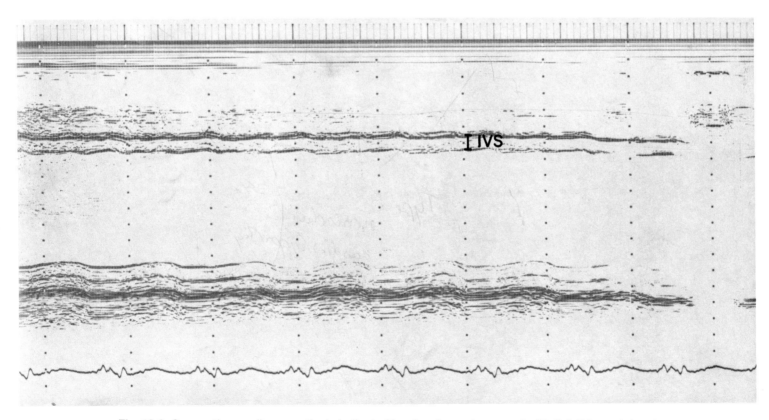

Fig. 13-3. Congestive cardiomyopathy is indicated by chamber enlargement with flat, thin septal and posterior wall motion.

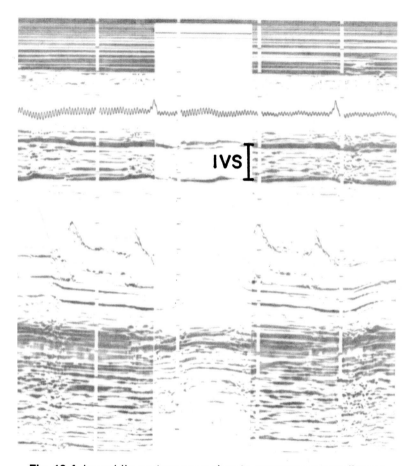

Fig. 13-4. Immobile septum secondary to coronary artery disease.

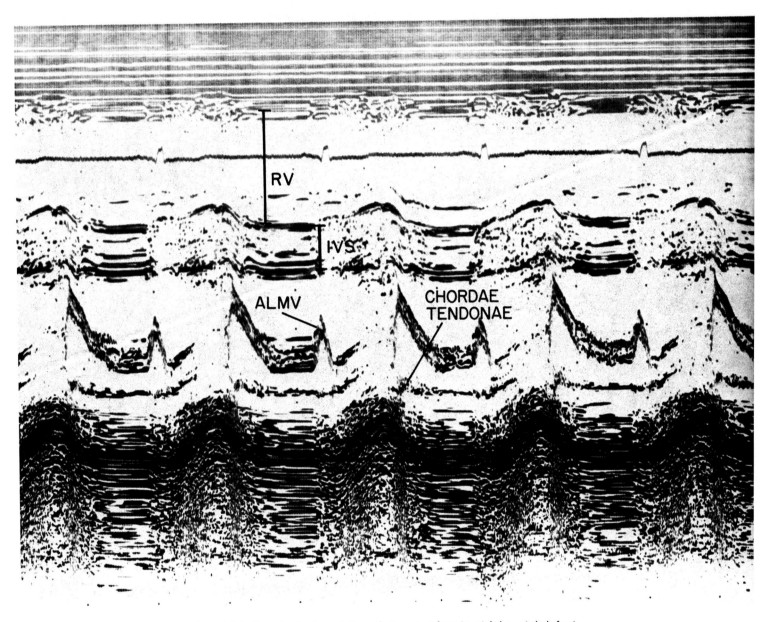

Fig. 13-5. Paradoxical septal motion secondary to atrial septal defect.

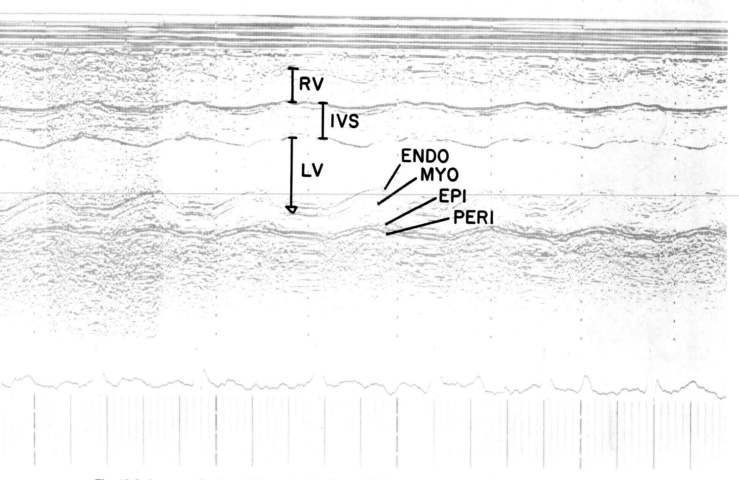

Fig. 13-6. Asymmetrical septal hypertrophy. Septal thickness measures 1.8 cm and the posterior wall 1.1 cm.

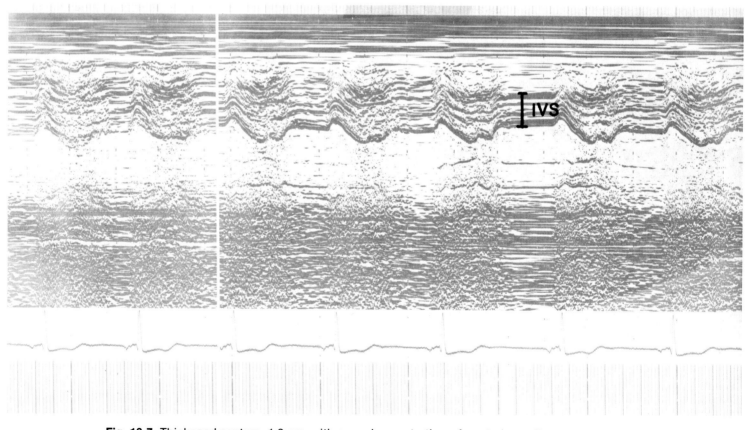

Fig. 13-7. Thickened septum, 1.9 cm, with poor demonstration of posterior wall to compare thickness.

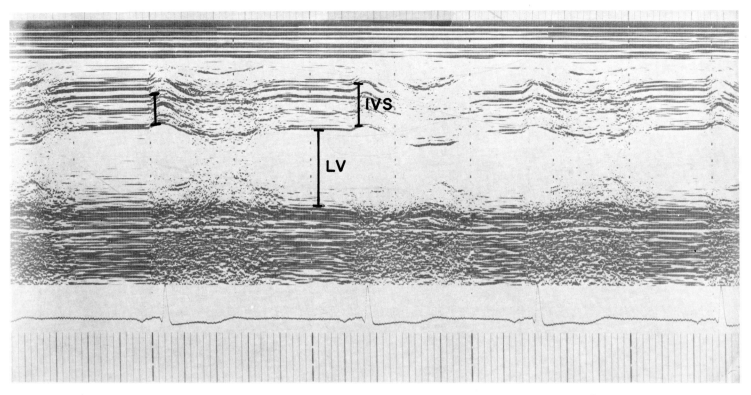

Fig. 13-8. Care must be used not to include chorade tendineae in measure comparisons. Septum is thickened here but measures 2.0 cm, not 2.5 cm.

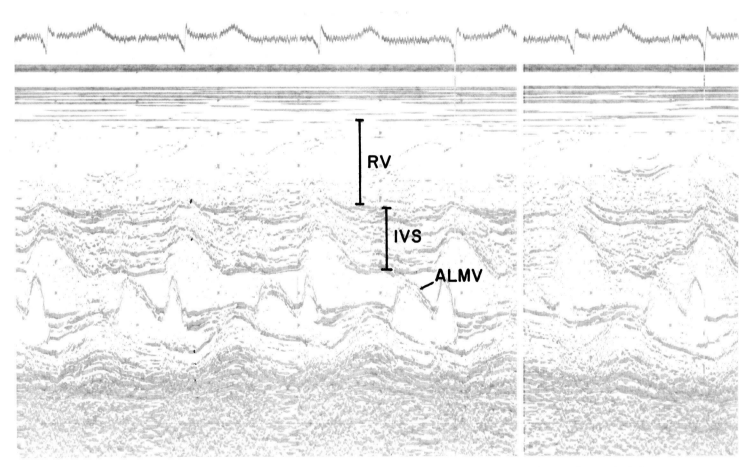

Fig. 13-9. Idiopathic diastolic thickening of the septum. This does not produce obstruction to the left ventricular outflow tract.

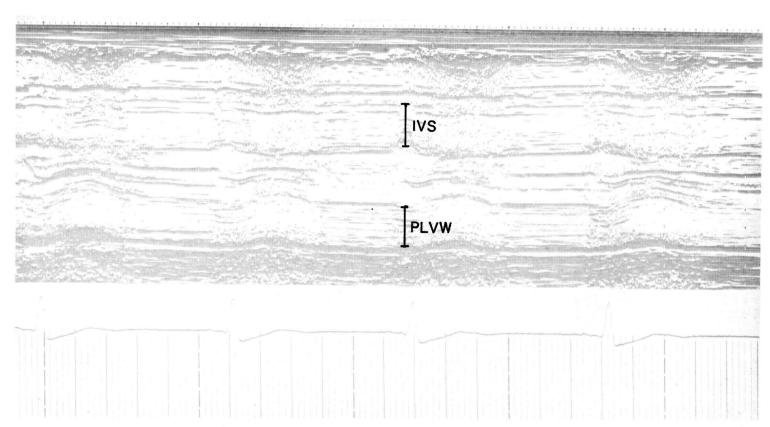

Fig. 13-10. Concentric hypertrophy of the septum and posterior left ventricular wall in a patient with hypertension.

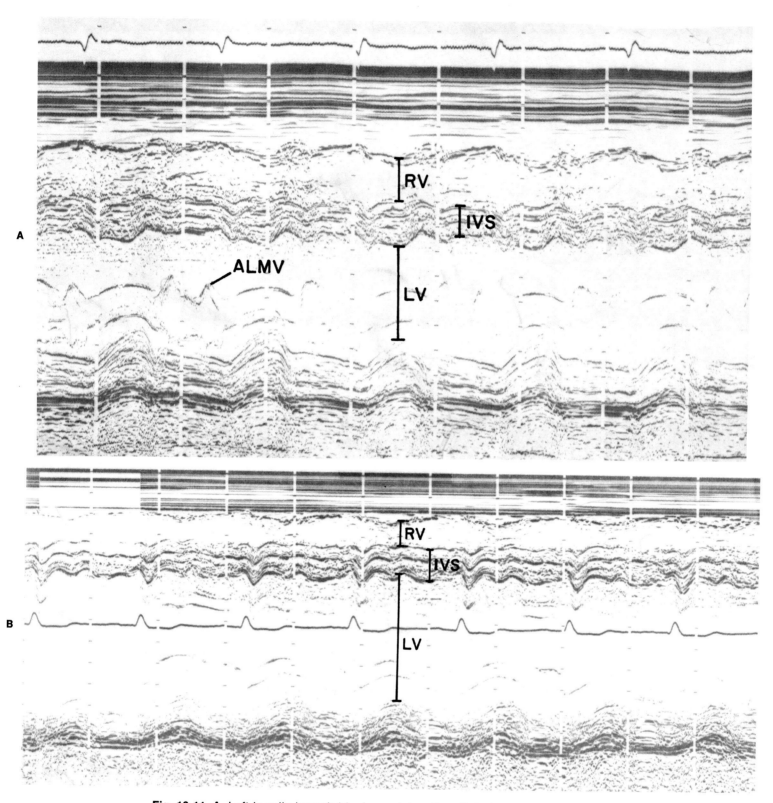

Fig. 13-11. A, Left bundle branch blocks septal motion. **B,** Left bundle branch block.

14 □ Left ventricle

Determination of left ventricular volume and function can be made with the routine M-mode sweep. The transducer should locate the anterior leaflet of the mitral valve and then direct the transducer inferior and slightly lateral to record the left ventricular chamber. Correct identification of this chamber may be made when both sides of the septum are seen to contract with the posterior heart wall. If the septum is not well defined or does not appear to move, medial placement of the transducer along the sternal border with a lateral angulation may permit better visualization. The three layers—endocardium (inside layer), myocardium (middle layer), and epicardium (outer layer)—should be identified separate from the pericardium. Sometimes it is difficult to separate epicardium from pericardium until the gain is reduced (unless the equipment has a special enhance control built into it). The

myocardium may appear echo free or echo producing, and care must be exercised to avoid mistaking it for pericardial fluid (the three layers of posterior wall must be *separated* from the pericardium in pericardial effusion). The endocardium is one of the most difficult structures to record, since it reflects a very weak echo pattern above the myocardium. Sometimes it is difficult to separate the multiple chordae tendineae from the endocardium, and careful evaluation of the posterior wall must be used to separate the two structures. The chordae are much denser structures than the endocardium. They generally are shown in the systolic segment along the anterior surface of the endocardium. As the ventricle contracts, the endocardial velocity is greater than that of the chordae tendineae. (See Figs. 14-1 to 14-11.)

Text continued on p. 184.

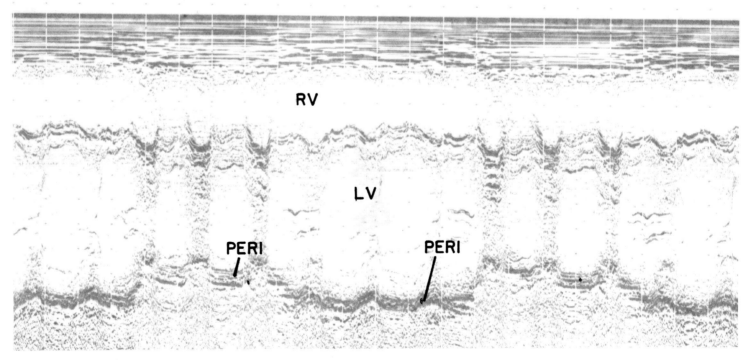

Fig. 14-1. Major-minor sweep, or T sweep, is used to record the maximum diameter of the left ventricle. Once the left ventricle is recorded in the normal position, a horizontal arc is made with the transducer across the minor axis of the ventricle.

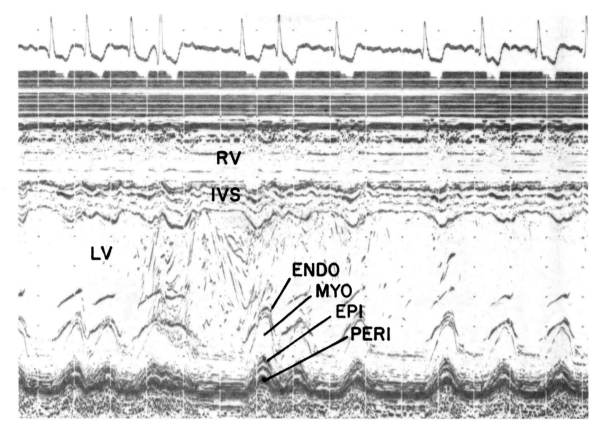

Fig. 14-2. Indocyanine green can be injected into the left ventricular cavity during cardiac catheterization. The dye causes the ventricular cavity to fill with echoes and thus differentiates the left side of the septum and the endocardial surface.

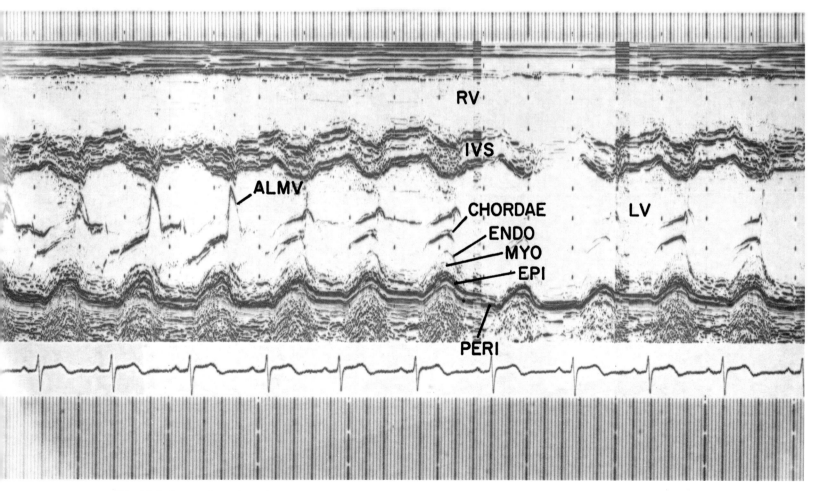

Fig. 14-3. Sweep from the mitral area into the left ventricle to differentiate chordae from the posterior wall. Decrease in gain further defines the pericardial layer.

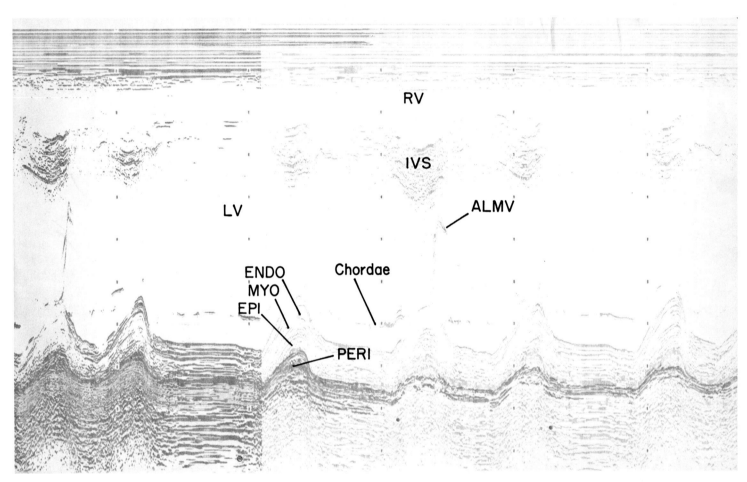

Fig. 14-4. Equipment with enhance capabilities defines the pericardium from the posterior heart wall. This allows definition without a change in gain settings.

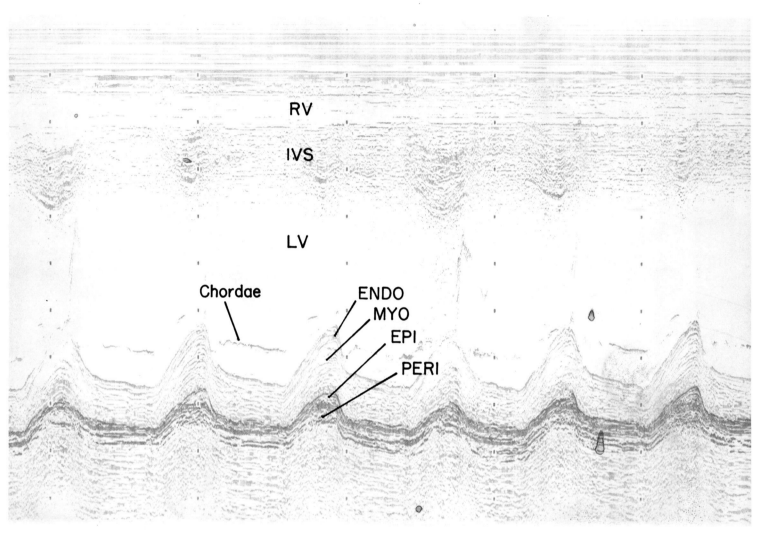

Fig. 14-5. Excellent visualization of the posterior wall with a poorly defined septum is generally the result of not positioning the transducer perpendicular to the septal wall.

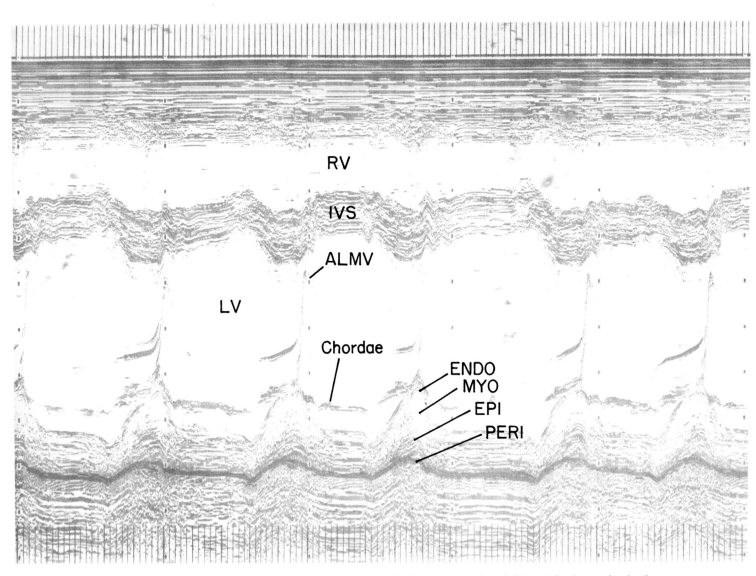

Fig. 14-6. Correct angulation of the transducer should demonstrate the right ventricular cavity, both sides of the septum, the left ventricular cavity (with pieces of the mitral apparatus within), and the posterior wall with pericardium.

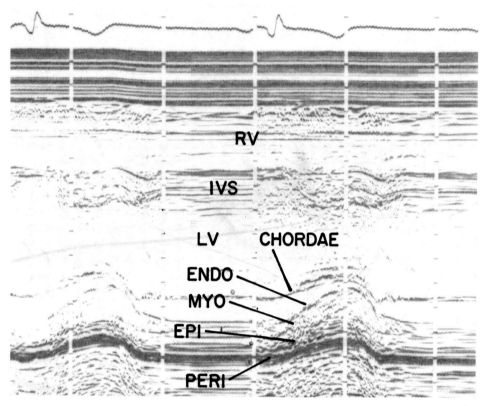

Fig. 14-7. Left ventricular study with fuzzy interventricular septum caused by respiratory artifacts.

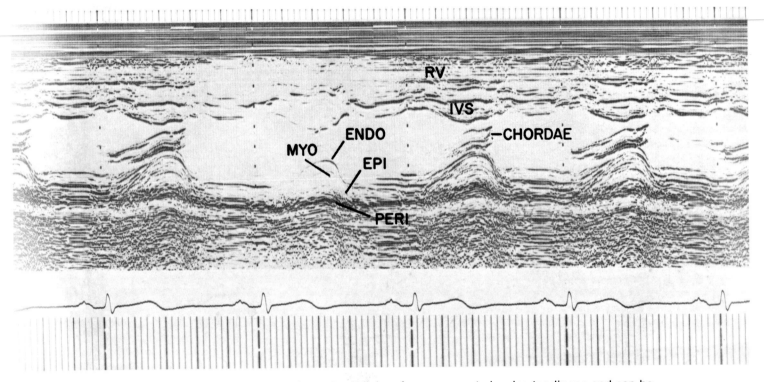

Fig. 14-8. Multiple echoes along the endocardial surface represent chordae tendineae and can be confusing in delineating the inner layer of the ventricle.

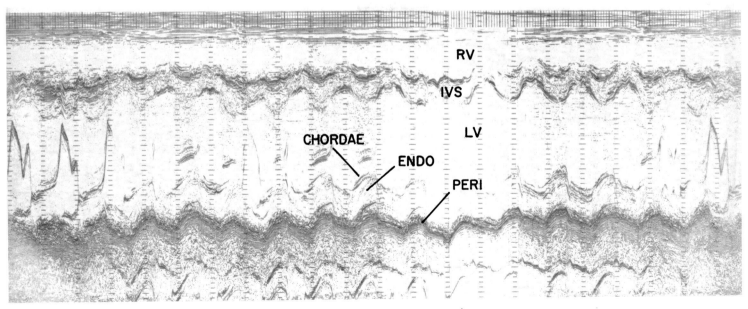

Fig. 14-9. Sweep is the best means of assuring proper transducer placement of the left ventricle.

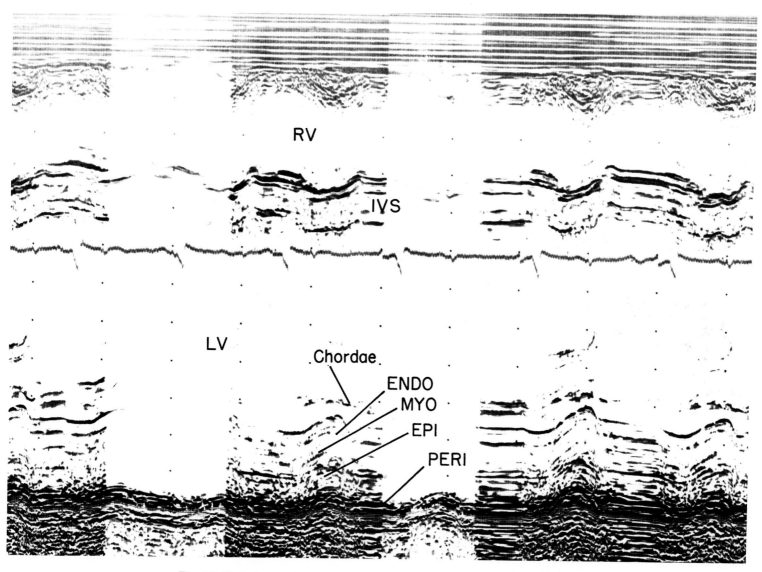

Fig. 14-10. Left ventricular enlargement is easily obtained in the echogram.

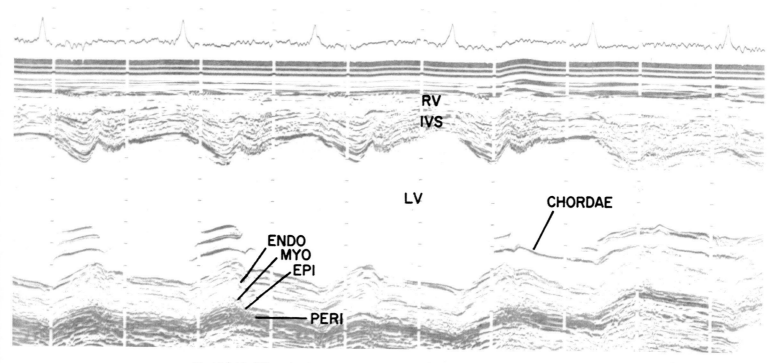

Fig. 14-11. Dilated left ventricle in a patient with mitral regurgitation.

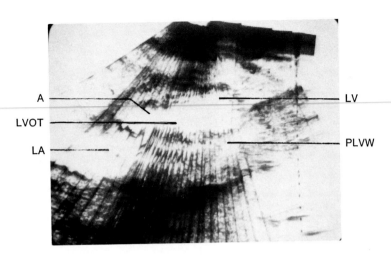

Fig. 14-12. B scan of a longitudinal cardiac scan in a patient with concentric hypertrophy shows symmetrical thickening of the septum and posterior wall.

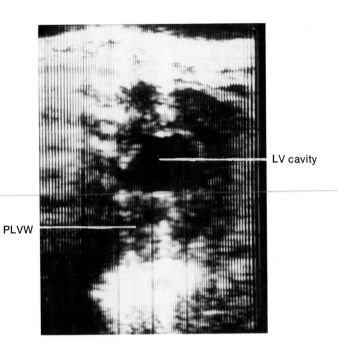

Fig. 14-13. Real-time horizontal view of the cardiac apex in a patient with concentric hypertrophy.

Small pieces of the mitral apparatus seen in the left ventricle ensure that the correct dimension is being evaluated. Posterior papillary muscles are shown near the apex of the ventricle. These appear as a dense, fuzzy echo band and make it difficult to evaluate the posterior wall. If ventricular volume is to be determined, these muscles are a clue that the transducer is directed inferior to the desired point of measurement.

The patient is generally examined in the supine position. If inadequate studies are shown in this position, the left semidecubitus position is used to define septal motion and posterior wall contraction.

Real-time evaluation of the cardiac structures allows excellent demonstration of the left ventricular contraction in the long axis from the mitral valve to its apex. The horizontal perspective affords a cross-sectional view of the left ventricular cavity, chordae, and papillary muscle function. A total picture of ventricular function is gained, which is not possible by M-mode techniques.

Appreciation of septal thickening with concentric hypertrophy may be seen on real-time equipment. Sometimes it is difficult to evaluate the right side of the septum, and the total view of the septum is useful in the long-axis view of the heart.

The evaluation of a left ventricular aneurysm can be made best by real-time evaluation. Areas of akinesis can be seen in contrast to the normal ventricular contraction. If real time is not available, the conventional M-mode sweep from the base of the heart to its apex at a very slow speed on the recorder can be made to evaluate areas of akinesis.

Concentric hypertrophy secondary to aortic stenosis or hypertensive heart disease may be shown with symmetrical thickening of the septum and posterior wall. Increased pressure in the left ventricle causes it to contract with more force, thus causing the thickening (Figs. 14-12 to 14-18).

Text continued on p. 190.

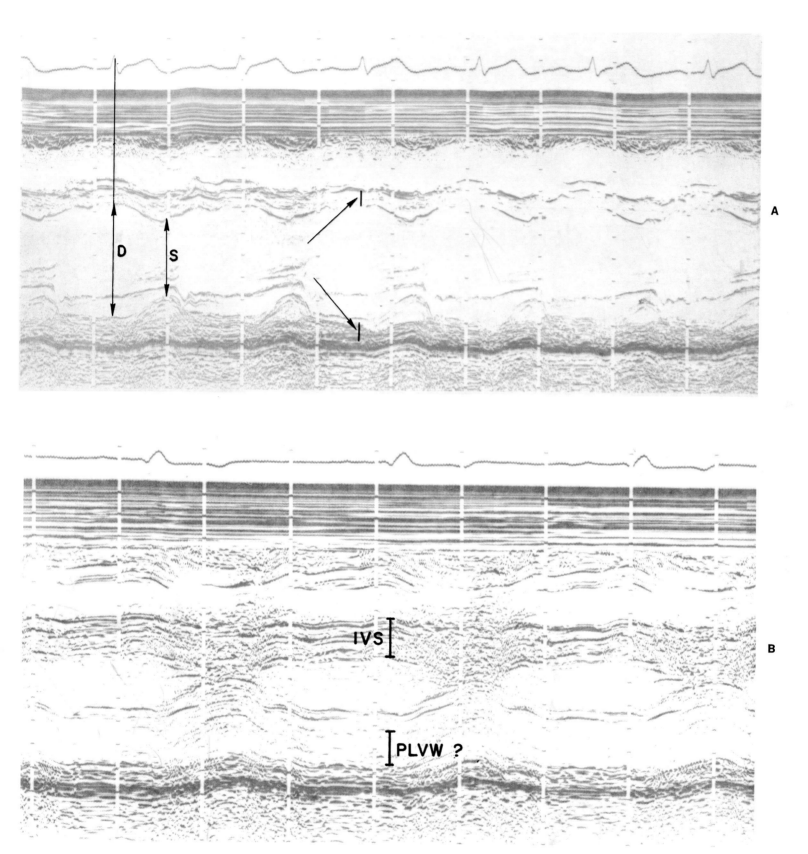

Fig. 14-14. A, Normally, the left ventricular dimension ranges from 4.0 to 5.5 cm. The septum and posterior wall thickness do not exceed a 1:1 ratio. **B,** In contrast, concentric hypertrophy shows decreased ventricular size with an increased mass due to symmetrical thickening of septum and posterior wall. In this patient with hypertension the PLVW is ill defined, thus making the diagnosis of concentric hypertrophy difficult with these gain settings.

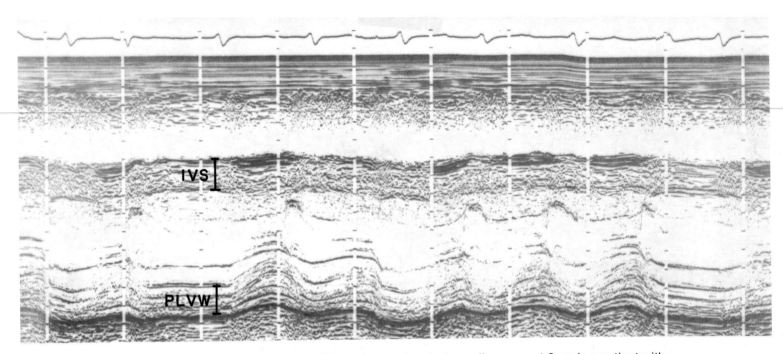

Fig. 14-15. Concentric hypertrophy. The septum and posterior wall measure 1.8 cm in a patient with hypertension.

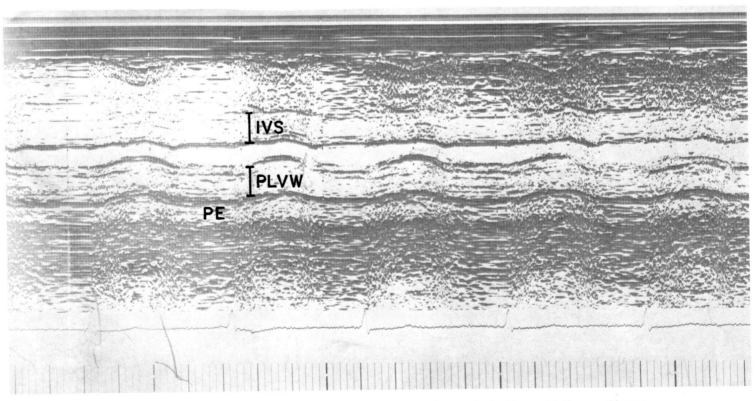

Fig. 14-16. Concentric hypertrophy and pericardial effusion in a patient with renal failure and hypertension.

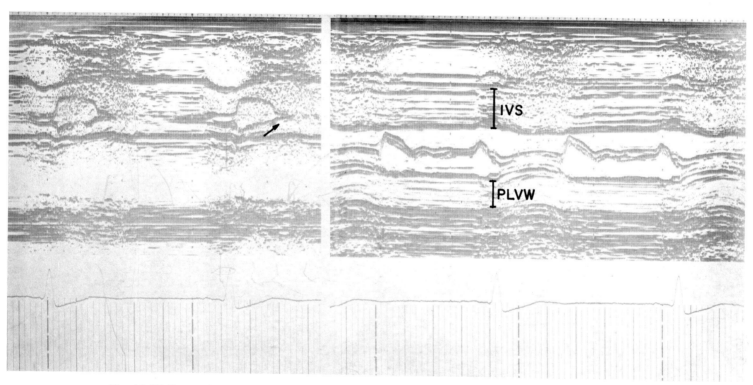

Fig. 14-17. Scan of a patient with renal failure and hypertension shows extremely thickened septum and posterior wall. The left ventricular outflow is narrow, and thus the cardiac output is reduced. Late systolic premature closing of the aortic cusps is seen with reduced cardiac output (see arrow).

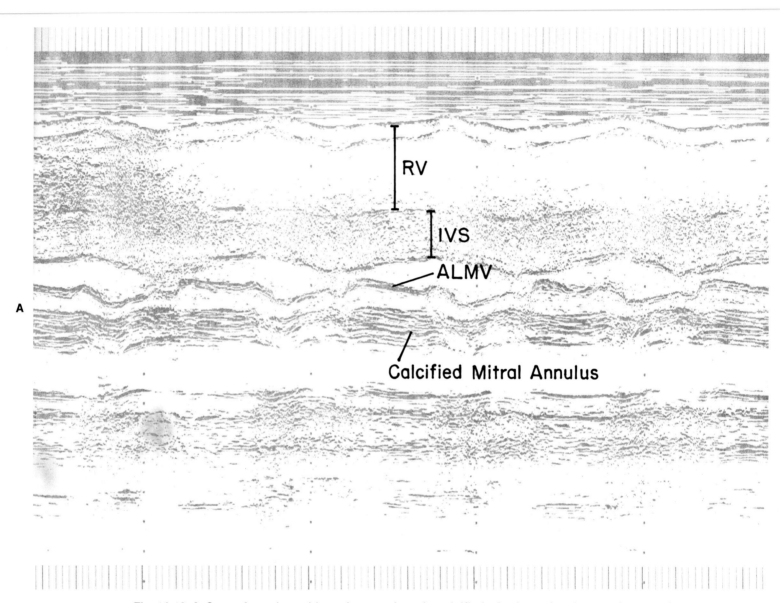

A

Fig. 14-18. A, Scan of a patient with aortic stenosis and a calcified mitral annulus shows a decreased mitral E-F slope and a thickened septum from concentric hypertrophy.

RVOT

AORTA

LA

Continued.

Fig. 14-18, cont'd. B, Calcified aortic root and cusps in the same patient.

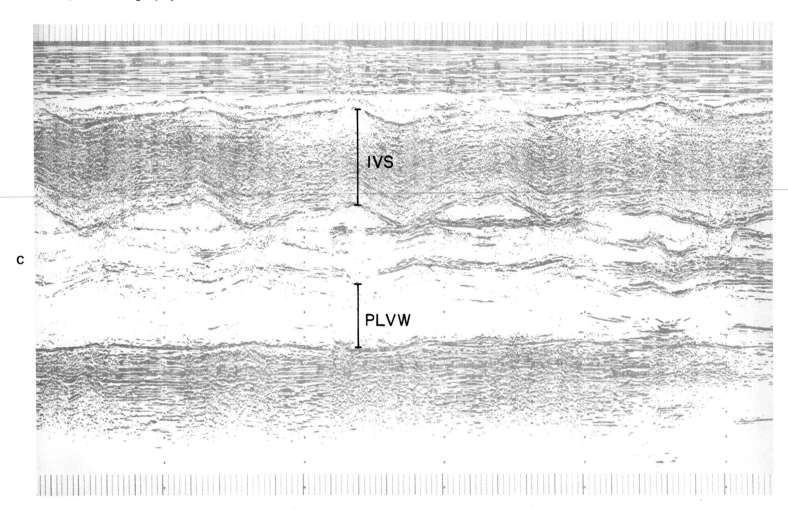

C

IVS

PLVW

Fig. 14-18, cont'd. C, Increased left ventricular mass with an extremely thickened septum and posterior wall.

CARDIOMYOPATHY
Alcoholic cardiomyopathy

It has been reported that alcohol and heart disease may be directly related because of the injurious effects produced by alcohol or its components. Indirectly, cardiac problems may result from lack of adequate diet or lowered resistance. The exact relationship between alcohol and heart disease is as yet unknown; however, an alcoholic history and primary myocardial disease are the basis for the diagnosis of alcoholic cardiomyopathy.

Clinical manifestations of cardiomyopathy are categorized depending on the dominance of either nutritional or toxic effects. Characteristically, the nutritional effect shows dilatation of the peripheral vascular system with low resistance, dilated veins, edema, and cardiac enlargement, sinus rhythm with abnormal ECG. The toxic manifestation are arrhythmias, myocardial hypertrophy, and heart failure.

By echography we have found the following characteristics of cardiomyopathy (Figs. 14-19 to 14-25):

1. Increased size of left ventricular outflow tract
2. C-D or D-E decreased
3. No thickening of cusps
4. Rapid E-F slope
5. Both leaflets recorded
6. Mitral valve echoes frequently reduplicated
7. Enlargement of left ventricular cavity
8. Thin walls
9. Diminished velocity of contraction

In our evaluation of patients with nonischemic cardiomyopathy, we obtained echograms in an attempt to determine characteristic findings. Diagnosis of nonischemic cardiomyopathy was based primarily on radiographic demonstration of cardiac enlargement in the absence of significant occlusive coronary artery disease or valvular disease by arteriography. The study demonstrated an increased size of the left ventricular cavity, both in systole and diastole, with a de-

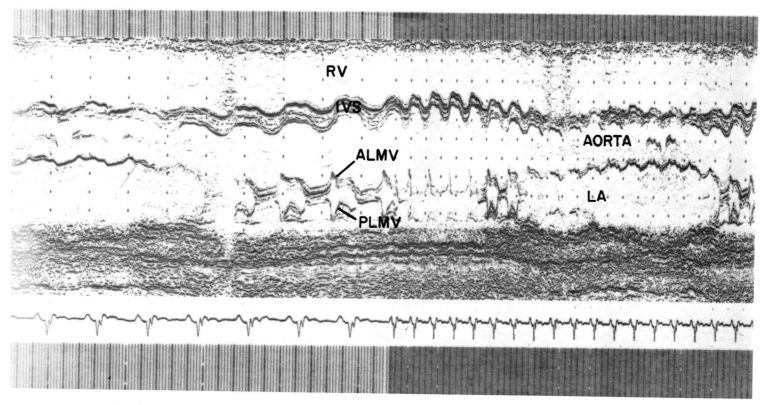

Fig. 14-19. Alcoholic cardiomyopathy shown by dilated cardiac chambers, with reduced amplitude of the mitral valve and multiple echoes in systole from the chordae tendineae.

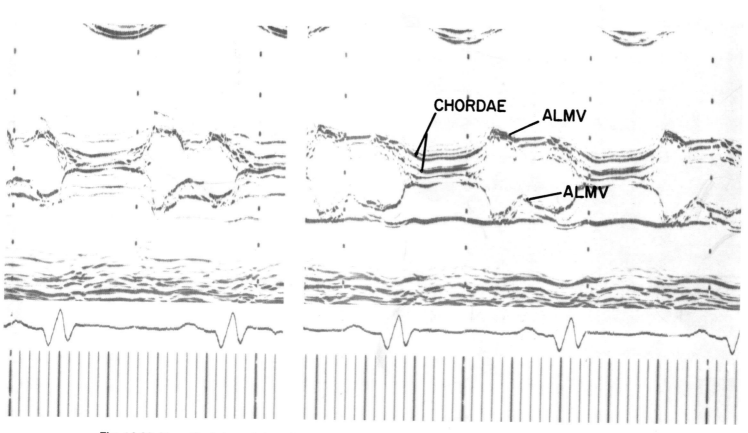

Fig. 14-20. Magnified view of the mitral valve shows a flat C-D slope, decreased C-E amplitude, and multiple echoes in systole.

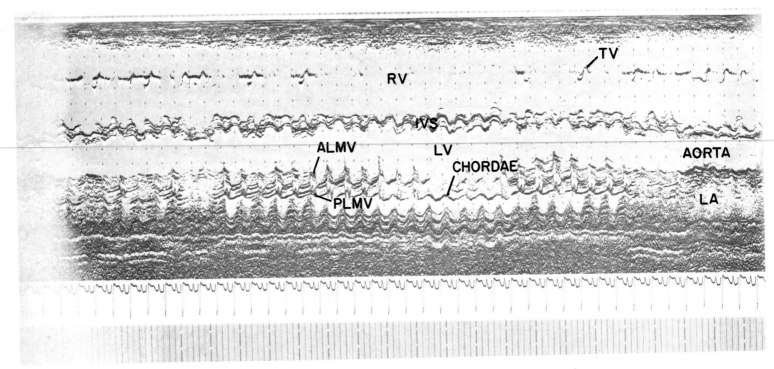

Fig. 14-21. Typical dilated heart seen in a patient with cardiomyopathy.

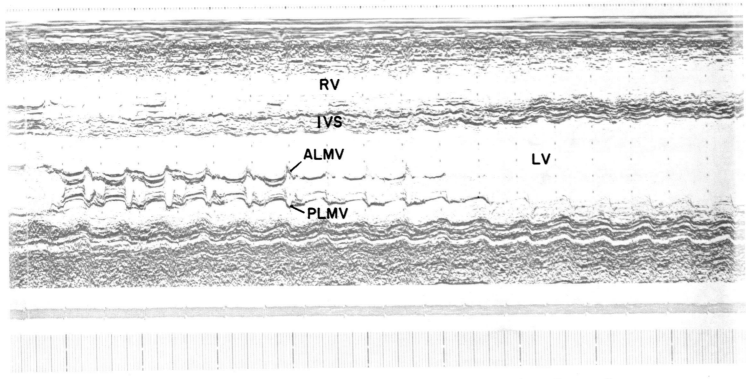

Fig. 14-22. Reduced contractility of the left ventricle is commonly seen in cardiomyopathy.

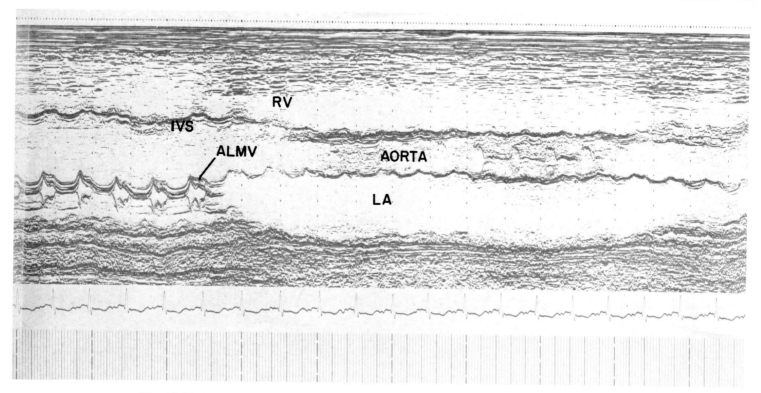

Fig. 14-23. Poor contractility of the aortic root is also demonstrated in cardiomyopathy.

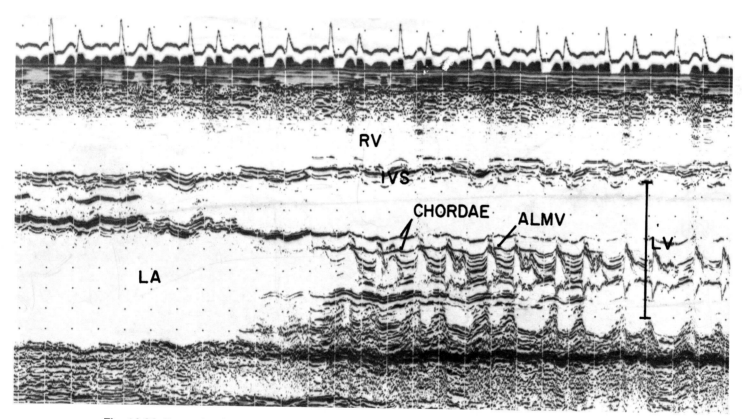

Fig. 14-24. Example of multiple chordae tendineae as seen in the systolic component of the dilated heart.

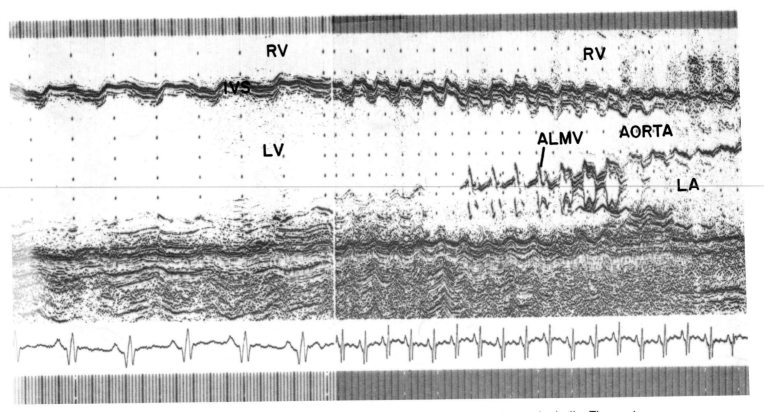

Fig. 14-25. Sweep from the left ventricle to the mitral valve to the aorta in an alcoholic. The septum and posterior wall are thin and contract poorly.

creased ejection fraction. Thickness of the posterior wall of the left ventricle was never increased, and the septum tended to be thin. Anterior and posterior leaflets of the mitral valve were readily discernible and demonstrated diminished opening and closing amplitudes. The aorta was small and the left atrium enlarged. These results were then compared with those of patients with ischemic cardiomyopathy in the absence of other disease, and no reliable differentiating features were found.

Hypertrophic cardiomyopathy

Asymmetrical septal hypertrophy (ASH) has been defined by the NIH group as a massive hypertrophied septum with abnormal cell groups found at autopsy. There is generally slow left ventricular filling during diastole, and there may be obstruction of the outflow tract during systole, commonly termed idiopathic hypertrophic subaortic stenosis (IHSS) or, as the British have termed it, hypertrophic obstructive cardiomyopathy (HOCM).

The left ventricular mass is increased, although there is no left ventricular dilatation. The septum is generally twice the size of the posterior wall thickness. Generally, the septum measures 1.8 to 2 cm. When its

thickness is divided by that of the posterior wall, the ratio should not exceed 1:3 in normal conditions. The maximum site of thickening is halfway between the aortic root and the apex of the ventricle. This septal hypertrophy accounts for the obstruction to the left ventricular outflow tract.

The mitral valve pathologically is essentially normal except for some anterior displacement and thickening. The left atrium may be dilated as a result of some degree of mitral regurgitation secondary to the disease.

The disease is hereditary and has various manifestations. Symptoms include dizziness, fainting, fatigue, and angina. Many patients are asymptomatic, with no obstruction to the outflow tract. Some experience pain, but no obstruction is found. The degree of obstruction depends on the narrowing of the left ventricular outflow tract at the onset of systole.

The disease is well recognized by echocardiography, although an initial attempt may present difficulty in recording the mitral apparatus. (See Figs. 14-26 to 14-32.) Careful definition of the septal thickness is very important. When compared to the left posterior wall thickness, the ratio of 1:3 is exceeded (the septum usually exceeds 1.8 cm). The left ventric-

Text continued on p. 199.

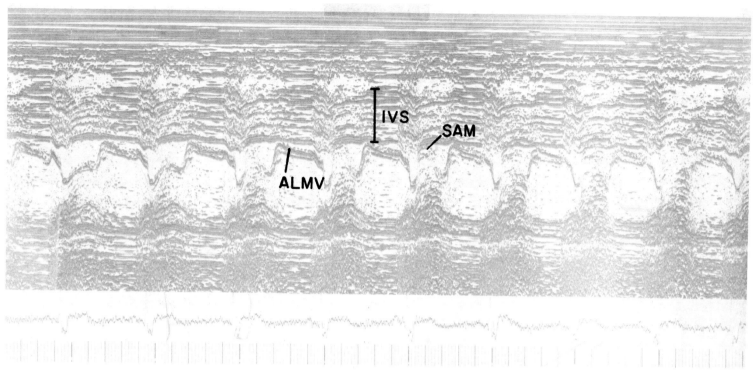

Fig. 14-26. Obstructive ASH (asymmetrical septal hypertrophy) in asymptomatic patient. Systolic anterior motion (SAM) is demonstrated during the Valsalva maneuver. Thickened septum and decreased mitral slope are also characteristic of the disease.

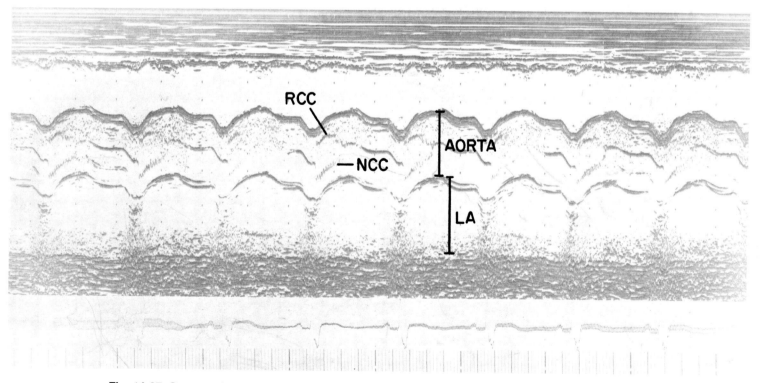

Fig. 14-27. Same patient as in Fig. 14-26 demonstrates no midsystolic closure of aortic cusps as is sometimes seen with obstructive ASH.

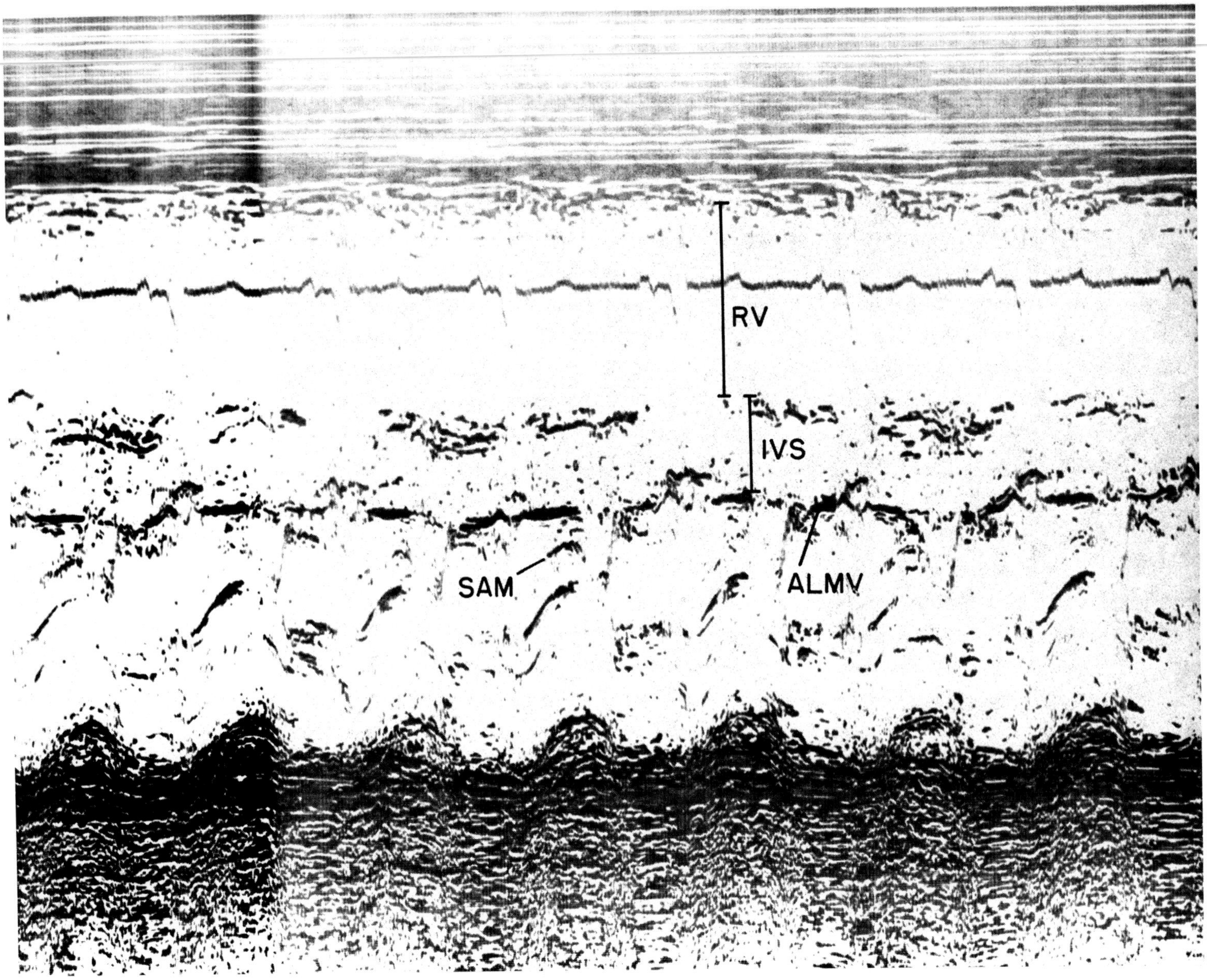

Fig. 14-28. Often patients with obstructive ASH are difficult to record adequately. Patience and perpendicularity of the transducer to the septum are necessary to record the correct septal thickness.

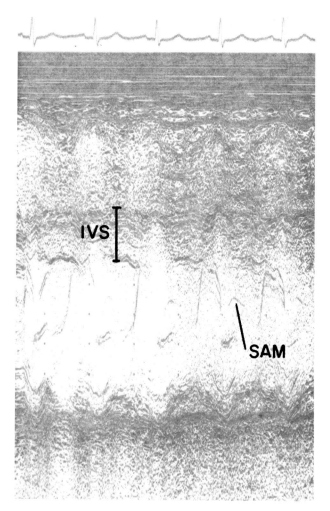

Fig. 14-29. Patient with mild obstructive ASH and mild mitral regurgitation with late systolic prolapse.

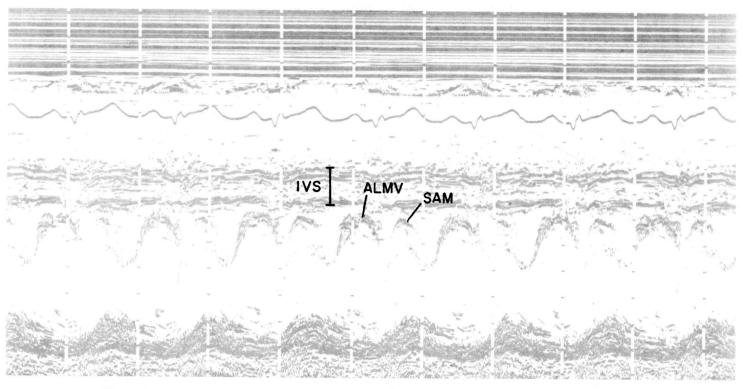

Fig. 14-30. Patient with symptoms of obstructive ASH. Without the ECG it becomes difficult to outline the systolic and diastolic components of the valve.

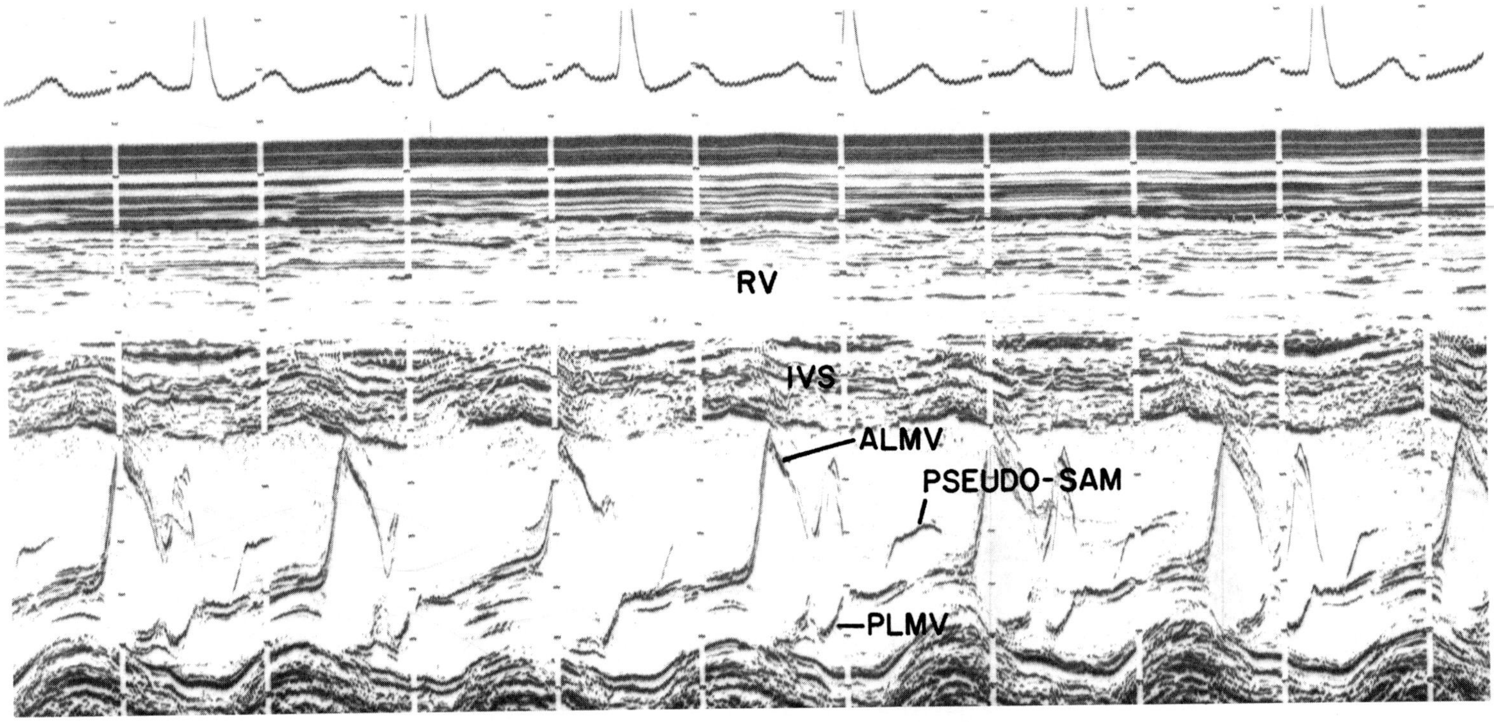

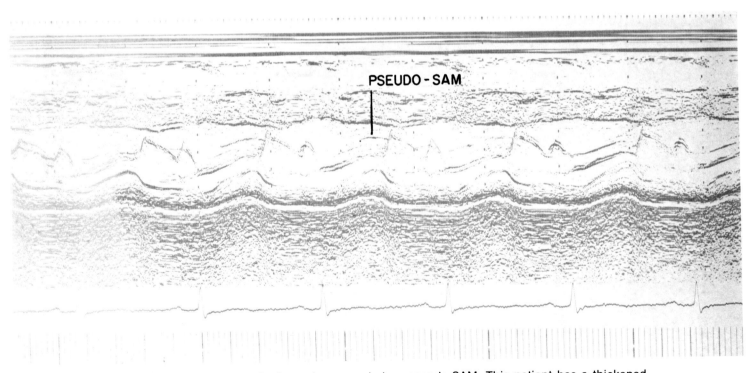

Fig. 14-31. Pseudo-SAM can be seen in patients with anterior prolapse of the posterior leaflet with the chordae swinging anterior in systole. Other patients with concentric hypertrophy have demonstrated this pseudo-SAM phenomenon.

Fig. 14-32. Pieces of the mitral annulus can mimic a pseudo-SAM. This patient has a thickened septum but no obstruction. The anterior echoes in systole are from the mitral annulus. Obstructive echoes take a more definitive anterior motion.

ular mass is increased, but the cavity is small. The anterior leaflet of the mitral valve touches the septum. The E-F slope is decreased, but the posterior leaflet is normal. In obstructive patients there is systolic anterior motion (SAM), which further obstructs the outflow tract. This movement has been attributed to the mitral apparatus itself as a display of abnormal motion and to redundant chordae tendineae, which interfere with the outflow of blood.

If obstructive disease is suspected, the patient should be provoked with a Valsalva maneuver or amyl nitrite to increase the degree of obstruction. Echo is an excellent method of following patients with obstructive ASH after medication has been given. The SAM may be initially measured and reevaluated on serial studies to note the decrease in obstruction.

CORONARY ARTERY DISEASE*

Coronary artery disease, as defined by Griffith, is any abnormal condition of the coronary arteries that interferes with the delivery of an adequate supply of blood to the structures of the heart. It is the most common cause of heart disease among adults in the United States.

Rare types of inflammation of the blood vessels caused by oversensitivity to certain substances and certain types of thickening and hardening in the blood vessel wall, such as Buerger's disease, may also affect the coronary arteries.

Atherosclerosis

There are several causes of coronary artery disease. The most common and most serious by far is atherosclerosis. Arteriosclerosis indicates disease of the larger arteries with narrowing of the blood vessels. Atherosclerosis is one particular form of arteriosclerosis that involves the arteries which carry blood to the heart, brain, kidneys, arms, and legs. It is a reversible disease and not necessarily an aging process.

An atheroma is a mass of fat that forms on the inside wall of a coronary artery, partly plugging the vessel. This mass of fat is made up of all the types of fat that normally circulate in the blood.

The presence of an atheroma on the lining of a coronary artery is bad in itself, but worse manifestations follow. Fibrous scar tissue grows into and around the mass of fat, binding it firmly to the wall of the artery. The atheroma, which starts as a soft rubbery mass of

fat, ends as a hard, rocklike, chalky plaque, like a piece of cement on the lining of the artery. An atheroma may grow to such a size that it blocks the coronary artery completely, similiar to a boulder completely damming a stream.

A blood clot is very likely to form any place in a blood vessel where the blood is partly dammed up. This often happens immediately "upstream" from an atheroma. Once the blood clot has formed, it extends down over and sometimes past the original atheroma. This is a thrombus. When a thrombus forms in a coronary artery, the condition is called coronary thrombosis, or stoppage of a coronary artery by a blood clot. Blood clots in the coronary arteries practically always form around an atheroma.

Sometimes there is bleeding in the tissue immediately under the atheroma. The bleeding tends to separate the plaque from the wall of the blood vessel, as if it had been dissected with a knife. The plaque then tends to lift out into the bloodstream and fall across the artery, blocking it completely.

Infection or necrosis of tissue under the atheroma may form an abscess in the wall of the artery immediately under the plaque. This will have the same effect as hemorrhage; the plaque will again lift off and block the artery completely.

Heart muscle extracts about four fifths of the oxygen supplied to it in the blood by the coronary arteries. This leaves an extremely small borrowing capacity, or reserve margin, if that blood supply is cut down. The collateral circulation between the coronary arteries is not good. When a coronary artery is blocked, however, there is usually death of tissue.

Complications of atherosclerosis

Angina pectoris (pain arising in the heart muscle). Angina pectoris is the mildest and earliest clinical symptom of heart disease caused by coronary atheromatosis. This is distress of some type, usually in the chest, brought on by increased heart work. It characteristically appears after physical exertion, large meals, emotional tension, or fear or anger, and it is usually relieved promptly by rest or by the use of nitroglycerin tablets.

Coronary insufficiency (myocardial ischemia without infarction). Coronary insufficiency is a more severe and prolonged form of disease than angina pectoris, and of the forms of coronary atheromatosis described so far, it can reduce the blood flow to an area of heart muscle to such a degree that the heart muscle actually does not receive enough blood to maintain life. Although there is still blood flow and the coronary artery

*Quoted with slight modification from Griffith, G. C.: Coronary artery disease. In Phibbs, B., editor: The human heart: a guide to heart disease, ed. 3, St. Louis, 1975, The C. V. Mosby Co.

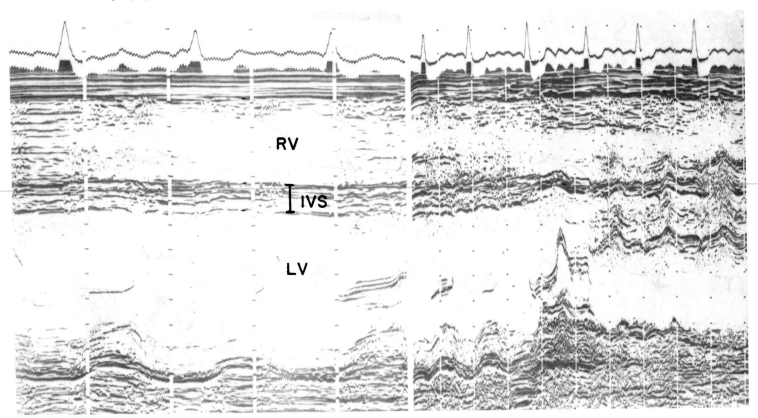

Fig. 14-33. Patient with coronary artery disease and anterior myocardial infarction shows flat septal motion with normal posterior wall contractility.

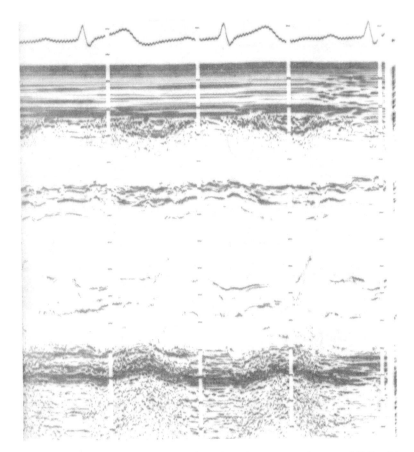

Fig. 14-34. Poor technique may cause a normal septum to appear abnormal if the transducer is not perpendicular. This patient was normal, but the echo appears with a flattened septum, suggesting coronary disease.

is not completely blocked, the blood supply to some areas of the heart muscle is so far below the requirements of the tissues that the cells are actually injured. The cells in the heart muscle are not dead. They can be brought back to normal function, but they do suffer some degree of injury because their blood supply is cut below the danger point. This might also be called reversible disease of the heart muscle produced by coronary atherosclerosis. (See Figs. 14-33 and 14-34.)

The patient often suffers pain typical of angina pectoris. The pain is still present, however, after the patient rests in a lying or sitting position or after two or three nitroglycerin tablets have been given at 5-minute intervals. The pain is finally relieved only after administration of a sedative. In this case it is likely that the heart muscle has been damaged.

To summarize, the second most serious type of disease produced by coronary atherosclerosis is prolonged coronary insufficiency, or myocardial ischemia without infarction. The word ischemia means a lack of adequate blood supply to maintain life in some area of tissue. The word infarct means that tissue has actually died because of complete blockage of blood flow. Ischemia means that an area of heart muscle, or myocardium, has not received enough blood supply but has not actually died, since the blood flow, although below the safe level, has not been cut off completely.

Myocardial infarction. Infarct is a term meaning that an area of tissue dies because its blood supply has been cut off. As a result of coronary artery disease, it often forms in the heart muscle or in the wall of the heart and is called a myocardial infarction. Once the blood supply to the heart muscle has been cut off and the infarct has formed, it takes a certain minimum amount of time for the tissue to die and to heal with strong scar formation. This never takes less than three weeks, and sometimes it takes longer. Finally, after this minimum period of time, a hard white scar forms in the wall of the heart.

A frequent complication of acute heart muscle injury, or myocardial infarction, is an irregularity of the heartbeat, or cardiac arrhythmia. Atrial or ventricular premature beats may appear. When atrial premature beats become very frequent, they may lead to the rapid forceful heart action called supraventricular tachycardia or to a totally irregular heart action called atrial fibrillation. Sometimes the ventricles may develop the same type of irregular beat with ventricular tachycardia or ventricular fibrillation. Sometimes a heart block will appear in the conducting system of the heart, and this again increases the risk sharply.

Another complication is acute congestion of the lungs, known as pulmonary edema. This happens when the left side of the heart, the ventricle, is so damaged by injury to heart muscle that blood dams up behind the ventricle in the lungs. The fluid in the lungs escapes from the small blood vessels, or capillaries, into the air-bearing cells, causing shortness of breath and often causing the patient to spit up a frothy fluid.

Finally, blood clots are an ever-present hazard. The infarct is often caused by the presence of a blood clot in a diseased part of a coronary artery. A mural, or wall, clot often forms inside the cavity of the left ventricle over the area of damaged muscle, much like a fungus growing on a tree. The prolonged rest in bed that goes with the early stages of myocardial infarction produces increased danger of blood clots in the veins of the lower extremities.

15 □ Pericardial disease

The pericardial sac is susceptible to various disease processes resulting in pericardial inflammation accompanied by pericardial effusion or pericardial thickening and constriction. The diseases most commonly afflicting the pericardial sac are acute pericarditis, constrictive pericarditis, and pericardial tamponade.

ACUTE PERICARDITIS

Acute pericarditis attacks the lining of the pericardium and results in inflammation and often a small pericardial effusion. There are several causes for acute pericarditis. The infective process associated with a viral or tuberculous organism may cause the pericardial inflammation. Often it is a complication of one of the collagen diseases such as rheumatic fever or systemic lupus erythematosus. Renal failure is commonly associated with pericardial effusion, and various neoplastic diseases may also cause pericarditis.

We have found the echographic diagnosis of pericardial effusion to be extremely useful in the clinical management of the patient. If a patient's heart or chest x-ray film indicates an enlargement, an echo can quickly distinguish ventricular enlargement from fluid in the pericardium. In renal patients with pericardial effusion, the fluid may be serially followed to note its increase or decrease in volume.

A systematic approach is followed to diagnose pericardial effusion. A routine scan is performed to locate the mitral valve area, aortic valve, and left ventricle. The left ventricle is examined closely to note its movement. In pericardial effusion the separation of the pericardium from the three layers of the heart wall by the fluid cause the pulsations of the heart to be dampened by the time they reach the pericardium. Thus one of the most obvious features of effusion is a nonmobile pericardium separated from the posterior heart wall by fluid. Sometimes the amount of fluid is so small that these pulsations are transmitted slightly to the pericardium, in which case the examiner would see diminished motion of the pericardium (Figs. 15-1 and 15-2).

Fluid generally accumulates in the most posterior-dependent area of the heart, accounting for the visualization of the posterior effusion before anterior fluid is seen. (See Figs. 15-3 to 15-7.) As the fluid accumulates in greater quantities (300 to 400 ml), separation of the anterior pericardium from the right ventricular wall will be noted. (See Figs. 15-8 to 15-12.)

The diagnosis of pericardial effusion can be very complex if the routine cardiac scan sweep is not performed. The technician must sweep the transducer in an oblique path to visualize the aortic root and mitral valve, carefully observing the continuity of the left atrial wall with the pericardium. Generally, the left atrial wall will be motionless in cases of moderate pericardial effusion. However, we have seen abrupt anterior movement of the left atrial wall in patients with a large pericardial effusion. As the sweep into the left ventricular cavity continues (the angle always toward the patient's left hip, inferior and lateral), the larger amount of fluid accumulates toward the apex of the heart.

We have found it very useful to document our cases of pericardial effusion with the real-time equipment. This allows us to visualize the total cardiac silhouette and permits a much clearer visualization of the amount and position of pericardial fluid. We look at the heart in a longitudinal and horizontal section with the patient in a supine position (Figs. 15-13 to 15-15). Small pericardial effusions that were difficult to diagnose on M-mode scans were easily demonstrated on the real-time equipment.

False negatives can only be made if technique is inadequate or if the proper sweep is not performed. Medial angulation of the transducer in the left ventricular cavity can give false reflections off the mediastinum. Pleural effusion can be confused with pericardial effusion if careful analysis of the left atrial-to-pericardial sweep is not made, or if the sensitivity is not dampened to demonstrate the posterior wall echoes from the pericardium.

Text continued on p. 210.

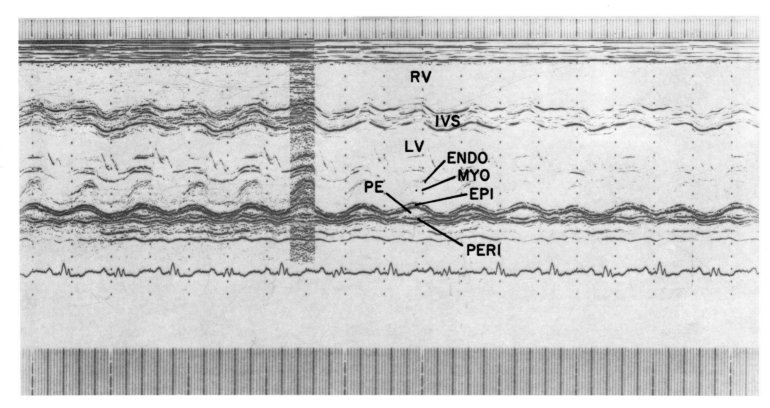

Fig. 15-1. Small pericardial effusion. A change in gain allows differentiation of the pericardium from the posterior heart wall.

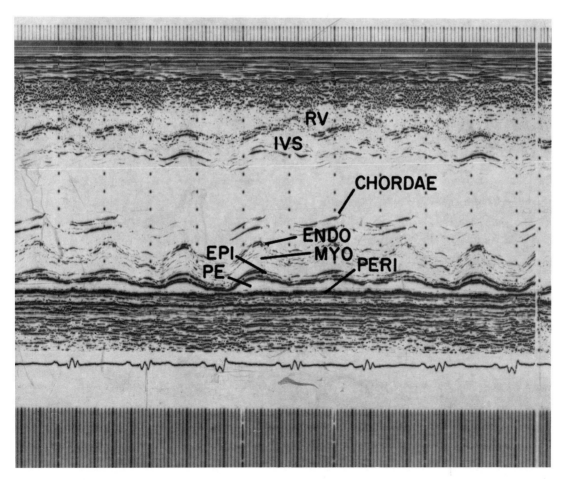

Fig. 15-2. Immobile pericardium dampened by a small pericardial effusion.

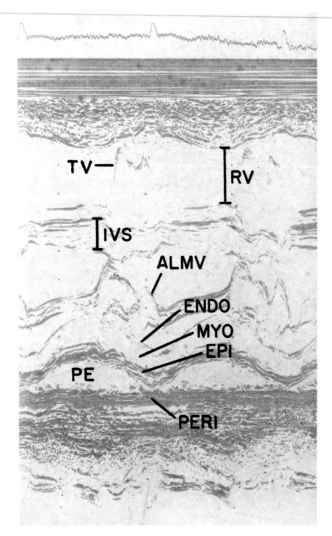

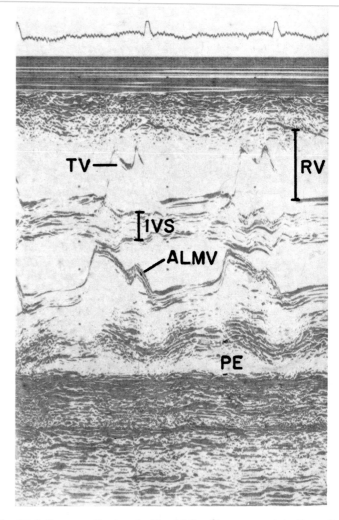

Fig. 15-3. Moderate pericardial effusion in a patient with an atrial septal defect.

Fig. 15-4. Same patient as in Fig. 15-3 with a sweep into the mitral valve area. Posterior effusion is still shown.

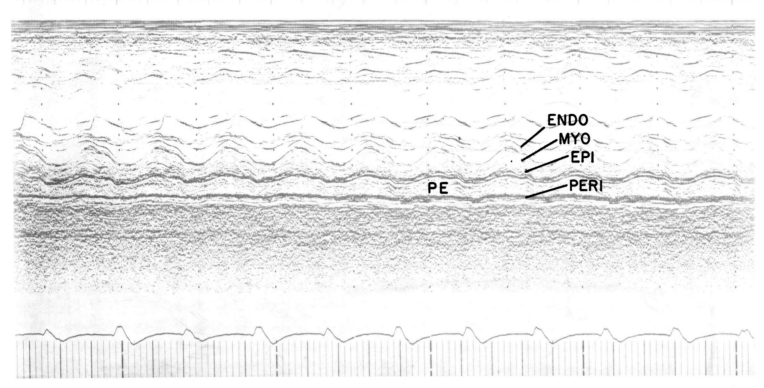

Fig. 15-5. Moderate posterior effusion in a patient with congestive cardiomyopathy.

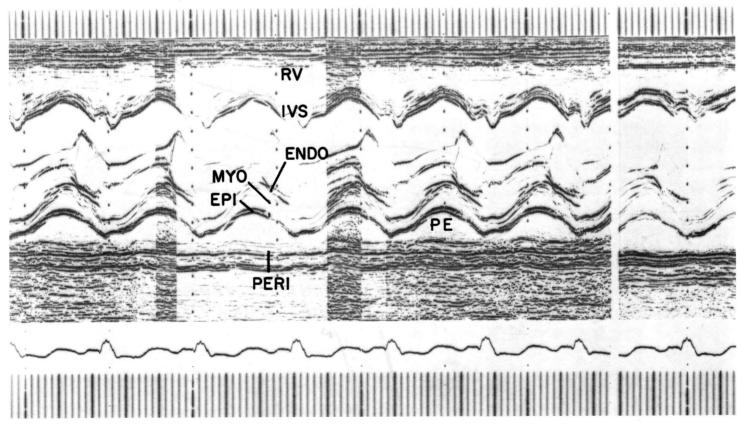

Fig. 15-6. Hyperdynamic heart with posterior effusion.

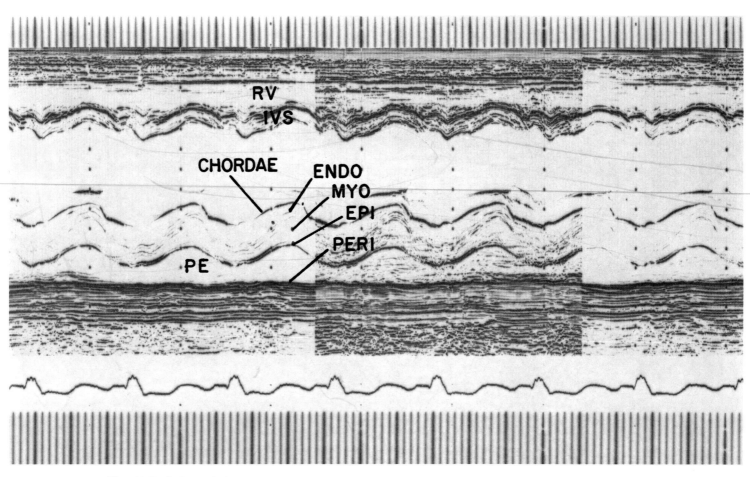

Fig. 15-7. Gain variations may show echoes within an effusion. Metastatic effusion or a bloody effusion may appear with multiple small echoes within, but usually these echoes persist with a decrease in gain.

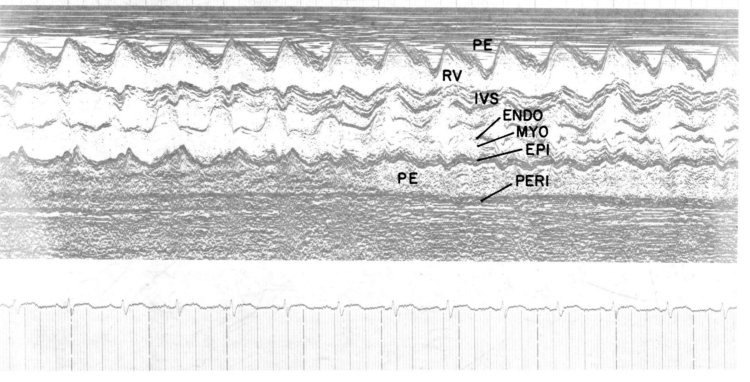

Fig. 15-8. Metastatic invasion into the pericardial sac with large effusions anterior and posterior.

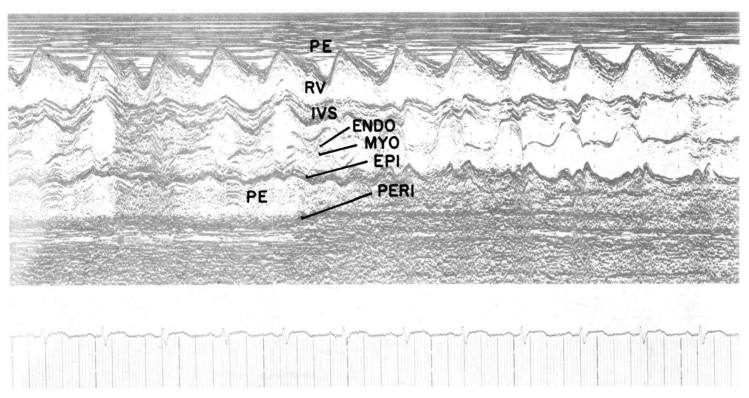

Fig. 15-9. Large effusions cause the heart to contract hyperdynamically.

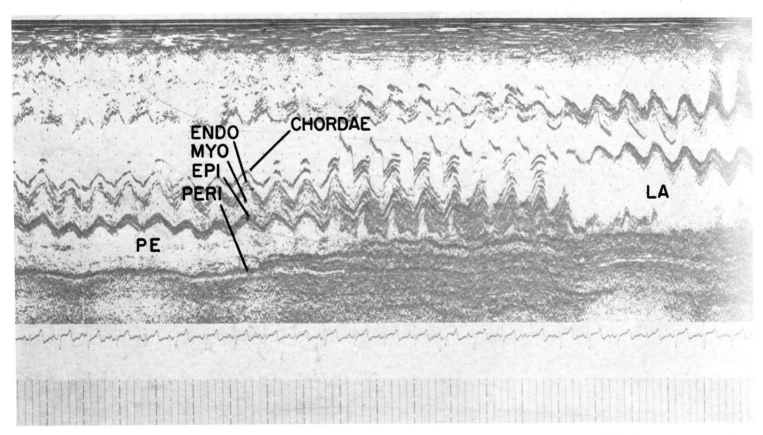

Fig. 15-10. Sweep from the ventricle to the aorta demonstrates a large posterior effusion, which does not persist behind the left atrial wall. Hyperdynamic wall motion is shown in the left atrium.

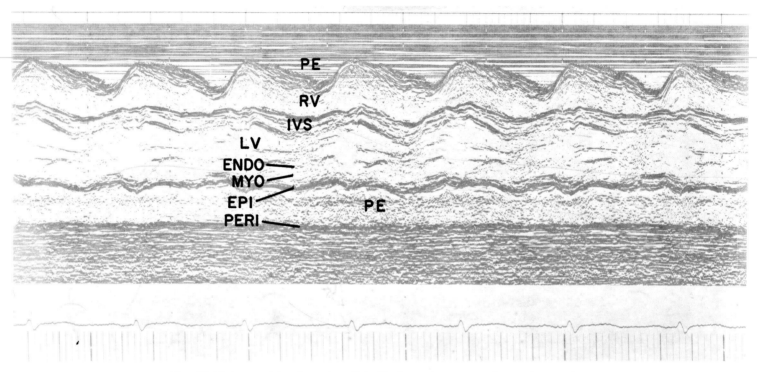

Fig. 15-11. Large, bloody pericardial effusions shown anterior and posterior.

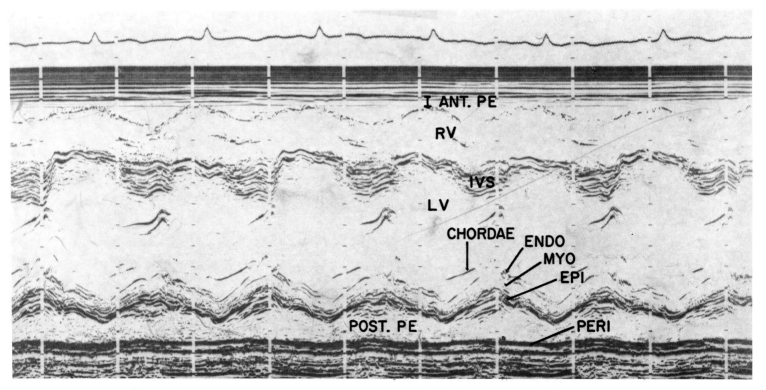

Fig. 15-12. Large effusion in a patient with mitral regurgitation and a dilated left ventricle.

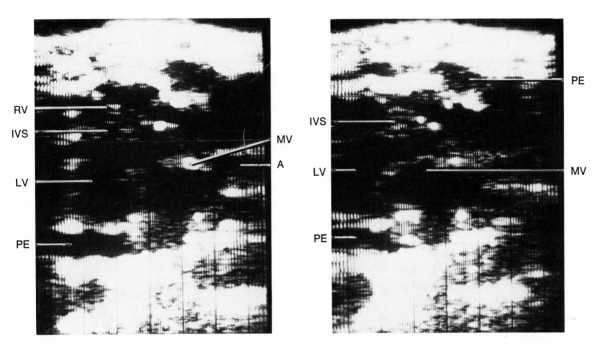

Fig. 15-13. Real-time longitudinal scan of a large effusion surrounding the heart.

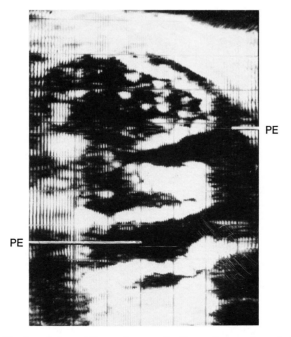

Fig. 15-14. Horizontal real-time demonstration of a pericardial effusion.

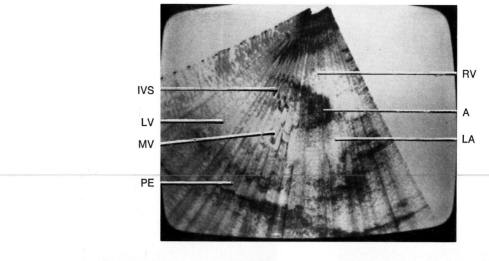

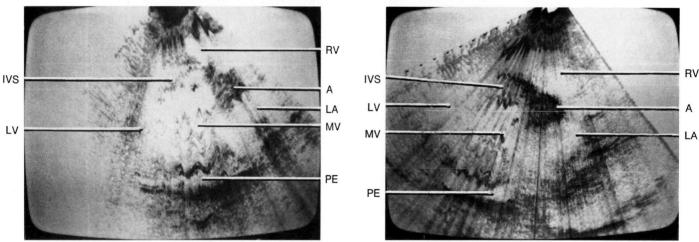

Fig. 15-15. If real-time equipment is not available, a conventional B-scan unit can image the cardiac silhouette. The sweep is made in an oblique path from the aorta to the left ventricle. A slow arc motion is made to record the cardiac contraction within the pericardial sac.

CONSTRICTIVE PERICARDITIS

Fibrosis of the pericardial lining may follow acute pericarditis, tuberculosis, or neoplastic invasion of the pericardium. The rigid pericardium affects ventricular contraction and results in reduced cardiac output.

We have found it difficult to echographically demonstrate constrictive pericarditis. The thickness of the pericardium is not effectively demonstrated, since the echo response may be increased or decreased with a change in sensitivity controls. Some investigators have reported a double reflection of the pericardial interface with reduced sensitivity settings in restrictive pericarditis. However, we have found this occurrence in patients without the disease and do not feel comfortable with this evaluation. Loss of motion of the pericardium can be seen in constrictive pericarditis and is probably one of the more definitive echographic features. Of course, restrictive motion is also seen in myocardial infarction and in cardiomyopathy diseases and is not specific in itself.

PERICARDIAL TAMPONADE

Excessive fluid in the pericardium can compress the heart, causing electrical alternans of the ECG. The excessive fluid in the pericardial sac causes inadequate filling of the ventricles during diastole. The heart begins contracting wildly to force the blood out, and an emergency situation arises. This fluid may accumulate after sudden cardiac trauma, a ruptured aneurysm, or after an attack of pericarditis.

Echographically a huge amount of fluid can be seen surrounding the heart anteriorly and posteriorly. There is a bizarre movement of the entire cardiac silhouette, which has been termed the "swinging" heart. The ECG demonstrates electrical alternans denoting poor ventricular compliance. Other cardiac

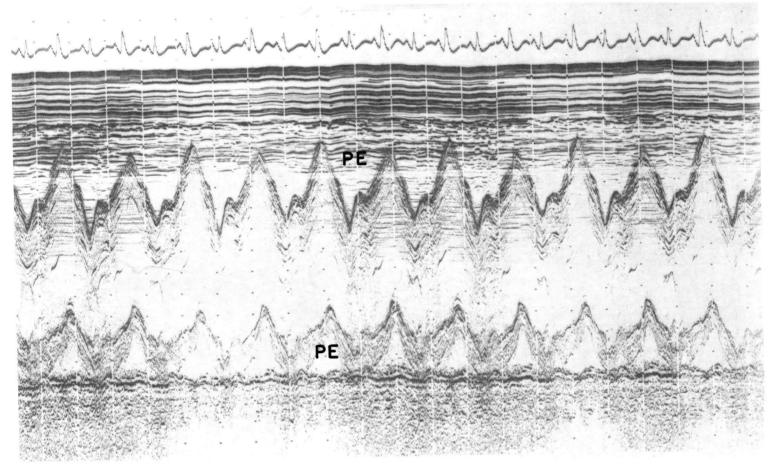

Fig. 15-16. Large pericardial effusion, or "swinging heart" syndrome, in a patient with pericardial tamponade.

findings of paradoxical septal motion and prolapse of the mitral valve have also been demonstrated to occur with tamponade and disappear after pericardial centesis (Fig. 15-16).

Subxyphoid aspiration techniques may be employed as a clinical tool in withdrawing the fluid from the pericardium. We have found it useful to locate the effusion in the normal position and slowly move the transducer toward the apex of the heart for localization for pericardial centesis.

16 □ Case presentations

CASE PRESENTATIONS

Case 1. Elderly woman in cardiac distress and renal failure.

Comment on
- Left atrial size
- Left ventricular cavity
- Aortic cusps
- Septum and posterior wall thickness

Diagnosis:

A

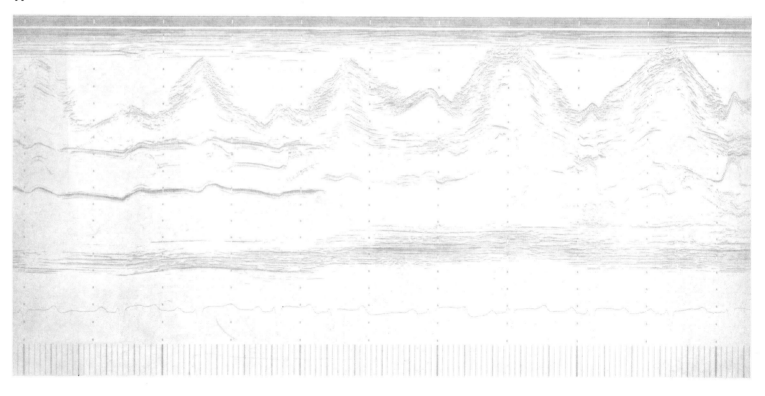

B

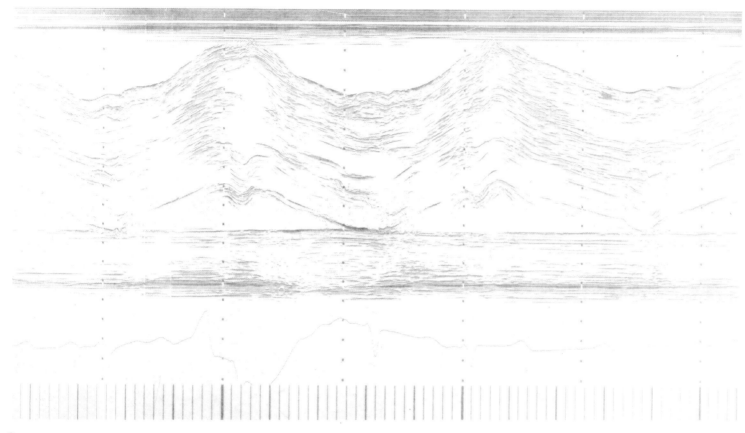

C

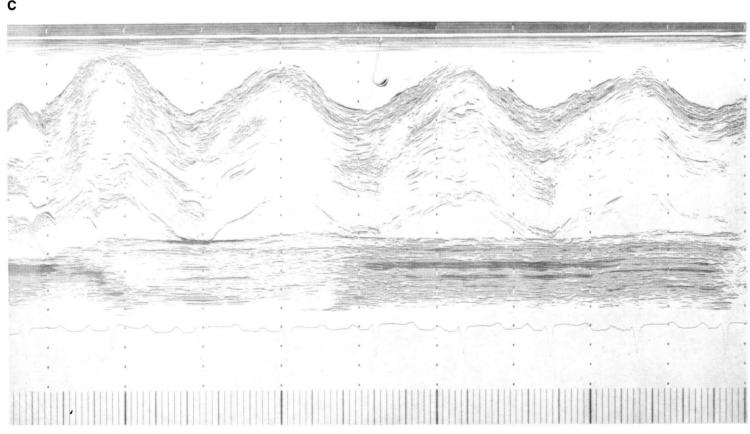

Case 2. Middle-aged woman with diastolic rumble and past history of rheumatic fever.

A. Measure the E-F slope.

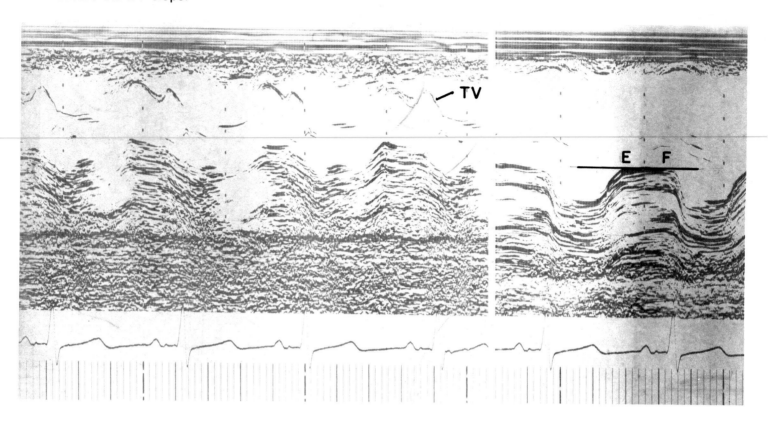

B. Differentiate stenosis from a myxoma.

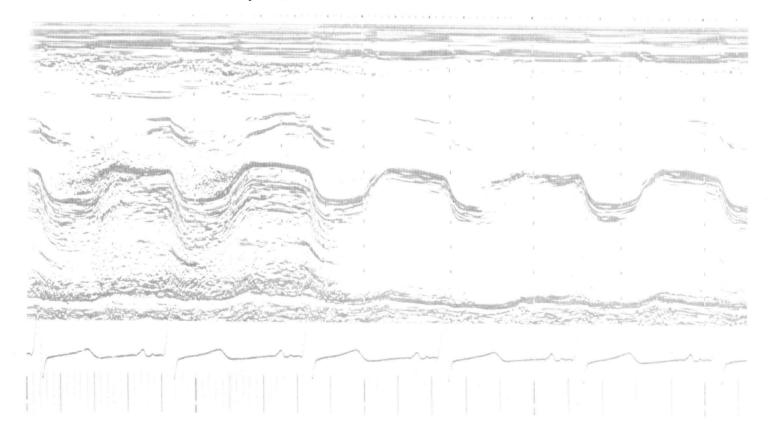

C. Evaluate the left atrial cavity.

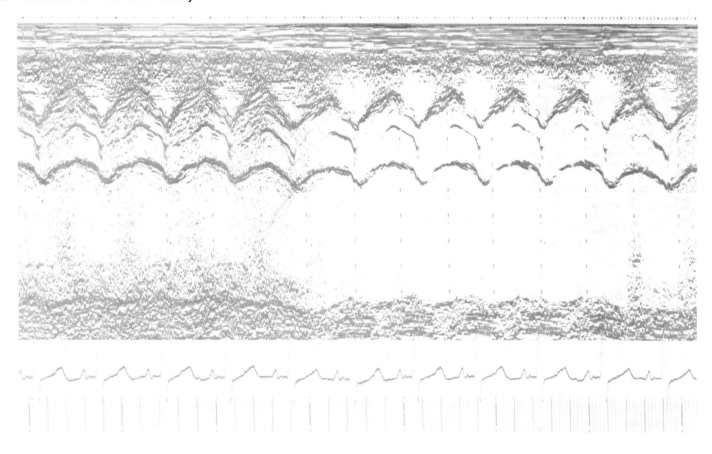

D. Evaluate the left ventricle.

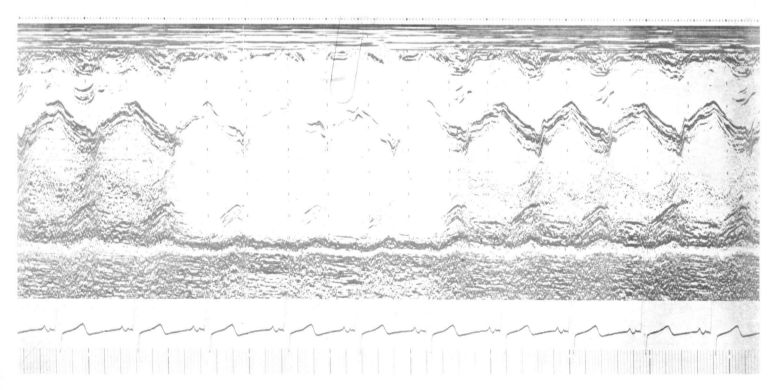

Case 3
● Is this a dissecting aortic aneurysm?

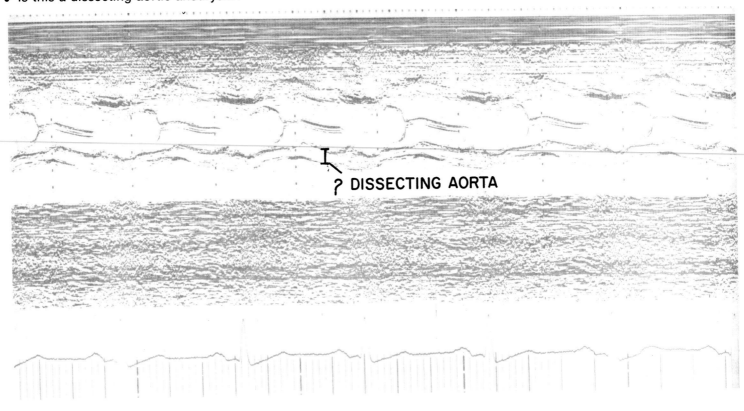

? DISSECTING AORTA

Case 4
● What does the echo posterior to the mitral valve represent?

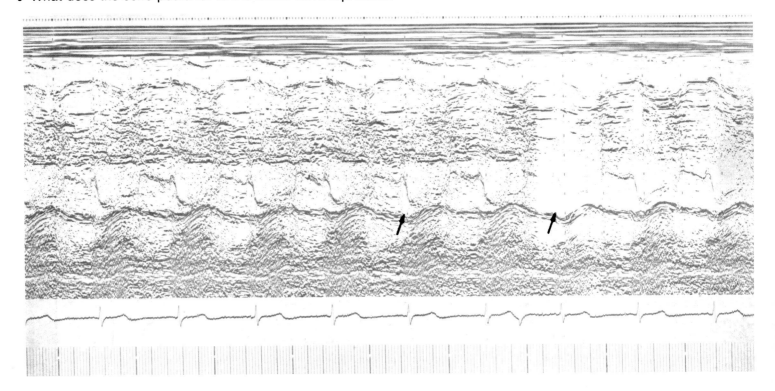

Case 5
• What could this enlarged right ventricle represent, and what does it measure?

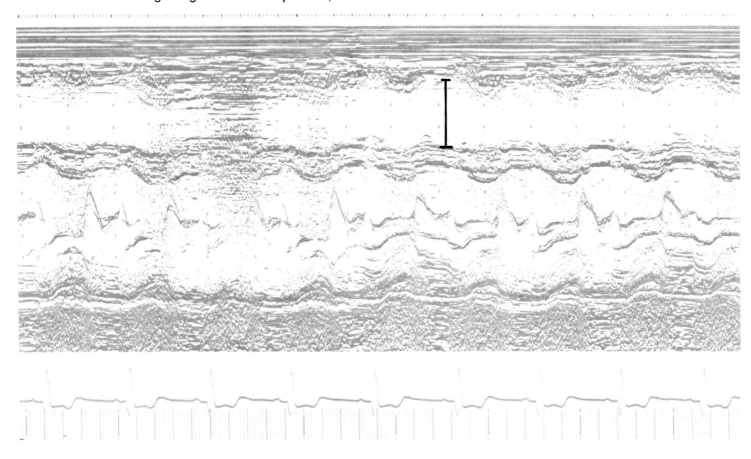

Case 6
• Comment on the ALMV. How would you measure the mitral velocity?

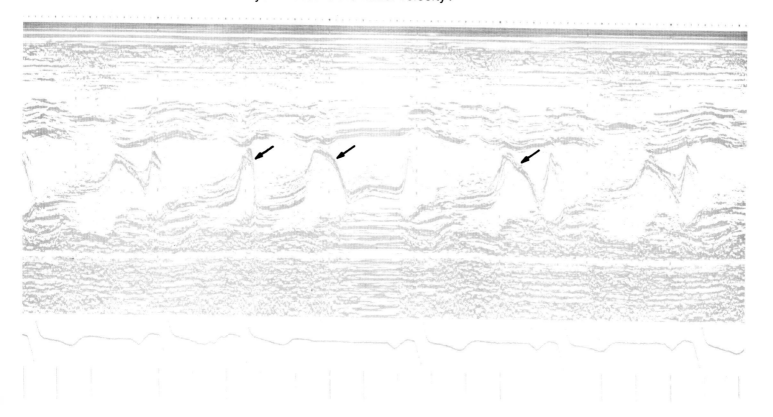

Case 7
● Comment on the aorta and left atrial cavity.

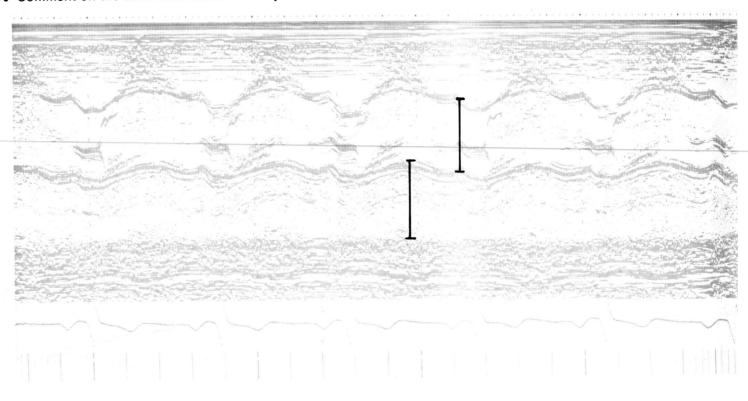

Case 8
● Are the aortic cusps normal?

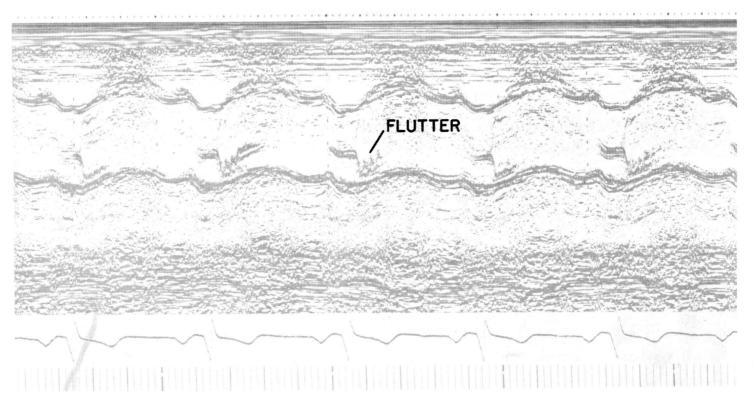

FLUTTER

Case 9. Tall, thin young man with double-jointed capabilities.

A. What is the size of the aortic root and left atrium?

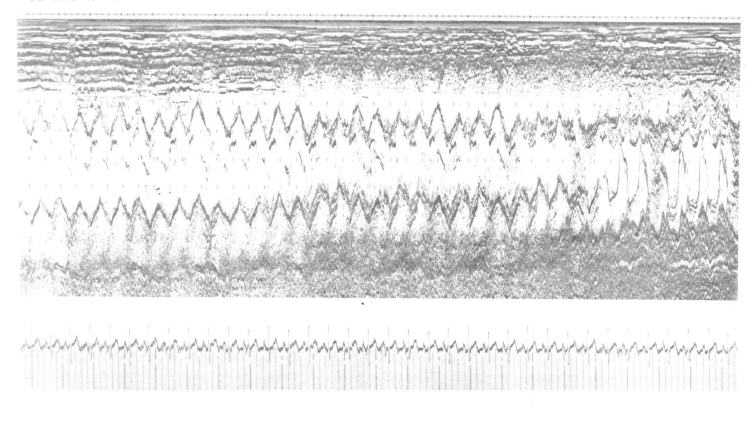

B. Comment on the mitral valve apparatus.

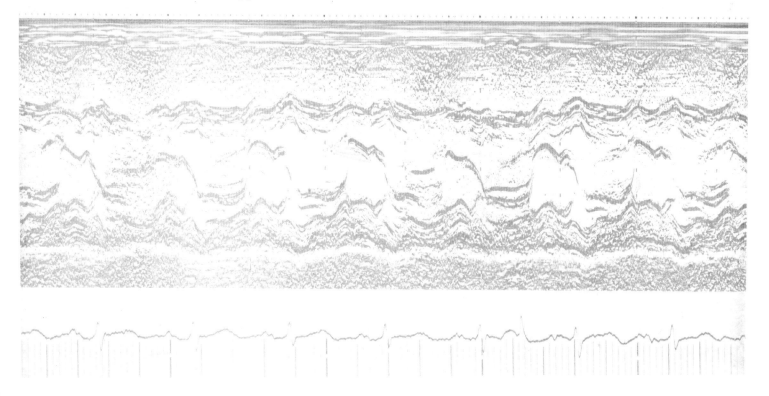

Case 10
- Diagnosis:

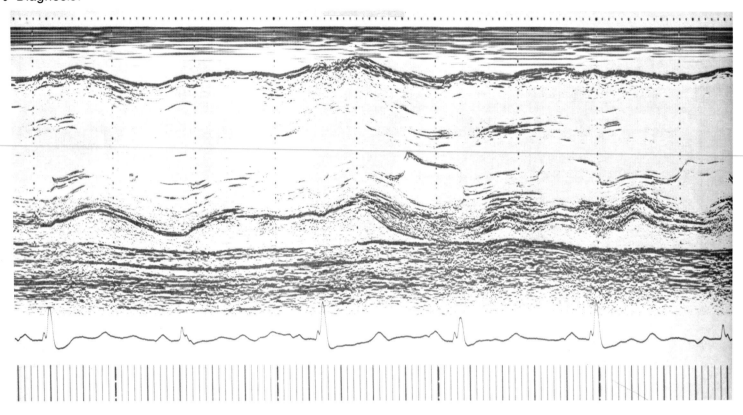

Case 11
- Does the group of echoes posterior to the mitral valve represent a myxoma?

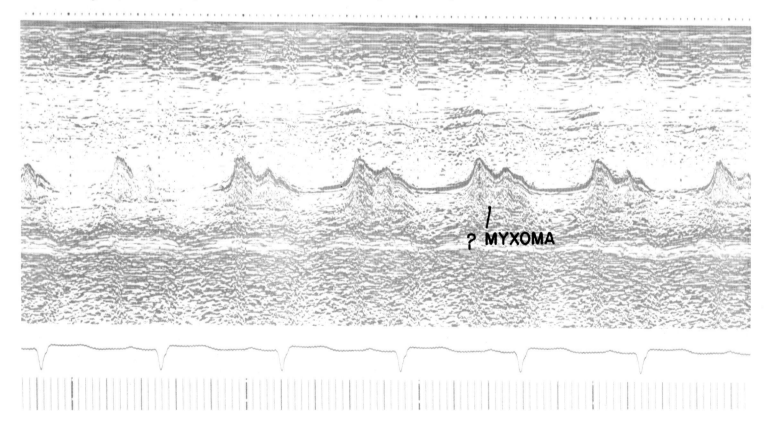

Case 12

A. Evaluate for IHSS.

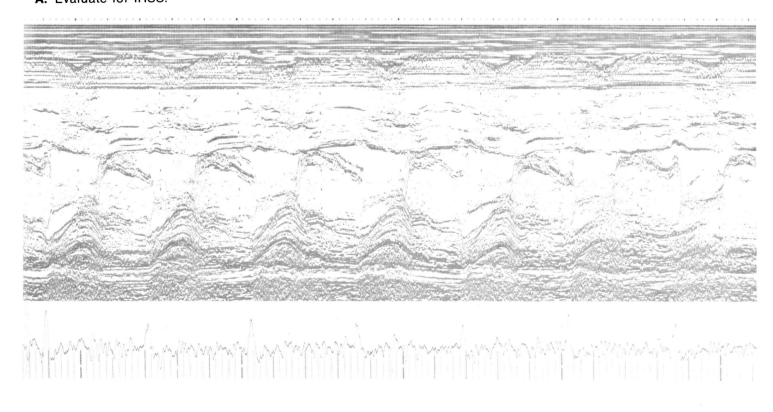

B. Measure the septum, the amplitude of the ALMV, and the E-F velocity.

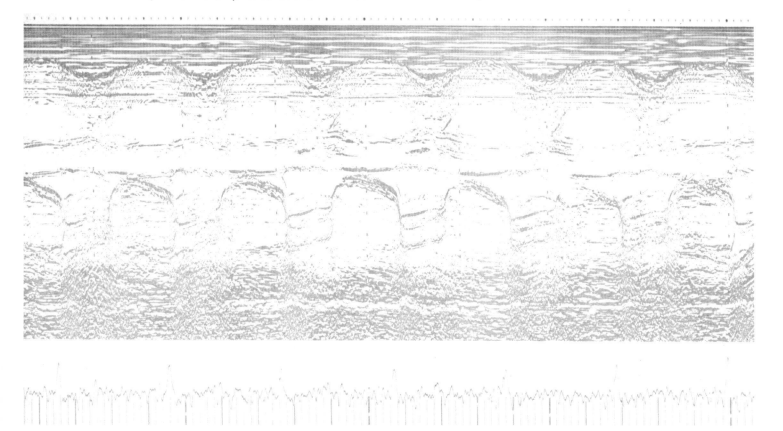

Case 13. Renal patient with dilated heart on x-ray examination; severe hypertension.

A. Comment on the mitral valve and left ventricular cavity.

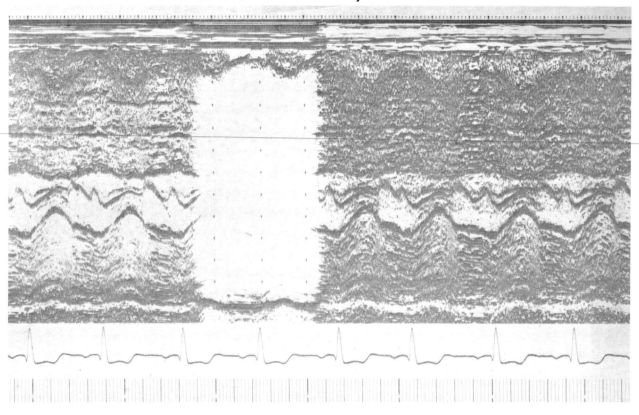

B. Comment on the aorta and cusps.

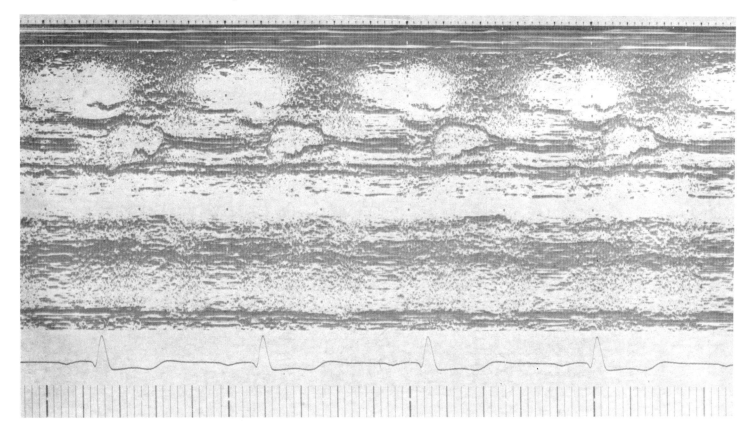

C. Rule out pericardial effusion. Measure the septum and posterior wall and comment.

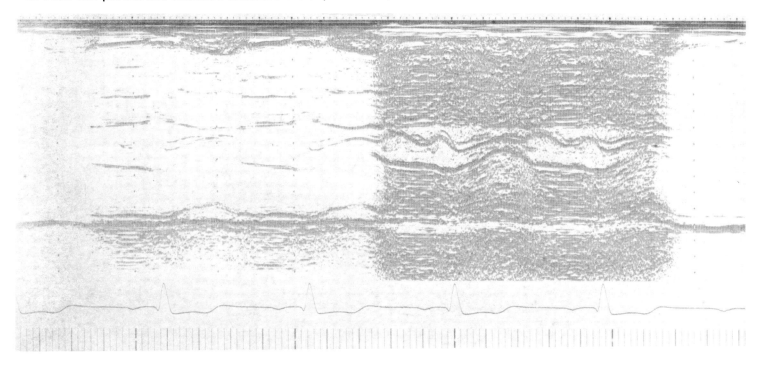

Case 14. Young patient with history of rheumatic fever and mild diastolic murmur.

- Comment on the mitral valve, ventricular size, and differential diagnosis.

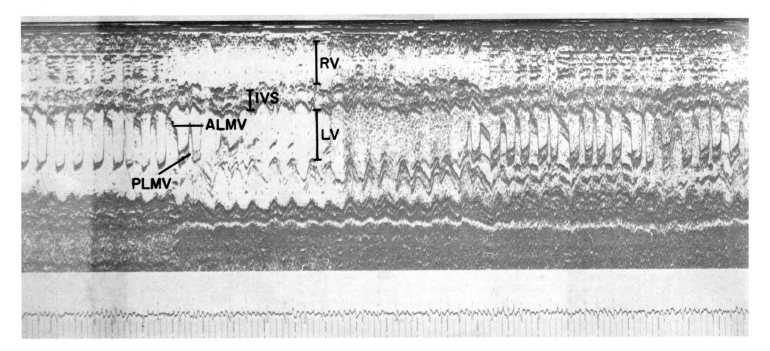

Case 15. Elderly patient with cor pulmonale and a systolic murmur over the second intercostal space.

Comment on
  A. ALMV

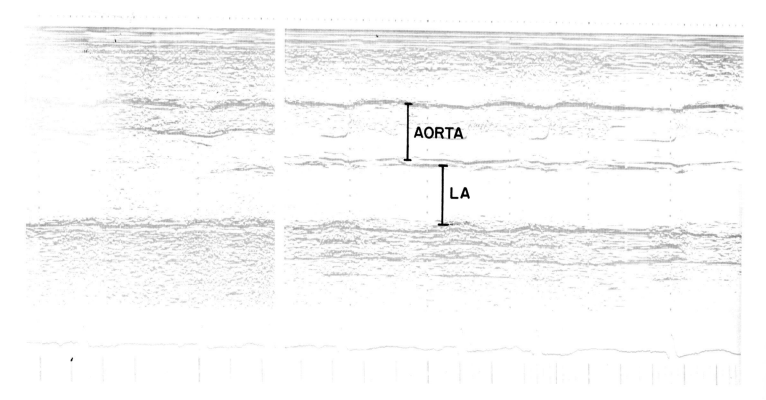

B. Aorta and left atrium

C. Pulmonary valve

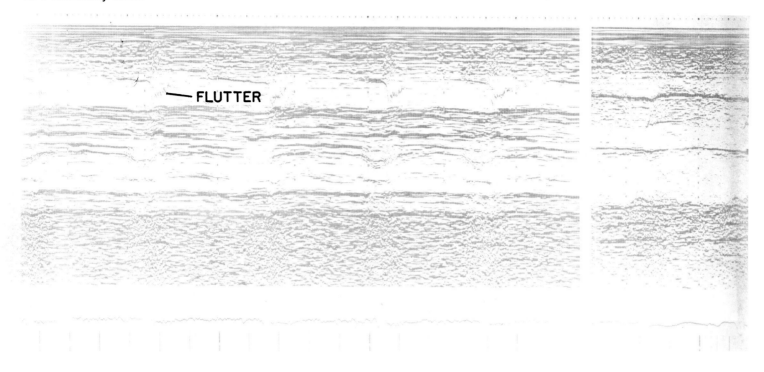

FLUTTER

Case 16. Young man with known drug addiction and fever of unknown origin.

Comment on
A. Left ventricle and mitral valve

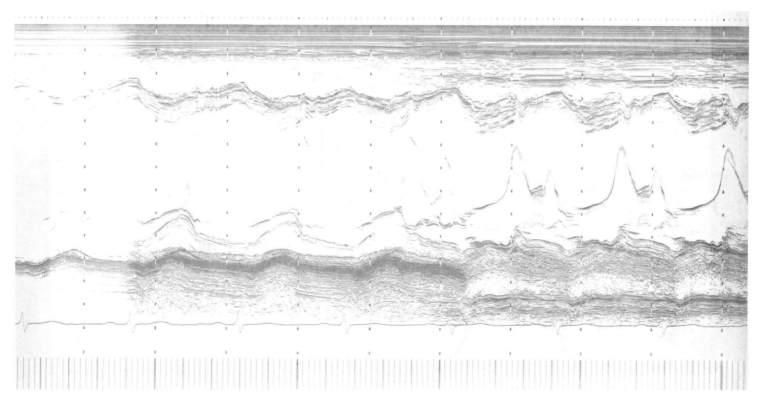

B. Aorta, cusps, and left atrium

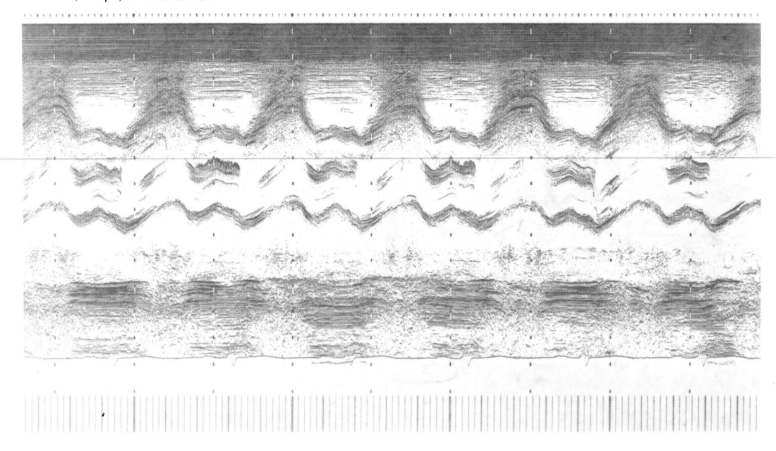

ANSWERS
Case 1
- Enlarged left atrium, 4.2 cm.
- Decreased left ventricular cavity.
- Early systolic closure of aortic cusps resulting from decreased cardiac output.
- Concentric hypertrophy of septum and posterior wall.

Diagnosis: Huge pericardial effusion with electrical alternans on ECG, "swinging" heart syndrome, most likely cardiac tamponade.

Case 2
- **A.** E-F slope = 3 to 4 mm/sec.
- **B.** This is a case of mitral stenosis, which can be confirmed by the decreased E-F slope and the calcification of both leaflets extending throughout the cardiac cycle. A myxoma would fall posterior to the mitral leaflet shortly after diastole occurred to cause multiple echoes behind the anterior leaflet.
- **C.** The left atrium is enlarged because of mitral valve disease and measures 5.2 cm.
- **D.** The left ventricle is normal. There is hyperdynamic septal motion.
  LVID ed = 4.8 cm
  LVID es = 2.4 cm

Case 3
- No; close evaluation will show a similar echo pattern on the anterior aortic wall. This wall thickness mea-

sures 0.8 cm, which is within normal limits. Asymmetrical thickening or widening of one wall more than 1.2 cm could represent a dissecting aneurysm.

Case 4
- Calcified mitral annulus, which commonly occurs when there is calcification of the aortic walls.

Case 5
- The right ventricle measures 3.0 cm at the *r* point on the ECG. This most likely indicates a right ventricular pressure overload. The septal motion appears to be normal in a sweep into the ventricular cavity to rule out volume overload. The most accurate diagnosis is ventricular septal defect or pulmonary stenosis.

Case 6
- The patient has multiple cardiac arrhythmias. To measure an accurate velocity, several "normal" E-F slopes should be measured and then an average value made.

Case 7
- There is a normal ratio shown between the aortic root and left atrial cavity, each measuring 3.2 cm.

Case 8
- Yes; normally the cusps show fine flutter in systole because of the high-pressure blood flow through them.

Case 9

A. The aortic root is enlarged (3.0 cm) in relation to the left atrial cavity.
B. Midsystolic sagging of the mitral apparatus represents prolapse.

Case 10

• Anterior and posterior pericardial effusion with electrical alternans on the ECG. The "swinging" heart is not as evident in this scan.

Case 11

• No; they most likely represent artifact echoes from the lung. As the sweep is made into the left atrial cavity, the echoes are lost. The tumor should be seen to flop back into the cavity during systole.

Case 12

A. From this scan it appears that the ALMV touches the septum, the E-F slope is decreased, and there is septal hypertrophy (2.0 cm). The anterior surface of the septum is ill-defined and should be further evaluated. The outflow tract of the left ventricle appears normal with no obstruction.
B. IVS measures 1 to 2 cm; C-E amplitude is 31 mm; E-F slope is 35 mm/sec. With better angulation of the transducer the septum is clearly defined and within normal limits. The mitral slope is decreased but is secondary to aortic stenosis and regurgitation. There is no IHSS.

Case 13

A. The mitral valve is well seen within the small left ventricular cavity. Although the amplitude is reduced, the E-F slope is normal. Decrease in gain separates the pericardium from the thickened posterior wall.

B. The aortic root is relatively flat, with early systolic closure of the aortic cusps caused by decreased cardiac output.
C. There may be minimal pericardial effusion in this patient with extreme concentric hypertrophy. The septum measures 1.8 cm, and the posterior wall measures 2.8 cm.

Case 14

• The mitral valve displays good C-E amplitude with a reduced E-F slope. The PLMV moves anterior, most likely representing mild mitral stenosis with good excursion. The possibility of mitral regurgitation should be considered. The left ventricle is within normal limits, and the right ventricle is top normal.

Case 15

A. Multiple echoes from lung interference make it difficult to record the mitral leaflet in its entirety. The E-F slope appears decreased, but that could be the effect of poor angulation.
B. The aortic root is flat with normal dimension compared with the left atrial cavity.
C. The pulmonary valve shows absent A wave and systolic flutter representing pulmonary hypertension secondary to cor pulmonale.

Case 16

A. Enlarged left ventricle with normal mitral valve apparatus.
B. Normal sized aortic root and left atrium, with increased echo formation in diastole most consistent with vegetations on the aortic valve. The enlarged left ventricle is secondary to aortic insufficiency, although no flutter was seen on the mitral apparatus.

PART THREE ABDOMEN

17 □ Anatomic relationships

The embryologic development of all abdominal organs occurs retroperitoneally, and many protrude into the peritoneum after full development has taken place. The kidneys and ureters remain retroperitoneal, whereas the other organs protrude into the peritoneum or become surrounded by it.

The peritoneum is subdivided into the omentum and the mesentery. The omentum is a double layer of peritoneum folded near the stomach; the mesentery is a double layer of peritoneum folded onto bowel. Parts of the colon become retroperitoneal as development progresses. The greater omentum covers the small bowel and large intestine like fatty glycerin.

The abdominal cavity (excluding the retroperitoneum and pelvis) is bounded superiorly by the diaphragm, anteriorly by abdominal wall muscles, posteriorly by vertebral column ribs and the iliac fossa, and inferiorly by the pelvis.

Liver

The diaphragmatic surface of the liver comprises the right and left lobes, with the falciform ligament separating each lobe. Within this ligament is a round fibrous cord, the teres ligament of the liver, which represents the old umbilical vein. The left lobe reaches to approximately 1 inch below the nipple. The visceral surface of the liver is subdivided into four lobes—right, left, anterior quadrate, and posterior caudate.

Vascular access to the liver is through the porta hepatis by the portal vein and hepatic artery. The portal triad that contains these two vessels also contains the common bile duct.

Pancreas

The pancreas is a retroperitoneal gland that is bounded anteriorly by the stomach and posteriorly by the prevertebral vessels.

Spleen

The spleen, a small organ, has a smooth, convex, diaphragmatic surface that fits under the diaphragm in the left upper quadrant. The hilus of the spleen contains the splenic artery and vein. It also has gastric, renal, and colic surface relationships.

Digestive tract

The esophagus descends from the thorax to enter the upper abdomen through the diaphragm and becomes continuous with the stomach. The stomach is a J-shaped structure anteriorly related to the thoracic cavity and muscles of the abdominal wall. It contacts the left lobe of the liver (the gastric area on the visceral surface of the liver). Posterior to the bed of the stomach lies the pancreas, with a layer of peritoneum separating the two structures. The greater curvature contacts the transverse colon. The stomach is divided into fundus, body, antrum and pyloric region, which turns into the duodenum. The duodenum remains retroperitoneal throughout development.

The intestine is suspended by the mesentery to give it greater mobility. The junction between the ileum and the cecum occurs on the right side of the abdomen. Much of the large ascending colon is retroperitoneal to the hepatic flexure. The transverse colon is a free structure, suspended by the mesentery, whereas the splenic flexure to the descending colon is retroperitoneal to the sigmoid mesocolon, which is surrounded by mesentery.

Thus the pancreas, duodenum, and ascending and descending colon are all retroperitoneal structures. The psoas muscles stretch into the lower pelvis to form the iliacus muscle, which outlines the true pelvic cavity.

Vessels

The major vessels are related to the posterior abdominal wall with branches to visceral organs. The blood supply for the gonads is near the renal artery throughout development. The left gonadal vein drains into the left renal vein.

Kidneys

The kidneys rest on the psoas and quadratus lumborum muscles in the retroperitoneal cavity. The left kidney contacts the spleen, pancreas, colon, and jejunum, and its superior medial pole holds the suprarenal gland. The right kidney contacts the liver, colon, and suprarenal gland. They are protected posteriorly by the eleventh and twelfth ribs. The inferior poles are not well protected, except for the quadratus lumborum muscles. On their medial surface is the exit of the renal veins and entrance of renal arteries. The renal pelvis is also at the hilus of the kidney to form the ureter that narrows to flow posteriorly into the pelvis to the bladder. The kidneys develop in the true pelvis and ascend into the abdomen. Occasionally, the inferior poles will fuse together, and the upper pole will ascend into the mesentery at the site of the inferior mesenteric artery to form a horseshoe kidney.

• • •

The sonographer must have a solid knowledge of gross anatomy, including cross-sectional and sagittal planes. Although "normal" anatomy is often illustrated throughout this book, the student must keep in mind the numerous variations that can occur in the anatomic structure. Thus organ and vessel relationships to neighboring structures should be carefully evaluated rather than memorizing at what point in the abdomen a particular structure should occur. For example, it is better to recall the location of the gallbladder as anterior to the right kidney and medial to the liver than to remember it is usually found at 6 to 8 cm above the umbilicus. The transverse anatomy guide should aid the reader in reviewing the illustrations throughout the abdominal chapters.

In Figs. 17-1 to 17-14 the transverse anatomic sections were obtained from an elderly woman with a number of pathologic disorders. Rheumatic disease of her heart left calcification on her aortic and mitral valves. The left atrial cavity was enlarged, and the left ventricular cavity demonstrated increased wall thickening. The pancreas was in an oblique lie and was huge, extending throughout several transverse sections yet maintaining its relationship to the prevertebral vessels. The gallbladder likewise was distended on several sections. The bowel was somewhat redundant, extending into the upper abdomen to the lower extent of the pelvis. Transverse cross sections were made at 2 cm increments. X = xyphoid; I = inferior; S = superior.

Text continued on p. 246.

TRANSVERSE ANATOMY GUIDE

AsA	Ascending aorta	**IVS**	Interventricular septum	**TL**	Teres ligament
DsA	Descending aorta	**D**	Diaphragm	**SMA**	Superior mesenteric artery
SVC	Superior vena cava	**L**	Liver	**SMV**	Superior mesenteric vein
MSB	Main-stem bronchus	**FL**	Falciform ligament	**RK**	Right kidney
E	Esophagus	**PC**	Peritoneal cavity	**LK**	Left kidney
OF	Oblique fissure	**CL**	Caudate lobe	**LRV**	Left renal vein
RL	Right lung	**RLL**	Right lobe of liver	**LRA**	Left renal artery
PA	Pulmonary artery	**LLL**	Left lobe of liver	**RRV**	Right renal vein
B	Bronchus	**VL**	Venous ligament	**RRA**	Right renal artery
LowLL	Lower lobe of left lung	**St**	Stomach	**I**	Ileum
PT	Pulmonary trunk	**LS**	Lesser sac	**Du**	Duodenum
PB	Pulmonary branch	**S**	Spleen	**GB**	Gallbladder
Stm	Sternum	**LGA**	Left gastric artery	**Py**	Pylorus
LA	Left atrium	**P**	Pancreas	**Ps**	Psoas
RAr	Right auricle	**PV**	Portal vein	**Du-J**	Duodenal-jejunal flexure
RA	Right atrium	**CBD**	Common bile duct	**GDA**	Gastroduodenal artery
PV	Pulmonary vein	**HA**	Hepatic artery	**SFC**	Splenic flexure colon
PS	Pericardial sac	**CT**	Celiac trunk	**DsC**	Descending colon
POT	Pulmonary outflow tract	**SA**	Splenic artery	**SmI**	Small intestine
RCA	Right coronary artery	**SV**	Splenic vein	**IMA**	Inferior mesenteric artery
MV	Mitral valve	**RSG**	Right suprarenal gland	**HF**	Hepatic flexure
RV	Right ventricle	**LSG**	Left suprarenal gland	**CA**	Celiac artery
TV	Tricuspid valve	**RF**	Retroperitoneal fat	**Ad**	Adrenal gland

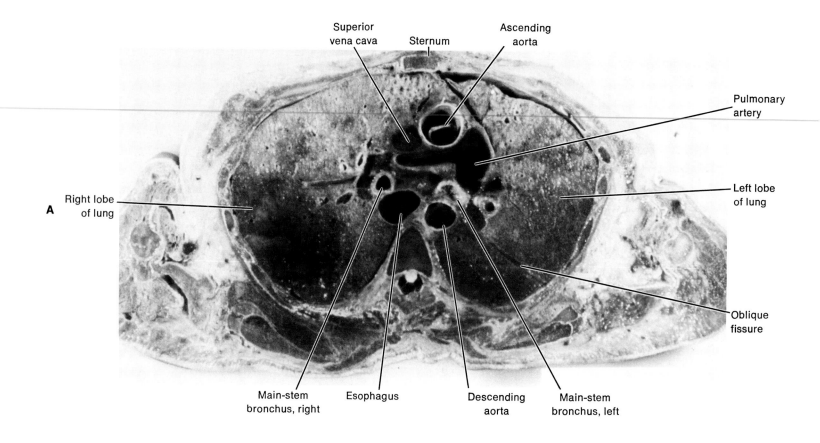

Superior vena cava   Sternum   Ascending aorta

Pulmonary artery

Right lobe of lung

A

Left lobe of lung

Oblique fissure

Main-stem bronchus, right   Esophagus   Descending aorta   Main-stem bronchus, left

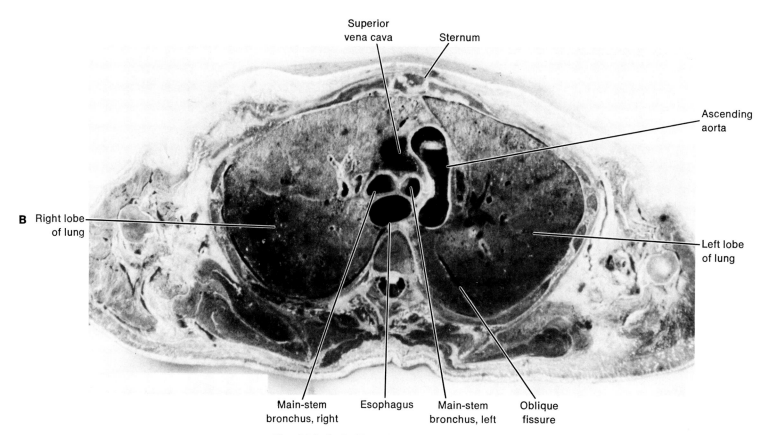

Superior vena cava   Sternum

Ascending aorta

B   Right lobe of lung

Left lobe of lung

Oblique fissure

Main-stem bronchus, right   Esophagus   Main-stem bronchus, left   Oblique fissure

Fig. 17-1. A, S; X + 10 cm. **B,** I; X + 10 cm.

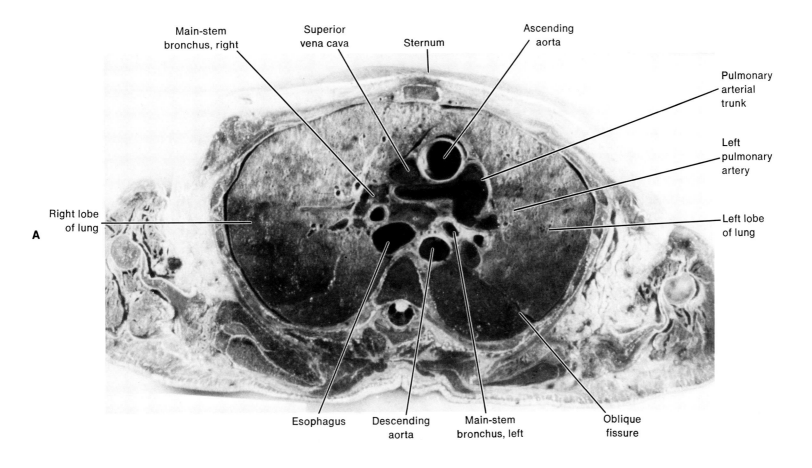

Main-stem bronchus, right
Superior vena cava
Sternum
Ascending aorta
Pulmonary arterial trunk
Left pulmonary artery
Right lobe of lung
Left lobe of lung
A
Esophagus
Descending aorta
Main-stem bronchus, left
Oblique fissure

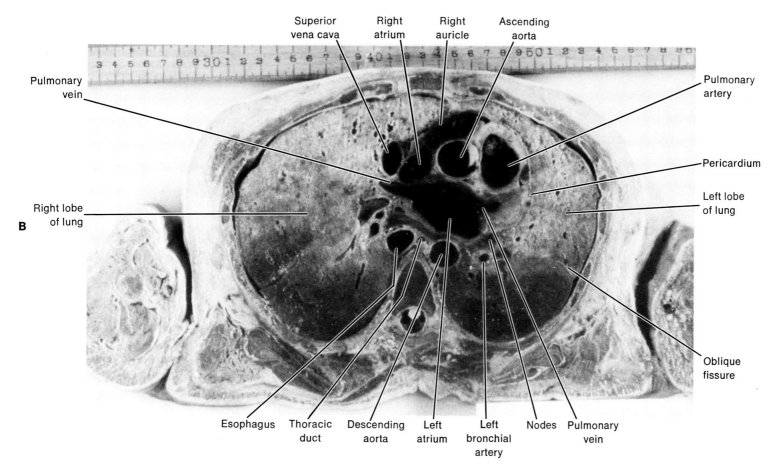

Superior vena cava
Right atrium
Right auricle
Ascending aorta
Pulmonary vein
Pulmonary artery
Pericardium
Right lobe of lung
Left lobe of lung
B
Esophagus
Thoracic duct
Descending aorta
Left atrium
Left bronchial artery
Nodes
Pulmonary vein
Oblique fissure

Fig. 17-2. A, S; X + 8 cm. **B,** I; X + 8 cm.

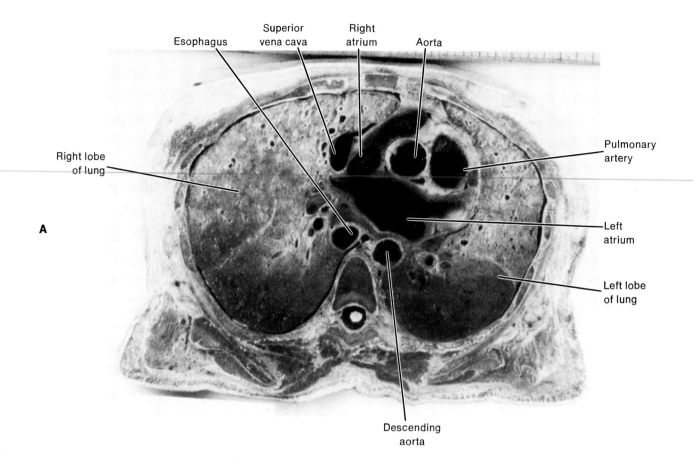

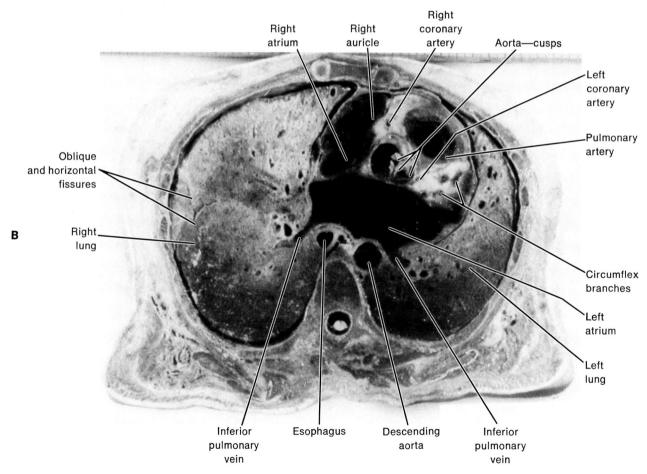

Fig. 17-3. A, S; X + 6 cm. **B,** I; X + 6 cm.

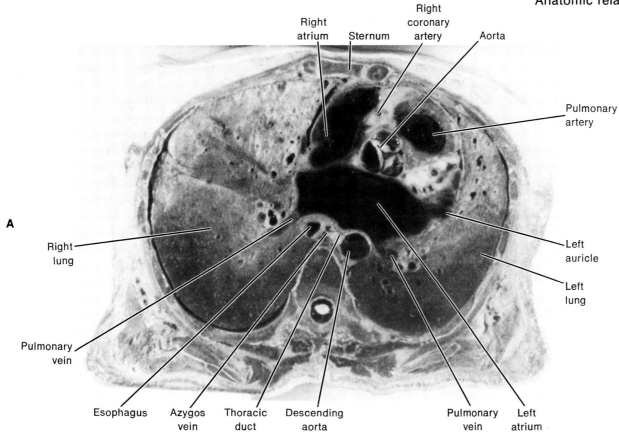

A

Right atrium
Sternum
Right coronary artery
Aorta
Pulmonary artery
Left auricle
Left lung
Right lung
Pulmonary vein
Esophagus
Azygos vein
Thoracic duct
Descending aorta
Pulmonary vein
Left atrium

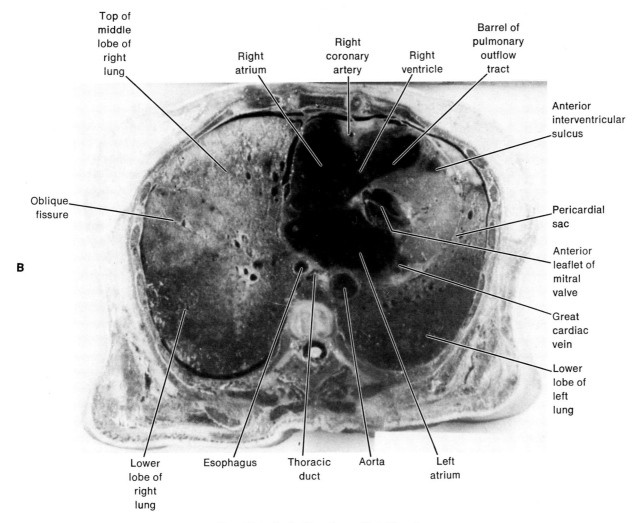

B

Top of middle lobe of right lung
Right atrium
Right coronary artery
Right ventricle
Barrel of pulmonary outflow tract
Anterior interventricular sulcus
Oblique fissure
Pericardial sac
Anterior leaflet of mitral valve
Great cardiac vein
Lower lobe of left lung
Lower lobe of right lung
Esophagus
Thoracic duct
Aorta
Left atrium

Fig. 17-4. A, S; X + 4 cm. **B,** I; X + 4 cm.

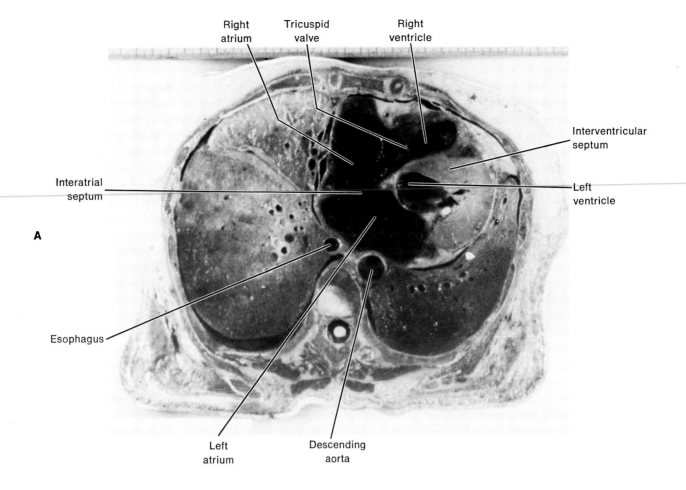

A

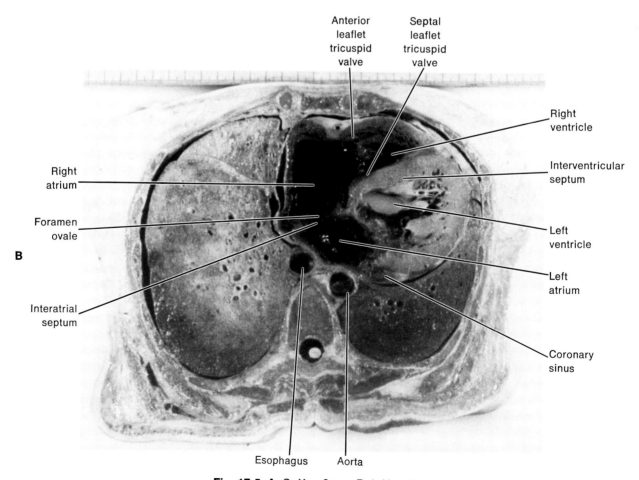

B

Fig. 17-5. A, S; X + 2 cm. **B,** I; X + 2 cm.

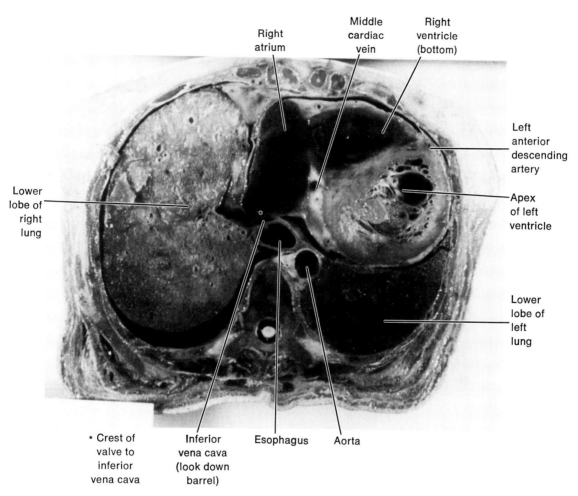

Right
atrium

Middle
cardiac
vein

Right
ventricle
(bottom)

Left
anterior
descending
artery

Lower
lobe of
right
lung

Apex
of left
ventricle

Lower
lobe of
left
lung

* Crest of
valve to
inferior
vena cava

Inferior
vena cava
(look down
barrel)

Esophagus

Aorta

Fig. 17-6. Xyphoid.

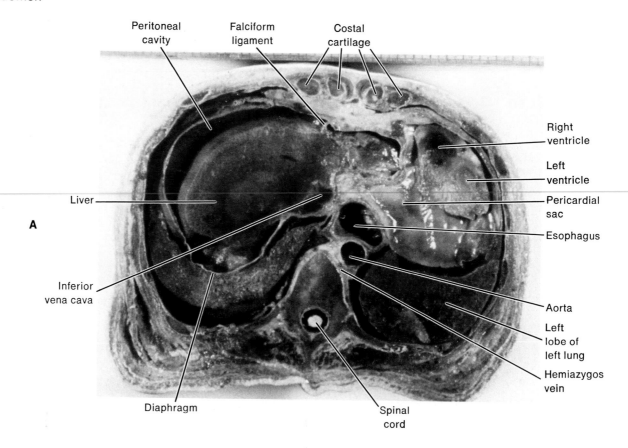

Peritoneal cavity

Falciform ligament

Costal cartilage

Right ventricle

Left ventricle

Pericardial sac

Esophagus

Liver

A

Inferior vena cava

Aorta

Left lobe of left lung

Hemiazygos vein

Diaphragm

Spinal cord

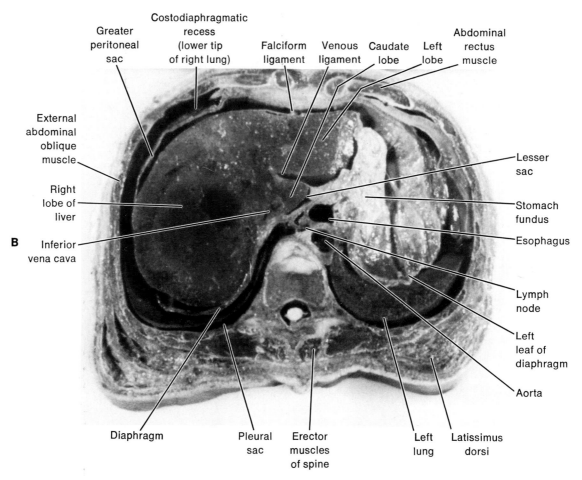

Costodiaphragmatic recess (lower tip of right lung)

Greater peritoneal sac

Falciform ligament

Venous ligament

Caudate lobe

Left lobe

Abdominal rectus muscle

External abdominal oblique muscle

Lesser sac

Right lobe of liver

Stomach fundus

B

Inferior vena cava

Esophagus

Lymph node

Left leaf of diaphragm

Aorta

Diaphragm

Pleural sac

Erector muscles of spine

Left lung

Latissimus dorsi

Fig. 17-7. A, S; X − 2 cm. **B,** I; X − 2 cm.

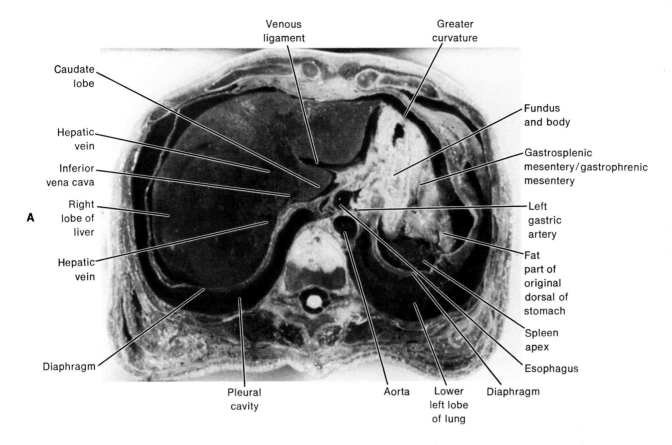

Venous ligament
Greater curvature
Caudate lobe
Hepatic vein
Inferior vena cava
Right lobe of liver
Hepatic vein
Diaphragm
Pleural cavity
Aorta
Lower left lobe of lung
Diaphragm
Esophagus
Spleen apex
Fat part of original dorsal of stomach
Left gastric artery
Gastrosplenic mesentery/gastrophrenic mesentery
Fundus and body

A

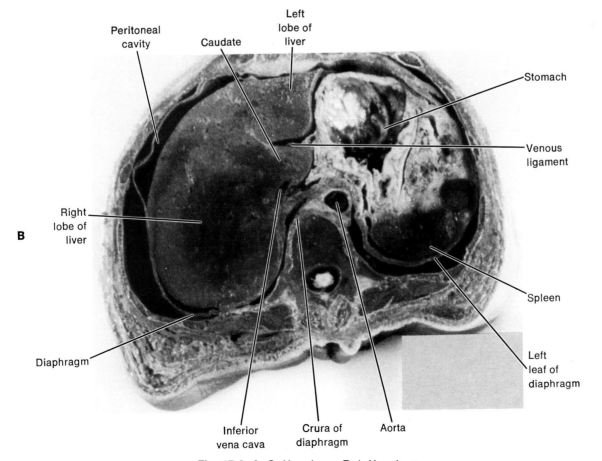

Left lobe of liver
Peritoneal cavity
Caudate
Stomach
Right lobe of liver
Venous ligament
Diaphragm
Spleen
Left leaf of diaphragm
Inferior vena cava
Crura of diaphragm
Aorta

B

Fig. 17-8. A, S; X − 4 cm. **B,** I; X − 4 cm.

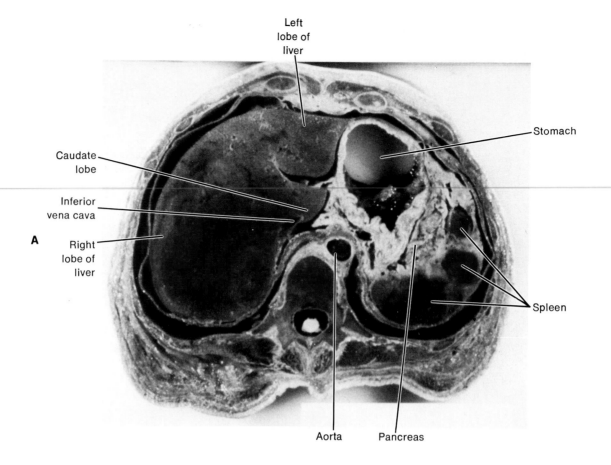

A

Left lobe of liver

Caudate lobe

Inferior vena cava

Right lobe of liver

Stomach

Spleen

Aorta   Pancreas

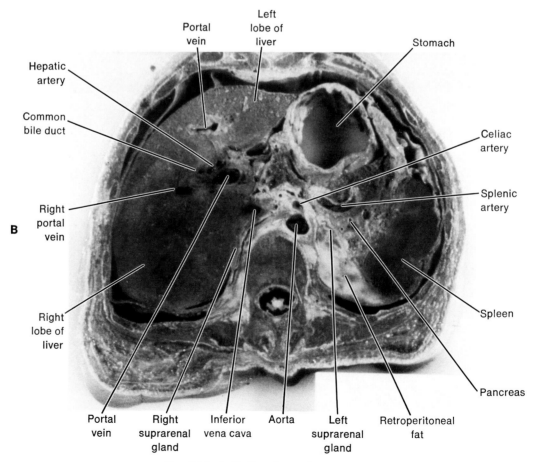

B

Portal vein

Left lobe of liver

Stomach

Hepatic artery

Common bile duct

Right portal vein

Right lobe of liver

Celiac artery

Splenic artery

Spleen

Pancreas

Portal vein

Right suprarenal gland

Inferior vena cava

Aorta

Left suprarenal gland

Retroperitoneal fat

Fig. 17-9. A, S; X − 6 cm. **B,** I; X − 6 cm.

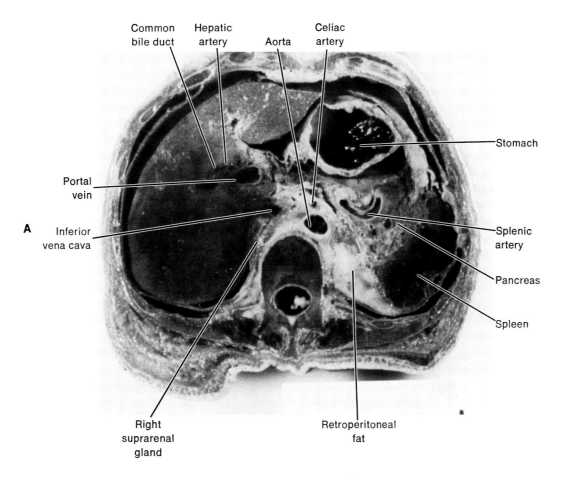

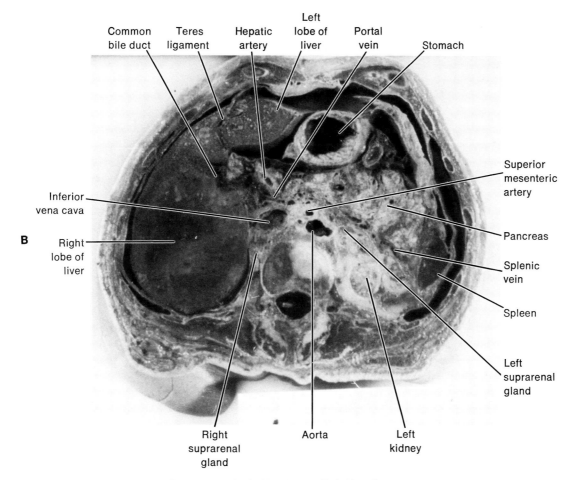

Fig. 17-10. A, S; X − 8 cm. **B,** I; X − 8 cm.

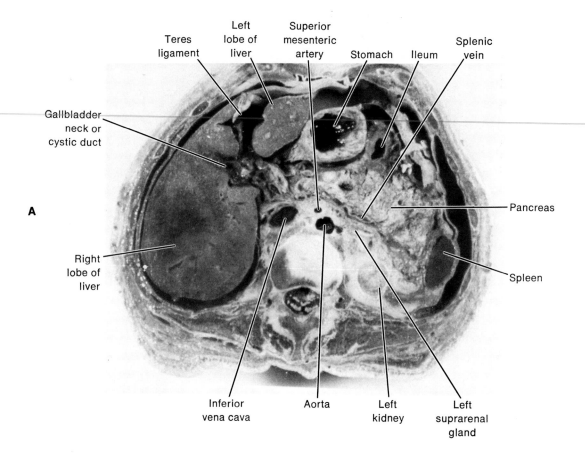

A

Teres ligament — Left lobe of liver — Superior mesenteric artery — Stomach — Ileum — Splenic vein

Gallbladder neck or cystic duct

Right lobe of liver

Pancreas

Spleen

Inferior vena cava — Aorta — Left kidney — Left suprarenal gland

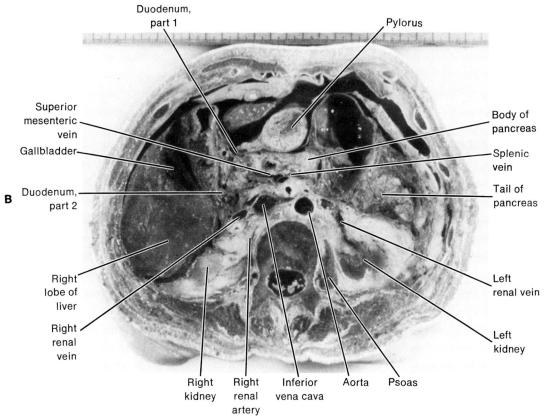

B

Duodenum, part 1 — Pylorus

Superior mesenteric vein

Gallbladder

Body of pancreas

Splenic vein

Duodenum, part 2

Tail of pancreas

Right lobe of liver

Right renal vein

Left renal vein

Left kidney

Right kidney — Right renal artery — Inferior vena cava — Aorta — Psoas

Fig. 17-11. A, S; X − 10 cm. **B,** I; X − 10 cm.

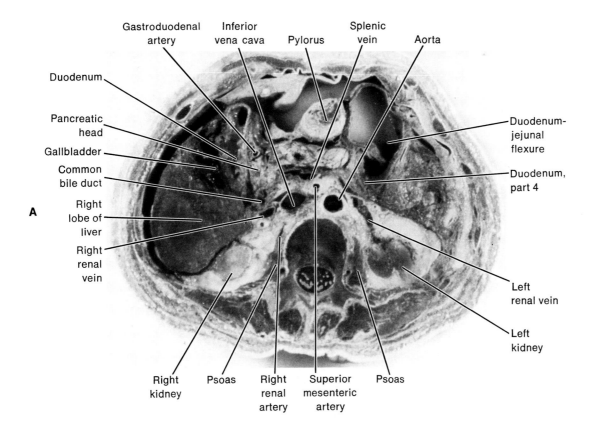

A

Gastroduodenal artery

Inferior vena cava

Pylorus

Splenic vein

Aorta

Duodenum

Pancreatic head

Gallbladder

Common bile duct

Right lobe of liver

Right renal vein

Duodenum-jejunal flexure

Duodenum, part 4

Left renal vein

Left kidney

Right kidney

Psoas

Right renal artery

Superior mesenteric artery

Psoas

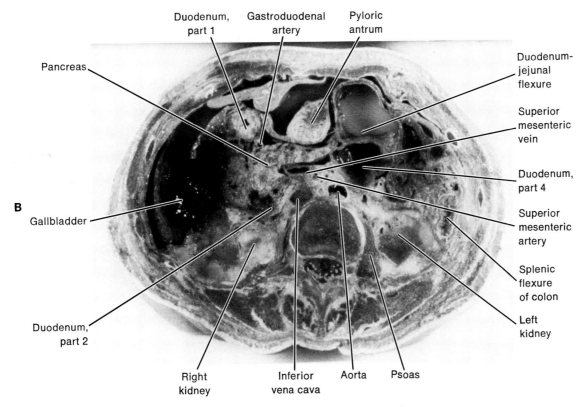

B

Duodenum, part 1

Gastroduodenal artery

Pyloric antrum

Pancreas

Gallbladder

Duodenum, part 2

Duodenum-jejunal flexure

Superior mesenteric vein

Duodenum, part 4

Superior mesenteric artery

Splenic flexure of colon

Left kidney

Right kidney

Inferior vena cava

Aorta

Psoas

Fig. 17-12. A, S; X − 12 cm. **B,** I; X − 12 cm.

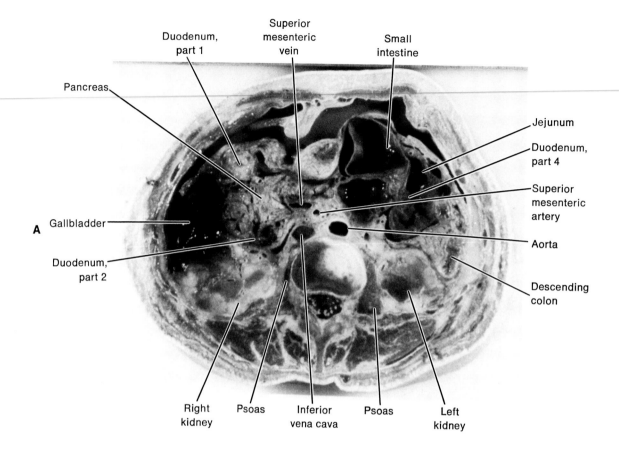

Duodenum, part 1

Superior mesenteric vein

Small intestine

Pancreas

Jejunum

Duodenum, part 4

Superior mesenteric artery

A Gallbladder

Aorta

Duodenum, part 2

Descending colon

Right kidney

Psoas

Inferior vena cava

Psoas

Left kidney

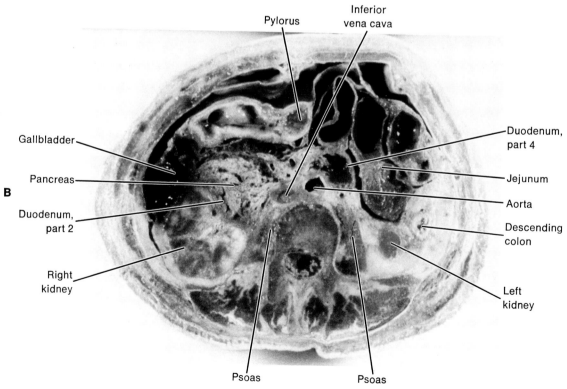

Pylorus

Inferior vena cava

Gallbladder

Duodenum, part 4

Pancreas

Jejunum

B

Aorta

Duodenum, part 2

Descending colon

Right kidney

Left kidney

Psoas

Psoas

Fig. 17-13. A, S; X − 14 cm. **B,** I; X − 14 cm.

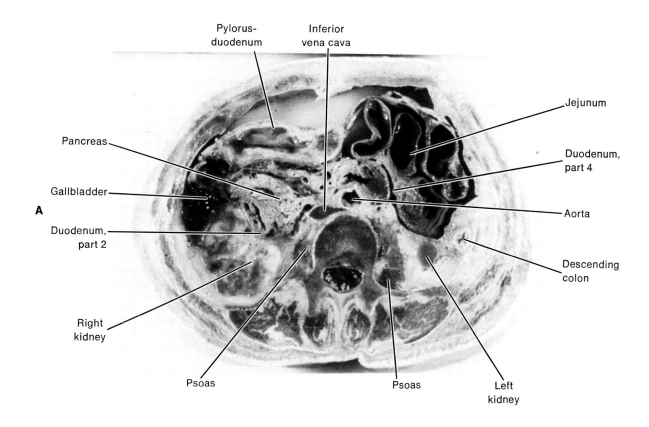

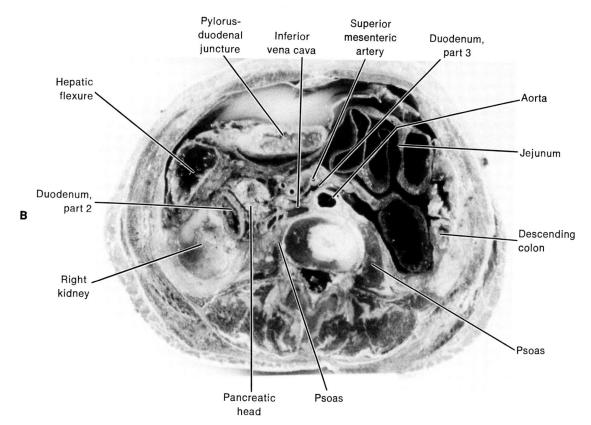

Fig. 17-14. A, S; X − 16 cm. **B,** I; X − 16 cm.

These longitudinal abbreviations apply to the sagittal sections and should be used to interpret the ultrasonic scans.

LONGITUDINAL ANATOMY GUIDE

S	Spleen	RA	Right atrium
C	Colon	SB	Small bowel
Ps	Psoas	U	Uterus
LK	Left kidney	PV	Portal vein
RK	Right kidney	B	Bladder
L	Liver	R	Rectum
H	Heart	Lg	Lung
IVC	Inferior vena cava	St	Stomach

The longitudinal gross anatomic sections were obtained from an elderly woman who had undergone a right thoracotomy. As a result of this surgery, the heart shifted its normal position to lie in the right thoracic cavity. She also had slight scoliosis, which shifted her spine to the right.

Fig. 17-15 begins at the right lateral border of the abdominal cavity. Figs. 17-16 to 17-24 are slices made approximately 2 cm apart. R = right; L = left.

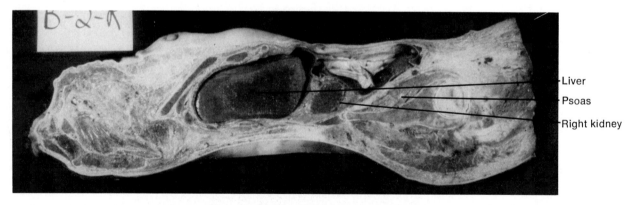

Fig. 17-15. R + 9 cm.

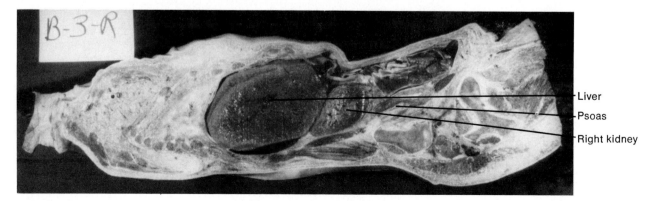

Fig. 17-16. R + 7 cm.

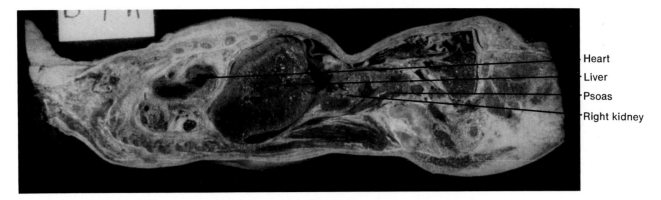

- Heart
- Liver
- Psoas
- Right kidney

Fig. 17-17. R + 5 cm.

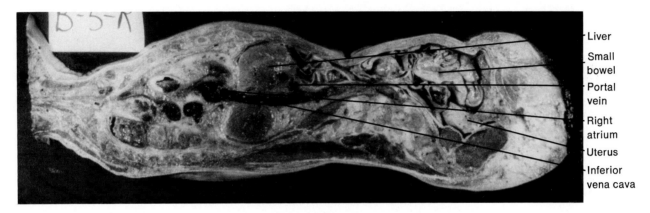

- Liver
- Small bowel
- Portal vein
- Right atrium
- Uterus
- Inferior vena cava

Fig. 17-18. R + 3 cm.

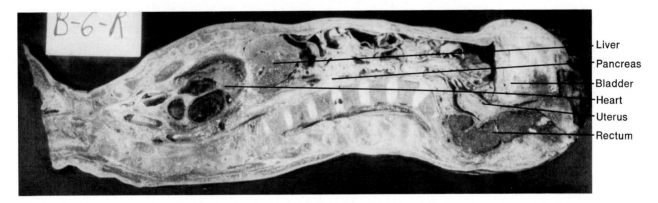

- Liver
- Pancreas
- Bladder
- Heart
- Uterus
- Rectum

Fig. 17-19. R + 1 cm.

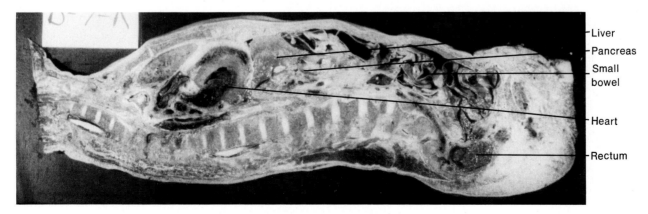

- Liver
- Pancreas
- Small bowel
- Heart
- Rectum

Fig. 17-20. L − 1 cm.

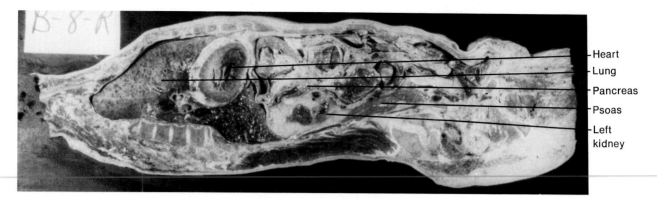

Heart
Lung
Pancreas
Psoas
Left kidney

Fig. 17-21. L − 3 cm.

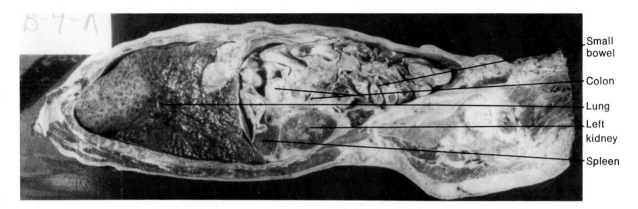

Small bowel
Colon
Lung
Left kidney
Spleen

Fig. 17-22. L − 5 cm.

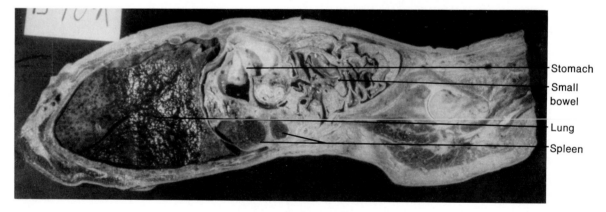

Stomach
Small bowel
Lung
Spleen

Fig. 17-23. L − 7 cm.

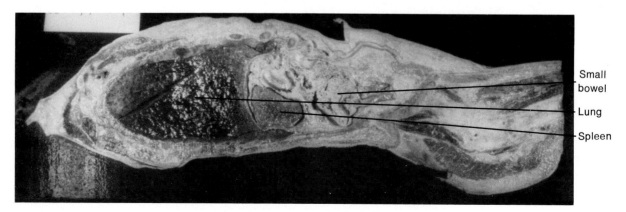

Small bowel
Lung
Spleen

Fig. 17-24. L − 9 cm.

18 □ Ultrasonic detection techniques

The state of the art of ultrasound demands a high degree of manual dexterity and hand-eye coordination. This applies to all branches currently making use of ultrasonic interpretation, that is, neurology, cardiology, abdominal studies, obstetrics, and gynecology. Specific applications of B scanning will be further discussed in this chapter, and other applications are discussed in later chapters.

To obtain expertise in scanning technique, the sonographer must be thoroughly familiar with anatomy, pathology, patient contours, machine capabilities, and transducer characteristics. Although it is difficult to appreciate scanning technique from a book, individual training in diagnostic ultrasound is part of the sonographer's experience in producing high-quality scans. The sonographer must be familiar with special scanning techniques, artifacts, and equipment malfunction to consistently produce quality scans. Automated ultrasonic equipment is currently being clinically evaluated for more efficient diagnostic results. Such units would replace the "art" in most of the scanning, in turn allowing the sonographer to fully concentrate on anatomy and pathology. However, until these units are commercially available, current contact scanners will have to be utilized.

With the advent of scan convertors for grey scale, some of the "art" in performing an adequate scan has been removed. By performing single scans with very slight sectoring motion, high-quality ultrasonograms can be made.

Ultrasound has the capability of distinguishing interfaces among soft tissue structures of different acoustic densities. The strength of the echoes reflected is dependent on the acoustic interface and the angle at which the sound beam strikes the interface. It is for this reason that a compound sector-scanning motion is used to record a maximum number of interfaces. If too much sectoring is used, the scan will lose much of its detail; therefore the sonographer must judge during the performance of the scan when the scan is completed.

ORIENTATION TO LABELING

An orderly procedure should be used to identify the anatomic position where the transverse and longitudinal scans have been taken. The illustrations in this book have used the umbilicus or the symphysis pubis in the transverse supine position; in the sagittal supine position the xyphoid and umbilicus are used; for the prone position the iliac crest is used as a landmark (Fig. 18-1).

All transverse supine scans are oriented with the liver to the left. Prone transverse scans orient the liver to the right. Longitudinal scans present the patient's head to the left and feet to the right of the scan.

The umbilicus or iliac crest is usually considered zero point for the upper abdomen. Scans cephalad from this point are labeled "+"; scans below this point are labeled "−". Longitudinal scans use the patient's xyphoid, umbilicus, and symphysis to denote the midline of the scan. Right of the midline is designated

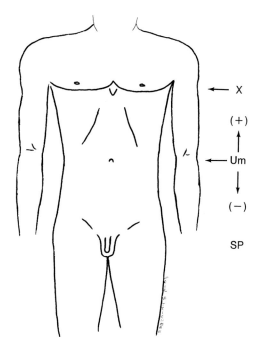

Fig. 18-1. Transverse labeling. *Um,* Umbilicus; *SP,* symphysis pubis; *X,* xyphoid.

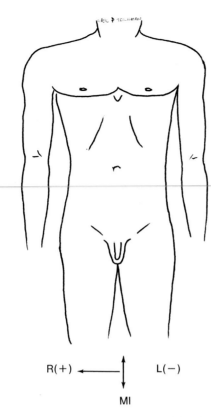

Fig. 18-2. Longitudinal labeling. *MI,* Midline.

"+," and a "−" is used for the left. For example, a scan made 2 cm to the right is R + 2 cm; a scan made 1.5 cm to the left is L − 1.5 cm (Fig. 18-2).

All scans should be appropriately labeled for future reference. This includes the patient's name, date, and anatomic position.

CRITERIA FOR AN ADEQUATE SCAN

Transverse scans

1. The horseshoe-shaped contour of the vertebral column should be well delineated to ensure that the sound is penetrating through the abdomen without obstruction from gas interference.

2. The prevertebral vessels should be well delineated anterior to the vertebral column. These are usually best demonstrated with a single "pie" sweep technique.

3. The posterior surface of the liver edge should be seen as the transducer is arced across the anterior abdominal wall. This ensures that the TGC is set correctly. If this posterior surface is not seen, the TGC may have to be broken earlier and the overall gain increased to allow adequate penetration. If there are too many echoes posterior to the liver, the overall gain should be decreased.

4. The individual organs should be well delineated with their specific echo patterns within their peripheral borders.

Sagittal scans

1. The diaphragmatic surface of the liver should be outlined to ascertain that the dome of the liver has been evaluated.

2. The posterior aspect of the liver should normally appear as the same fine echo pattern as the anterior surface. Gain adjustments should be made for overall penetration, or a lower-frequency transducer could be used for increased penetration to its posterior surface.

3. The prevertebral vessels should be outlined with a single sweep technique.

Abdominal scans are probably the most difficult to produce because of the multiple interfaces and curved surfaces within the abdominal cavity. Some laboratories will require the complete abdominal contour on each scan. Precise scanning technique is required to be able to demonstrate the vessels in the midline with a single "pie" sweep. Careful sector scanning along the lateral margin is necessary to outline the liver, the lateral and medial margins of both kidneys, and the spleen. Avoidance of the ribs is important to eliminate rib artifacts that may destroy necessary information. Quick sector scans over their borders usually work well to avoid these ring-down artifacts.

Automated equipment and real-time devices provide uniformity in scans for the unskilled sonographer. However, most of these complex machines provide so much detail and resolution that the sonographer must be well qualified in the areas of anatomy and pathology to produce optimum scans.

PROTOCOL PROCEDURE

Most laboratories will establish specific protocol procedures for each examination. This protocol provides uniformity and reproducibility in each examination performed. An example of our protocol follows, with brief notations on specific organ structures. All examinations are performed with their specific protocol. In addition, special or extra views of the area of interest may be included for individual examinations.

Aorta	Supine, longitudinal (midline, 0.5 cm intervals)
	Transverse (umbilicus, 2 cm intervals)
	If there is an aneurysm, define renal arteries on transverse; see if there is extension into the iliac; define thrombus.
Vessels	"Single sweep" transverse (xyphoid, 0.5 to 1 cm intervals); longitudinal (0.5 cm from midline to R + 5 cm and L − 3 cm)
	Deep inspiration
Liver	Supine, longitudinal (2 cm increments, deep inspiration)
	Transverse (xyphoid, 2 cm increments)
	Be sure gain is set for homogeneous stippling throughout liver

Gallbladder	Supine, transverse (xyphoid, 2 cm increments until area of GB is seen; then 0.5 cm increments)
	Oblique
	Longitudinal
	Decubitus
	Erect
Pancreas	Supine, transverse (xyphoid to area of aorta, SMA, SMV, splenic artery and vein to see area of pancreas; then scan at 0.5 cm increments)
	May have to angle cephalad or caudad
	Oblique 30° scan to determine entire outline of pancreas (if pancreas falls in this particular lie)
	Longitudinal (midline, 0.5 cm increments to demonstrate IVC, portal vein, aorta, SMA)
	Prone, transverse, and longitudinal to see left kidney, pancreas, and stomach relationship and size
Spleen	Supine, transverse (umbilicus, 2 cm increments)
	Longitudinal, for splenic size along length of spleen
	Prone, transverse (from top of spleen and left kidney caudad at 1 cm increments)
	Oblique, decubitus (between ninth and tenth ribs to see spleen, left kidney, and diaphragm)
Kidney	Localize renal area on intravenous pyelogram
	Prone, transverse (from iliac crest cephalad at 1 cm increments)
	Mark upper, middle, lower pole of kidney to define axis for complete view of longitudinal axis
	Longitudinal, midline of longitudinal axis (0.5 cm to either side of each kidney)
	Be sure to record kidney in longitudinal of three major areas: (1) pedicle, (2) calyceal system, (3) outer lateral border
	Full bladder
Gynecologic	Longitudinal (midline, 1 cm increments to either side until iliopsoas muscle is shown)
	Transverse cephalad angle to visualize bladder, uterus, and mass interface
	Full bladder
Obstetric	Longitudinal (midline, 2 to 3 cm increments to either side to cover full extent of uterus)
	Show fetal position, placenta, fetal trunk, and other areas of interest
	Transverse (3 cm increments to show BPD and thickness of placenta)
	Show head/thorax ratio
Thyroid (with and without water bath)	Transverse (sternal notch, 0.5 cm increments)
	Longitudinal (0.5 cm increments to visualize carotid and jugular with and without Valsalva maneuver)
Extremities (leg)	Prone, transverse (at knee joint, both legs together, 1 cm increments)
	Longitudinal (1 cm increments, both legs)
Breast	Check with staff first for area of interest
	Use bedstand: patient seated with breast on table
	Transverse (1 cm increments)
	Longitudinal (1 cm increments)

PHYSIOLOGIC ARTIFACTS

The examiner should recognize scanning artifacts and try to avoid them if possible. Slight alterations in normal scanning technique will be discussed for the multiple possibilities of artifacts.

Bowel and gas interference. Since air is a very strong reflector of sound, in the event of bowel gas interference it is best to postpone the examination and rescan the patient when this problem has been resolved. Gas is probably the most frequent problem encountered in scanning. The air reflects virtually all the sound, thus eliminating penetration to the deeper structure (Fig. 18-3). In our experience we have found it more practical to examine the abdominal patients early in the morning, eliminating most of the gas problems. Gentle pressure with the transducer can help to dissipate gas interference.

The patient may also be scanned in the prone position to avoid gas interference. Although most commercially available equipment does not allow the patient to be examined from the anterior abdominal surface while lying prone, the automated Octoson is helpful. This equipment houses eight transducers in a water bath tank. The plastic membrane across the open tank on the top of the machine allows excellent coupling with the anterior abdominal wall. The patient lies prone across the tabletop; thus the oil-coated membrane serves as an excellent coupler to the an-

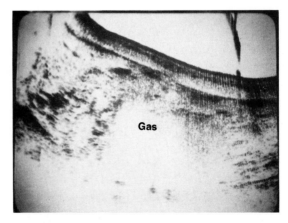

Fig. 18-3. Sagittal scan with gas shadow eliminating sound penetration.

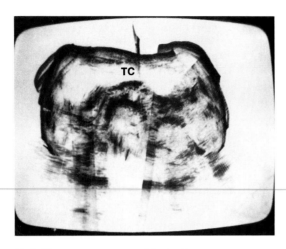

Fig. 18-4. Transverse scan of fluid-filled transverse colon.

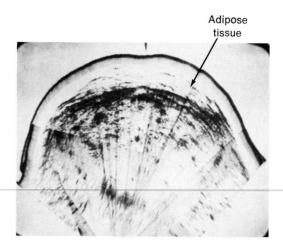

Fig. 18-5. Transverse scan of adipose tissue beneath crystal artifact extending 4 to 5 cm into the abdominal cavity.

terior wall, as well as a gas dissipator. The transducers are then directed to move along the anterior abdominal surface to record soft tissue images.

Simethicone (Mylicon-80) is the drug option to eliminate gas and has been used by several ultrasound laboratories in cases where repeat visualization proved unsuccessful.

Dilated loops of bowel may appear as a mass within the abdomen and may be mistaken for an abnormal growth. Several scans may outline the pattern of a fluid-filled loop of bowel. The transverse colon appears as a circle on the sagittal scan but drapes across the midline on transverse scans (Fig. 18-4). The descending and ascending colons appear as circles on most scans with a dark central core representing the mucosal folds with a sonolucent border. In the lower pelvic cavity dilated or obstructed bowel may be confused with a complex pelvic mass. Delineation of normal pelvic structures or evaluation of other diagnostic modalities (radiography) may help in the separation of a pelvic mass from a dilated bowel.

Barium. It has been clinically proved by Leopold and associates (1970) that barium contrast material has an adverse effect on the quality of abdominal and pelvic scans. Since barium causes significant attenuation, the ultrasound examination should be completed prior to the radiologic procedures when barium contrast material is being used. The other contrast materials used in intravenous pyelography, cholecystography, or arteriography do not affect the echogram quality.

Dehydration. Ultrasound travels better through a liquid medium than solid tissue. Therefore a patient suffering from dehydration may present difficulty in visualizing normal structures, since the lack of body fluids prevents changes in acoustic impedance to separate one structure from another.

Adipose tissue. Excessive obesity will present ultrasonically as a lightly stippled homogeneous echo pattern just beneath the crystal artifact. At first it appears as if the near gain is incorrectly adjusted. However, fine echoes will be seen throughout the fatty layer to allow the sonographer to identify the band as adipose tissue (Fig. 18-5).

Too full bladder. All pelvic scans should be performed with a distended bladder. If the bladder becomes too distended, the normal anatomy will be compressed and difficult to evaluate. Early pregnancy is especially difficult to evaluate in this condition. The patient should be told to void until she feels comfortable; thus enough urine should be retained to perform an adequate examination (Figs. 18-6 and 18-7).

EQUIPMENT ARTIFACTS

Gain control. Since each machine has its own particular sensitivity, or gain control, the sonographer should understand the complexity of these knobs to produce a quality scan. If the far gain is not set correctly, the echoes from the posterior aspect of the abdomen appear to fade out. This is usually corrected by adjusting the overall gain (attenuation, output, coarse gain) and time- and depth-gain compensation (TGC and DGC) until the near echoes are balanced with the far echoes. The slope of the curve should break just anterior to the deepest structure (Figs. 18-8 to 18-11). The near gain is independently controlled and should be adjusted to outline the anterior abdominal wall, muscles, and organ structures (Figs. 18-12 and 18-13). A higher-frequency transducer will produce a sharper near field, allowing more control with the near gain adjustment, but a decrease in penetration.

Contrast controls. Each ultrasonic machine with a scan convertor is capable of displaying the number of

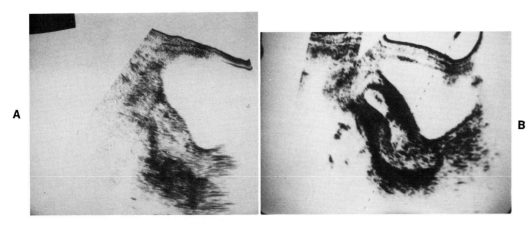

Fig. 18-6. **A,** Longitudinal scan of full bladder pressed against anterior uterine wall. **B,** Longitudinal scan of eight-week gestational sac compressed by full bladder.

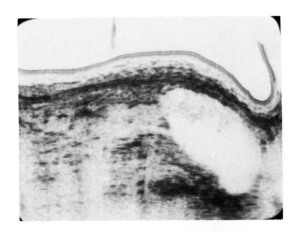

Fig. 18-7. If bladder is too full or gain too high, the uterine structures will not be identified.

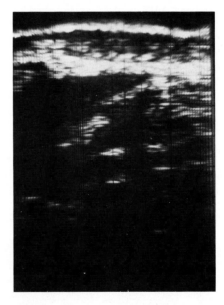

Fig. 18-8. Inadequate far gain barely allows outline of abdominal aorta.

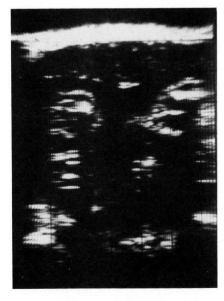

Fig. 18-9. Fetal extremities are barely delineated with inadequate far gain and low overall gain.

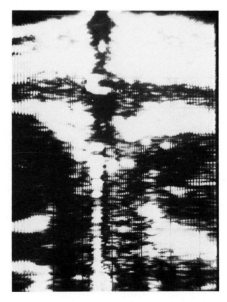

Fig. 18-10. Overcompensation of the gain controls destroys the fine detail information of the fetal skull and trunk.

shades of grey it can produce. A test pattern can be displayed on the monitor in an effort to photograph this grey scale (Fig. 18-14). The darkest to the lightest shade should be distinguishable; then compare the photographic results with the image on the monitor. Photographically the brightness and contrast controls may need to be adjusted to obtain an adequate image on the film. The background should be a light shade of grey to produce optimum grey scale on the Polaroid film.

Other contrast controls found on the equipment are *enhance* and/or *balance*. The enhance control may vary the image from very dark to very light, and thus the correct balance of echoes must be found to visualize low-level information (Fig. 18-15). Generally, it is best to leave this enhance control in a midway position. Some machines have a balance control that allows the operator to adjust the image presentation. If this is incorrectly set, the image will appear very

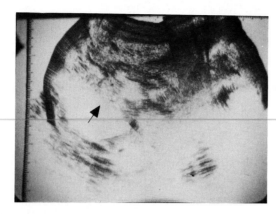

Fig. 18-11. Posterior liver is sometimes difficult to stipple in with fine echoes. Care must be taken not to mistake this "hole" for a mass. Rib artifacts can be seen lining the anterior surface of the "mass" (arrow). A lower-frequency transducer (1.6 MHz, 19 mm) may be used to stipple in fine echoes.

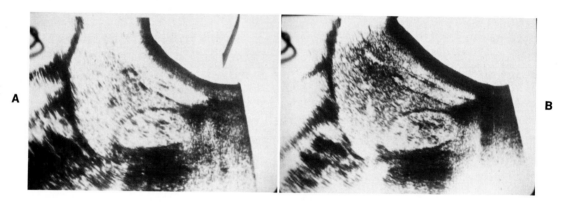

Fig. 18-12. A, Longitudinal scan of right upper quadrant with decreased near gain prohibits visualization of anterior peripheral tissue. B, Corrected gain allows uniform visualization of the liver and right kidney.

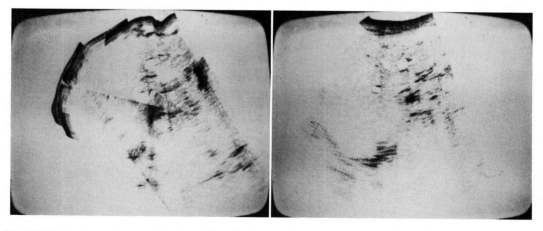

Fig. 18-13. Inadequate overall gain setting limits the diagnostic value of the scan. Both scans show limited liver and vessel detail.

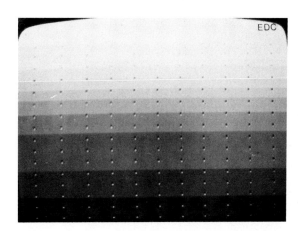

Fig. 18-14. Grey-scale test pattern to illustrate various shades of grey.

harsh. The balance control does not need to be re-adjusted once the optimum setting is attained.

Linear overwrite. The scan convertors are built to process only new information as the transducer sweeps across the abdomen. Several problems can occur with the scan convertor that will appear as visual signs on the monitor. If the transducer is moved too fast, linear blankout lines will appear throughout the scan (Fig. 18-16).* Conversely, if the transducer is held in one area too long "overwrite" will occur, demonstrated as a linear artifact (Fig. 18-17). Smooth continuous sweeps will eliminate these problems and allow the sonographer to obtain a diagnostic scan.

Scan convertor focus. The internal focus control on the scan convertor should be adjusted at the time of installation. This control allows the individual echo

*Each machine has its own writing speed with lines of information displayed on the monitor. Thus the sonographer must determine the optimum scan speed to produce a quality image.

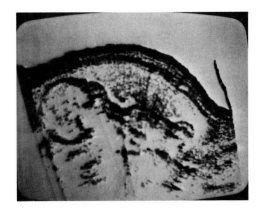

Fig. 18-15. Longitudinal scan of a third trimester pregnancy with poorly adjusted contrast controls. Grey-scale definition is lost.

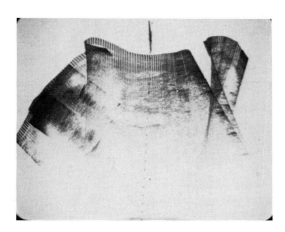

Fig. 18-16. Poor scanning technique. Initial pie sweep is performed too fast, leaving white blankout areas in the midline. Multiple rib artifacts are made along the lateral borders with no attempt to make the scan appear as a continuous skin layer.

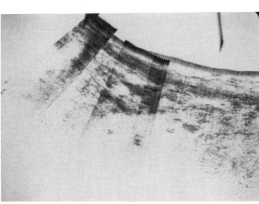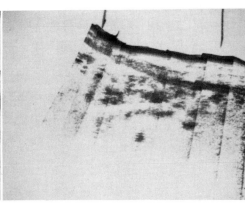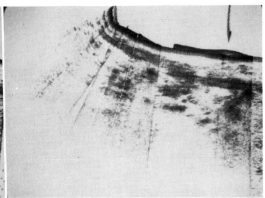

Fig. 18-17. Jerky sector technique with hesitation causes multiple dark lines throughout the longitudinal scan.

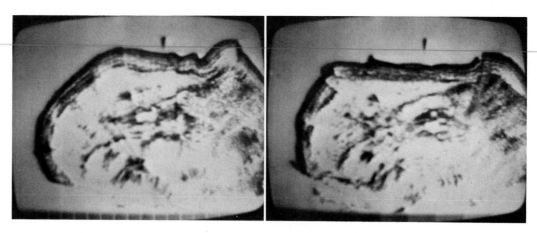

Fig. 18-18. Upper abdominal scans with scan convertor out of focus.

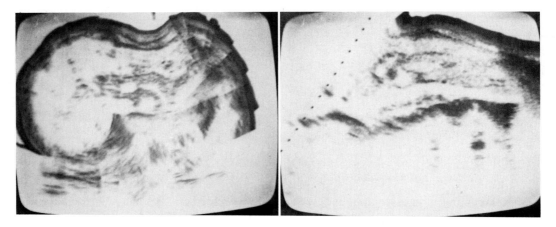

Fig. 18-19. Slight distortion of focus controls causes the image to appear blurred without sharp detail.

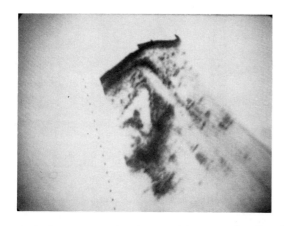

Fig. 18-20. Fetal scan with the machine out of calibration.

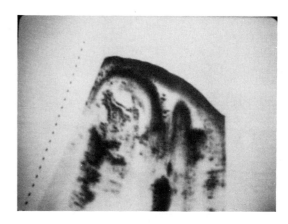

Fig. 18-21. Fetal thorax appears somewhat distorted because the machine is out of calibration.

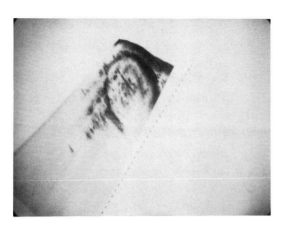

Fig. 18-22. Distorted fetal head with the machine out of calibration.

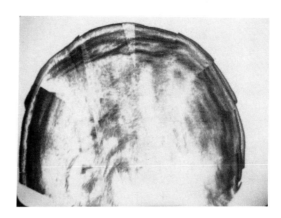

Fig. 18-23. Abdomen appears to be distorted in the vertical axis in comparison with the patient's size.

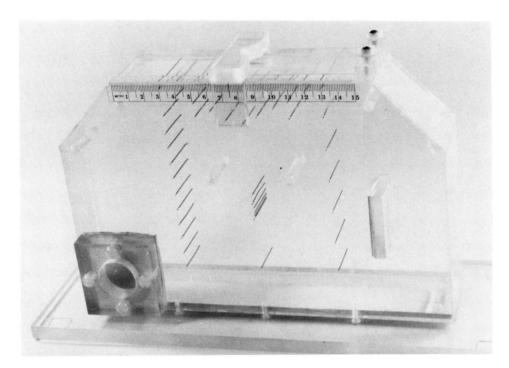

Fig. 18-24. American Institute of Ultrasound in Medicine (A.I.U.M.) test phantom.

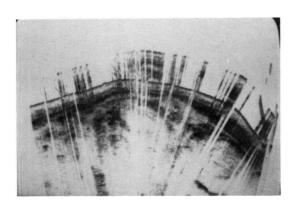

Fig. 18-25. Irregular artifact shown in longitudinal fetal scan.

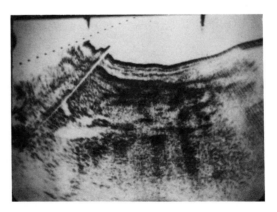

Fig. 18-26. "Swizzle stick" artifact caused by the internal function of the equipment.

reflection dots to be round and sharply focused. If this control is not adjusted properly or is knocked out of calibration from excessive moving of the equipment or electronic drifting, the image becomes very fuzzy and out of focus (Figs. 18-18 and 18-19). Detail will be lost as the machine loses its focus, and the service department should be called to adjust this control.

Equipment calibration. Each machine has x-y potentiometers within the scanning arm to plot the two-dimensional image on the screen. If these potentiometers become loose, broken, or damaged from extreme movement of the scanning arm, the third arm calibration of the machine is affected. The image will appear distorted, and depth measurements will be inaccurate. The sonographer may note the contour of the abdomen to appear egg-shaped. It is difficult to scan either side of the abdomen without irregular contours appearing on the monitor (Figs. 18-20 to 18-23).

The calibration may be evaluated more precisely by scanning the test phantom. (The American Institute of Ultrasound in Medicine recommends a standard test phantom that is commercially available.) This phantom is a device with several wires mounted within its water-filled central core. An acoustic gel is applied to the outside of the phantom, and the transducer is directed along the top and side borders to record reflections from the wire interfaces. The gain should be reduced to obtain a sharp image. One complete pass is made along the three walls of the phantom; the transducer is then angled the opposite way, and a repeat pass is made in the opposite direction. The end product should appear as perfect Xs throughout the phantom. If calibration is off, these Xs on the screen will appear as Ys, or pigeon feet.

Other artifacts. The sonographer can attain a feeling for what is real and reproducible from what is artifact as the scan is being performed (Figs. 18-24 and 18-25). Careful angulation to allow transducer perpendicularity to each structure without rib interference is necessary to produce a good scan (Fig. 18-26).

19 □ Liver

with assistance of
MARCIA LAVERY, R.T., R.D.M.S.

GROSS ANATOMY

The liver is the largest gland in the body, occupying almost all of the right hypochondrium, the greater part of the epigastrium, and usually extending into the left hypochondrium as far as the mammillary line (Fig. 19-1). The liver's greatest transverse measurement is 20 to 22.5 cm, and its vertical measurement near the lateral or right surface is 15 to 17.5 cm. The anteroposterior diameter near the level of the upper end of the right kidney is 10 to 12.5 cm.

Lobes

The liver can be subdivided into four lobes—right, left, caudate, and quadrate (Fig. 19-2). Each will be discussed separately.

Right lobe. The right lobe is the largest of the four lobes of the liver. In proportions it exceeds the left lobe size by a 6:1 ratio. It occupies the right hypochondrium. The left lobe is bordered on its upper surface by the falciform ligament, on the posterior surface by the left sagittal fossa, and in front by the umbilical

notch. The inferior and posterior surfaces of the right lobe are marked by three fossae—the porta hepatis, the gallbladder fossa, and the inferior vena cava fossa. A congenital anomaly of the right lobe of the liver, Riedel's lobe, can sometimes be seen as a downward projection of the liver.

Left lobe. This lobe is smaller and thinner than the right lobe. It lies in the epigastric and left hypochondriac regions. The upper surface is convex and molded onto the diaphragm. Its undersurface includes the gastric impression and omental tuberosity.

Caudate lobe. This small lobe is situated on the posterior surface of the right lobe, opposite the tenth and eleventh thoracic vertebrae. It is bounded below by the porta hepatis; on the right by the fossa for the

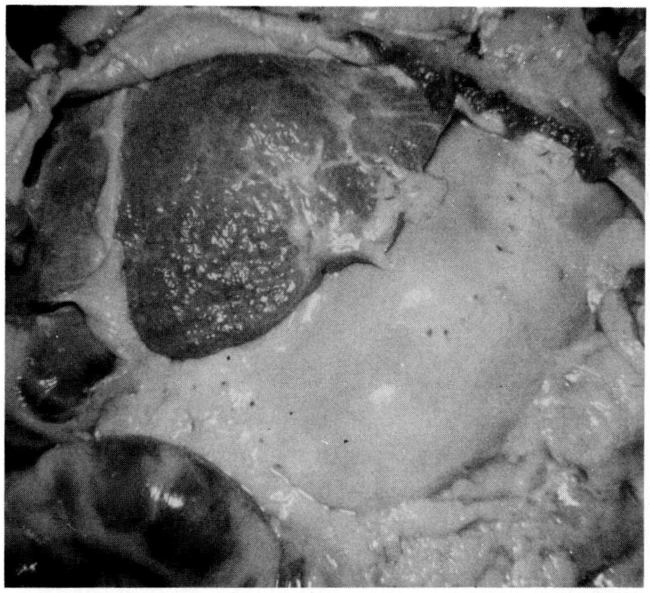

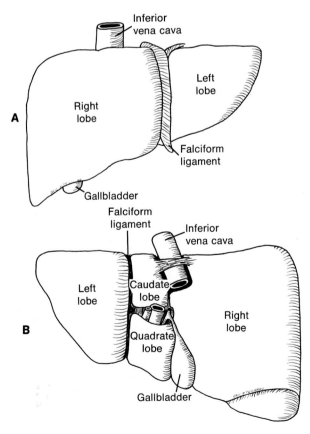

Fig. 19-2. A, Anterior view of the liver. **B,** Posterior view of the four lobes of the liver with the medial attachment of the gallbladder.

Fig. 19-1. Gross anatomic specimen of the upper abdominal cavity. The liver can be seen to the left of the stomach. The falciform ligament divides the right and left lobes.

inferior vena cava, and on the left by the fossa for the venous duct.

Quadrate lobe. This lobe is oblong and situated on the posterior surface of the right lobe of the liver. It is bounded in front by the anterior margin of the liver, behind by the porta hepatis, on the right by the fossa for the gallbladder, and on the left by the fossa for the umbilical vein.

Fossae

The left sagittal fossa separates the right and left lobes of the liver. The porta hepatis joins it at right angles and divides it into two parts.

The shallow, oblong gallbladder fossa is located on the undersurface of the right lobe. It extends from the anterior free margin of the liver to the right extremity of the porta hepatis.

The inferior vena cava fossa is a short depression on the posterior surface between the caudate lobe and bare area of the liver. The caudate lobe separates it from the portahepatis, a short deep fissure extending transversely across the undersurface of the left portion of the right lobe. It separates the quadrate lobe in front from the caudate lobe behind. The fossa transmits the portal vein, the hepatic artery and nerves, and the hepatic duct and lymphatics.

Vessels

An integral part of the hepatic system is composed of the venous, arterial, and biliary systems involved in hepatic function (Fig. 19-3).

Portal vein. The portal vein is formed by the junction of the splenic and superior mesenteric veins. It branches into the right and left portal veins shortly after entering the liver and then continues to branch until entering microscopic hepatic sinusoids (Fig. 19-4).

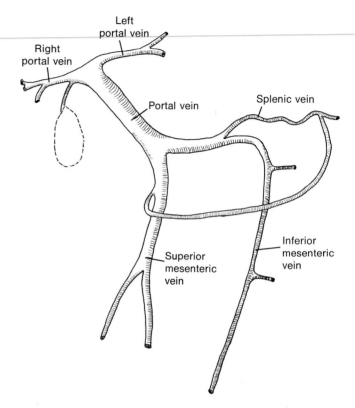

Fig. 19-3. Formation of the portal system with major contributions from the splenic and superior mesenteric veins.

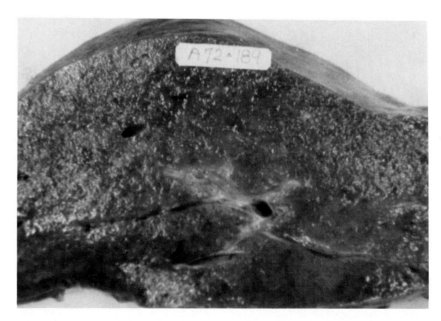

Fig. 19-4. Gross specimen of the liver. The dense vascular structures represent portal vessels and the smaller tubular structures the hepatic veins.

Hepatic vein. The hepatic vein commences in the substance of the liver, in the terminations of the portal vein and hepatic artery. The hepatic sinusoids empty into one vessel, the intralobular vein. These veins unite to form larger trunks and end at last in the hepatic veins. The hepatic veins converge to form three large trunks that open into the inferior vena cava located in its fossa on the posterior surface of the liver.

Hepatic artery. The hepatic artery enters the liver with the portal vein, and the hepatic duct ramifies with these vessels through the portal canals (Fig. 19-5).

Bile ducts

The bile ducts begin as communicating passages between two hepatic cells. They radiate to the circumference of the lobule and open into the interlobular ducts that run with the hepatic artery and portal vein back to the porta hepatis. The small ducts join to form the two main trunks, which leave the liver and then join to form the hepatic duct. The cystic duct joins the hepatic duct to form the common bile duct, which then enters the duodenum.

CROSS-SECTIONAL ANATOMY

Superior surface. The superior surface of the liver is convex and comprises a part of both lobes of the liver. Fitting under the vault of the diaphragm and lying behind the xyphoid process, it is completely covered by the peritoneum except along the line of attachment of the falciform ligament, which separates the right and left lobes.

Inferior surface. This surface is uneven and concave and is directed downward, backward, and to the left. It sits in relation to the stomach, duodenum, right colic flexure, right kidney, and right adrenal gland. It is also

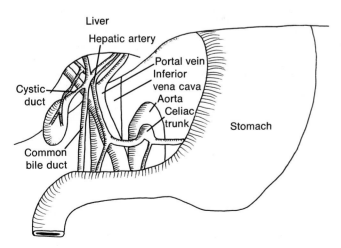

Fig. 19-5. Formation of the porta hepatis by the hepatic artery, portal vein, and common bile duct.

covered by peritoneum except where the gallbladder is attached and at the area of the porta hepatis.

Posterior surface. Behind the right lobes of the liver the posterior surface is round and broad, whereas behind the left lobe the surface is narrow. A large extent of the posterior surface is not covered by peritoneum. It is in direct contact with the diaphragm. The central part is concave and is molded on the vertebral column and the crura of the diaphragm. The inferior vena cava lies to the right of the vertebral column. The posterior surface also forms part of the posterior boundary of the porta hepatis.

Anterior surface. The anterior surface is thin and sharp. It is marked opposite the attachment of the falciform ligament by the deep, umbilical notch and opposite the cartilage of the ninth rib by the notch for the fundus of the gallbladder.

SAGITTAL ANATOMY

The superior border of the liver fits snugly into the diaphragm. The lower border of the pleural cavity often covers this section of the dome of the liver. The posterior surface is bounded by the right kidney and adrenal, the porta hepatis, and the inferior vena cava.

FUNCTION

The liver is considered the chemical factory of the body and has several functions. It is responsible for the metabolism of products of carbohydrate and protein digestion conveyed through the portal vein.

The liver also has an important role in the formation and destruction of red blood cells. It is the storage depot for vitamin B_{12}, which passes to the bone marrow for the normal development of red blood cells. It removes bilirubin, formed from broken-down red blood cells, from the blood and excretes this bilirubin through the bile duct into the duodenum. If this excretory pathway fails, the bilirubin accumulates in the blood and jaundice develops. The liver manufactures plasma proteins and forms blood clotting factors.

Besides storing glycogen, amino acids, fats, vitamins A, D, and B complex, iron, and copper, the liver is essential in maintaining the blood glucose level. It forms urea from ammonia, which results from the deamination of the surplus amino acids. This enables the carbon and hydrogen parts of these amino acids to be used for heat and energy. The bile salts produced by the liver aid in the digestion and absorption of fat.

LABORATORY TESTS FOR LIVER EVALUATION

There are several laboratory tests to help in the assessment of liver function. The two primary tests are for serum glutamic oxaloacetic transaminase (SGOT) and serum glutamic pyruvic transaminase (SGPT), both of which increase with hepatocellular disease. Direct bilirubin increases with obstruction, whereas indirect bilirubin increases with hepatocellular disease. Serum protein levels as well as prothrombin time decrease with hepatocellular disease. The fetal antigen is present in over 50% of patients with hepatomas.

CLINICAL SIGNS AND SYMPTOMS
Right upper quadrant pain

Cancer of the liver may cause pain in the right upper quadrant of the abdomen, associated with jaundice and loss of appetite but usually not with nausea or vomiting. Fever and weight loss may be present if the cancer is advanced. Physical examination reveals the enlarged liver with irregular tumor masses.

Pain in the right upper quadrant may be caused by cirrhosis of the liver, a complication of long-term heavy alcohol consumption. The patient reports a long history of heavy drinking and poor food intake, and there may be evidence of vitamin deficiency such as split lips or sore tongue. Jaundice may be present, but there is usually no fever. The liver may be sore to the touch. The pain of cirrhosis is a mild dull ache rather than the episodic, severe, crampy pain of gallstones.

A liver abscess causes severe pain in the right upper quadrant and is associated with fever and prostration.

Jaundice

Jaundice is characterized by the presence of bile in the tissue with resulting yellow-green color of the skin. In dark-skinned persons jaundice may be evident only in the white of the eye.

Enlarged liver

An enlarged liver may be the result of cancer, which may be either primary or spread from other areas. In both cases palpation reveals irregular areas due to the tumor. As productive liver tissue is replaced by tumor, loss of appetite and nausea ensue. As the liver cancer progresses, weight loss and extreme fatigue are noted.

Jaundice may be present early if a tumor mass blocks the outflow of bile, and in advanced disease jaundice is often intense. If the liver cancer has spread from other areas, such as the lung or stomach, there is evidence of tumor in those sites. There is no effective treatment. Successful surgical removal of a liver tumor is rare, and prognosis is unfavorable.

Chronic congestive heart failure is a common cause of liver enlargement, since back pressure from the heart causes the blood to pool in the liver. The patient demonstrates other evidence of heart failure, such as swollen ankles, weight gain, and shortness of breath when lying flat. The enlarged liver and congestive heart failure should respond promptly to treatment with digitalis, diuretics, and salt restriction.

ULTRASONIC EVALUATION

The time gain compensation should be set according to normal soft tissue attenuation, that is, 1dB/cm/MHz. Generally, this means that the slope of the gain curve can be slowly elevated so that the gradual break-off occurs around 15 cm from the initial main bang reflection. This means the near gain will be reduced and the far gain amplified to obtain an adequate scan. Most patients, front to back, measure approximately 15 cm to their posterior liver edge, which allows this technique to work consistently. The output should be adequate to produce low-level echoes of liver parenchyma on grey-scale equipment.

Various transducers may have to be used to obtain the optimum balance of echoes in the liver. Most average patients can be scanned with a 2.25 MHz transducer with a long focus (10 cm). Smaller patients may require a shorter focus and/or a higher-frequency transducer for maximum resolution. The larger, more muscular patients require the 1.6 MHz transducer for adequate penetration.

Supine transverse scans

The patient is generally positioned supine for the initial transverse liver scan. The transducer head should be angled slightly cephalad to obtain good con-

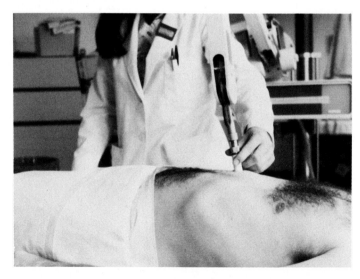

Fig. 19-6. Supine transverse scans of the abdomen should begin at the xyphoid. The transducer head should be angled slightly to visualize structures under the costal margin. A small-diameter transducer allows better penetration through the costal margin.

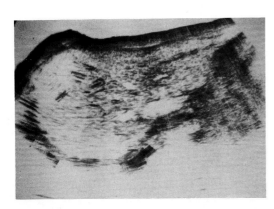

Fig. 19-7. Full scan of the liver parenchyma with slight sectoring along the lateral abdominal wall to fill in the right side of the liver wall and lateral margin of the spine.

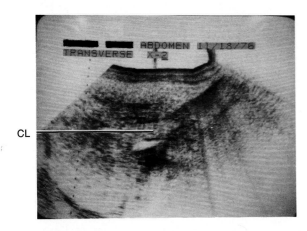

Fig. 19-8. Single sweep of the liver with normal liver pattern. The caudate lobe is shown just anterior to the inferior vena cava. This small lobe can vary in size and may be mistaken for an abnormal mass in the liver if careful evaluation is not made.

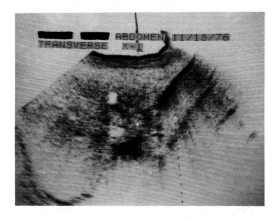

Fig. 19-9. Normal liver parenchyma with single scan technique.

tact between the patient's skin and the transducer. We have found it best to begin at the level of the xyphoid and move caudally by 2 cm intervals until the bottom of the right lobe of the liver is shown (Fig. 19-6). The patient should be scanned in full inspiration to record maximum detail of the liver parenchyma and vessels.

In transverse scans two separate techniques should be used to record maximum information. One is a compound scanning technique in which the transducer is sectored perpendicular to multiple interfaces to record the entire abdominal interface (Fig. 19-7). The sonographer should pie sweep the midline area and sector along the side of the abdomen while always angling the transducer back toward the spine. Often this technique can be done rapidly with the patient in suspended respiration. This allows a total view of the liver parenchyma and often helps in orientation purposes. Single scans are also very useful and often give maximum resolution when performed correctly. These scans are pie single sweeps. With the patient in full inspiration, the transducer is severely angled to one side of the abdomen and slowly arched across to a severe angle on the other side. It is important not to move the transducer across the abdomen; rather, arc the beam severely enough to record a large area in the sweep. This generally gives excellent visualization of the smaller vessels within the liver (Figs. 19-8 and 19-9).

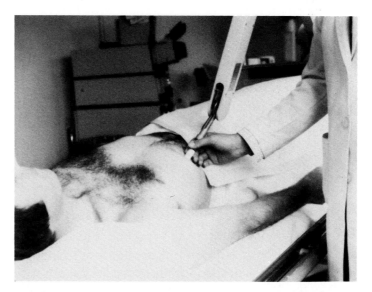

Fig. 19-10. Sagittal scan is thought to be the best way to fully see the entire liver parenchyma. The transducer scans along the anterior abdominal wall until the costal margin is reached. At this point the transducer is swept under the ribs to record the dome of the liver and the diaphragm from a perpendicular angle.

Supine longitudinal scans

Generally, the sagittal scan better outlines the liver parenchyma than does the transverse scan. This is because the transducer can be swept under the patient's costal margin perpendicular to the diaphragm and the dome of the liver. In the transverse scan the overlying lung tends to interfere with adequate visualization in the dome of the liver, and thus the longitudinal scan becomes the scan of choice for liver detail (Fig. 19-10).

Usually, the scan is centered midway between the umbilicus and xyphoid in the midline of the patient. Smaller increments of 0.5 or 1.0 cm are made in the prevertebral area to outline the smaller vessels posterior to the liver. As the sweep moves out of this area, larger increments of 1 to 2 cm complete the series. The transducer should be directed under the rib cage and angled cephalad as much as possible with the patient in full inspiration. With a continuous sweep the beam should slowly be angled caudally to record the lower segment of the right lobe.

Supine oblique subcostal scans

For a supine oblique scan the transducer is placed just beneath and parallel to the right costal margin using a 10° to 15° cephalad angle of the transducer head. This technique usually enables examination of serial sections of the liver with greater ease than in the straight transverse plane. The beam can be directed under the costal margin to avoid reflections and reverberations from the rib interfaces.

Another technique that works well with dehydrated patients is to ask the patient to expand the abdomen to make the path of the anterior abdominal wall smooth in relation to the costal margin.

Right anterior oblique scans

Right anterior oblique scans require that the patient roll slightly to the right; a 45° sponge is placed under the left hip for support. Again, this allows better visualization of the lower liver segment, usually displacing the duodenum and transverse colon out of the field of view (Fig. 19-11).

Normal echographic patterns

Formerly, with bistable equipment, the liver was thought to be anechoic except for the few branching echoes in the area of the porta hepatis. With high-gain settings the liver filled in with multiple weak echoes evenly distributed throughout.

Grey-scale equipment has demonstrated, with transverse scans, homogeneous low-level echoes in the left lobe and medial aspect of the right lobe (Fig.

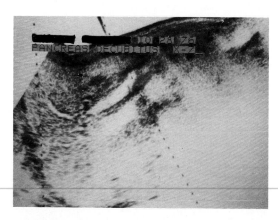

Fig. 19-11. Slight right decubitus position allows the liver to fall slightly anterior for better penetration, since the transducer can angle under the costal margin to avoid the rib artifacts and attenuation problems.

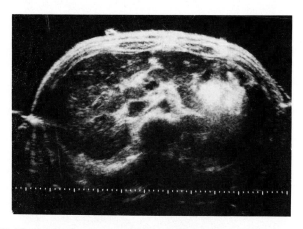

Fig. 19-12. Transverse scan of the right upper quadrant as seen with the eight transducers of the Octoson. The combination of multiple transducer and water bath contact allows good penetration of the ultrasound beam.

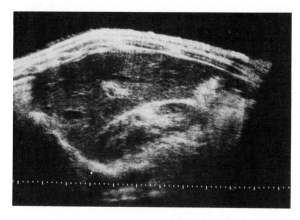

Fig. 19-13. Longitudinal Octoson scan of the liver and right kidney.

19-12). Usually, rib artifacts cause an inconsistent pattern in the lateral aspect of the right lobe. The portal vein is clearly shown as a tubular structure in the midaspect of the liver and the falciform ligament as a linear area of increased echoes between the right and left lobes. The posterior part of the right lobe is often

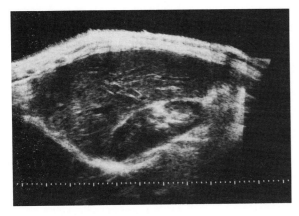

Fig. 19-14. Longitudinal scan with hepatic veins shown within the central portion of the liver.

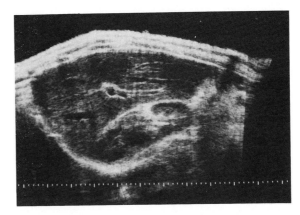

Fig. 19-15. Octoson's water bath allows better penetration through the ribs causing little, if any, reverberation.

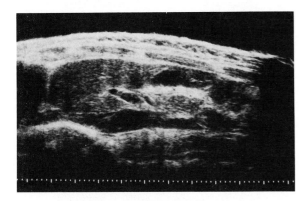

Fig. 19-16. Longitudinal scan of the liver with the inferior vena cava, portal vein, and gallbladder.

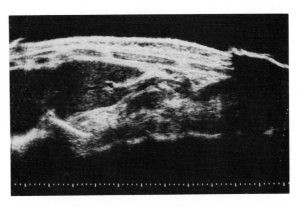

Fig. 19-17. Sometimes a large pulsatile cystic mass can be seen anterior to the left lobe of the liver. This is the heart.

difficult to routinely stipple in with normal gain settings, and the examiner may have to change to a lower-frequency transducer (1.6 MHz) to adequately record echoes in this area.

On longitudinal scans the homogeneous low-level echoes throughout the entire liver are visible. Multiple fluid-filled circular or short linear structures throughout the liver represent various vessels. Usually, these small thick-walled vessels are part of the portal system, but the hepatic system is shown as finer thin-walled structures (Figs. 19-13 to 19-22).

PATHOLOGIC PATTERNS DETECTED BY ULTRASOUND

Evaluation of the liver parenchyma includes assessment of its size, configuration, and contour. Determination of liver volume can be made from serial scans. As in other organ systems, the liver's parenchyma pattern changes with disease. The detection of cirrhosis, ascites, and the cause of jaundice may be accomplished by ultrasound. Recognition of intra-

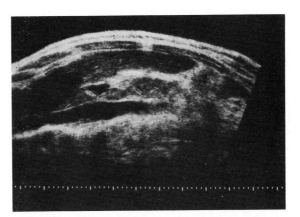

Fig. 19-18. Single transducer technique with the Octoson showing fine echo detail in the normal liver parenchyma, with the portal vein and inferior vena cava.

hepatic, extrahepatic, subhepatic, or subdiaphragmatic masses can be outlined and internal composition (cystic, solid, or abscess) recognized by specific echo patterns.

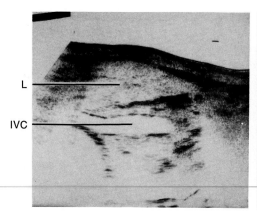
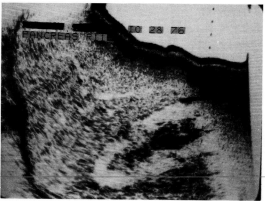

Fig. 19-19. Longitudinal scans of a normal liver. The large tubular structure is the inferior vena cava. The thin-walled, tubular, small vessels are hepatic veins; portal veins appear as thicker-walled vessels. The right kidney may be seen posterior to the liver.

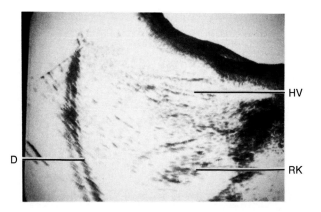

Fig. 19-20. Double echo pattern superior to the dome of the liver represents diaphragmatic motion. The patient should take a deep breath before the single scan is made from the right lobe toward the diaphragm. Then the patient expels the breath and the scan is repeated from the top of the diaphragm down to the right lobe of the liver.

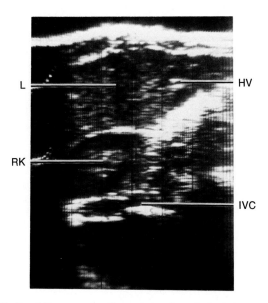

Fig. 19-21. Real-time evaluation of the liver is helpful to evaluate venous structures, diaphragmatic motion, and internal consistency of the liver.

Localized masses (cystic patterns)

There are two types of liver cyst patterns—simple and multiple. A simple hepatic cyst may present as a palpable mass, hepatomegaly, or be completely asymptomatic. Laboratory data reveal normal liver function. Its echo appearance is an echo-free mass that is smooth-walled and has good through-transmission. Simple cysts usually are solitary. The other pattern, that of multiple cysts, demonstrates clinical signs like those of a simple cyst. Laboratory data usually reveal normal liver function, but occasionally they present minimal hepatocellular abnormalities. Echo appearance is the same as for a simple cyst, except that multiple cysts are noted throughout the parenchyma. Multiple cysts are usually associated with polycystic renal disease. It has been reported that approximately 35% to 40% of these patients develop liver cysts as well (Figs. 19-23 and 19-24).

Solid patterns

A hepatoma of the liver may produce a variety of clinical signs: palpable mass, hepatomegaly, jaundice, liver failure, weight loss, ascites, and splenomegaly. Laboratory data show abnormal hepatocellular function, increased alkaline phosphatase, and a positive fetal antigen. Its echo appearance may be more or less echo producing than normal liver parenchyma but is isolated as a single discrete mass. Generally, the enlarged, somewhat irregular shape of the liver is first recognized by ultrasound. With increased sensitivity the normal parenchyma will stipple in with echoes, whereas the hepatoma may present as a more complex pattern within the liver.

Metastatic carcinoma presents ultrasonically various patterns depending on the cell type of the tumor. Thus

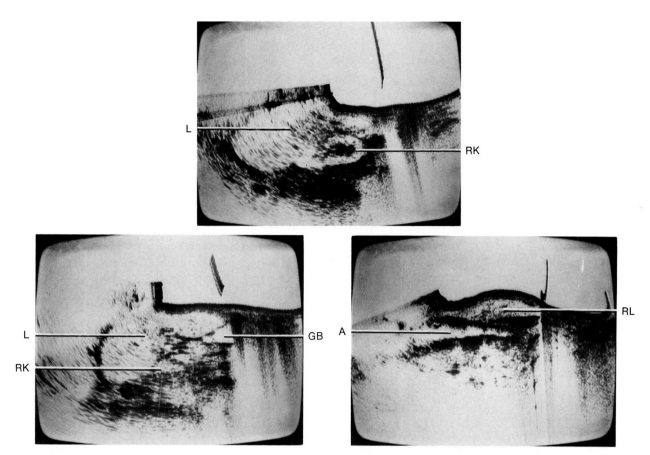

Fig. 19-22. Evaluation of Riedel's lobe of the liver can be made on multiple scans. As one moves toward the midline, the long extension of liver can still be seen anterior to the great vessels.

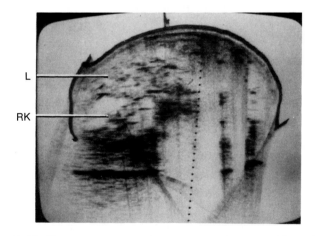

Fig. 19-23. Transverse scan of polycystic kidneys with multiple scattered cysts within the liver.

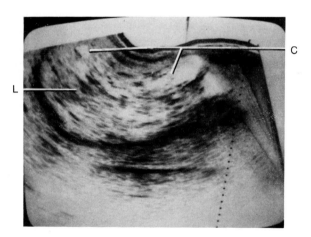

Fig. 19-24. Longitudinal scan better demonstrates multiple cysts within the kidneys and liver.

its pattern may be more or less echo producing than the normal parenchyma. Adenocarcinoma presents a dense central echo pattern surrounded by a less echo–producing halo and hence has been called "bull's-eye" sign. It may manifest as a single lesion or multiple lesions within the liver (Figs. 19-25 and 19-26).

The pattern of lymphoma is a homogeneous tumor. It generally is less echo producing than normal pa-renchyma and can be distinguished as a separate mass with distinct borders. The A-mode presentation is helpful in evaluating the consistency of a lymphoma. The through transmission will be reduced, and, as the gain is increased, small internal echoes will be shown along its internal dimension (Figs. 19-27 and 19-28). Sarcoma tumors generally produce more echo patterns within the liver.

Other patterns of liver metastasis are homogeneous

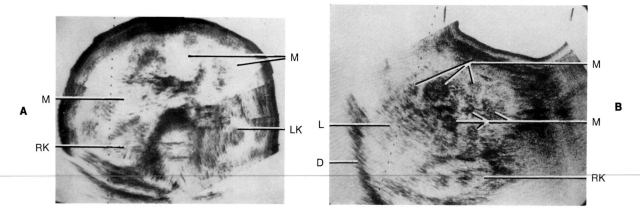

Fig. 19-25. Transverse **(A)** and longitudinal **(B)** scans of metastatic adenocarcinoma to the liver from the colon. Multiple bull's-eye patterns are seen throughout the liver. Adenocarcinoma may appear as sonolucent areas if the transducer is not directly perpendicular to the tumor. Large masses are seen throughout the enlarged liver.

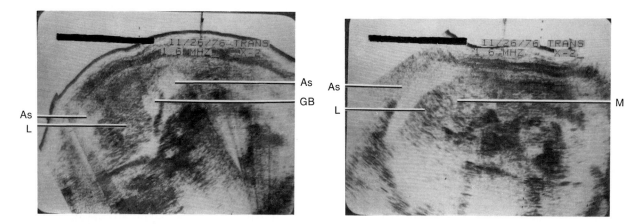

Fig. 19-26. Middle-aged woman with Hodgkin's disease demonstrates hepatosplenomegaly and ascites. Multiple filling defects are seen within the liver parenchyma, representing a tumor.

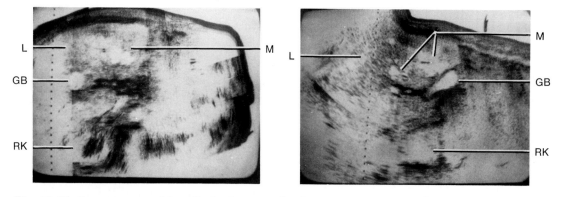

Fig. 19-27. Transverse and longitudinal scans of a homogeneous tumor found in a patient with Hodgkin's disease.

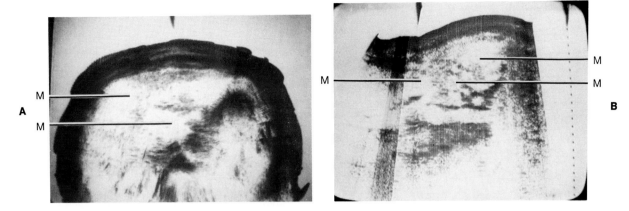

Fig. 19-28. A, Transverse scan of homogeneous echo masses within the liver due to necrotic tumor formation. **B,** Longitudinal scan of metastases.

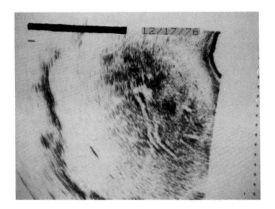

Fig. 19-29. Longitudinal scan of a liver with a dense echo pattern within the porta hepatis.

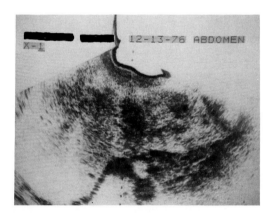

Fig. 19-30. Transverse scans of liver in Fig. 19-29 showing dense echo formations within the liver. The dense tumor may not have borders as well-defined as the homogeneous or complex tumor patterns.

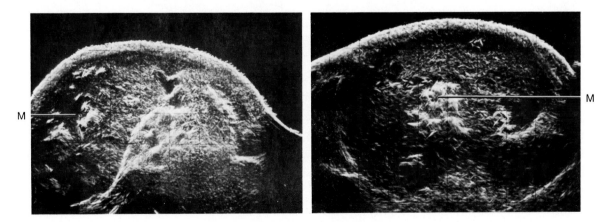

Fig. 19-31. Transverse and longitudinal scans of liver metastasis show intense, irregular echo pattern lateral to the normal liver parenchyma. The sonolucent echo pattern in the left lobe of the liver also represents tumor.

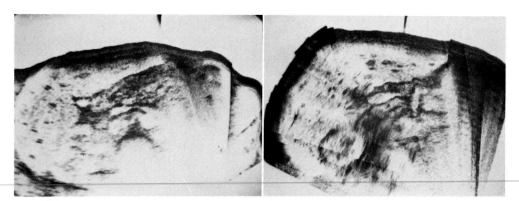

Fig. 19-32. Transverse scan of liver metastases shown as dense echoes throughout the liver parenchyma. The abnormal echoes are larger than vessel reflections.

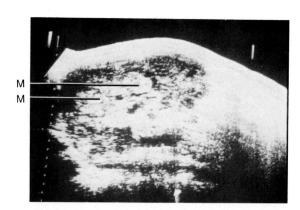

Fig. 19-33. Longitudinal scan of liver metastases. Intense echoes throughout the liver represent tumor.

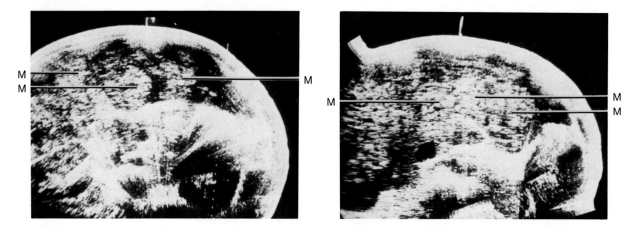

Fig. 19-34. Transverse scans of the liver in Fig. 19-33 showing hepatomegaly and intense echoes throughout.

masses caused by necrosis of the tumor, dense echo reflections as a result of the attenuation of sound by the tumor (Figs. 19-29 to 19-35), or combinations of the homogeneous and dense patterns (Figs. 19-36 to 19-42). We do not classify specific tumors by ultrasonic patterns but describe their appearance, number, and location if a biopsy is performed. Research is currently underway to associate specific ultrasonic patterns with tumor types by means of A-mode tissue analysis with computer programing. Clinical signs for metastasis are the same as for a hepatoma. Laboratory data indicate abnormal hepatocellular function and increased alkaline phosphatase.

Complex patterns

A liver abscess may be clinically suspected if the patient has fever, chills, and right upper quadrant pain. Foreign travel may also be directly related, es-

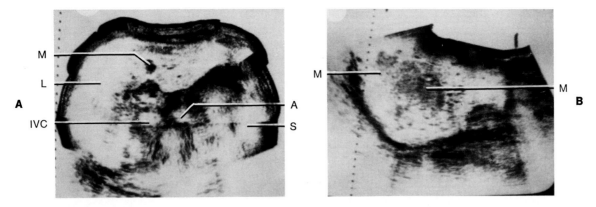

Fig. 19-35. Transverse and longitudinal scans of the liver metastases sometimes demonstrate complex patterns. **A,** Bull's-eye pattern. **B,** Mass of dense echoes within the liver parenchyma.

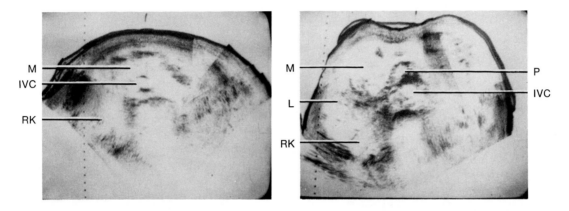

Fig. 19-36. Lymphoma is shown within and without the hepatic structure. The inferior vena cava is completely surrounded by enlarged lymph nodes, lifting it off the anterior surface of the spine.

pecially with the development of amebic abscess. Laboratory data may indicate occasional hepatocellular abnormalities.

The echo appearance generally represents hepatomegaly. As the gain is increased, the area of abscess remains fairly echo free, but the normal parenchyma fills in. The mass generally has irregular borders and may have internal echoes from the debris within the abscess. There is good through-transmission posterior to the mass. Ultrasound is an effective means of following such an abscess after treatment. It is a safe noninvasive way to monitor the shrinkage and final disappearance of the abscess. (See Figs. 19-43 to 19-44.)

Diffuse abnormalities

Biliary obstruction proximal to the cystic duct can be carcinoma of the common bile duct or hepatic metastases in the porta hepatis. In the former, jaundice and pruritus are the clinical signs. Laboratory data show an increase in direct bilirubin and alkaline

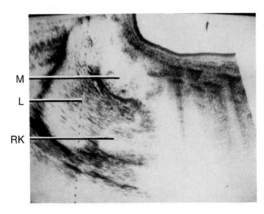

Fig. 19-37. Longitudinal scans of the area in Fig. 19-36 show a somewhat complex echo pattern within the liver parenchyma representing the tumor.

phosphatase. The echo appearance of carcinoma of the common bile duct is tubular branching, fluid-filled structures (dilated hepatic ducts) that are best seen in the periphery of the liver on longitudinal scans. No mass is visualized. The gallbladder is normal in size, even after a fatty meal (Fig. 19-45).

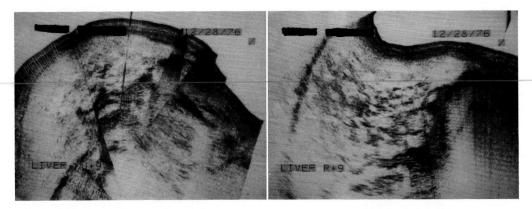

Fig. 19-38. Transverse and longitudinal scans of the area in Fig. 19-36 showing complex patterns within the liver parenchyma.

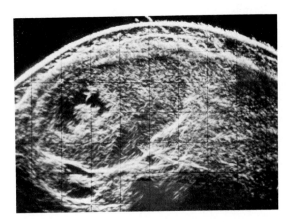

Fig. 19-39. Octoson scan of a large complex liver tumor in the right lobe.

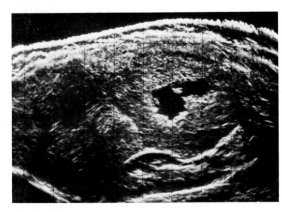

Fig. 19-40. Longitudinal scan clearly shows the complexity of the liver tumor.

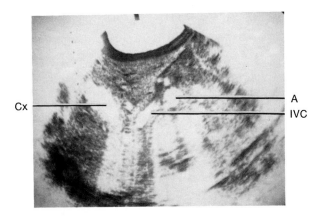

Fig. 19-41. Mass within the liver appears cystic in character on transverse scans.

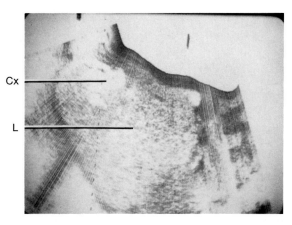

Fig. 19-42. Longitudinal scans show organized echoes within the mass that could represent a multiloculated cyst, a cyst that was bled into, or a necrotic tumor. At surgery a hemangioma was found.

Hepatic metastases in the porta hepatis present the same clinical signs and laboratory data, except that there is abnormal hepatocellular function. The echo appearance is an intrahepatic mass in the area of the porta hepatis that may be more or less echo producing than its normal parenchyma. The dilated hepatic bile ducts are best seen on the longitudinal scans. It is usually associated with other hepatic metastases in other areas of the liver. The gallbladder is normal in size, even after a fatty meal.

Biliary obstruction distal to the cystic duct may be caused by common duct stones, extrahepatic masses in the porta hepatis, or common duct stricture. Common duct stones cause right upper quadrant pain, jaundice, and pruritus as well as an increase in direct bilirubin and alkaline phosphatase. The echo appearance, best seen on sagittal scans, shows the dilated hepatic bile ducts in the periphery of the liver. The gallbladder size is variable, usually small. Gallstones are usually present and appear as dense echoes along the bed of the gallbladder with an acoustic shadow posterior. The stones within the duct may be seen if they are large enough; a shadow may also be present.

Clinical signs of the extrahepatic masses at the porta hepatis include jaundice and symptoms referable to primary disease, and laboratory data are the same as for a stone in the common duct. The echo appearance shows an extrahepatic mass in the area of the porta hepatis, which could be lymph node enlargment or pancreatitis, a pseudocyst, or carcinoma in the head of the pancreas. The tubular branching, fluid-filled, dilated hepatic ducts are seen on longitudinal and transverse scans. The gallbladder is dilated, with no change in size after a fatty meal.

Common duct stricture can be diagnosed by jaundice and past history of cholecystectomy. Direct bilirubin is increased, as is alkaline phosphatase. The echo appearance is dilated hepatic ducts with no porta hepatic mass.

Passive hepatic congestion is another diffuse hepatic abnormality. Generally it develops secondary to congestive heart failure, showing clinical signs of hepatomegaly. Laboratory data indicate normal or slightly abnormal hepatocellular function. The echo appearance shows dilated hepatic and portal veins that are more prominent centrally than peripherally. These structures are usually nonbranching (as the hepatic ducts are) and may decrease in size with expiration or increase with inspiration. The inferior vena cava is usually dilated, as are the superior mesenteric and splenic veins.

Diffuse hepatocellular disease is manifested in hepatitis and cirrhosis (Figs. 19-46 and 19-47). The clinical signs of hepatitis are jaundice, loss of appetite, nausea, and fatigue, with a sharp increase in SGOT and SGPT.

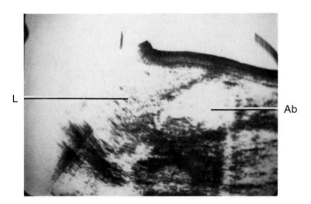

Fig. 19-43. Subhepatic abscess. This complex structure can be seen separate from the liver structure. Generally, the patient develops a spiking fever postoperatively.

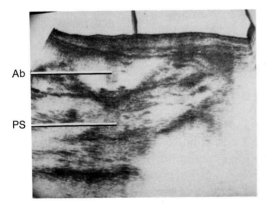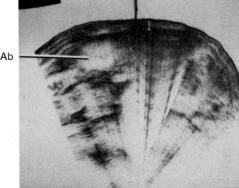

Fig. 19-44. Common location for postoperative abscesses is along the psoas muscle or in the posterior part of the pelvis. A complex structure may be seen anterior to the right kidney and psoas muscle.

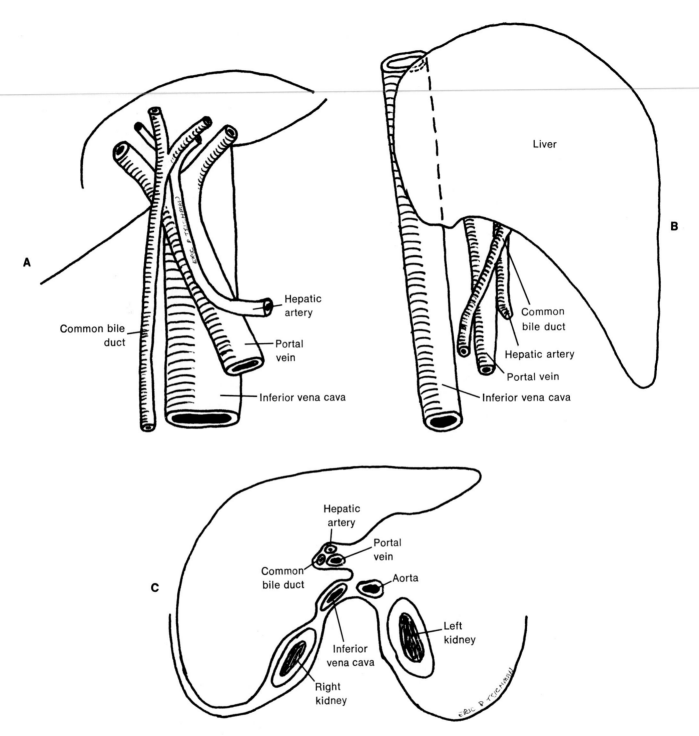

Fig. 19-45. Anterior **(A)** and posterior **(B)** views of the porta hepatis. **C,** Cross-sectional view of the common bile duct, hepatic artery, and portal vein.

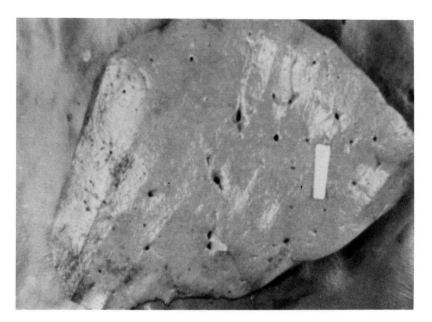

Fig. 19-46. Gross specimen of an enlarged fatty liver.

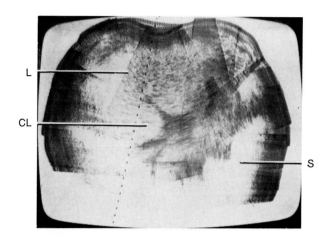

Fig. 19-47. Enlarged liver and spleen, with the fine parenchymal detail, may be due to hepatitis or early cirrhosis. *CL,* Caudate lobe.

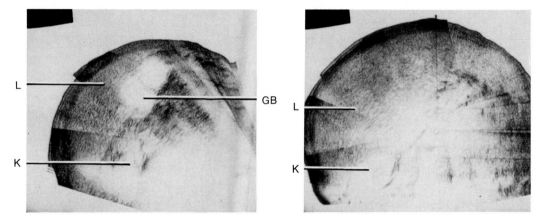

Fig. 19-48. Transverse scans show enlarged liver, poor sound transmission (cirrhosis), and enlarged, thick-walled gallbladder.

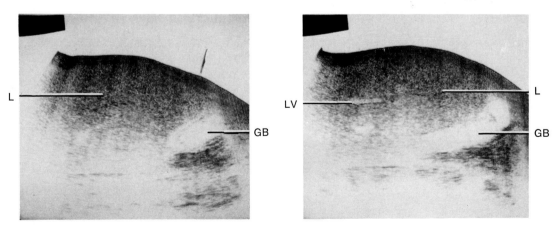

Fig. 19-49. Longitudinal scans of area in Fig. 19-48 show the hepatomegaly with diffuse internal echoes and dilated gallbladder.

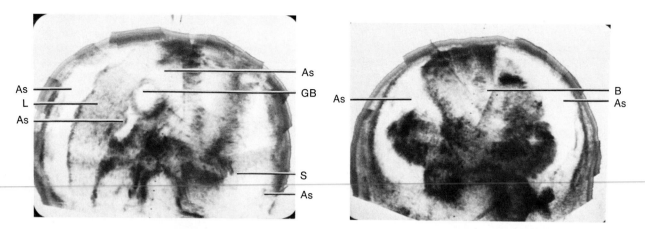

Fig. 19-50. Transverse and longitudinal scans of liver cirrhosis, massive ascites, and thick-walled gallbladder. The ascites is shown bilaterally and anterior to the right kidney. Multiple loops of bowel are seen inferior to the liver.

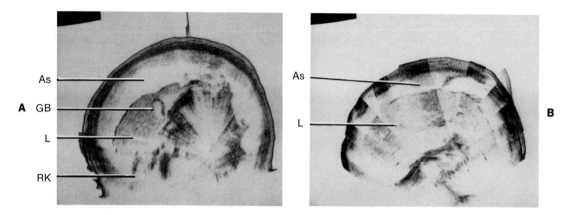

Fig. 19-51. A, Transverse scans of massive ascites and advanced cirrhosis of the liver. **B,** The falciform ligament can be seen as it hangs from the peritoneal wall.

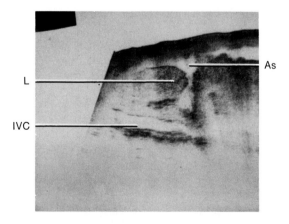

Fig. 19-52. Longitudinal scan of shrunken liver completely surrounded by massive ascites.

The echo appearance shows hepatomegaly with normal or increased parenchymal echoes. The sound attenuation may be normal or increased by the hepatocellular disease. The spleen may be normal or increase in size (Fig. 19-48).

Clinical signs of cirrhosis include jaundice, ascites, gastrointestinal bleeding, decreased alertness, spider angiomas of the face, and palmar erythema. The laboratory data show abnormal hepatocellular function. The echo appearance of early cirrhosis is enlarged liver and spleen with multiple fine echoes throughout the periphery. The sound attenuation is demonstrated along the posterior border because of the fatty degeneration (Figs. 19-49 and 19-50). As the cirrhosis advances, the liver begins to shrink in size. Sound transmission is dramatically reduced through the liver parenchyma. Internal echo patterns become more intense and diffuse throughout the liver. Ascites may be seen separating the anterior and lateral margins of the liver and spleen from the abdominal cavity (Figs. 19-51 to 19-52).

20 □ Gallbladder and biliary system

EXTRAHEPATIC BILIARY APPARATUS

The extrahepatic biliary apparatus consists of the right and left hepatic ducts, the common hepatic duct, the common bile duct, the gallbladder, and the cystic duct (Fig. 20-1).

Hepatic duct. The right and left hepatic ducts emerge from the right lobes of the liver and the porta hepatis and unite to form the common hepatic duct. Each duct is formed by the union of bile canaliculi from the liver lobules.

The common hepatic duct is approximately 4 cm long and descends within the edge of the lesser omentum. It is joined on the right side by the cystic duct from the gallbladder to form the common bile duct.

Common bile duct. This duct is 8 cm long and lies in the right free edge of the lesser omentum in the first part of its course. It is situated posterior to the first part of the duodenum in the second part of its course, and it lies in a groove on the posterior surface of the head of the pancreas in the third part of its course.

The common bile duct ends by piercing the medial wall of the second part of the duodenum about halfway down its length. It is usually joined by the main pan-creatic duct, and together they open into a small ampulla into the duodenal wall called the ampulla of Vater. The end parts of both ducts and the ampulla are surrounded by circular muscle fibers known as the sphincter of Oddi.

Gallbladder. The gallbladder is a pear-shaped sac lying on the visceral surface of the liver (Fig. 20-2). It is divided into the fundus, body, and neck. The rounded fundus usually projects below the inferior margin of the liver, where it comes in contact with the anterior abdominal wall at the level of the ninth right costal cartilage. The body generally lies in contact with the visceral surface of the liver and is directed upward, backward, and to the left. The neck becomes continuous with the cystic duct, which turns into the lesser omentum to join the right side of the common hepatic duct to form the common bile duct (Fig. 20-3).

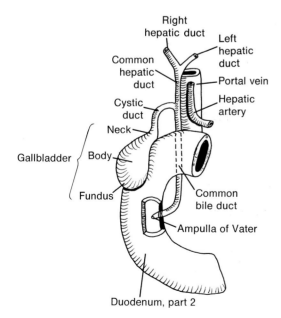

Fig. 20-1. Extrahepatic biliary apparatus.

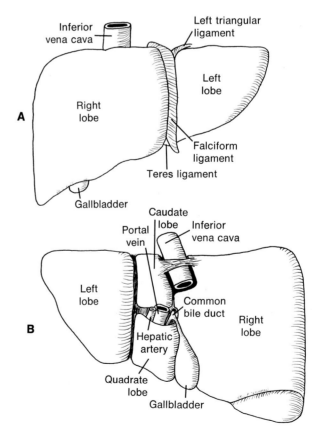

Fig. 20-2. Anterior **(A)** and posterior **(B)** projections of the liver and gallbladder.

277

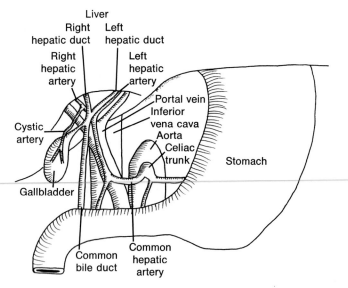

Fig. 20-3. Structures entering and leaving the porta hepatis.

The gallbladder serves as a reservoir for bile with a capacity of 50 ml. It also has the ability to concentrate the bile. To aid this process its mucous membrane contains folds that unite with each other, giving the surface a honeycomb appearance.

The arterial supply of the gallbladder is from the cystic artery, which is a branch of the right hepatic artery. The cystic vein drains directly into the portal vein. A number of smaller arteries and veins run between the liver and the gallbladder.

Cystic duct. The cystic duct is about 4 cm long and connects the neck of the gallbladder to the common hepatic duct to form the common bile duct. It is usually somewhat S-shaped and descends for a variable distance in the right free edge of the lesser omentum.

BILIARY SYSTEM

Bile is secreted continually by the parenchymal cells of the liver. It enters minute channels in the liver (bile canaliculi), through which it flows to a converging system of small ducts into the common bile duct, which enters the duodenum at or near the site where the pancreatic duct joins the liver.

When there is no food in the upper digestive tract, most of the bile secreted by the liver is diverted into the gallbladder, where it is stored and concentrated by the absorption of fluid. Following a meal the amount of bile entering the duodenum is increased as a result of contraction of the gallbladder and enhanced secretion by the liver.

Bile is essential in the intestinal absorption of fat and is the vehicle for the excretion of certain end products of hemoglobin metabolism.

Composition of bile

The amount of bile secreted every day by the human liver ranges from 250 to 1000 ml.

The bile salts are the major secretory components of bile, and the bile pigments are the chief excretory components. Other organic constituents produced in lesser amounts are cholesterol, lecithin, fatty acid, and mucin. During the time bile is stored in the gallbladder, inorganic salts and water are absorbed across the wall of the organ into the blood. The result of this removal of fluid from bile is that the organic constituents, which are not absorbed, are concentrated fivefold to tenfold in the gallbladder.

Bile salts. The parenchymal cells of the liver possess an active transport system for the secretion of bile salts, and this enables these cells to secrete bile salts in a concentration a hundred times greater than that of the blood from which they are derived.

Following their appearance in the small intestine, the bile salts play an essential role in the absorption of fat. After that function has been served, the bile salts are absorbed from the terminal ileum by an active process specialized for the transport of these substances. They are then returned by the portal vein to the liver, where they are removed from the blood and resecreted in the bile. This recycling of biles salts between liver and small intestine is called the enterohepatic circulation of bile salts.

Bile pigments. The reticuloendothelial system contains cells distributed throughout the body that dispose of senescent red blood cells. Bile pigments are an end product of the degradation of the free hemoglobin resulting from the destruction of red blood cells by this system. The major pigment of bile is bilirubin. The 0.5 to 2 gm of bilirubin produced in humans every day is extracted from the blood by the liver cells and secreted into the bile. Intestinal bacteria convert bilirubin into other pigments, and small quantities of these are absorbed from the intestine and excreted by the kidneys. Most of the pigments are excreted in the feces, to which they impart a characteristic brown color.

Control of bile secretion

Any substance that stimulates an increased secretion of bile is a choleretic, and the process by which this occurs is known as choleresis. Choleretics may be chemical, hormonal, or neural. The bile salts are potent chemical choleretics and are the major stimuli for the secretion of bile. These substances act directly on the secretory cells of the liver to stimulate secretion of bile in proportion to their concentration in the portal venous blood. When the portal venous concentration of bile salts is increased, there is a greater transport of bile salts and a greater flow of bile.

Between meals, most of the bile salts of the body pool are stored in the gallbladder, the portal venous concentration of these substances is low, and stimulation of bile flow by bile salts is minimal. When food is being digested, the bile salts are delivered into the small intestine by contractions of the gallbladder and are returned to the liver by the portal circulation. This raises the portal venous concentration of bile salts, and liver bile flow is stimulated. Any stimulus that releases secretin from the intestinal mucosa and causes the pancreas to secrete also stimulates the secretion of bile. The role of secretin in the stimulation of liver secretion is secondary to that of the bile salts, since the increase in bile flow produced in response to secretin release is small compared with that produced by bile salts. The response of the liver to secretin consists of an increased output of water and electrolytes, particularly sodium bicarbonate, without any increase in the output of organic constituents.

Filling and evacuation of the gallbladder

A smooth muscle sphincter, the sphincter of Oddi, surrounds the common bile duct where it enters the duodenum. During fasting, this sphincter is usually closed and offers enough resistance to divert into the gallbladder most of the bile secreted by the liver. Following a meal, the gallbladder is emptied over a period of time by a series of contractions of the smooth muscle in the wall of this organ, and gallbladder bile is delivered into the duodenum whenever the pressure exerted by these contractions is sufficient to overcome sphincteric resistance.

Contraction of the gallbladder occurs reflexly during the cephalic phase of digestion. The efferent limb of the reflex arcs involved is in the vagus nerve. In addition, the hormone cholecystokinin, which is released from the duodenal mucosa into the blood, stimulates contraction of the gallbladder. Release of this hormone occurs particularly in response to fat and protein digestion products in the intestine.

Abnormalities

Cholelithiasis—the presence of gallstones in the gallbladder or bile ducts—is one of the most common diseases of the gastrointestinal system. Cholesterol, a normal constituent of bile, is the major component of most gallstones. Cholesterol is virtually insoluble in water. Two other constituents of bile, the bile salts and lecithin, together possess the capacity to dissolve cho-

lesterol by forming water-soluble aggregates that contain all three of these molecules. Whenever cholesterol precipitates out of solution, small crystals of cholesterol are formed, and these can grow gradually into large gallstones. This can happen when the capacity of the bile salts and lecithin to dissolve cholesterol is exceeded, for example, when the liver secretes higher than normal quantities of cholesterol or the amount of bile salts secreted is less than normal.

When the bile ducts are obstructed either by a gallstone or by a tumor, the flow of bile into the small intestine is retarded or stopped. Since secretion by the liver continues, pressure in the biliary system rises to higher than normal levels, and severe pain may be experienced as the result of stimulation of receptors in the wall of the biliary tree. High pressures also result in the leakage of bile from the biliary system back into the circulation, and the bile pigments, rather than being excreted, accumulate in the blood and tissues, giving the skin a yellow color (jaundice). Another consequence of obstructed flow of bile into the intestine is excessive excretion of fat in the feces, since the quantity of intestinal intraluminal bile salts is not sufficient to ensure the normal absorption of fat.

CLINICAL SYMPTOMS

The most classic symptom of gallbladder disease is right upper quadrant abdominal pain, usually occurring after ingestion of greasy foods. Nausea and vomiting may occur in gallbladder disease and may indicate the presence of a stone in the common bile duct. A gallbladder attack may cause pain in the right shoulder, with inflammation of the gallbladder often causing referred pain in the right shoulder blade.

Gallstones. After a fatty meal the gallbladder contracts to release bile, and if the outflow tract is blocked by gallstones, pain results. As bile is stored in the gallbladder, small crystals of bile salts precipitate and may form gallstones varying from pinhead size to the size of the organ itself. There may be a single large gallstone or hundreds of tiny ones. Resolution capabilities of most ultrasonic equipment make it very difficult to visualize gallstones under 2 to 3 mm in diameter. These tiny stones are the most dangerous, since their small size permits them to enter the bile ducts and obstruct the outflow of bile.

Jaundice. Jaundice is characterized by the presence of bile in the tissues with resulting yellow-green color of the skin. It may develop when a tiny gallstone blocks the bile ducts between the gallbladder and the intestines, producing pressure on the liver and forcing bile into the blood.

ULTRASONIC EVALUATION

A normal gallbladder is approximately 3 cm in width and 7.5 to 10 cm in length. In the evaluation of our own cases, we have found the normal size of the gallbladder to vary in width in the anteroposterior diameter from 1 to 4 cm, with the average being 2 to 3 cm. In the longitudinal direction the length of the gallbladder varied from 5 to 11 cm, with the average being 6 to 7 cm. Sometimes it is difficult to evaluate what is a top normal gallbladder with good contractility versus an

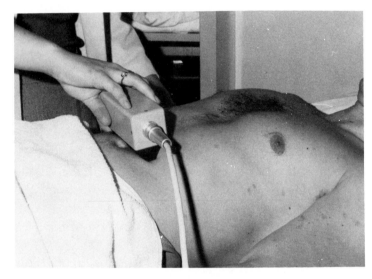

Fig. 20-4. Real-time evaluation of the abdomen aids in the visualization and localization of the gallbladder. The scan may be initiated at the xyphoid or iliac crest with special attention to the costal margin, under which the gallbladder lies.

abnormal gallbladder. If this question should arise, we would administer a fatty meal to the patient, wait 40 minutes, and rescan the patient to see if contractility resulted.

All patients should fast at least 8 to 12 hours prior to the examination to ensure the maximum dilatation of the gallbladder. The patient is scanned in the supine position, using the costal margin as a reference point (Fig. 20-4). We have found that transverse scans prove most successful in the localization of the gallbladder apparatus. A line may be drawn along the patient's costal margin with a marking pencil as an initial starting point. Each scan should be made at 0.5 cm increments from this costal margin in the cephalad and caudal directions to visualize the sonolucent structure medial to the liver and anterior to the right kidney. Once identified, marks should be made on the patient's skin over the neck, body, and fundus to aid the sonographer in locating the organ in the longitudinal plane. Generally, these marks will fall in an oblique path perpendicular to the costal margin (Fig. 20-5). With careful scanning evaluation there should be little difficulty in distinguishing the gallbladder from the head of the pancreas, the inferior vena cava, or the portal vein. Generally, on the transverse plane, the gallbladder lies inferior to the pancreas and the portal vein and medial to the inferior vena cava. Difficulties may be encountered if the costal margin is obstructing the field of view, causing shadowing as the scan moves along the anterior abdominal wall. There are

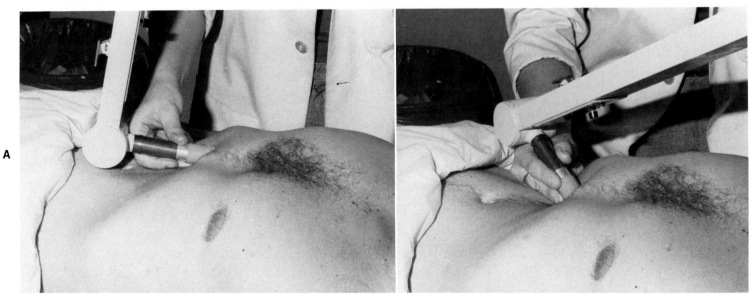

Fig. 20-5. A, Longitudinal oblique scans of the gallbladder area are performed with the patient in deep inspiration. The transducer is arced under the costal margin to record the gallbladder and liver.
B, Reverse oblique scan to record the hepatic artery and biliary system.

several ways to overcome this problem. The patient may be rolled in a semidecubitus position and the scans made in an oblique fashion along the costal margin, thus throwing the gallbladder slightly anterior; or the angle could be increased on the transducer head to scan in a more cephalic presentation along the anterior abdominal wall; or the patient could take a deep breath, thus pushing the liver and gallbladder into the area of view. The patient also could be scanned in an upright position, thus causing the gallbladder to fall to a more inferior position. In our experience the water bath real-time method has proved quite effective in locating gallbladders that are very difficult to localize by conventional grey-scale techniques. The water bath facilitates the sound transmission through the costal margin without any problem and thus aids in visualization. In addition, we have obtained better visualization with the use of the Octoson, with patients lying in a prone position and the transducer directed along the anterior abdominal wall. Again, the water bath presentation aids in the visualization of the gallbladder area with little bowel gas or rib interference. Patients who have been difficult to visualize through conventional grey-scale techniques have been visualized with the Octoson.

A normal gallbladder may assume any one of various shapes and sizes. Since most gallbladders take on a somewhat oblique path in the right upper quadrant, transverse scans demonstrate a small, circular, echo-free area anterior to the right kidney and medial to the

liver (Figs. 20-6 to 20-10); longitudinal scans made along the oblique path perpendicular to the costal margin demonstrate a somewhat pear-shaped sonolucent structure under the lip of the liver and anterior to the right kidney (Figs. 20-11 to 20-13). Gallbladders that have a transverse lie are more difficult to visualize and are probably best seen in the transverse presentation (Fig. 20-14). In a few cases we have seen patients whose scan demonstrated more than one gallbladder, with one normal-sized gallbladder and a smaller echo-free area beside it.

A dilated gallbladder may be top normal in some individuals because of their fasting state (Fig. 20-15). The fatty meal should be administered and further

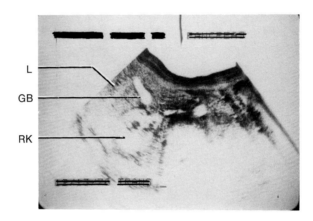

Fig. 20-6. Transverse scan of the gallbladder shown as a small sonolucent structure medial to the liver and anterior to the right kidney.

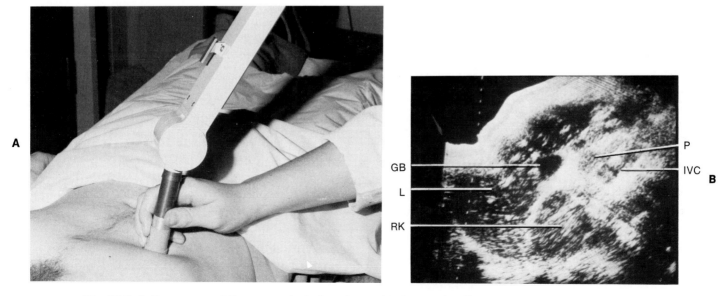

Fig. 20-7. A, Transverse oblique scan technique is used to better visualize the gallbladder under the costal margin. **B,** Representative transverse oblique scan of the gallbladder with high-gain technique.

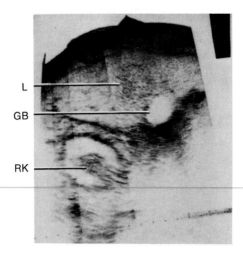

L
GB
RK

Fig. 20-8. Lateral decubitus transverse scan demonstrates the liver, gallbladder, and right kidney.

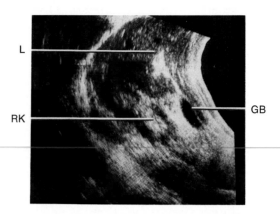

L
RK
GB

Fig. 20-10. Longitudinal upright scan of the liver, gallbladder, and right kidney.

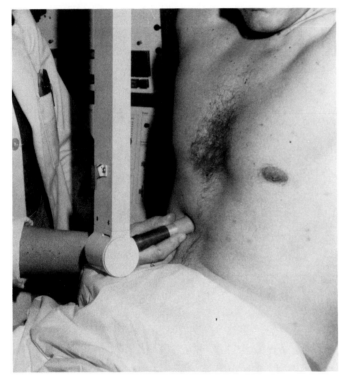

Fig. 20-9. Upright scan performed to evaluate the internal echoes within the gallbladder. Normally the bile should be echo free, but with disease, increased echoes appear. Change in position should alter these echoes to prove they are real structures within the gallbladder parenchyma.

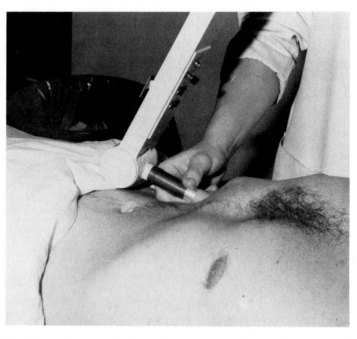

Fig. 20-11. Longitudinal supine scan technique for the gallbladder.

ultrasonic evaluation made to detect if it is a large gallbladder or a normal gallbladder. If the gallbladder fails to contract during examination, further investigation of the pancreatic area should be made. Courvoisier's sign indicates an extrahepatic mass compressing the common bile duct, which can produce an enlarged gallbladder. In addition, the liver should be carefully examined to detect the presence of dilated bile ducts.

Evaluation of the internal structure of the gallbladder may be made by ultrasound. Our experience has shown that cholecystitis is demonstrated as a slightly enlarged sonolucent structure with thickening of the gallbladder wall. The thickening appears to be symmetrical without cause for shadowing, as would be found in gallstones (Figs. 20-16 to 20-18).

It has now been clinically proved that the detection of gallstones by ultrasound is accurate, and, in most

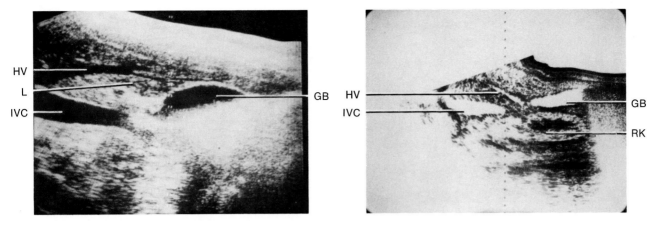

Fig. 20-12. Longitudinal supine scan of the gallbladder.

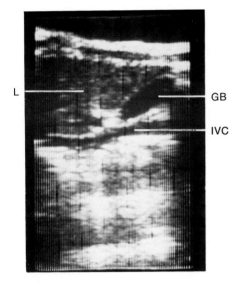

Fig. 20-13. Real-time longitudinal scan demonstrates the normal gallbladder just under the lip of the liver and anterior to the inferior vena cava.

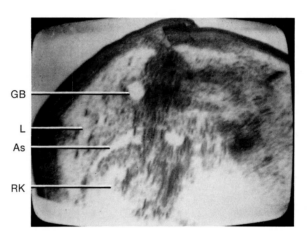

Fig. 20-14. Transverse supine scan of the gallbladder in its anterior and medial positions in a patient with cirrhosis and ascites.

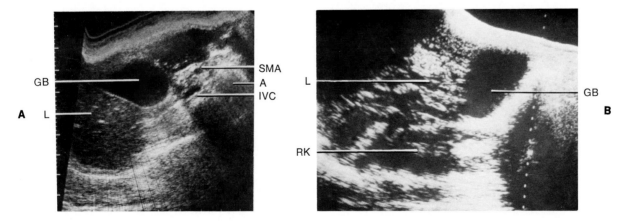

Fig. 20-15. Enlarged noncontractile gallbladders scanned before **(A)** and after **(B)** fatty meal ingestion.

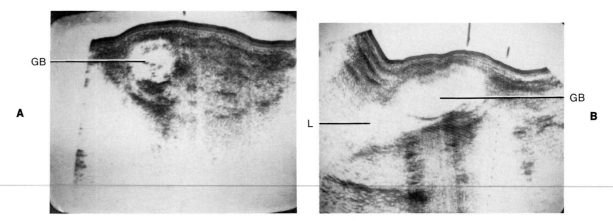

Fig. 20-16. A, Enlarged gallbladder with symmetrical thickening of its walls. **B,** Longitudinal scan of the gallbladder with some thickening of the walls shown on a scan performed with moderate-gain settings.

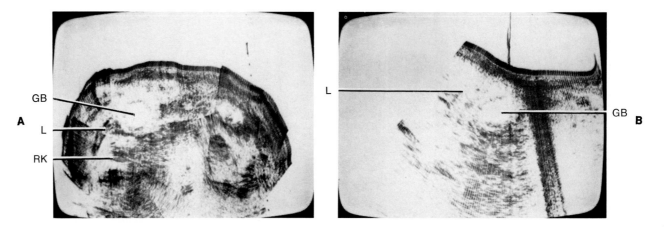

Fig. 20-17. A, Transverse scan of the thickened gallbladder in a patient with cholecystitis. **B,** Longitudinal scan of the thickened gallbladder under the lip of the liver.

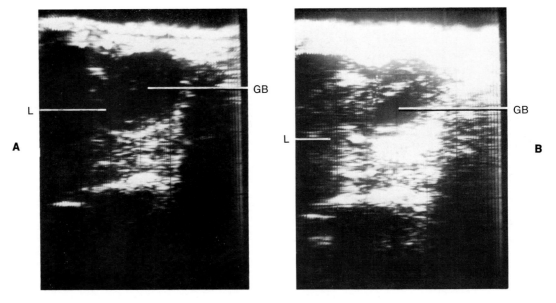

Fig. 20-18. A, Low-gain study of an enlarged gallbladder in the longitudinal axis. **B,** Increased gain demonstrates symmetrical thickening of the walls.

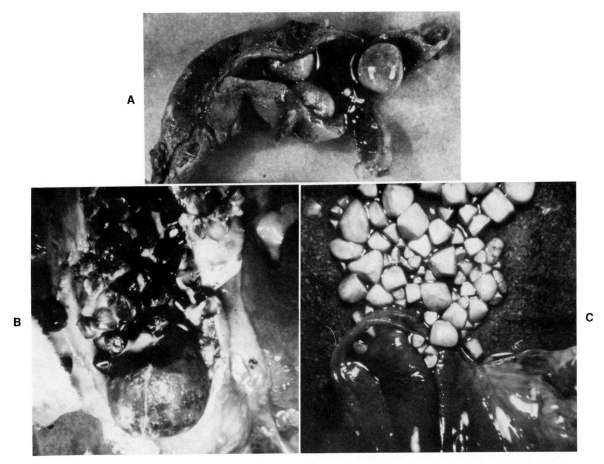

Fig. 20-19. A, Gross specimen of a diseased gallbladder with multiple large gallstones. **B,** Gross specimen of a diseased gallbladder with multiple small gallstones. **C,** Gross specimen of gallstones from within the gallbladder.

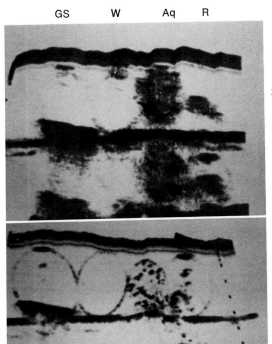

Fig. 20-20. Experimental study was performed with a simulated gallbladder (a balloon) filled with sand to represent gallstones *(GS)*, water to represent bile *(W)*, Aquasonic to represent thickened bile *(Aq)*, and an actual gallstone *(R)*. Scans were performed with a 2.25 and 5.0 MHz transducer to evaluate resolution capabilities of the equipment. Low sensitivity (36 dB) and high sensitivity (42 dB) were used to evaluate transmission quality.

W

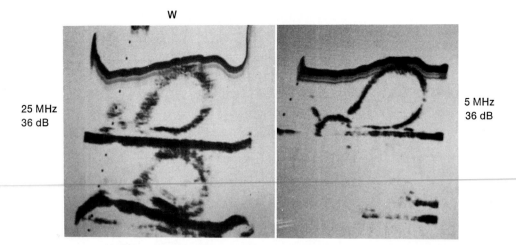

25 MHz
36 dB

5 MHz
36 dB

Fig. 20-21. Water-filled balloon simulating bile in normal gallbladder as seen with a low- and high-frequency transducer. Much sharper resolution can be seen with the higher-frequency transducer.

institutions, patients who cannot be diagnosed through radiography will undergo ultrasonic evaluation for gallstones. We have found 50% of the patients who developed gallstones had a dilated gallbladder. Stones as small as 2 to 3 mm have been detected and can be separated as single or multiple stones within the floor of the gallbladder (Fig. 20-19). They are generally thought to cause dense echoes within the sonolucent gallbladder and may be accompanied by a sonic shadow. (See Figs. 20-20 to 20-27.) However, we have also found that 50% of the patients with gallstones have no dropout of sound posterior to the gallbladder (Fig. 20-28). In comparing densities of gallstones, we have found that 45% of the patients had gallstones the same density as the anterior gallbladder wall; another 45% developed gallstones denser than the anterior gallbladder wall; and 10% had gallstones

GS

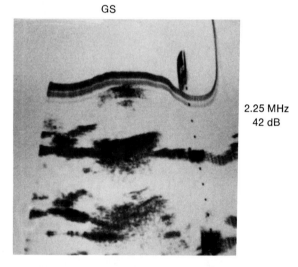

2.25 MHz
42 dB

Fig. 20-22. Sand-filled balloon representing gravel or small stones within the gallbladder as seen with a low-frequency transducer at high-sensitivity settings demonstrates poor resolution quality.

GS   GS

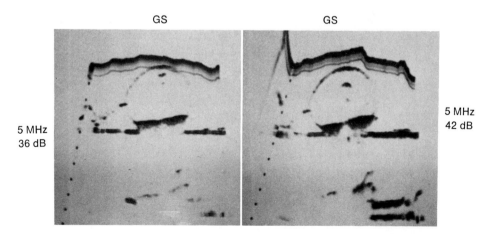

5 MHz
36 dB

5 MHz
42 dB

Fig. 20-23. Higher-frequency transducer sharpens the image of the fine echoes within the gallbladder bed.

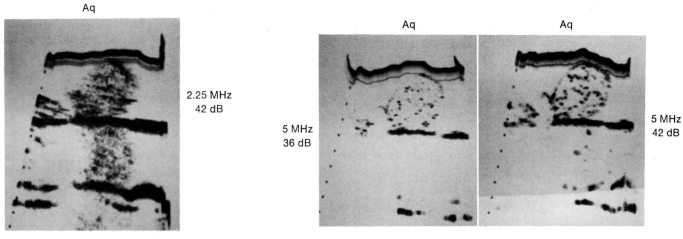

Fig. 20-24. Aquasonic-filled balloon to simulate a gallbladder with thick bile as scanned with low frequency and high gain. Multiple increased echoes are shown within the gallbladder.

Fig. 20-25. With the higher-frequency transducer the smaller pockets within the Aquasonic gel can be clearly detected within the balloon.

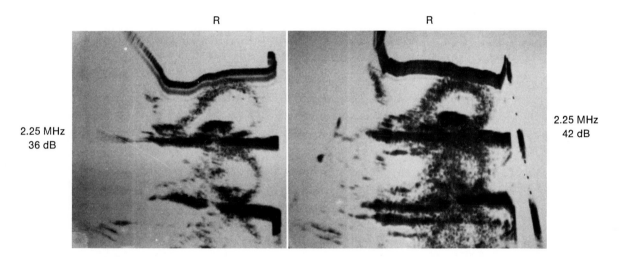

Fig. 20-26. Actual gallstone within the gallbladder is very coarsely outlined with a low-frequency transducer with no shadow behind.

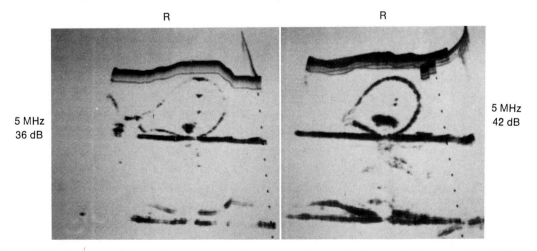

Fig. 20-27. As the transducer frequency was increased, the resolution quality improved to delineate the size of the stone much more accurately. A definite posterior shadow is difficult to appreciate in this water bath study.

lighter than the anterior gallbladder wall. Direct correlation with the type of stone and the ultrasonic pattern has not yet been clinically evaluated.

Shadowing effect of the gallstones is caused by the attenuation of the sound beam by the stone. Care must be exercised in evaluating the gallbladder by using a single sweep technique and always remaining perpendicular to the gallbladder and the stone. Slight sectoring will almost certainly fill in the shadow posterior to the stone and thus cause the stone to be overlooked by ultrasound (Figs. 20-29 to 20-34).

The patient's position should be shifted during the procedure to further demonstrate the presence of the stones. Patients should be scanned in the right decubitus, right lateral, and upright positions. Scans should be made along the right costal margin to see if the stones will shift. The stones should shift to the most dependent area of the gallbladder. In some cases, when the bile has a thick consistency, the stones may remain near the top of the gallbladder; thus the density of the stones and the shadow behind will be the ultrasonic evidence of stones.

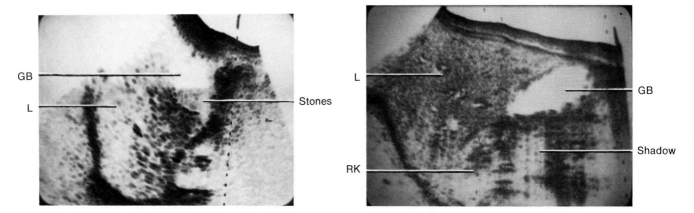

Fig. 20-28. Very small stones along the gallbladder bed may be difficult to distinguish from thickening of the gallbladder wall, an artifact caused by increased gain settings, or poor resolution of the transducer. Higher-frequency transducers should be used with the patient rotated in different positions to see if the echoes change.

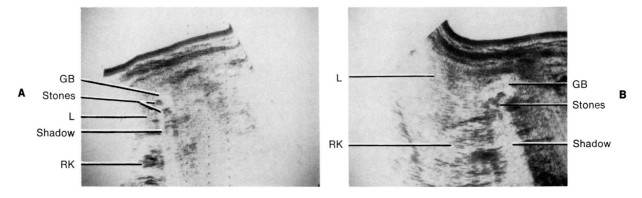

Fig. 20-29. A, Transverse scan of gallstones with shadow posterior. **B,** Longitudinal view of the gallstones with the shadow posterior.

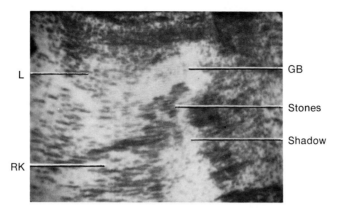

Fig. 20-30. Transverse view of gallstones with shadow.

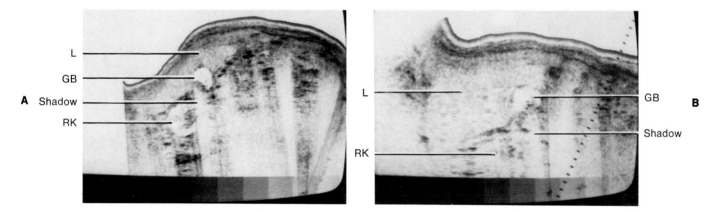

Fig. 20-31. A, Transverse view of gallstones with shadow running into the right kidney. **B,** Longitudinal view of the gallstones with shadow.

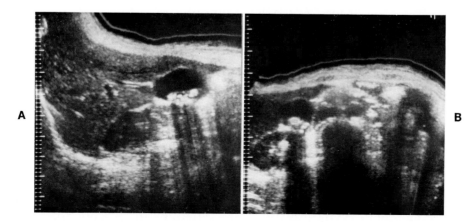

Fig. 20-32. A, Transverse view of gallstones with shadow. **B,** Longitudinal view of gallstones with shadow.

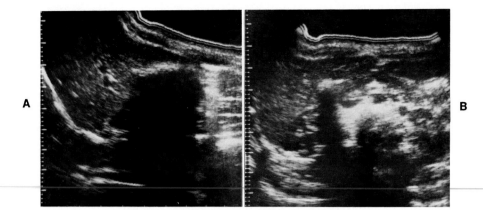

Fig. 20-33. A, Transverse view of gallstones with shadow. **B,** Longitudinal view of gallstones with shadow.

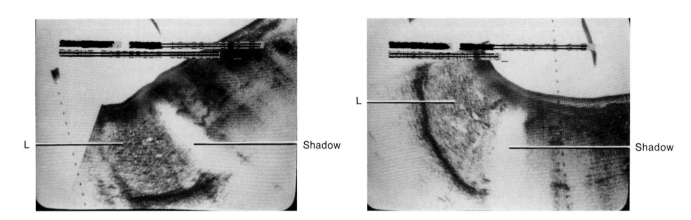

Fig. 20-34. Oblique views of gallstones.

BILIARY TRACT

Generally, the cystic and common bile ducts are beyond the limits of resolution for most ultrasonic equipment. Transverse scans, however, may demonstrate small circular areas anterior to the inferior vena cava and superior mesenteric vein (Fig. 20-35). If two small circular areas are seen at the same time, the most lateral circle represents the common bile duct, and the medial circle represents the common hepatic artery. The examiner may follow the course of each of these structures with a mark on the patient's abdomen so that they may be visualized in the longitudinal direction. A slight oblique path is required, slightly to the right of midline. With a single sweep technique the transducer should be directed toward the right shoulder and carefully guided along the marks toward the patient's left hip.

The dilated bile ducts we have scanned varied in size from 1 to 3 cm. Of course, the larger the ducts, the easier they are to visualize. We evaluated the ducts' curvature within the liver. Most ducts were found to curve posteriorly near the portal triad as the bile duct emptied into the duodenum (Figs. 20-36 to 20-41) or were found in a horizontal plane. As the ducts were followed distal to the portal triad, they tended to curve in the anterior position, whereas veins were shown to dip posteriorly. Most of the ducts were found to stop at the midline. If the patient has right-sided heart failure or liver failure giving rise to increased hepatic veins, the sonographer will have to carefully distinguish the hepatic veins from the dilated bile ducts. Real-time equipment with high resolution has made it possible to trace the cystic duct and common bile duct into the gallbladder and the hepatic system. Of course, venous structures will dilate with a Valsalva maneuver, and ducts will remain constant.

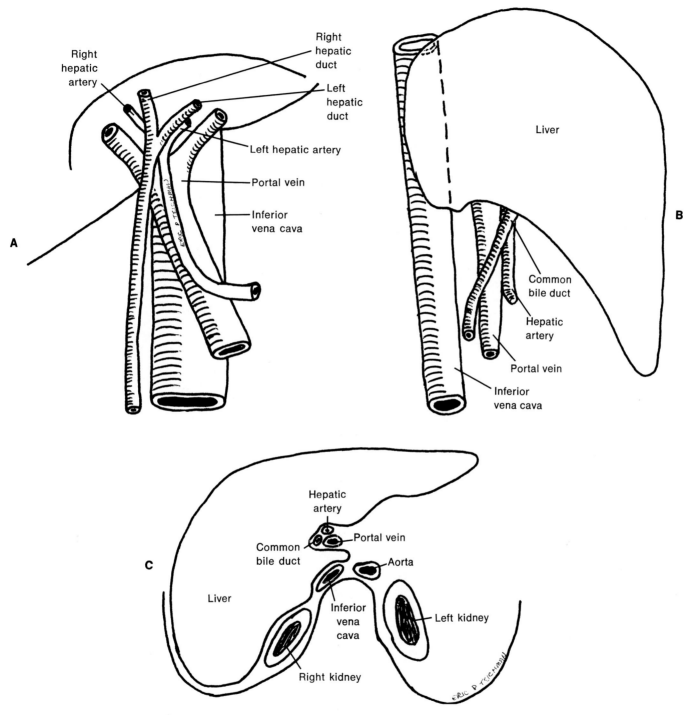

Fig. 20-35. A, Anteroposterior view of the biliary apparatus as it enters the porta hepatis. **B,** Posterior view of the biliary apparatus. **C,** Transverse view of the upper abdomen to show the common bile duct lateral to the hepatic artery.

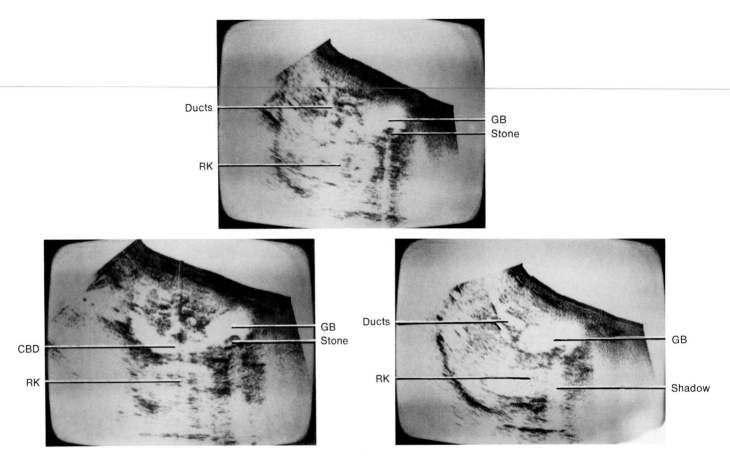

Fig. 20-36. Longitudinal view of dilated gallbladder, gallstones, and dilated ducts.

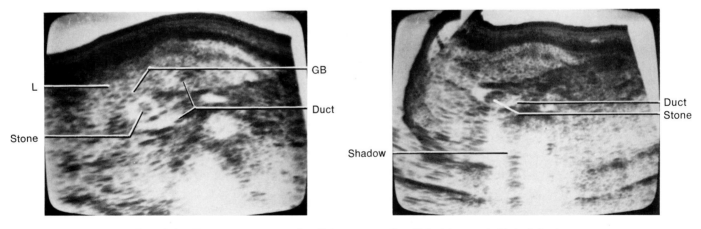

Fig. 20-37. Transverse scans of gallstones, small gallbladder, and dilated ducts.

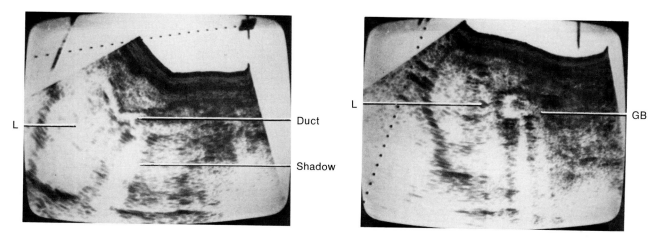

Fig. 20-38. Longitudinal scans of area in Fig. 20-37 showing dilated ducts and the gallstone within the gallbladder. Small stones are also shown within the dilated duct, with shadow behind.

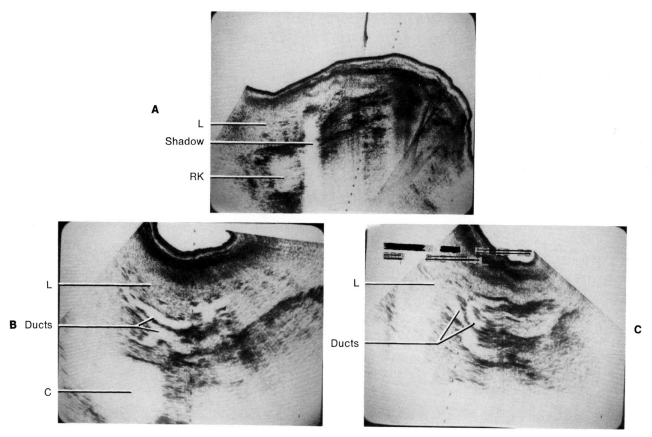

Fig. 20-39. A, Transverse scan of gallstones with shadow. **B,** Transverse scan of dilated ducts and gallstone with a renal cyst posterior. **C,** Transverse scan of the same patient above the area of the renal cyst.

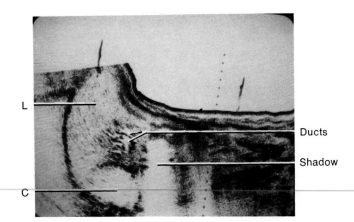

Fig. 20-40. Longitudinal scan of the area in Fig. 20-39 showing dilated ducts with a stone. Complete shadowing is seen posterior to the gallbladder.

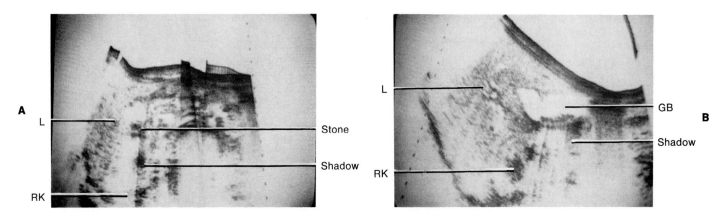

Fig. 20-41. A, Transverse scan of dilated duct with stone. **B,** Longitudinal scan of the same area showing dilated ducts with stones.

21 □ Prevertebral vessels

ANATOMY OF POSTERIOR ABDOMINAL WALL ARTERIES

Aorta. The descending aorta enters the abdomen through the aortic opening of the diaphragm in front of the twelfth thoracic vertebra in the retroperitoneal space. It descends anteriorly to the bodies of the lumbar vertebrae. At the level of the fourth lumbar vertebra it divides into the two common iliac arteries. The abdominal aorta is usually 2 to 4 cm in width. Although the diameter may vary slightly along the aortic contour as it branches to the visceral organs, it is generally believed to be uniform in contour. The aorta has four main branches that it supplies to other visceral organs and to the mesentery. These branches are the celiac trunk, the superior and inferior mesenteric arteries, and the renal arteries (Fig. 21-1).

The common iliac arteries arise at the bifurcation of the aorta and run downward and laterally along the medial border of the psoas muscle. At the level of the sacroiliac joint the iliac artery bifurcates into external and internal iliac arteries. The external iliac artery runs along the medial border of the psoas following the pelvic brim. This artery gives off the inferior epigastric and deep circumflex iliac branches before it passes under the inguinal ligament to become the femoral artery. The internal iliac artery enters the pelvis in front of the sacroiliac joint, at which point it is crossed anteriorly by the ureter. It also divides into anterior and posterior divisions to supply the pelvic viscera, peritoneum, buttock, and sacral canal.

Celiac trunk. The celiac trunk originates within the first 2 cm of the abdominal aorta. It is surrounded by the liver, spleen, inferior vena cava, and pancreas. The celiac trunk immediately branches into the left gastric artery, the splenic artery, and the common hepatic artery (Fig. 21-2). The left gastric artery further divides into the short gastric, splenic, and left gastroepiploic arteries. The splenic artery is the largest of the three branches of the celiac trunk. From its origin in the celiac trunk the splenic artery takes a somewhat tortuous course horizontally to the left, usually along the upper margin of the pancreas. At a variable distance

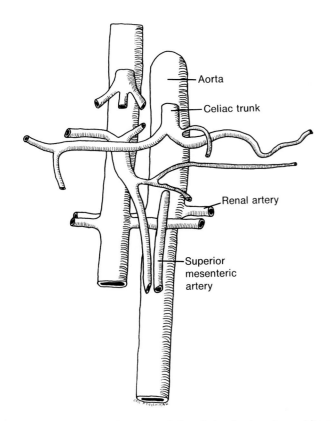

Fig. 21-1. Anteroposterior view of the abdominal aorta and its superior major branches. The inferior mesenteric artery (not shown) branches from the SMA to the left of the abdomen.

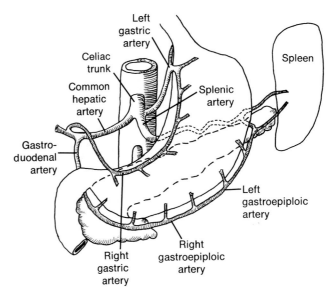

Fig. 21-2. Celiac trunk and its branches into the left gastric artery, splenic artery, and common hepatic artery, with further branching to the stomach and pancreatic area.

from the spleen it divides into two branches. One branch runs caudally into the greater omentum toward the right gastroepiploic artery. This branch is the left gastroepiploic artery. The other branch runs cephalically and divides into the short gastric artery, which supplies the fundus of the stomach and several splenic branches that supply the spleen. Several small branches originate at the splenic artery as it runs along the upper border of the pancreas. The dorsal pancreatic, great pancreatic, and caudal pancreatic, three of the larger arteries, are pertinent. The dorsal pancreatic artery (also known as the superior pancreatic artery) usually originates from the beginning of the splenic artery but may also arise from the hepatic artery, celiac trunk, or aorta. It runs down behind and in the substance of the pancreas, dividing into right and left branches. The left branch comprises the transverse pancreatic artery. The right branch constitutes an anastomotic vessel to the anterior pancreatic arch and also a branch to the uncinate process. The great pancreatic artery originates from the splenic artery further to the left and passes downward, dividing into branches that anastomose with the transverse or inferior pancreatic artery. The caudal pancreatic artery supplies the tail of the pancreas and divides into branches that anastomose with terminal branches of the transverse pancreatic artery. The transverse pancreatic artery, usually the left branch of the dorsal pancreatic artery, courses behind the body and tail of the pancreas close to its lower border. It may originate from or communicate with the superior mesenteric artery.

The common hepatic artery comes off the celiac trunk and courses to the right of the aorta at a close 90° angle. It courses along the upper border of the head of the pancreas, behind the posterior layer of the peritoneal omental bursa, to the upper margin of the superior part of the duodenum, which forms the lower boundary of the epiploic foramen. It ascends into the liver with the hepatic duct, which lies to its right, and the portal vein, which lies posterior to it. It then divides into two major branches at the portal fissure that subdivide as they enter the liver to supply the right and left lobes.

The right hepatic branch supplies the gallbladder via the cystic artery. The smaller left branch of the hepatic artery serves both the caudate and left lobes of the liver. Within the liver parenchyma the hepatic arterial branches further divide repeatedly into progressively smaller vessels eventually supplying the portal triad.

The terminal ends of the hepatic artery form a plexus of interlobular branches outside each liver lobe to supply the walls of the inner lobular meshwork of veins and accompanying bile ducts. From this plexus, lobular branches enter the lobe and end in a network of sinusoids between the cells.

The head of the pancreas, the duodenum, and parts of the stomach are supplied by the gastroduodenal artery coming off the common hepatic artery.

Superior mesenteric artery. The superior mesenteric artery arises anteriorly from the abdominal aorta approximately 1 cm below the celiac trunk. It runs posterior to the neck of the pancreas, passing over the uncinate process of the pancreatic head anterior to the third part of the duodenum, where it enters the root of the mesentery and colon. It has five main branches: the inferior pancreatic artery, the duodenal artery, the colic artery, the ileocolic artery, and the intestinal artery. These branches to the small bowel consist of ten to sixteen branches arising from the left side of the superior mesenteric trunk. They extend into the mesentery, where adjacent arteries unite to form loops or arcades. Thus their distribution is to the proximal half of the colon and small intestine (Fig. 21-3).

Inferior mesenteric artery. This artery arises approximately at the level of the third or fourth lumbar vertebra. It proceeds to the left to distribute arterial blood to the descending colon, the sigmoid colon, and

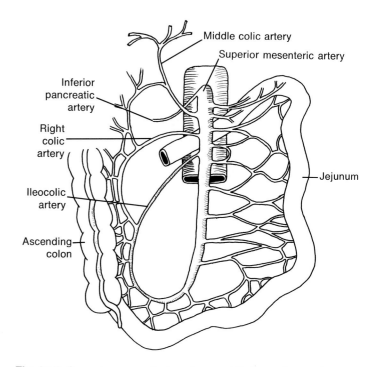

Fig. 21-3. Superior mesenteric artery and its branches to the small bowel and colon.

to the rectum. It has three main branches: the left colic artery, the sigmoid artery, and the superior rectal artery.

Renal arteries. The right and left renal arteries arise anterior to the first lumbar vertebra and inferior to the superior mesenteric artery. They divide into anterior and inferior suprarenal branches.

ULTRASONIC EVALUATION OF ARTERIAL VESSELS

Aorta. The abdominal aorta is ordinarily one of the easiest abdominal structures to visualize by ultrasound because of the marked change in the acoustic impedance produced by the elasticity of its walls and its blood-filled internal structure. Early detection of the abdominal aorta was noted by A-mode techniques. Approximate localization of the aorta was made by manual palpation, and the transducer was then placed over the area suspected to be aneurysmal. Since the aorta demonstrated parallel pulsatile movement of its anterior and posterior walls, it became fairly easy to recognize by A-mode techniques. Increased echoes within the aortic walls represented a thrombus, or clot, within the aorta. Of course, patients with arteriosclerotic disease demonstrated decreased motion in the aorta, and thus the vessel became more difficult to recognize in A mode. Calcification of the abdominal aorta demonstrated denser echoes than did a noncalcified aorta.

Grey-scale sonography provides diagnostic information needed to visualize the entire abdominal aorta and to accurately predict the diameter of the aorta, thus making it possible to detect abnormalities.

The patient is routinely scanned in the supine position, since the vertebral column prevents visualization from the prone position. Gas-filled loops of bowel sometimes may prevent adequate visualization of the aorta, but this may be overcome by applying pressure with the transducer to the area of interest or by changing the angle of the transducer to a slight medial angulation to permit the sound to be unobstructed by air-filled bowel. Prior to scanning, the abdomen should be palpated to predetermine the course of the abdominal aorta. Initial scans should be made in the longitudinal plane to outline the course of the vessel (Fig. 21-4). Each longitudinal scan should include the area from the xyphoid to well below the area of the umbilicus, which is usually the level of the bifurcation. The longitudinal scans are made beginning at the midline with successive scans made every 0.5 to 1 cm increment to either side for several centimeters. Single sweep techniques are best utilized to demonstrate the aorta without artifacts. It is important that the

transducer follow a perpendicular path along the entire curvature of the aorta, since the aorta follows the anterior course of the vertebral column. Slight sectoring motion may be needed if echoes are not recorded from all borders. However, as the sectoring motion is begun, the sensitivity should be decreased to avoid overwriting the area of interest. If artifact echoes persist within the lumen of the aorta, the TGC or the overall sensitivity should be decreased. The anterior and posterior walls of the abdominal aorta should be easily seen as a thin line for accuracy in measuring the diameter. This facilitates the anteroposterior diameter of the aorta, which is made from the leading edge of the anterior aortic wall to the leading edge of the posterior aortic wall.

In an effort to measure the anteroposterior width of the abdominal aorta, transverse scans are usually made every 2 cm, from the umbilicus to the xyphoid. The normal aorta is visualized as a circular structure anterior to the spine and slightly to the left of the midline. In some cases the transverse diameter of the aorta may differ from the longitudinal measurements; thus it is important to identify the vessel in two dimensions. If the patient has a very tortuous aorta, scans may be difficult to obtain in one plane. As one scans in the longitudinal plane, the upper part of the abdominal aorta may be well visualized, but the lower portion of the vessel may be out of the plane of view. In this case

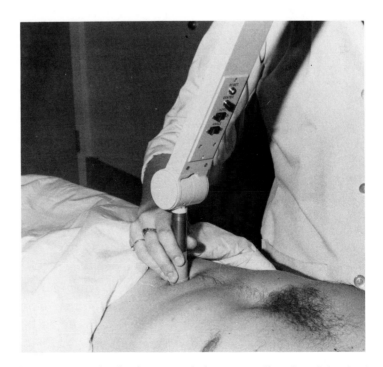

Fig. 21-4. Longitudinal scan technique to outline the abdominal aorta. The transducer should follow a perpendicular course to the aortic wall to record maximum information.

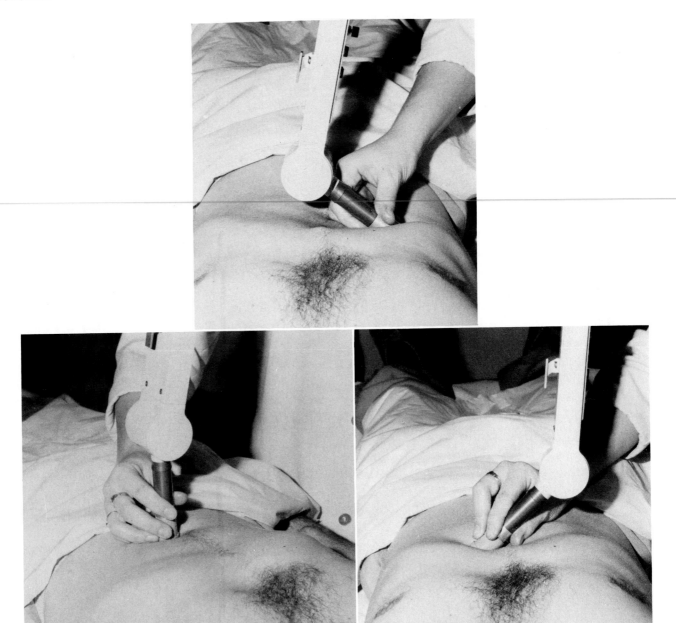

Fig. 21-5. Transverse pie sweep to demonstrate the aorta and prevertebral vessels.

the examiner should obtain a complete scan of the upper part of the vessel and then concentrate fully on the lower segment of the vessel. Sometimes it is helpful to mark the areas of the aorta on the abdomen by using a wax pencil so that proper alignment can be obtained with the transducer and an oblique scan made. (See Figs. 21-5 to 21-7.) However, if it is difficult to outline the aorta in the longitudinal plane, transverse scans may be used in an effort to follow its course. In our experience we have seen the abdominal aorta stretch from the far right of the abdomen to the far left of the abdomen in certain patients. However, if the examiner palpates the abdomen prior to the examination, much time can be saved in searching for the aorta. (See Figs. 21-8 to 21-10.) Arteriosclerosis usually

causes decreased pulsation of the aortic walls with intense aortic wall echoes demonstrated on sonography (Figs. 21-11 and 21-12).

The greatest value of ultrasonography in the aortic area is the assessment of an abdominal aneurysm. Aneurysms are generally diagnosed if the internal lumen diameter is greater than 3 cm. A good rule to remember for evaluating an abdominal aneurysm is to look for any abnormal bulging of the vessel that may be greater in diameter than the rest of the aorta. Generally, aneurysms occur at the level of the bifurcation near the umbilicus. Careful attention should be given to this area (Fig. 21-13).

Longitudinal scans are performed first with subsequent transverse scans recorded over the greatest

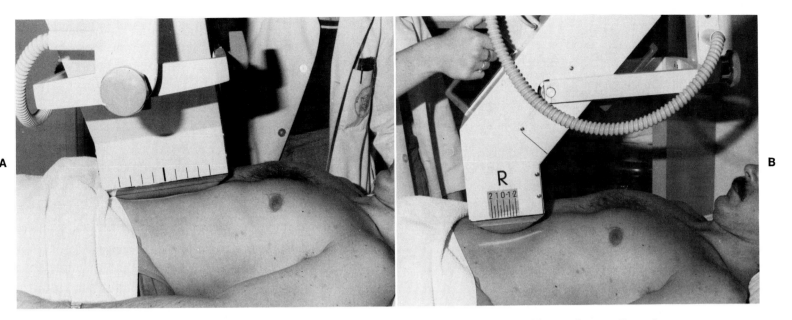

Fig. 21-6. A, Vidoson real time has proved a useful technique in the recognition and separation of vascular structures from other structures within the abdominal cavity. **B,** Transverse position of the real-time unit.

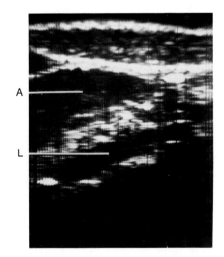

Fig. 21-7. Longitudinal scans of the abdominal aorta using real time.

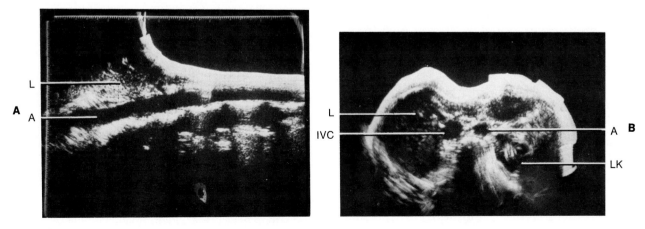

Fig. 21-8. Longitudinal **(A)** and transverse **(B)** scans of the abdominal aorta.

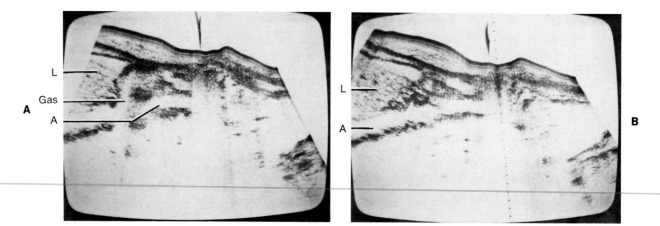

Fig. 21-9. A, Longitudinal scan of aorta partially obscured by bowel gas. **B,** Slight angulation of the transducer allows better penetration of the aortic lumen.

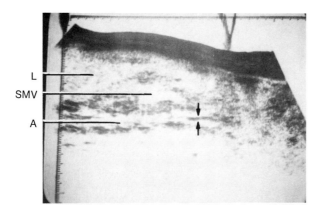

Fig. 21-10. Longitudinal scan of the abdominal aorta with bifurcation of the iliac arteries (arrows).

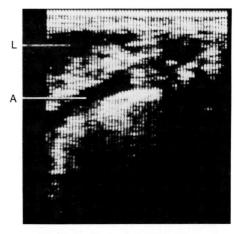

Fig. 21-11. Gross specimen of arteriosclerotic disease of the aorta and iliac vessels.

diameter of the aneurysm. High-gain technique should be used to record internal echoes within the aneurysm in an effort to visualize the exact lumen diameter of the vessel as well as the aneurysmal vessel. Thrombus echoes within the lumen can be easily detected with higher gain. These echoes can be seen in the anterior or posterior portion of the vessel and have a distinct margin (Figs. 21-14 and 21-15). In contrast, anterior reverberation echoes diminish in intensity from the source and do not have a distinct margin. Calcification with the walls of the vessels often produces dense, sharp contours. Serial examinations for abdominal aneurysms can be performed as indicated, evaluating for aneurysmal growth. In our past experience at the University of California, San Diego, most patients with aneurysm varying in size from 4 to 6 cm in diameter did not show any significant change subsequent on follow-up examinations of three to six months. Of the 88 patients studied, two went on to develop dissecting aneurysms, whereas the re-

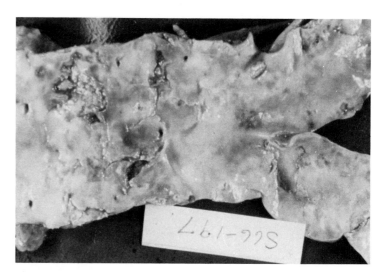

Fig. 21-12. Increased echoes along the anterior and posterior walls represent calcification. Real-time analysis will indicate reduced motion of the aortic pulsations.

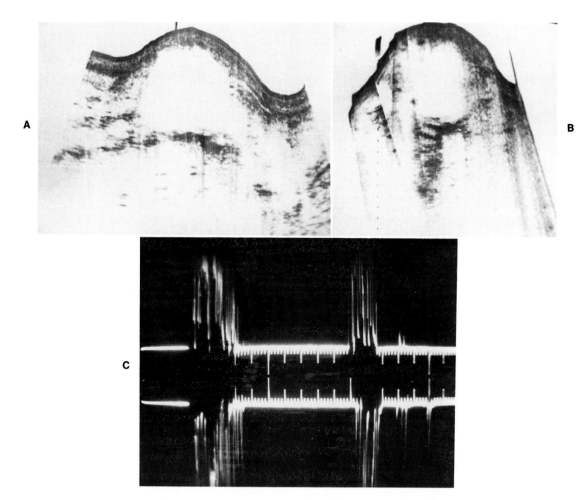

Fig. 21-13. A, Longitudinal scan of a large abdominal aneurysm at the level of the umbilicus. No internal echoes are seen within the vessel to indicate thrombosis. **B,** Transverse section at the level of the umbilicus shows the greatest dimension of the aorta is found in the anteroposterior direction. **C,** A-mode tracing can be made to accurately record the anterior and posterior walls of the aneurysm.

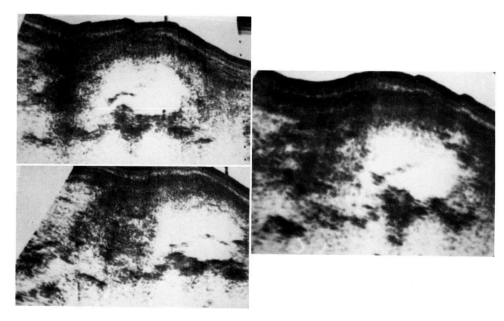

Fig. 21-14. Longitudinal scans of a tortuous aorta with a large aneurysm. The internal line represents part of the clot formation within the vessel.

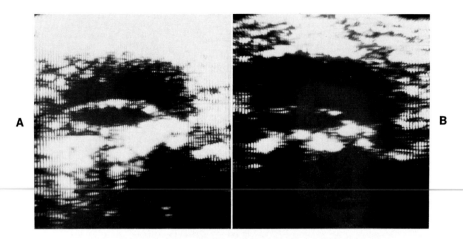

Fig. 21-15. Real-time longitudinal scans performed at high and low sensitivity demonstrate the aneurysm with thrombus formation. **A,** High gain. **B,** Low gain.

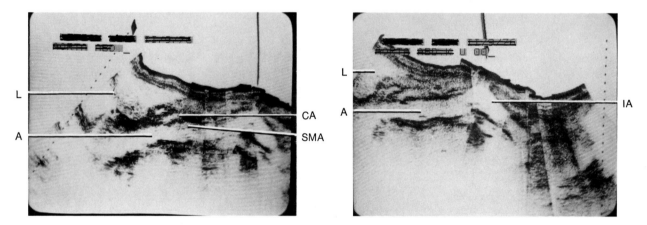

Fig. 21-16. Longitudinal scans of an aortic aneurysm extending into the iliac artery.

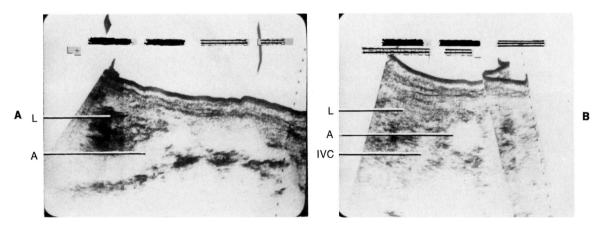

Fig. 21-17. A, Uniform enlargement of the abdominal aorta on the longitudinal scan. **B,** Transverse scan of an aneurysm.

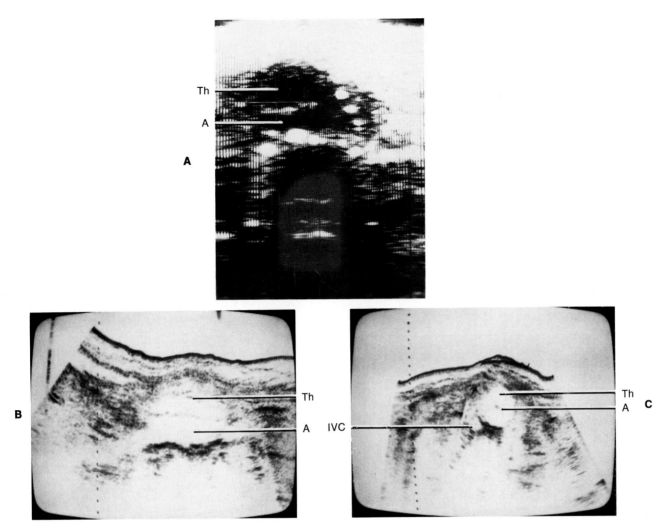

Fig. 21-18. A, Real-time longitudinal scan of the aneurysm with thrombus *(Th).* **B,** Longitudinal scan of the same area. **C,** Transverse scan of the aneurysm with thrombus.

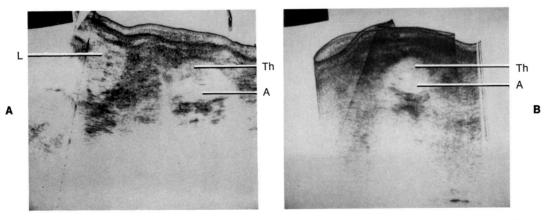

Fig. 21-19. A, Longitudinal scan of a tortuous aortic aneurysm near the level of the umbilicus. **B,** Transverse scan of the aneurysm with thrombus.

mainder of the patients demonstrated no significant growth. Thus ultrasound provides a very accurate clinical evaluation of patients with abdominal aneurysms. (See Figs. 21-16 to 21-20.)

An abdominal aortic aneurysm may be surgically repaired with a flexible graft material attached to either end of the remaining aorta (Fig. 21-21). Postsurgically the attached walls may swell at the site of attachment and form another aneurysm. Ultrasound is useful for postsurgical aneurysm studies as well as follow-up studies to visualize the graft and normal aortic attachment. The graft usually produces a dense echo reflection compared with the normal aortic walls.

A dissecting aneurysm may be detected with ultrasound and generally displays one or more of these characteristic signs. Generally, these patients are known to have an abdominal aneurysm and may develop sudden back pain due to a dissecting aneurysm. Since most aneurysms enlarge fairly symmetrically in the anteroposterior and width dimensions, an irregular enlargement with scattered internal echoes may represent an aneurysm with clot. Real-time techniques may be used to detect the actual flap or site of the dissection along the abdominal wall. If real time is not available, the A mode or M mode may be held over the site of dissection for observation of the irregular movement of the flap of the abdominal aortic wall. (See Figs. 21-22 to 21-24.)

Celiac trunk. The celiac trunk is best visualized ultrasonically by the longitudinal view where the aorta pierces the diaphragm and extends into the abdominal cavity. It is most commonly seen as a small vascular structure arising anteriorly from the abdominal aorta. Since the trunk is only 1 to 2 cm in length, it is sometimes difficult to record unless very careful evaluation near the midline of the aorta is made. Sometimes the celiac trunk can be seen to extend in a cephalic rather than a caudal presentation (Figs. 21-25 and 21-26). The superior mesenteric artery is usually seen just inferior to the origin of the celiac trunk and may be used as a landmark in locating the celiac trunk. Transversely one can differentiate the celiac trunk as a small vessel that arises directly anterior to the abdominal aorta. The splenic artery may be seen to flow from the celiac trunk toward the splenic area. Since the splenic artery is so tortuous, it is very difficult to follow its course routinely in the transverse direction. Generally, small pieces of the splenic artery may be seen as it weaves in and out the

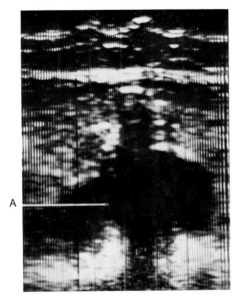

Fig. 21-20. Real-time longitudinal scan of the aortic aneurysm.

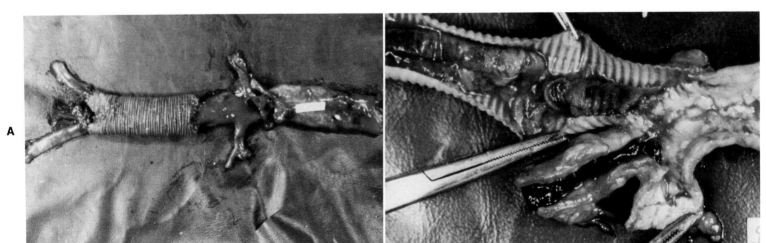

Fig. 21-21. A, Gross specimen of the abdominal aorta with a graft attached below the renal arteries and above the iliac arteries. **B,** Thrombus and clot are shown within the vessel at dissection.

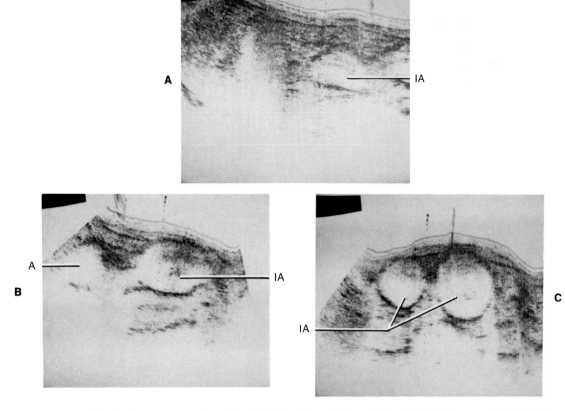

Fig. 21-22. Abdominal aneurysm extending into the iliac arteries. **A,** Longitudinal scan slightly to the right of midline. **B,** Longitudinal scan slightly to the left of midline. **C,** Transverse scan demonstrating both iliac arteries greatly enlarged. Real time can be a tremendous aid in the localization of the iliac arteries, especially if they are slightly enlarged.

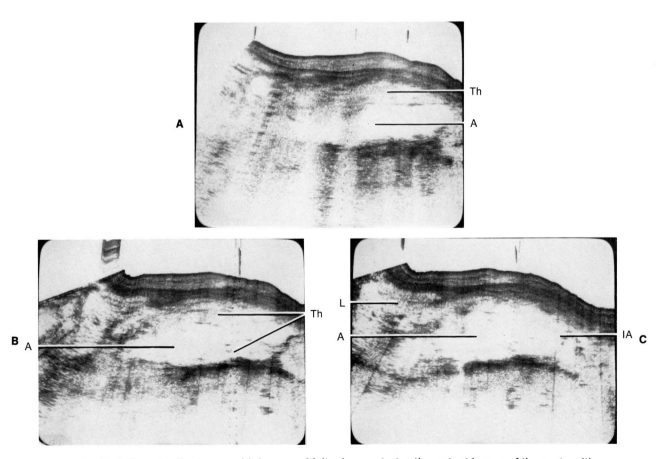

Fig. 21-23. A, Longitudinal scan with low sensitivity demonstrates the patent lumen of the aorta with anterior thrombus within the aorta. **B,** As the transducer is placed more perpendicular to the aortic area, thrombus can be seen anterior and posterior. **C,** Low sensitivity barely allows visualization of the aneurysm with thrombus formation.

left upper quadrant (Figs. 21-27 and 21-28). The hepatic artery may be seen to flow anterior and to the right of the celiac trunk, where it then divides into the right and left hepatic arteries (Figs. 21-29 to 21-31). The left gastric artery is very small in diameter and often difficult to visualize by ultrasound. It becomes difficult to separate the splenic artery from the left gastric artery unless separate structures are seen in the area of the celiac trunk branching to the left of the abdominal aorta.

Superior mesenteric artery. This vessel is well seen on both transverse and longitudinal scans. Single sweep technique should demonstrate the superior mesenteric artery arising from the anterior aortic wall. It may follow a parallel course along the abdominal aorta or may branch off at a slight angle to the anterior wall of the aorta and then follow its parallel course. If the angle is severe, adenopathy should be considered. The artery generally arises from the aorta and takes an anterior course as it moves inferiorly to branch to the

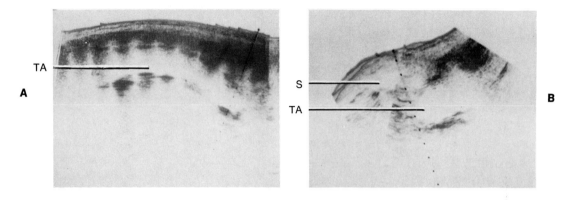

Fig. 21-24. A, Longitudinal prone scan demonstrates the thoracic aorta just beneath the vertebral column. **B,** Transverse scan to show the enlarged thoracic aorta just medial to the spleen.

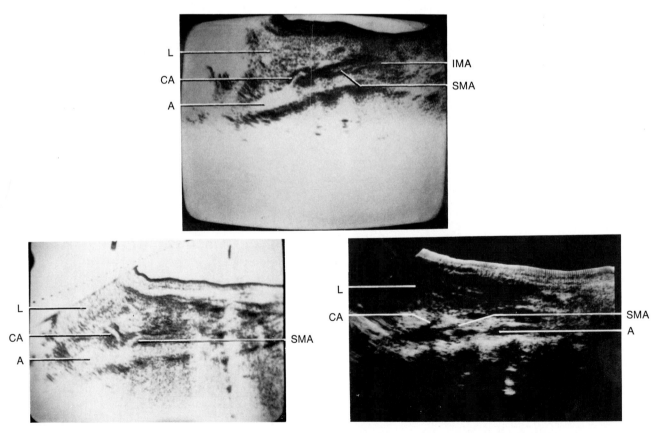

Fig. 21-25. Longitudinal scans of the celiac trunk shown to arise from the anterior wall of the abdominal aorta, just above the superior mesenteric artery. It may take a cephalic or caudal course as it flows from the aortic wall.

mesentery and colon. Transversely the superior mesenteric artery can be seen as a separate small circular structure anterior to the abdominal aorta and posterior to the pancreas. In some instances it can be anterior to the uncinate process of the pancreas and posterior to the body. (See Figs. 21-32 and 21-33.)

Renal arteries. Both renal arteries are best seen on transverse scans. The right renal artery passes behind the inferior vena cava and into the right kidney (Fig.

21-34). The left renal artery has a direct course from the aorta to the left kidney (Fig. 21-35).

Inferior mesenteric artery. This artery is more difficult to visualize, but when seen it is generally identified on the longitudinal scan as a small structure inferior to the superior mesenteric artery and celiac trunk. On transverse scans it is difficult to separate the inferior mesenteric artery from small loops of bowel within the abdomen (Fig. 21-36).

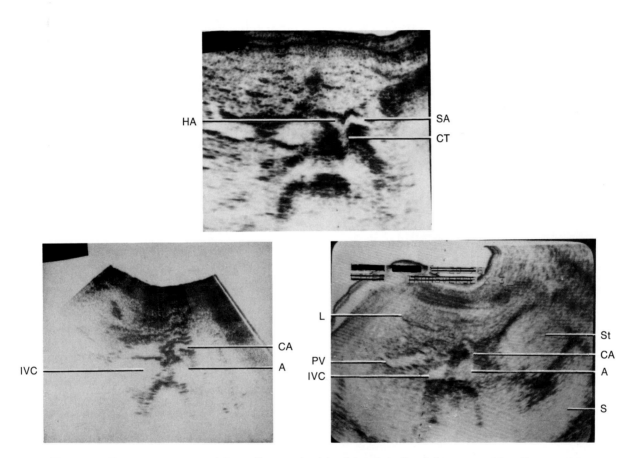

Fig. 21-26. Transverse scans of the celiac trunk with a branch to the right representing the common hepatic artery and the branch to the left of the splenic artery.

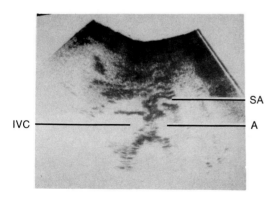

Fig. 21-27. Transverse scan of the splenic artery as it arises from the celiac trunk and courses to the left of the midline to the spleen.

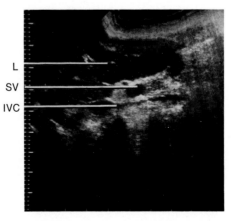

Fig. 21-28. Longitudinal scan of the splenic artery (small circular dot just superior and anterior to the splenic vein).

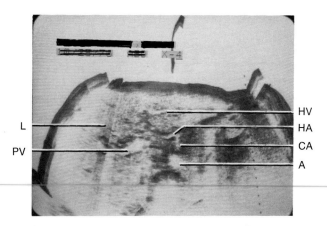

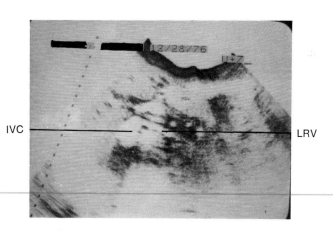

Fig. 21-29. Transverse scan of the hepatic artery as it courses to the right of the midline into the porta hepatis.

Fig. 21-30. Sometimes the hepatic artery is seen as a circle on the transverse scan after it branches off the celiac trunk. It may be seen lateral to the other small circle of the common bile duct and anterior to the portal vein and inferior vena cava.

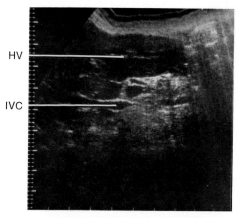

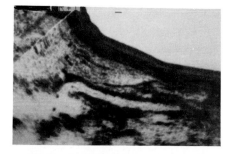

Fig. 21-31. Longitudinal scan of the hepatic artery anterior to the portal vein.

Fig. 21-32. Longitudinal scans of the superior mesenteric artery as it courses from the anterior aortic wall just beneath the celiac trunk.

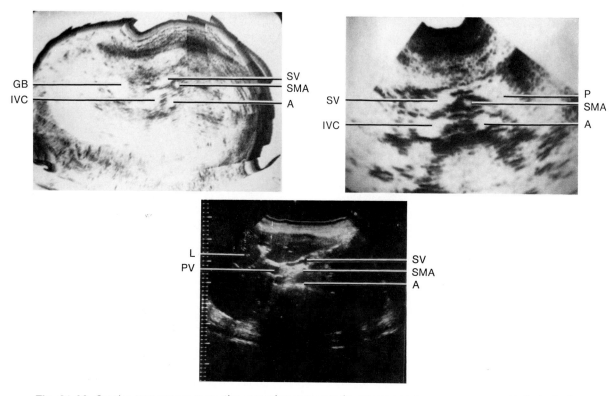

Fig. 21-33. On the transverse scan the superior mesenteric artery can be seen as a small circle just anterior to the aorta.

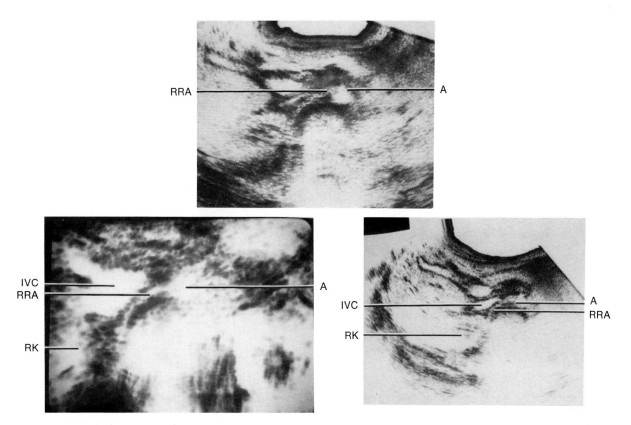

Fig. 21-34. Right renal artery can be seen to flow from the lateral margin of the aorta, posterior to the inferior vena cava, and to the right kidney.

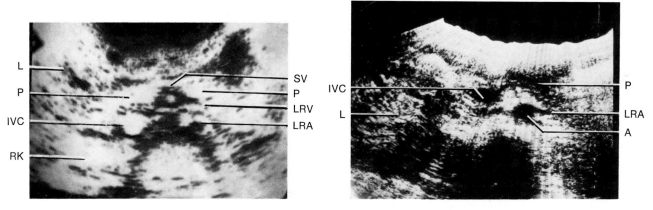

Fig. 21-35. Left renal artery takes a direct course from the aortic lateral wall to the left kidney.

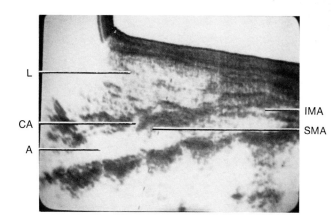

Fig. 21-36. Inferior mesenteric artery can sometimes be seen to course just anterior to the aorta beneath the superior mesenteric artery.

ANATOMY OF POSTERIOR ABDOMINAL WALL VEINS

Inferior vena cava. This vessel is formed by the union of the common iliac veins behind the right common iliac artery. It ascends vertically through the retroperitoneal space on the right side of the aorta

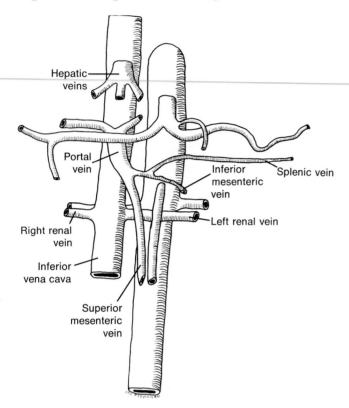

Fig. 21-37. Venous structures and their major branches.

posterior to the liver. It pierces the central tendon of the diaphragm at the level of the eighth thoracic vertebra and enters the right atrium of the heart. The entrance into the lesser sac separates the inferior vena cava from the portal vein.

The tributaries of the inferior vena cava correspond closely to the branches of the abdominal portion of the aorta (Fig. 21-37). The venous blood from the abdominal portion of the venous tract drains to the liver by means of the tributaries of the portal vein. The left suprarenal and gonadal veins drain first into the left renal vein.

The tributaries of the inferior vena cava are the hepatic veins, the right suprarenal vein, the renal veins, the right testicular or ovarian vein, the inferior phrenic vein, the four lumbar veins, the two common iliac veins, and the median sacral vein.

Inferior mesenteric vein. This vein is a tributary of the portal circulation. It begins midway down the anal canal as the superior rectal vein. It runs up the posterior abdominal wall on the left side of the inferior mesenteric artery and duodenojejunal junction and joins the splenic vein behind the pancreas. It receives many tributaries along its way, including the left colic vein.

Splenic vein. The splenic vein is also a tributary of the portal circulation. It begins at the hilus of the spleen as the union of several veins and is then joined

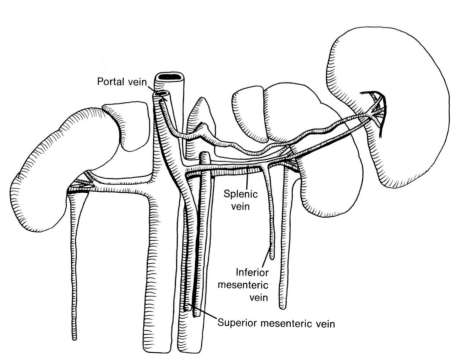

Fig. 21-38. Superior and inferior mesenteric veins join the splenic vein to form the portal vein.

by the short gastric and left gastroepiploic veins. It passes to the right within the lienorenal ligament and runs posterior to the pancreas below the splenic artery. It then joins the superior mesenteric vein behind the neck of the pancreas to form the portal vein. It is joined by veins from the pancreas and the inferior mesenteric vein (Fig. 21-38).

Superior mesenteric vein. The superior mesenteric vein is also a tributary of the portal circulation. It begins at the ileocolic junction and runs upward along the posterior abdominal wall within the root of the mesentery of the small intestine and on the right side of the superior mesenteric artery. It passes anterior to the third part of the duodenum and posterior to the neck of the pancreas, where it joins the splenic vein to form the portal vein. It also receives tributaries that correspond to the branches of the superior mesenteric artery, joined by the inferior pancreoduodenal vein to the right and the right gastroepiploic vein from the right aspects of the greater curvature of the stomach.

Portal vein. This vein is formed posterior to the pancreas by the union of the superior mesenteric and the splenic veins. Its trunk is approximately 5 to 7 cm in length. It runs upward and to the right, posterior to the first part of the duodenum, and enters the lesser omentum. It then ascends in front of the opening into the lesser sac to the porta hepatis, where it divides into right and left terminal branches. The right branch of the portal vein divides into interlobular veins, and the left branch supplies the caudate and quadrate lobes of the liver. The portal vein drains blood out of the gastrointestinal tract from the lower end of the esophagus to the upper end of the anal canal, from the pancreas, gallbladder, and bile ducts, and from the spleen. It has an important anastomosis with the esophageal veins, rectal venous plexus, and superficial abdominal veins.

The portal venous blood transverses the liver and drains into the inferior vena cava by way of the hepatic veins.

Hepatic veins. These veins are the largest visceral tributaries of the inferior vena cava. They originate in the liver and drain into the inferior vena cava, bringing blood back from the liver that was brought in by the hepatic artery and portal vein. Its minor tributaries, the right hepatic vein in the right lobe, the middle hepatic vein in the caudate lobe, and the left hepatic vein in the left lobe, empty into the inferior vena cava at the level of the diaphragm.

ULTRASONIC EVALUATION OF THE VENOUS STRUCTURE

Inferior vena cava. The inferior vena cava may be clearly seen during a Valsalva maneuver to the right of the abdominal aorta. Differentiation of the inferior vena cava from the aorta can easily be made. The vena cava has a horizontal course with the proximal portion curving slightly anterior, whereas the aorta follows the curvature of the spine with the distal portion going more posterior. The inferior vena cava is slightly to the right of the midline, as much as 3 to 4 cm. As is true with venous structures, the Valsalva maneuver causes dilatation, making the vena cava easier to demonstrate in both transverse and sagittal sections. The proximal portion can often be seen to enter the right atrium on the longitudinal scan as it pierces the diaphragm (Figs. 21-39 to 21-43). It serves as a landmark for many other structures in the abdomen and should be routinely visualized on all abdominal scans. On transverse scans it serves as a landmark for localization of the superior mesenteric vein, which is generally found anterior and slightly to the right or slight medial to the inferior vena cava (Fig. 21-44). On longitudinal scans it serves as a

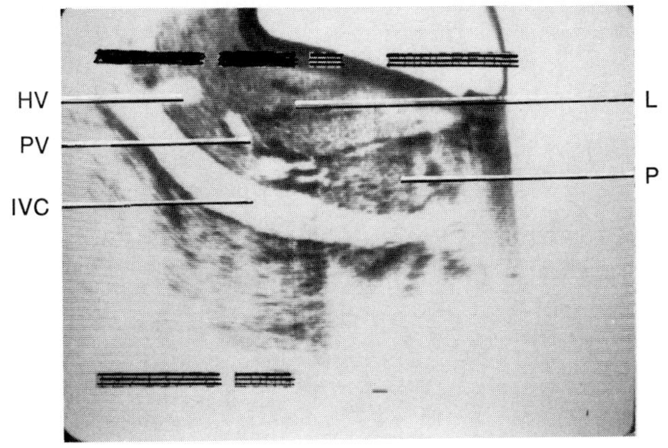

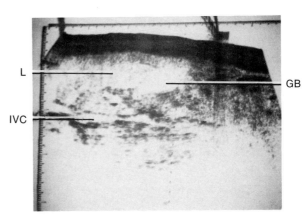

Fig. 21-39. Longitudinal view of the liver and inferior vena cava in full inspiration.

Fig. 21-40. Longitudinal view of the inferior vena cava during respiration demonstrates the somewhat collapsed vessel.

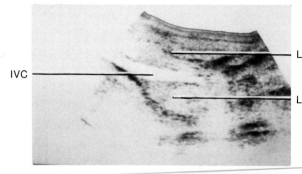

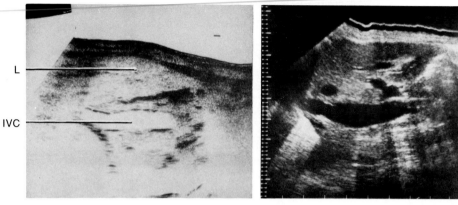

Fig. 21-41. Longitudinal view of the inferior vena cava with the patient performing a Valsalva maneuver.

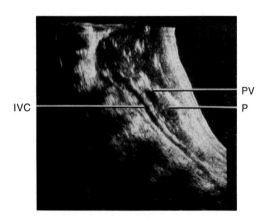

Fig. 21-42. Upright view of the inferior vena cava during normal respiration.

landmark for the portal vein, which is located just anterior to and midway down the inferior vena cava. It is also useful in locating the pancreas, which is found just inferior to the portal vein and anterior to the inferior vena cava, making a slight impression or indentation on the anterior wall of the vena cava.

Inferior mesenteric vein. This venous structure is difficult to recognize because of its anatomic location and small diameter. It is generally covered by small bowel tissue and has no major vascular structures posterior to it to aid in its recognition.

Splenic vein. The splenic vein is best seen in the transverse scans as it crosses the abdomen from the hilus of the spleen to join the portal vein slightly to the

right of midline. Single sweep technique should be used, with the patient performing a Valsalva maneuver or in suspended respiration. It crosses anteriorly to the aorta and the inferior vena cava and generally serves as the medial-to-superior posterior border of the pancreas (Fig. 21-45). On longitudinal scans the splenic vein can be visualized posterior to the left lobe of the liver and anterior to the major vascular structures. The pancreas may be seen inferior and slightly anterior to the splenic vein (Fig. 21-46).

Superior mesenteric vein. This venous structure is somewhat variable in its anatomic location. Generally, it is related to the inferior vena cava in an anterior position. Often it is seen slightly to the right or slightly

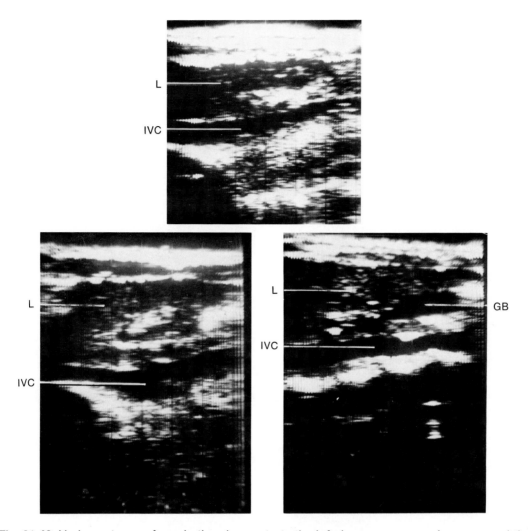

Fig. 21-43. Various stages of respiration demonstrate the inferior vena cava as shown on real-time equipment.

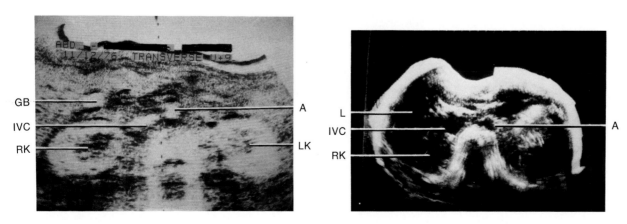

Fig. 21-44. Transverse scans demonstrate the inferior vena cava anterior to the spine and slightly to the left of the aorta.

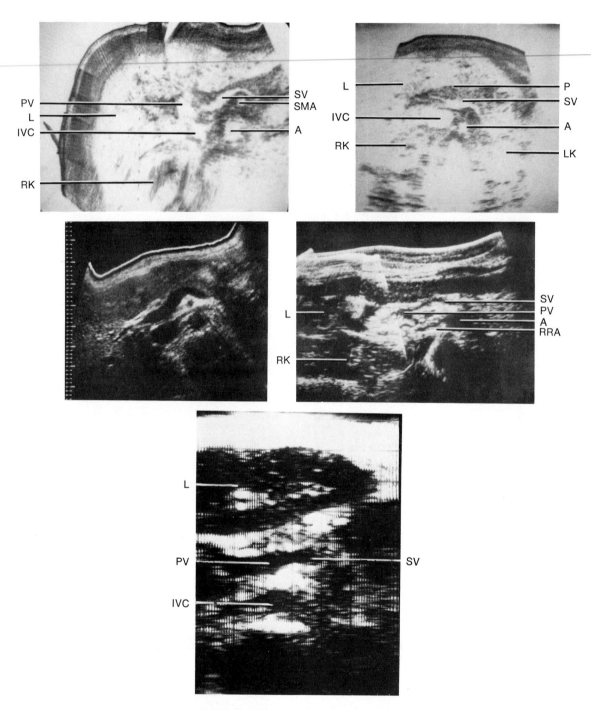

Fig. 21-45. Transverse scans of the splenic vein as it drapes over the superior mesenteric artery, aorta, and inferior vena cava to form the portal vein.

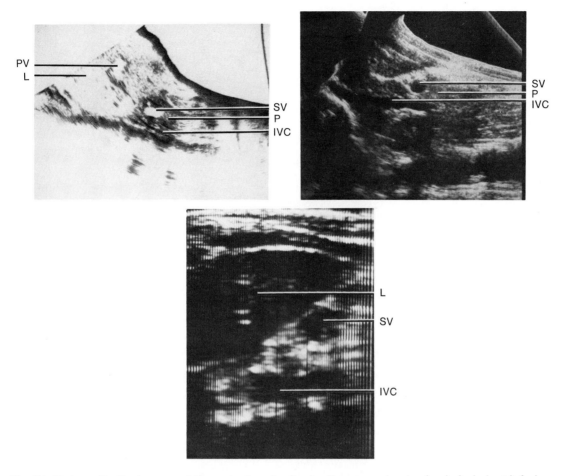

Fig. 21-46. Longitudinal scans of the splenic vein display it as a moderate sized circle just inferior to the liver and anterior to the major vessels. The pancreatic tissue can be seen surrounding this vessel in many scans.

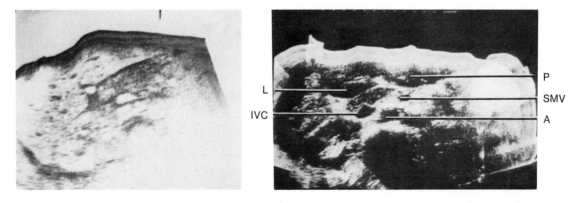

Fig. 21-47. Transverse view of the superior mesenteric vein as it appears in deep inspiration—a fairly large circular structure adjacent to the inferior vena cava and to the right of the superior mesenteric artery.

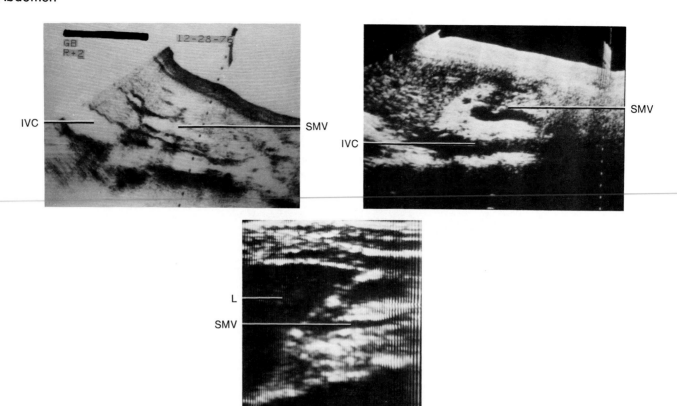

Fig. 21-48. Longitudinal scans of the superior mesenteric vein display it as a tubular structure usually anterior to the inferior vena cava or aorta. Pancreatic tissue can be seen anterior and posterior to this vessel in many scans.

to the left of the inferior vena cava and to the right of the superior mesenteric artery (Fig. 21-47). Since the superior mesenteric vein drains into the portal vein, as does the splenic vein, the sonographer should not be able to demonstrate these three structures together on a single transverse scan. Thus it doubles as the posterior border of the neck of the pancreas and as the anterior border where it crosses over the uncinate process of the pancreatic head. On longitudinal scans it is seen as a long tubular structure generally anterior to the inferior vena cava (Fig. 21-48). Often, with correct oblique angulation, the scan can follow the path of the superior mesenteric vein as it enters the portal system.

Portal vein. The portal vein is clearly seen on both transverse and longitudinal scans. On transverse scans it is a thin-walled circular structure, generally lateral and somewhat anterior to the inferior vena cava. With single sweep technique it is often possible to record the splenic vein as it crosses the midline of the abdomen to join the portal trunk. Thus a long section of the portal vein can be visualized. Often the right or left portal vein can be seen coming off the portal trunk in the hilus of the liver (Fig. 21-49). In the longitudinal

plane, slightly to the right of midline, the portal vein is situated between the inferior vena cava and the liver. It is anterior to the inferior vena cava and posterior to the liver. A landmark for localizing the pancreas can be established with the demonstration of these vessels. The pancreas is anterior to the inferior vena cava and caudad to the portal vein (Fig. 21-50).

Portal vein dilatation can be seen with many forms of hepatic disease, especially with cirrhosis.

Hepatic veins. Hepatic veins are best seen on longitudinal scans with single sweep technique. The venous structure is seen entering the vena cava near the level of the diaphragm. Again, with various forms of hepatic disease these venous structures may dilate, making them easier to see on both longitudinal and transverse scans (Figs. 21-51 and 21-52).

Renal veins. The right renal vein is seen best on the transverse scan with single sweep technique. It can be seen to flow directly from the kidney into the inferior vena cava (Fig. 21-53). The left renal vein may not be seen so easily. However, when seen, it takes a course anterior to the abdominal aorta and posterior to the superior mesenteric artery to enter the inferior vena cava (Fig. 21-54).

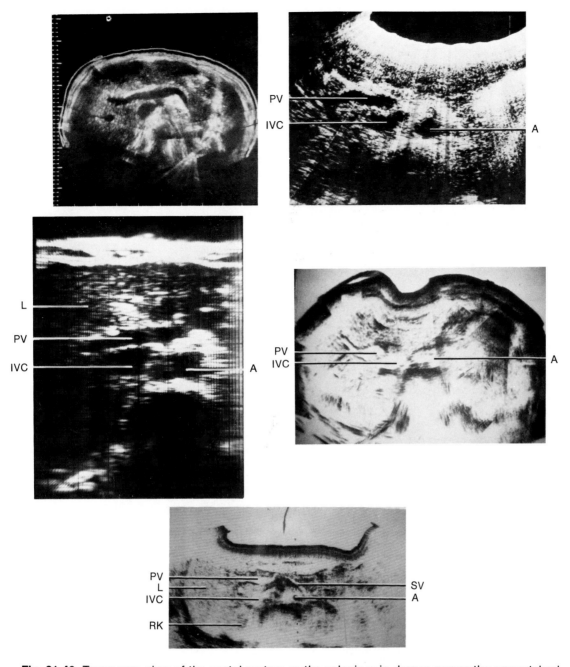

Fig. 21-49. Transverse view of the portal system as the splenic vein drapes across the prevertebral vessels to form the trunk of the portal vein. Often the right and left portal branches may be seen as the patient suspends respiration.

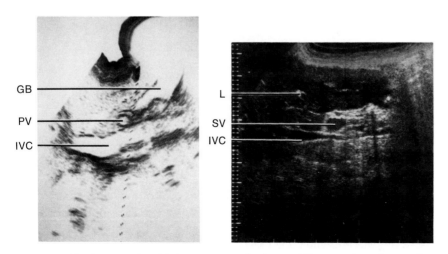

Fig. 21-50. Longitudinal scans should demonstrate the base of the portal trunk as a circular structure just anterior to the inferior vena cava.

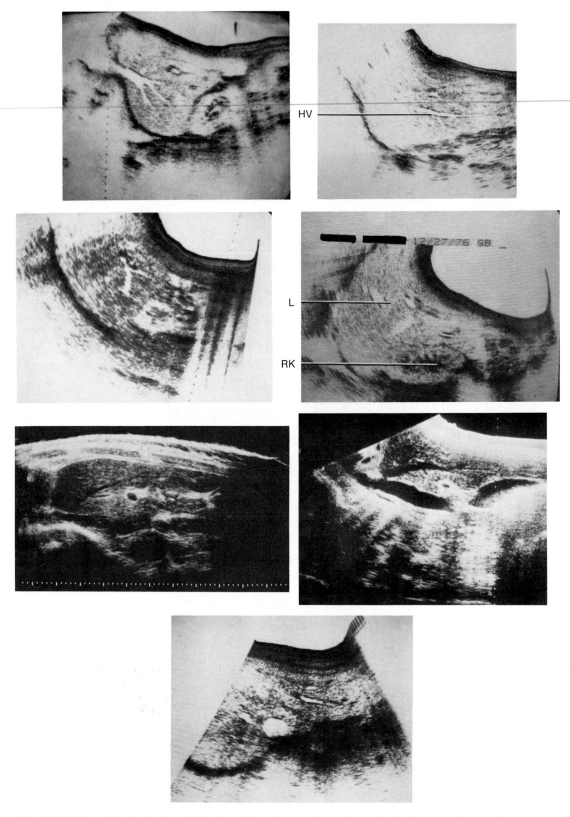

Fig. 21-51. Longitudinal view of the hepatic veins are best shown in full inspiration as the venous structures drain into the inferior vena cava. They can be distinguished from the portal structures within the liver as finer tubular structures within the liver parenchyma, whereas the portal system presents denser vessel patterns within the liver.

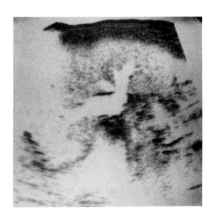

Fig. 21-52. Transverse view of a dilated hepatic system draining into the inferior vena cava.

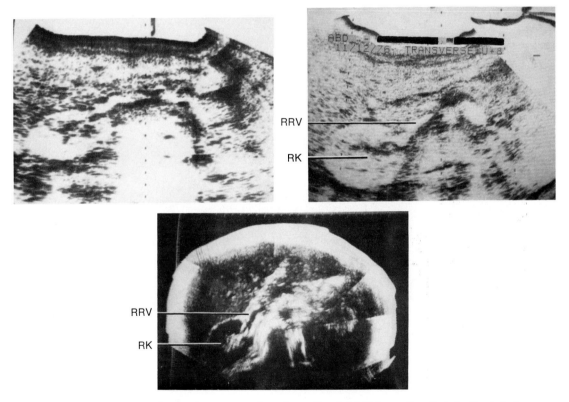

Fig. 21-53. Right renal vein can be seen to flow from the right kidney directly into the inferior vena cava.

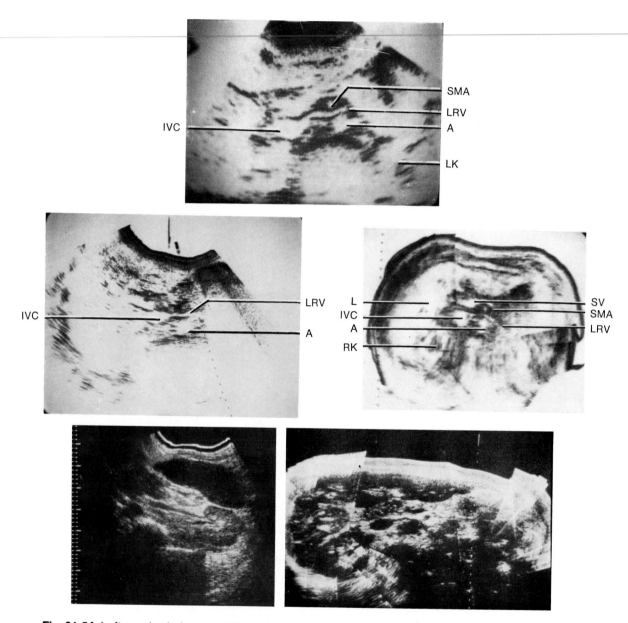

Fig. 21-54. Left renal vein is more difficult to recognize but is shown to flow over the aorta and under the superior mesenteric artery into the inferior vena cava.

22 □ Pancreas

with assistance of
BRENDA MANICH, M.A., R.N.M.

NORMAL PANCREATIC ANATOMY

The pancreas lies in the retroperitoneal area. The pancreatic gland is usually 10 to 15 cm long and approximately 13 cm at its greatest depth, at the head (Fig. 22-1). Generally, it is found in an oblique lie, extending from the concavity of the duodenum to the hilus of the spleen. Other variations of the gland are the transverse lie and the S-shaped lie.

The pancreas is seen anterior to the first or second vertebral body, deep in the epigastrium and left hypochondrium and behind the lesser omental sac. Thus it is hidden from direct physical examination.

The pancreas is divided into three major areas: the head, body, and tail (Fig. 22-2).

Head. The head is a globular shape on the right of the gland and lies in the lap of the duodenum. Picture the gland as a crowbar shape, with the head as the end of the crowbar. The very tip to the left of the head is the lingula (uncinate process) and is crossed anteriorly by the superior mesenteric vessels. The head is covered anteriorly by the pylorus of the stomach and the transverse colon (Fig. 22-3). The common bile duct passes either through a groove or through the substance of the gland (Fig. 22-4). The posterior surface of the head touches the inferior vena cava, the left renal vein, and the aorta.

The gastroduodenal artery serves as the anterolateral border of the pancreas (Fig. 22-5). The second part of the duodenum is deeper than the head of the pancreas. The second and third parts of the duodenum run between the superior mesenteric vessels, and the pancreas lies anterior to these vessels (Fig. 22-6).

The upper anterior part of the head uses the accessory pancreatic duct of Santorini, which enters the duodenum at a small accessory papilla.

Body. The head narrows to form the body of the pancreas, which is usually shown draping over the vertebral body and the prevertebral vessels. It lies on an angle from caudad right to cephalad left behind the stomach and in front of the origin of the portal vein and is the largest part of the gland. The right half of the body almost reaches the level of the celiac trunk. The

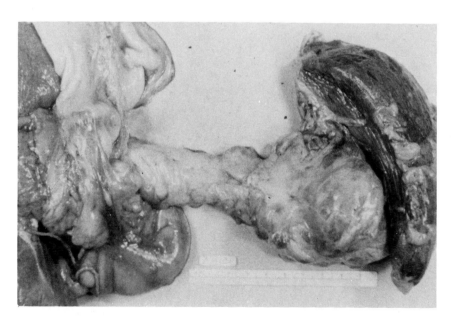

Fig. 22-1. Gross anatomic specimen of the pancreas and its relation to the hilus of the spleen and the medial aspect of the liver.

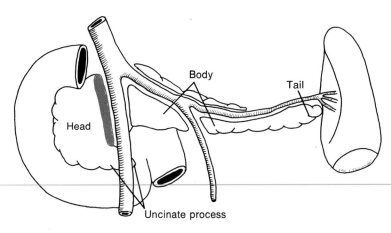

Fig. 22-2. Four parts of the pancreas: head, uncinate process, body, and tail.

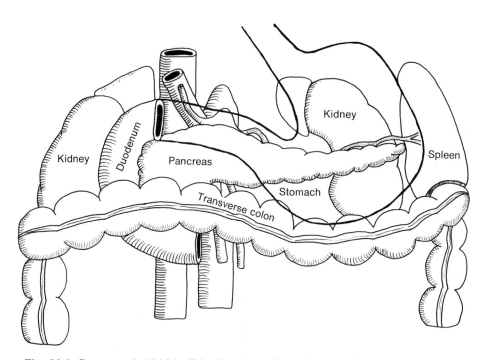

Fig. 22-3. Pancreas is "hidden" by the stomach, pylorus, and transverse colon.

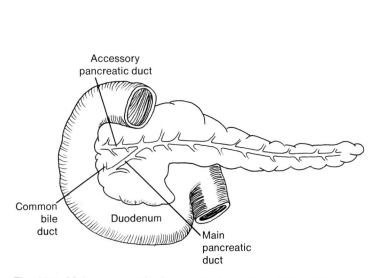

Fig. 22-4. Main pancreatic duct runs along the middle of the pancreatic gland. The common bile duct is shown along the lateral wall of the head of the gland.

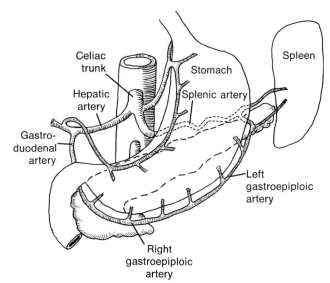

Fig. 22-5. Gastroduodenal artery serves as the anterior lateral border of the pancreatic head.

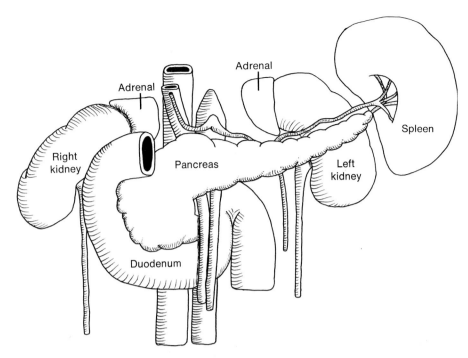

Fig. 22-6. Relationship of the pancreas to the other retroperitoneal structures.

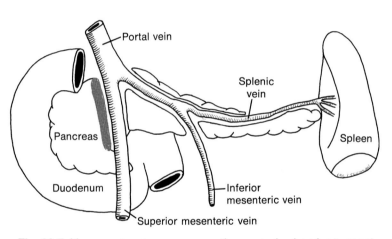

Fig. 22-7. Venous structures serve as the posterior border to most of the pancreatic tissue.

superior border of the body is important because the somewhat tortuous splenic artery extends along its upper surface. Its anterior surface is separated by the omental bursa from the posterior wall of the stomach. The inferior surface, below the attachment of the transverse mesocolon, is related to the duodenojejunal junction and to the splenic flexure of the colon. The posterior surface is in contact with the aorta, splenic vein, and left kidney (Fig. 22-7).

Tail. The body tapers off into a short tail, which is generally in contact with the hilus of the spleen.

The pancreatic duct of Wirsung begins in the tail of the gland and extends into the head. At this point it turns downward and backward to approximate the infraduodenal portion of the common bile duct. It terminates at the papilla in the duodenum.

Relational anatomy. The important structures related to the posterior surface of the gland include the inferior vena cava, the aorta, the superior mesenteric vessels, the splenic and portal veins, and the common bile duct. The splenic artery runs along the superior border of the pancreas, and the tail of the gland lies in contact with the hilus of the spleen.

Because of the unyielding nature of the posterior abdominal wall, any enlargement of the gland will extend anteriorly. The anterior surface of the pancreas is related to the lesser peritoneal cavity, whereas the inferior surface is related to the greater peritoneal cavity.

PHYSIOLOGY

The pancreas is both an exocrine and an endocrine gland. Its exocrine function is to produce pancreatic juice, which enters the duodenum together with bile. The exocrine secretions of the pancreas and the liver, both of which are delivered into the duodenum through duct systems, are essential for normal intestinal digestion and absorption of food. Pancreatic secretion is under the control of the vagus nerve and the two hormonal agents secretin and pancreozymin, which are released when food enters the duodenum. The endocrine function is the production of the hormone insulin. Failure of the pancreas to produce sufficient amounts of insulin leads to diabetes mellitus.

The components of the pancreatic juice are the enzymes lipase, amylase carboxypeptidase, trypsin, and chymotrypsin. The latter three are secreted as inactive enzyme precursors to be activated when they have entered the duodenum. The pancreas contains acinar cells, exocrine secretory cells that are arranged in saclike clusters (acini) and are connected by small intercalated ducts to larger excretory ducts. The excretory ducts converge into one or two main ducts, which deliver the exocrine secretion of the pancreas into the duodenum.

Pancreatic juice is the most versatile and active of the digestive secretions because its enzymes are capable of almost completing the digestion of food in the absence of all other digestive secretions. Because the digestive enzymes that are secreted into the lumen of the small intestine require an almost neutral pH for best activity, the acidity of the contents entering the duodenum must be reduced. Thus the pancreatic juice contains a relatively high concentration of sodium bicarbonate, and this alkaline salt is largely responsible for the neutralization of gastric acid.

The nervous secretion of pancreatic juice is thick and rich in enzymes and proteins. The chemical secretion resulting from pancreozymin activity is thin, watery, and is also rich in enzymes. Pancreatic juice is alkaline and becomes more so with increasing rates of secretion. This is due to a simultaneous increase in bicarbonates and decrease in chloride concentration.

The proteolytic enzyme, trypsin, may hydrolyze the protein molecule to polypeptides. Chymotrypsinogen is activated by trypsin. Amylase causes hydrolysis of starch with the production of maltose, which is further hydrolyzed to glucose. Lipase is capable of hydrolyzing some fats to monoglycerides and some to glycerol and fatty acids. Although lipases are also secreted by the small intestine, what is secreted by the pancreas accounts for 80% of all fat digestion. Thus impaired fat digestion is an important indicator of pancreatic dysfunction.

PATHOLOGIC CONDITIONS OF THE PANCREAS
Congenital anomalies

Ectopic pancreatic tissue. This is the most common anomaly, usually in the form of intramural nodules, and may be found in various places in the gastrointestinal tract. The most common sites are the stomach, duodenum, small bowel, and large bowel. On palpation they may seem polypoid and characteristically have a central dimple. The lesion is composed of elements of the pancreas, usually the acinar and ductal structures and less frequently the islets of Langerhans. They are usually small (0.5 to 2 cm). Acute pancreatitis or tumor may occur in these ectopic tissues.

Annular pancreas. Annular pancreas is a rare anomaly in which the head of the pancreas surrounds the second portion of the duodenum. More common in males than in females, all grades, from an overlapping of the posterior duodenal wall to a complete ring, may be found. The annular pancreas may be associated with complete or partial atresia of the duodenum and is susceptible to any of the diseases of the pancreas.

Fibrocystic disease of the pancreas. This is a hereditary disease of the exocrine glands seen frequently in children and young adults. The pancreas is usually firm and of normal size. Cysts are very small but may be present in the advanced stages. The acini and ducts are dilated. The acini are usually atrophic and may be totally replaced by fibrous tissue in many of the lobules. Nausea and vomiting may also occur, thus leading to the patient's malnourishment. The pancreatic secretion is gradually lost. With developing pancreatic fibrosis, jaundice may develop from the common duct obstruction. A late manifestation is diabetes. Grossly, the pancreas is found to be somewhat nodular and firm. One may see edema and fat necrosis, but gradually fibrous replacement occurs in much of the parenchyma. Ducts may dilate and contain calculi. Calcification of the gland may be seen in as high as 50% of the patients by radiography.

Pancreatic cysts

There are two types of pancreatic cysts—true cysts and pseudocysts. Both may be either unilocular or multilocular.

True cysts can be congenital or acquired. They arise from within the gland, usually in the head, then in the body and the tail. They have a lining epithelium (which may be lost with inflammation) and contain pancreatic enzymes or are found to be continuous with a pancreatic duct.

In contrast, pseudocysts are always acquired, resulting from trauma to the gland or secondary to acute pancreatitis. Encapsulated collections of pancreatic juice, blood, and debris form the pseudocyst. They usually present few symptoms until they become large and cause pressure on other organs.

Both kinds of cysts may protrude anteriorly in any direction, although the true cyst is generally associated directly with the pancreatic area. Pseudocysts most commonly develop through the lesser omentum, displacing the stomach or widening the duodenal loop. The majority of pseudocysts are found in the head and body but have been reported in the mediastinum and in the groin.

Benign tumors

The most frequent benign tumors of the pancreas are islet cell tumors. They are usually small (1 to 2 cm in diameter), may be multiple, and may develop in ectopic pancreatic tissue. They are well encapsulated and have a strong vascular supply. About 70% are associated with hyperinsulinism and hypoglycemia. Insulin shock, psychic disturbances, dizziness, nausea, and vomiting are common symptoms. Many of these tumors are found in the tail of the gland.

Neoplasms

Adenocarcinoma. The most common primary neoplasm of the pancreas is adenocarcinoma, which usually occurs in the head. It is more commonly found in middle-aged men than in women. Symptoms usually appear late, the most common being pain radiating to the back or a dull, steadily aching midepigastrium pain. Weight loss, painless jaundice, nausea and vomiting, and changes in stools are also clinical symptoms. The painless jaundice usually appears first, followed by nausea and vomiting. The presence of a dilated gallbladder and a palpable mass is strongly suggestive of carcinoma (Courvoisier's law). A cyst or pancreatitis may occur behind the neoplastic obstruction of the duct. With obstruction of the pancreatic ducts, enzymes will be absent or present only in small amounts.

Cystadenoma and cystadenocarcinoma. The cystadenoma is a rare benign neoplasm arising from the pancreatic ducts, usually in the tail of the pancreas. Occurring more commonly in women, it ranges anywhere from 2 to 15 cm or more in diameter.

Cystadenocarcinoma may be difficult to separate from a carcinoma arising in a true cyst or cystic degeneration of a solid carcinoma. It is as an irregular, lobulated cystic tumor, with thick cellular walls. Metastases arise most commonly in the lymph nodes and liver. The course of this tumor may be slowly progressive with a tendency for the recurrent disease to remain localized.

ULTRASONIC EVALUATION

The pancreas is one of the most, if not the most, inaccessible of abdominal organs to the ordinary methods of physical examination.

With the advent of each new medical procedure, efforts to visualize the pancreas have met with varying degrees of success. Prior to the relatively recent use of diagnostic ultrasound, other noninvasive procedures were unsuccessful in accurate visualization of the pancreas. The plain film of the abdomen is diagnostic of pancreatitis if calcification is visible in the pancreatic area; however it does not occur in all cases. Localized ileus ("paralyzed gut," gas and fluid accumulation near the area of inflammation) may be shown on the plain radiography in patients with pancreatitis. The upper gastrointestinal test series provides indirect information about the pancreas when the widened duodenal loop is visualized. Other diagnostic methods such as hypotonic duodenography, isotope examination, arteriography, fiberoptic gastroscopy, and intravenous cholangiography all provide indirect information about the pancreas or prove limited in their diagnostic ability. Thus investigators have been striving to develop an examination that will be accurate, readily repeatable, and safe. Diagnostic ultrasound appears to be such an examination.

Of course, at the present time there are still a few problems in pancreatic visualization with the ultrasonic technique. Familiar impediments are the reflections and absorptions caused by bone, gas, and air. If this occurs over the area of interest, it becomes impossible to outline prevertebral vessels, and thus visualization of the pancreas is limited. Obesity presents a problem in some cases. The far gain and/or the overall gain of the equipment may have to be adjusted to properly penetrate these patients. Normal organ movement makes exact repetition difficult in some cases, and several scans may have to be made before a confident analysis is possible. However, the real-time ultrasonic equipment has aided in this problem, enabling the sonographer to accurately follow the course of the vessels and delineate the borders of the pancreas with more precise accuracy.

The pancreas may be a more difficult organ to visualize than the liver, gallbladder, spleen, or kidneys for many reasons. Filly and Freimanis (1970) have presented evidence that the normal pancreas is difficult to visualize by the conventional bistable ultrasonic equipment, since the gland produces many echoes even at normal sensitivity because of the multiple interfaces within it. With grey-scale ultrasound, low-level echoes have been reported from the pancreatic region appearing as a uniform snowflake or stippled pattern anterior to the prevertebral vessels. The frequency of such echo patterns in our laboratory will be discussed.

Scanning techniques

We generally use a commercially available grey-scale contact scanner, with a 2.25 MHz, 13 mm long-focus or a 2.25 MHz, 19 mm long-focus transducer. When greater penetration is needed, a 1.6 MHz, 19 mm long-focus transducer is used. Commercially available real-time equipment is also employed to locate the prevertebral vessels as a preliminary to the contact scanner. The patient's skin is covered with a layer of mineral oil to ensure proper sonic contact with the ultrasonic system.

The patient is routinely scanned in the supine position after full inspiration. Commencing at the level of the xyphoid and moving caudal at 1 cm intervals, the sonographer carefully searches for the pancreatic area by the recognition of the prevertebral vessels (Fig. 22-8). The pancreas varies in location from 2 to 14 cm above the umbilicus. Thus, because of the anatomic variation of the body, it is difficult to predetermine the exact location of the pancreas. However, when it is viewed in relation to its surrounding anatomy, its location can be accurately and consistently demonstrated.

For maximum resolution, each scan is performed using the single pie sweep technique (Fig. 22-9). The initial movement of the transducer is angled almost perpendicular to the costal margin. Extremely slowly the transducer is arced toward the midline, moving gradually across the abdomen until it becomes possible to arc the transducer perpendicular to the other costal margin. Thus the single sweep pie scan allows the sonographer to visualize the prevertebral vessels in detail.

Anatomic identification

Head. The head of the pancreas is generally the easiest to outline, since it lies near the hilus of the liver. It is found inferior to both the portal vein and the caudate lobe of the liver. The inferior vena cava is its posterior border, and the superior mesenteric vein crosses anterior to the uncinate process and then descends posterior to the head of the gland. The superior mesenteric vein can be identified by dilatation with a Valsalva maneuver.

Body. The body of the pancreas may be seen draping across the prevertebral vessels. Adequate identification of the aorta, inferior vena cava, and superior mesenteric artery and vein is needed to accurately locate this part of the gland. The sonolucent tubular vessel structures may be distinguished from the more echo-producing structure of the pancreas. The splenic vein can follow a posterior course just below the superior aspect of the pancreas. Identification of this vein is helpful, since the pancreatic tissue above and below the tubular venous structure can be recognized. One can also follow the course of the splenic vein as it empties into the portal vein.

Tail. The tail of the pancreas fits snugly into the hilus of the spleen, and the stomach serves as the anterior border. Thus, as may be surmised, visualization is most difficult in this region because the sound is being attenuated by air and gas in the stomach. Often

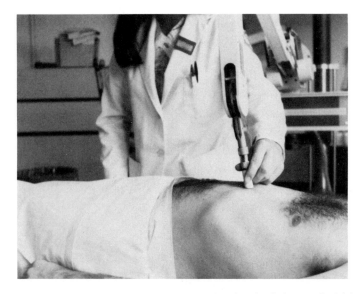

Fig. 22-8. Initial scans are made at the level of the xyphoid in search for the prevertebral vessels and pancreatic tissue.

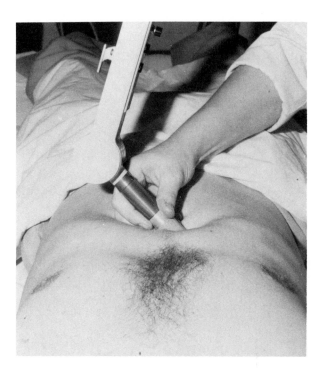

Fig. 22-9. Single pie sweep technique is used for better visualization of the midline structures such as the vessels and pancreas.

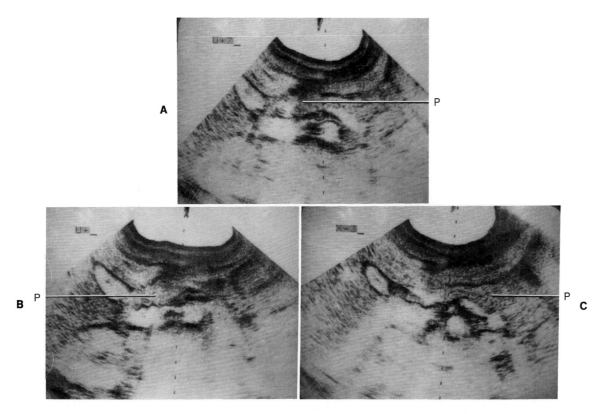

Fig. 22-10. A, Transverse scan of the body and tail of the pancreas draping over the splenic vein and great vessels. B, Transverse scan of the pancreatic head just medial to the gallbladder. C, Transverse scan of the tail of the gland under the left lobe of the liver.

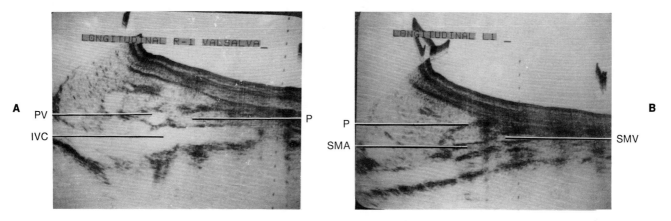

Fig. 22-11. A, Longitudinal scan of the pancreas inferior to the portal vein and superior to the inferior vena cava. B, Longitudinal scan of the pancreas anterior to the superior mesenteric artery shown coming off the aorta.

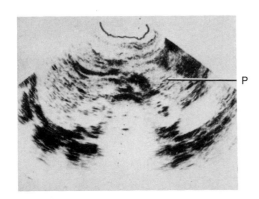

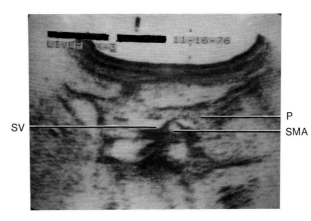

Fig. 22-12. Transverse view of the body and tail of the pancreas, which is anterior to the left kidney. Good visualization of the tail of the gland is shown.

Fig. 22-13. Transverse scan of body and tail draping over the splenic vein.

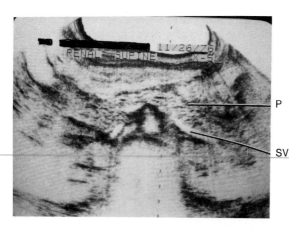
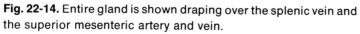

P

SV

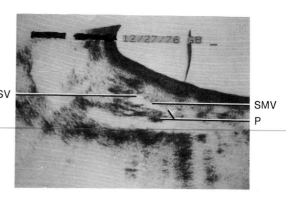

SV

SMV

P

Fig. 22-14. Entire gland is shown draping over the splenic vein and the superior mesenteric artery and vein.

Fig. 22-15. Longitudinal view of the superior mesenteric vein running through the pancreatic head and uncinate process.

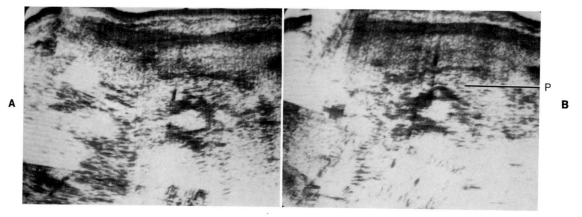

A

B

P

Fig. 22-16. A, Transverse scan of the body of the pancreas anterior to the prevertebral vessels. **B,** Body and tail of the pancreas draping over the superior mesenteric artery.

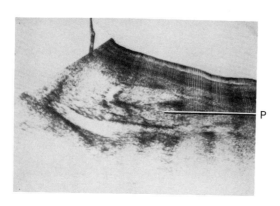

P

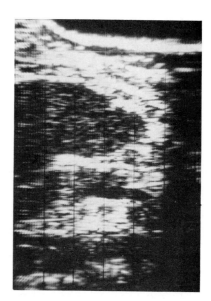

Fig. 22-17. Longitudinal scan of the pancreas anterior to the inferior vena cava and inferior to the portal vein.

Fig. 22-18. Real-time longitudinal scan of the superior mesenteric vein running through the substance of the pancreas.

it is possible to place the patient in the prone position, thus eliminating the gas factor, and search for the tail of the pancreas anterior to the left kidney and posterior to the stomach.

Transducer angle

Because of the variety of positions the pancreas may occupy, it may be difficult to record the entire gland on the cross-sectional view. If part of the gland is outlined on several transverse scans, a mark may be made on the patient's skin so that the proper oblique path can be used to fully outline the pancreas. (See Figs. 22-10 to 22-24.)

The right anterior oblique view has also proved effective in demonstrating the head and body of the gland. The sonographer is able to scan under the costal

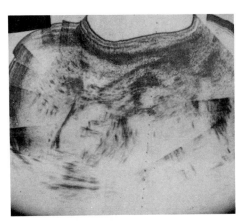

Fig. 22-19. Head and body of the pancreas seen anterior to the prevertebral vessels.

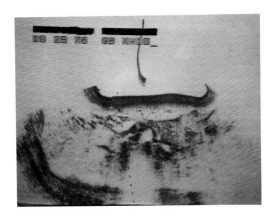

Fig. 22-20. Tail of the pancreas shown anterior to the renal vein and left kidney.

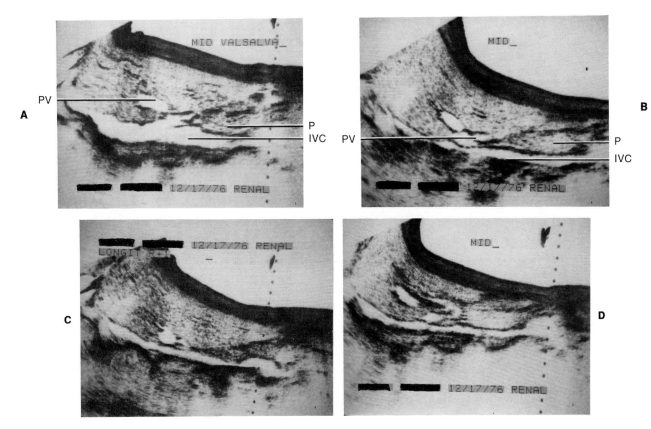

Fig. 22-21. A, Longitudinal scan of the pancreas shown slightly indenting the inferior vena cava. **B,** Pancreas is well shown anterior to the inferior vena cava and inferior to the portal vein. **C,** Small piece of the pancreas shown on the longitudinal scan superior to the splenic vein. **D,** Pancreas well seen on this longitudinal scan inferior to the portal vein.

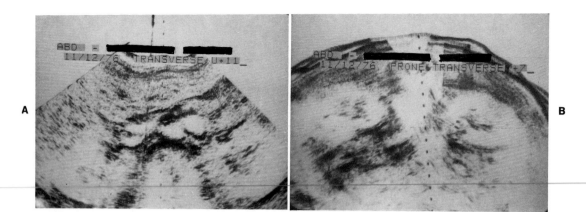

Fig. 22-22. A, Transverse scan of the tail of the pancreas anterior to the left kidney. **B,** The tail can also be shown well in the prone position, just beneath the left kidney and posterior to the stomach.

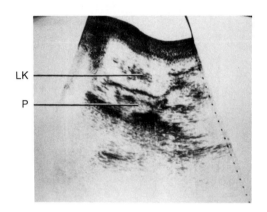

Fig. 22-23. Prone scan of the left kidney and tail of the pancreas.

margin to permit an easy access to the liver, prevertebral vessels, and pancreatic region.

On the sagittal view the portal vein and the vena cava can be identified slightly to the right of the patient's midline. The head of the pancreas lies just inferior to the portal vein and anterior to the inferior vena cava. Normally, the pancreas leaves a slight depression on the inferior vena cava. If the patient performs a Valsalva maneuver, the superior mesenteric vein can be demonstrated as a long tubular structure running through the gland. The body and tail are more difficult to visualize on the sagittal sections because the pancreas may appear quite thin in these areas (1 to 2 cm). However, proper identification of the prevertebral vessels can greatly aid in its identification.

ECHOGRAPHIC VISUALIZATION OF NORMAL PANCREAS TISSUE PATTERNS

It should be noted that in cases where the pancreas is not well visualized in the normal subject, in this same person "the edematous organ of pancreatitis, the tumors within the pancreas, and especially the fluid-containing pancreatic cyst and pseudocyst often are clearly apparent" (Stuber, 1974).

Freimanis (1970) states that although the pancreas is generally an echogenic organ, in many cases it is possible to have the pancreas appearing as a relatively transonic organ in comparison with the surrounding irregular connective tissue structures.

Failure or success in demonstrating the pancreas does not necessarily mean it is abnormal. The diagnosis of abnormalities relies on increased transonance, enlargement, or abnormal shape of the organ (Freimanis, 1970).

With currently available grey-scale ultrasound equipment, the normal pancreas can be visualized 75% to 95% of the time. (Varying degrees of success depend on individual experience and scanning technique.) The echographic appearance of the pancreas has been reported as more echogenic than the liver parenchyma. Stuber and associates (1974) report that "the pancreas, probably because of its numerous ducts and blood vessels and its lobular structures, belongs to the category of heavily echo-producing organs. The relative thinness and irregularity of the organ, as well as its lack of a dense capsule, further encourages its appearance into the indefinable echoes of the retroperitoneum."

Often we have noted the normal pancreas to be inconsistent in this echogenic pattern. Thus we are conducting an ongoing survey of normal subjects to evaluate these echographic patterns of the pancreas. At this time, we have collected data on twenty-two young adults in an effort to evaluate the normal pancreas. Visualization of the gland was possible in 90% of the subjects. Protocol demanded utilization of the pie sweep technique to visualize the prevertebral vessels.

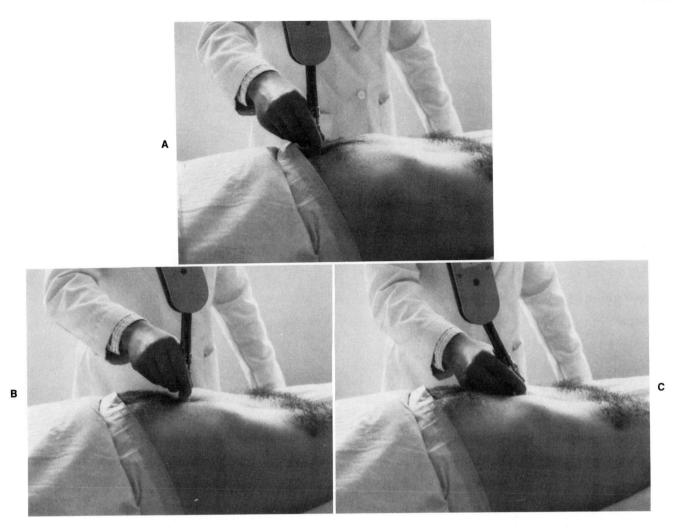

Fig. 22-24. A, Sagittal scans should be performed in full inspiration to outline the vessels for pancreatic location. **B,** Single sweep should be used for maximum resolution. **C,** Slight arc motion of the transducer allows the beam to sweep under the xyphoid or costal margin.

Methods

The splenic vein takes a posterior course from the spleen, joining the superior mesenteric vein to form the portal vein. This venous structure serves as the medial to superior border of the pancreas and can be identified as a sonolucent tubular structure flowing over the prevertebral vessels on the transverse scan. The sagittal scan shows the splenic vein as a small circular structure with echo-producing pancreatic tissue either surrounding it or inferior to it.

The superior mesenteric artery is most commonly shown as a small circular vessel on the transverse scan immediately anterior to the abdominal aorta, and the superior mesenteric vein medial to the superior mesenteric artery or anterior to the inferior vena cava. The body of the pancreas is shown anterior to these vessels. As the scan moves more caudal to the body of the pancreas, the uncinate process of the head is shown posterior to the superior mesenteric vessels.

This is an important relationship and enables the examiner to understand why the pancreatic tissue appears to be surrounding the superior mesenteric vein on transverse scans.

The sagittal scan is performed in full inspiration, allowing the sonographer to fully demonstrate the superior mesenteric vein as the posterior (near the body) and anterior (near the uncinate process) border of the gland. The superior mesenteric artery can often be seen arising from the anterior aortic wall, just inferior to the celiac axis. The body of the pancreas is best shown anterior to these structures, between the celiac axis and the superior mesenteric artery.

Results

Frequency of echo patterns. The frequency of echo patterns was classified into four types: (1) type a, densely echoic; (2) type b, slightly echoic; (3) type c, anechoic; and (4) type d, nonvisualization.

Approximately 72% of the subjects' pancreases demonstrated densely to slightly echoic patterns in comparison with the liver parenchyma. It was interesting to note that 18% of the pancreases were normal in size (less than 3 cm in the anteroposterior transverse dimension) but anechoic. Nonvisualization of the pancreas was demonstrated in 9% of the subjects due to gas interference.

Distance from left lobe of liver. The mean distance from the anterior edge of the left lobe of the liver to the anterior edge of the pancreas was 2.5 cm.

Drinking habits. The subjects' drinking habits ranged from none (9%), occasional (9%), social (50%), to often (32%).

Pitfalls of pancreatic echography

Pancreatic echography may be obscured for any of the following reasons:

1. A small echo-free area medial to the liver could be fluid-containing duodenum and could be mistaken for the pancreas. Slight right anterior oblique decubitus scans should enable the sonographer to distinguish the duodenum from the pancreas (Fig. 22-25).

2. The pancreas may be difficult to visualize because of overlying structures such as the stomach, fat, muscles, and costal cartilage.

3. Other echo-free areas in the region of the pancreas could be the splenic vein, which usually runs through the posterior aspect of the pancreas. This structure may cause some confusion because of its

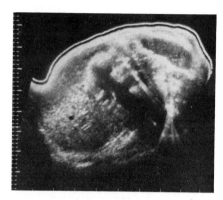

Fig. 22-25. Duodenum causes a shadow posterior, which prohibits visualization of the head of the pancreas.

Table 22-1. Subjects' data

Case	Age	Height	Weight	BSA(m²)	Drinking habits*	Neighbor organs†	Echo patterns‡	Distance d§
1	23	5'8''	125	1.65	Occasionally	SV through	c	3.0
2	29	5'10''	150	1.83	Socially	SV under	c	3.5
3	21	5'4''	170	1.82	None	SV through	a	3.0
4	27	5'0''	165	1.72	None	SV (gallstone)	a	3.2
5	21	5'3''	182	1.85	Often	SV through	b	4.5
6	27	5'5''	113	1.55	Often	Nonvisualized	b	2.0
7	21	5'8''	180	1.93	Often	Nonvisualized	d	—
8	21	5'10''	180	1.98	Often	Nonvisualized	d	—
9	21	5'6''	96	1.44	Often	Prominent LLL	b	—
10	20	5'5''	125	1.61	Socially	SV under	b	2.5
11	27	5'2''	113	1.50	Socially	—	b	—
12	21	5'11''	140	1.79	Socially	SV under	c	1.8
13	27	5'1''	108	1.44	Socially	—	b	2.0
14	23	5'2''	100	1.42	Socially	SV under	c	2.5
15	28	5'11''	148	1.85	Often	SV through	a	2.0
16	22	5'5''	127	1.61	Occasionally	SMV seen	b	2.5
17	18	5'8''	143	1.75	Socially	SMV seen	a	3.5
18	19	5'4''	102	1.46	Socially	SV under	a	1.3
19	18	5'10''	142	1.78	Socially	SV through	b	3.5
20	19	5'6''	190	1.95	Socially	SV through	a	3.5
21	22	5'0''	126	1.52	Socially	SV under	a	2.0
22	26	5'1''	105	1.42	Often	SV through	a	2.0

*Drinking habits: occasionally (less than socially), socially (once in a while), and often (few times a week).
†Neighbor organs: organs well seen around the pancreas.
‡Echo patterns: type *a*, densely echoic; type *b*, slightly echoic; type *c*, anechoic; type *d*, nonvisualized.
§Distance d: distance from anterior edge of liver to anterior edge of pancreas.

close relationship to the gland, although it is useful when taken as another landmark to identify the pancreas. Doust (1976) states that the boundary between the splenic vein and the pancreas is obscured in cases of pancreatitis.

4. Other solid masses in the retroperitoneal region, such as that caused by lymphadenopathy, may cause some confusion in the identification of the pancreatic region, since the lymph nodes drape across the prevertebral vessels within the region where the pancreas may lie.

Conclusions

After performing twenty-two ultrasound abdominal examinations for the pancreas on normal subjects, we reached the following conclusions:

1. The pancreas was best visualized in the transverse or decubitus position anterior to the prevertebral vessels.

2. There did not seem to be any relationship between the subject's dimensions (body surface area) and the visualization of the gland. Obesity did not limit the penetration or resolution in the pancreatic area.

3. In most cases the splenic vein appeared to run through the posterior body of the pancreas, although some cases demonstrated the vein inferior to the pancreas and anterior to the prevertebral vessels.

4. The pancreas was visualized in 90.9% of the cases.

Interpretation of the data

A. Frequency of echo patterns

Type a (densely echoic):	8 subjects	(36.4%)
Type b (slight echoic):	8 subjects	(36.4%)
Type c (anechoic):	4 subjects	(18.2%)
(Type d (nonvisualized pancreas):	2 subjects	(9.0%)
	22	(100.0%)

B. Mean distance d (from anterior edge of liver to anterior edge of pancreas): 2.5 cm

C. Classification of drinking habits

Occasionally:	2 subjects	(9.1%)
Socially:	11 subjects	(50.0%)
Often:	7 subjects	(31.8%)
None:	2 subjects	(9.1%)
	22	(100.0%)

D. Visualization of the pancreas

Visualization of the gland:	20 subjects	(90.9%)
Nonvisualization of the gland:	2 subjects	(9.1%)
	22	(100.0%)

Table 22-1 contains a detailed breakdown of the subjects' data.

ULTRASONIC EVALUATION OF ABNORMAL PANCREAS

The major abnormalities that affect the pancreas—pancreatitis, pseudocyst, and carcinoma—often have characteristic ultrasonic patterns. Difficulties in distinguishing these patterns will also be discussed and are shown in Table 22-2.

Pancreatitis

In a case of pancreatitis the swollen gland causes increased sonolucency (Fig. 22-26). The borders become distinct and only occasionally have irregular margins with normal or increased sound transmission. It it easiest to record this pattern in the head of the pancreas, since it lies beneath the liver, the homogeneity of which allows good penetration of the ultrasonic beam. The fibrous tissues may still be apparent within the gland and account for the scattered echoes seen sonographically (Figs. 22-27 to 22-36). If visualization is difficult in the supine position, the patient may be rolled into a right semilateral decubitus position to permit a better view of the pancreatic area. The normal thickness of the pancreas is usually less than 3 or 4 cm. With pancreatitis the pancreas enlarges due to edema. Patients with pancreatitis will often have an unusual amount of bowel gas as a result of ileus. This can prevent penetration of the ultrasonic beam. When this condition is present, a repeat examination should be performed.

Table 22-2. Difficulties of pancreatic visualization

Echographic results of pancreatic visualization	Number of patients
Pancreatic echograms	
Pancreas well demonstrated	61
Pancreas shown with ill-defined borders	5
Pancreas not well shown	16
Total	82
Pancreatic visualization (76%)	
Normal pancreas, well defined	54
Normal, but ill-defined borders	5
Calcified pancreas	1
Pancreatitis	2
Pancreatic carcinoma	1
Pancreatic pseudocyst	3
Total	66
Pancreatic nonvisualization (24%)	
Abdominal distension, gas	8
Lymphadenopathy	1
Anterior renal cyst	1
Huge gallbladder	1
No prevertebral vessels seen	4
Recent surgery	1
Total	16

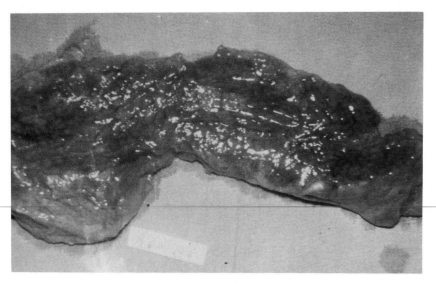

Fig. 22-26. Gross specimen of pancreatitis.

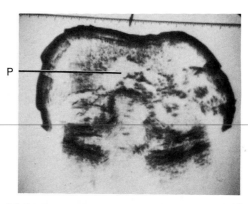

Fig. 22-27. Transverse scans of edematous pancreatic tissue draping over the prevertebral vessels.

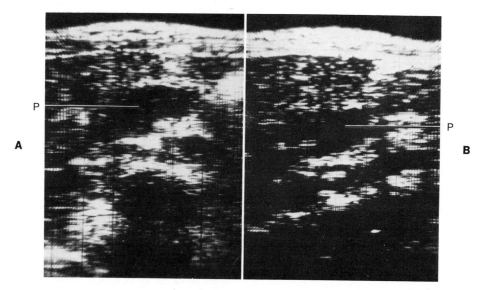

Fig. 22-28. Transverse (A) and longitudinal (B) views of a swollen pancreas as seen anterior to the prevertebral vessels.

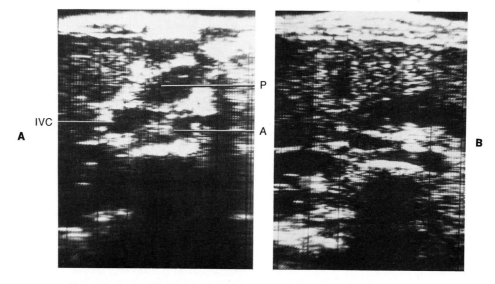

Fig. 22-29. A, Transverse real-time scans of pancreatitis anterior to the inferior vena cava and aorta. B, Real-time transverse scans of the swollen body of the pancreas.

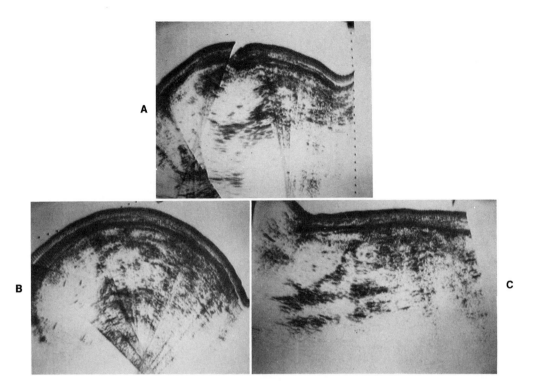

Fig. 22-30. A and **B,** Transverse scans of pancreatitis as seen in the swollen head of the gland. Multiple internal echoes represent the multiple interfaces within the gland. **C,** Longitudinal scan shows an enlarged pancreas just under the liver and anterior to the aorta.

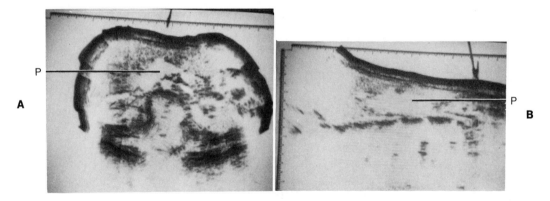

Fig. 22-31. Transverse **(A)** and longitudinal **(B)** scans of pancreatitis.

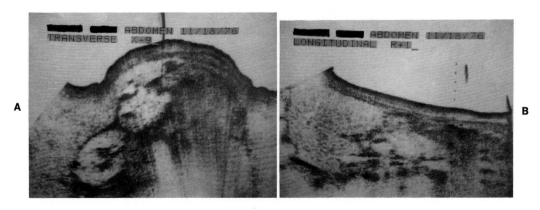

Fig. 22-32. A, Transverse section of a swollen pancreas. The gland shows very irregular borders with internal echoes. **B,** Longitudinal scan.

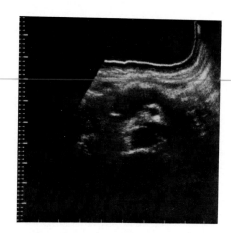

Fig. 22-33. Swollen pancreas anterior to the superior mesenteric artery and aorta.

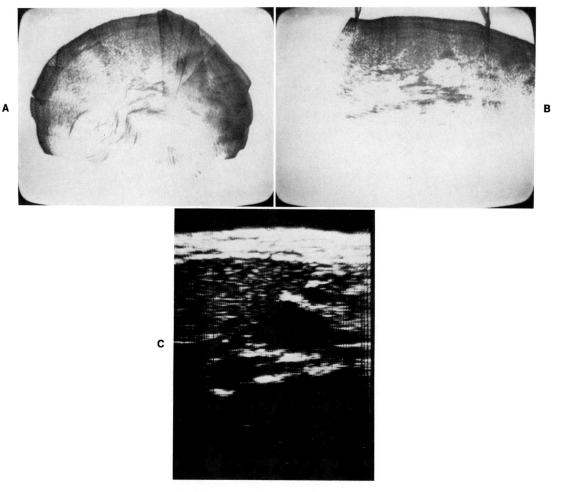

Fig. 22-34. A, Transverse scan of pancreatitis in the body of the gland. **B,** Longitudinal scan of pancreatitis anterior to the aorta and superior mesenteric artery. **C,** Real-time scan.

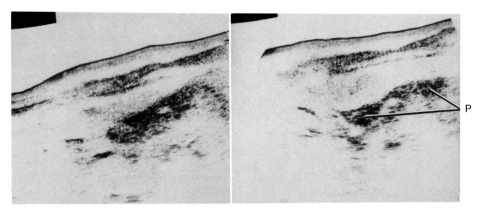

Fig. 22-35. Multiple scans over the pancreatic area demonstrate increased echoes within the gland, most likely representing chronic pancreatitis with calcification.

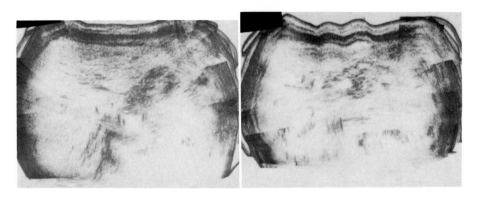

Fig. 22-36. Increased echo pattern most consistent with calcification of the pancreatic area.

Chronic versus acute pancreatitis

It is virtually impossible to distinguish acute from chronic pancreatitis on a single examination. With uncomplicated acute pancreatitis the ultrasonic pattern generally reverts to normal in time, whereas with chronic pancreatitis, patients may have a persistently enlarged pancreas on serial echograms, even during asymptomatic periods. When the ultrasonic pattern changes in patients with chronic pancreatitis, the diagnosis of pancreatic pseudocyst formation, carcinoma, or superimposed acute pancreatitis should be considered.

Pancreatic pseudocysts

A pseudocyst develops when pancreatic enzymes escape from the gland and break down tissue to form a sterile abscess somewhere in the abdomen. Its walls are not true cyst walls—hence its name pseudo, or false, cyst. Pseudocysts may develop anywhere in the abdominal cavity and have even been found as far as the groin and as high as the mediastinum. They generally takes on the contour of the available space around them and therefore are not always spherical, as are normal cyst. There may be more than one pseudocyst, so the sonographer should search for other daughter collections when performing an echogram.

Sonographically pseudocysts usually appear as well-defined masses with essentially echo-free interiors. (See Figs. 22-37 to 22-40.) Because of debris, scattered echoes may sometimes be seen at the bottom of the cyst. When a suspected pseudocyst is located near the stomach, the stomach should be drained so that the cyst is not mistaken for a fluid-filled stomach. If the patient has been on continual drainage prior to the ultrasonic examination, this problem is eliminated.

Sokoloff (1974) has described results of the problem of false positive diagnosis of a pseudocyst of the pancreas. If the gland is so edematous and transonic, it may be impossible to distinguish pancreatitis from a pseudocyst formation, particularly when the head of the gland is involved.

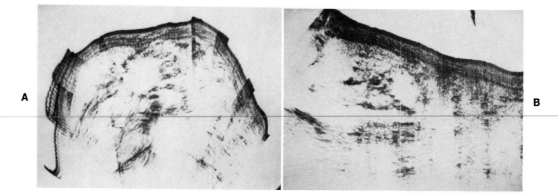

Fig. 22-37. A, Supine transverse scan of a pancreatic pseudocyst shown in the head of the gland. B, Supine longitudinal scan of the swollen head of a pancreas anterior to the IVC.

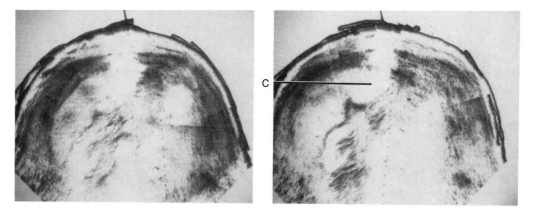

Fig. 22-38. Double-sided pancreatic pseudocyst. Longitudinal and oblique scans would separate this from an enlarged gallbladder.

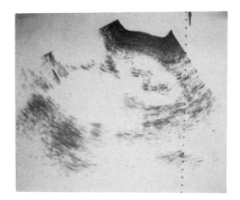

Fig. 22-39. Large pseudocyst anterior to the left kidney in the prone position. A fluid-filled stomach must be further evaluated in such cases.

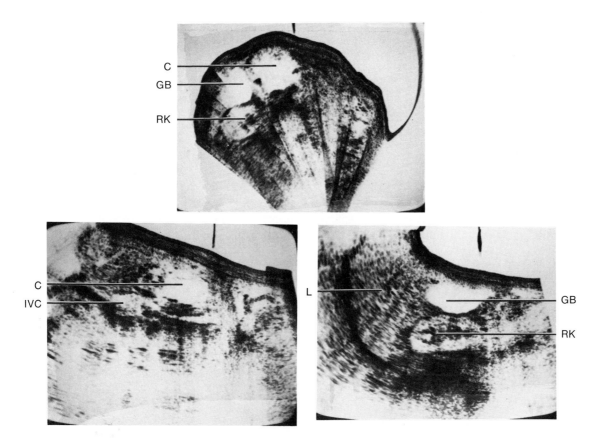

Fig. 22-40. Pseudocyst with enlarged gallbladder due to obstruction from the head of the pancreas.

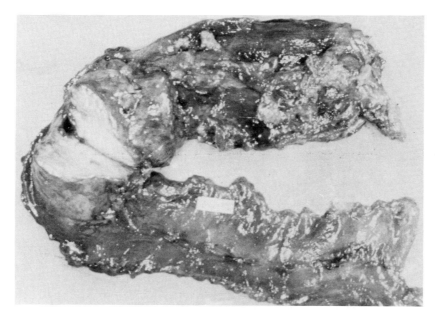

Fig. 22-41. Gross specimen of pancreatic tumor in the body of the gland.

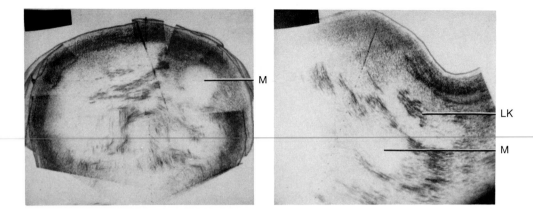

Fig. 22-42. Left upper quadrant mass separate from stomach and consistent with tumor or pseudocyst. Some necrotic tumors may appear very homogeneous and transmit sound well.

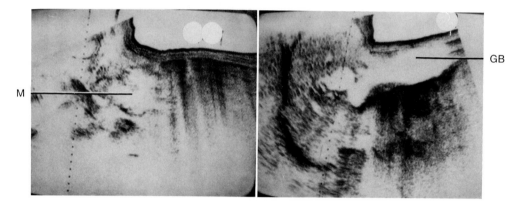

Fig. 22-43. Carcinoma of the pancreas with compression of the common bile duct produces an enlarged gallbladder.

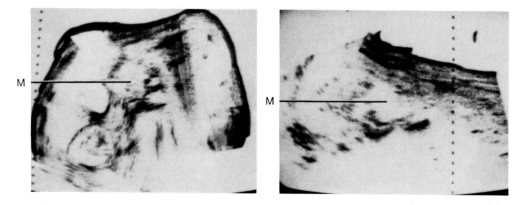

Fig. 22-44. Carcinoma of the head of the pancreas. Gallbladder is top normal in size.

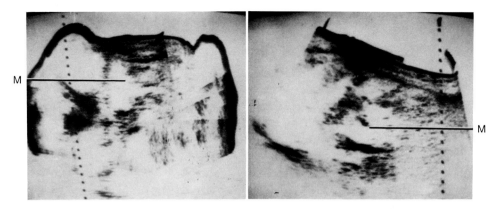

Fig. 22-45. Carcinoma of the head of the pancreas with enlarged gallbladder just lateral to the mass.

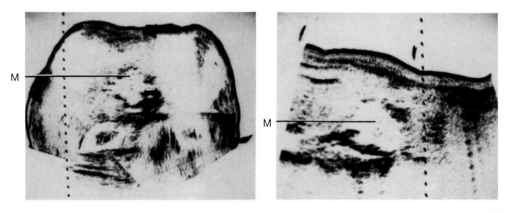

Fig. 22-46. Carcinoma of the head of the pancreas presenting with fine internal echoes and fairly good borders.

Carcinoma

Carcinoma of the pancreas often appears as an irregular mass with ill-defined borders and scattered internal echoes. (See Figs. 22-41 to 22-46.) The detection of carcinoma of the pancreas can be very difficult, especially if the tumor is infiltrating, and therefore the examiner should be aware of other echographic findings. A large noncontracting gallbladder, in association with a mass in the head of the pancreas, is suggestive of carcinoma. A large gallbladder may be tested with a fatty meal to note contraction. After waiting 40 minutes from the administration of the fatty meal, rescan the patient to note the full contraction of the gallbladder. Sokoloff and colleagues (1974) state that typically large, unobstructed gallbladders are seen in fasting normal and/or vagotomized patients, in the presence of diabetes mellitus, or in association with contiguous inflammatory process.

Lymph node enlargement, secondary to lymphoma or metastatic carcinoma, may be confused with pancreatic carcinoma or pancreatitis. This diagnosis can be made by considering splenic enlargement or the presence of nodes elsewhere in the abdomen. It is often difficult to differentiate carcinoma from pancreatitis. With pancreatitis the borders tend to be well-defined, whereas with carcinoma they are often poorly defined. If the pancreas is diffusely involved, this is highly suggestive of inflammatory disease. However, these findings, in association with a mass in the region of the head of the pancreas, do not exclude carcinoma, since pancreatitis and tumor can coexist. In these cases serial examinations can be very helpful in the evaluation of size changes in the gland.

SUMMARY

The normal pancreas can be outlined in a majority of patients by using the surrounding paravertebral vessels for localization purposes. The normal gland, by grey-scale B-scan imaging, appears generally as an echo-producing mass anterior to the aorta and inferior to the splenic vein. Its position is quite variable, but it is seen best in an oblique or transverse path across the abdomen. Difficulties encountered in making proper diagnoses have been presented to give the sonographer a better understanding of the diagnostic signs of pancreatic disease.

23 ☐ Retroperitoneum

The retroperitoneal cavity is the area posterior to the peritoneal cavity. The kidneys, ureters, aorta, lymph chain, and pancreas lie within this cavity. This discussion will concern the lymphatic system and other masses in the retroperitoneal space that are unattached to an organ structure.

The lymphatic chain follows the course of the thoracic aorta, abdominal aorta, and iliac arteries (Fig. 23-1). Normal lymph nodes are smaller than the tip of a finger (less than 1 cm) and are not visualized by current ultrasound techniques. However, if these nodes enlarge because of infection or tumor, they become easier to visualize.

Since the nodes lie along the lateral and anterior margins of the aorta, the best scanning is done with the patient in the supine position. It is important to examine the patient in two planes, since enlarged nodes seen in the longitudinal plane may mimic an abdominal aneurysm at lower-gain settings. As the transverse scan is completed, the differential of an aneurysm versus lymphadenopathy can be made. The aneurysm will enlarge fairly symmetrically, whereas enlarged lymph nodes drape over the prevertebral vessels.

Longitudinal scans may be performed first to outline the aorta and to search for enlarged lymph nodes. The aorta provides an excellent background for the somewhat sonolucent nodes. Longitudinal scans should be performed beginning at the midline with scans recorded both to the left and to the right at 0.5 cm increments. If an abnormality is noted on these sagittal scans, the area should be marked with a grease pencil for proper identification in the transverse plane. Transverse scans are made from the xyphoid to the symphysis at 2 cm intervals (Fig. 23-2). Careful identification of the great vessels, organ structures, and muscle patterns should be accomplished. Problems with a fluid-filled duodenum or bowel patterns may make it difficult to outline the great vessels or cause confusion in diagnosing lymphadenopathy.

Scans performed below the umbilicus may be more difficult to perform because of small bowel interference. Careful attention should be given to the psoas and iliacus muscles within the pelvis, since the iliac arteries run along their medial border. Both muscles serve as a sonolucent border along the pelvic sidewall.

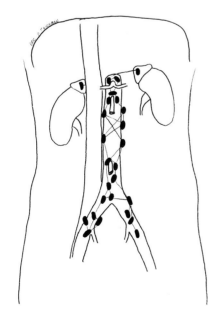

Fig. 23-1. Lymphatic chain along the aorta and iliac artery.

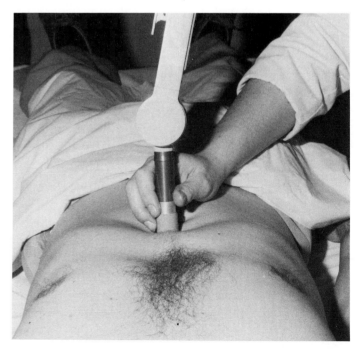

Fig. 23-2. Transverse scans of the lymph node area should be performed in a single sweep maneuver. Moderate to high gain should be used to evaluate the preaortic area.

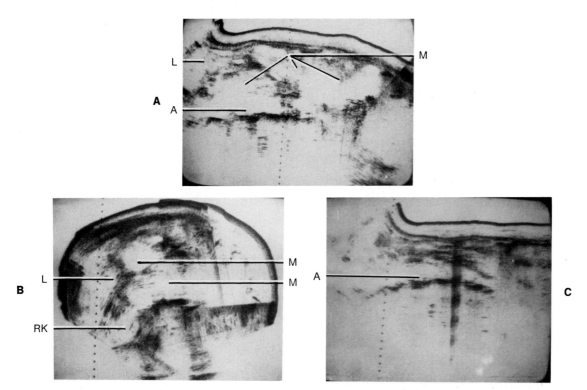

Fig. 23-3. A, Longitudinal scan of patient with lymphosarcoma shows an irregular clump of enlarged nodes anterior to the abdominal aorta. This echo silhouette sign may be produced when a group of nodes lie adjacent to the abdominal aorta. Because of the acoustic similarity of the aorta and lymph nodes, no distinct echo border can be detected. B, The transverse scan shows multiple nodes surrounding the abdominal aorta. C, Repeat scan made post–radiation therapy demonstrates normal aorta with shrinkage of enlarged lymph nodes.

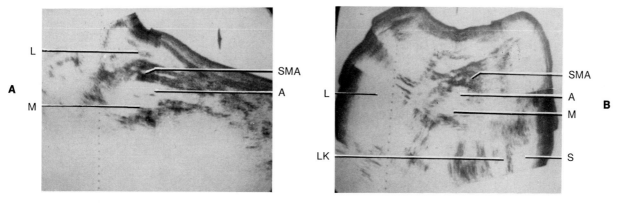

Fig. 23-4. A, Longitudinal scan of patient with enlarged retroperitoneal nodes. The aorta is anteriorly displaced. B, Transverse scan shows anterior displacement of the aorta by lymphadenopathy. Higher sensitivity would outline the aortic wall as separate from the node.

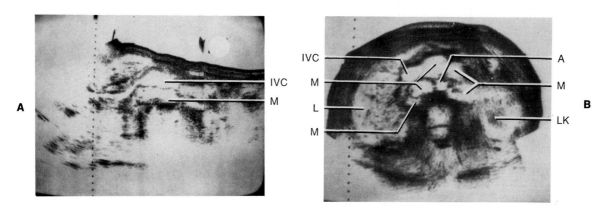

Fig. 23-5. A, Longitudinal scan of retroperitoneal nodes in a patient with breast carcinoma. The inferior vena cava is displaced anteriorly by enlarged nodes. B, Transverse scan shows multiple well-defined nodes surrounding the great vessels.

Enlarged lymph nodes can be identified anterior and medial to these margins. The smooth sharp border indicates no node involvement. The bladder should be filled to help push the small bowel out of the pelvis.

Splenomegaly should also be evaluated in lymphadenopathy. As the scanner moves from the xyphoid in a caudal direction, attention should be on the splenic size and great vessel area.

In our experience we have found lymph nodes to remain as consistent patterns, whereas bowel and duodenum present changing patterns. As gentle pressure is applied with the transducer in an effort to displace the bowel, the lymph nodes remain constant. The echo pattern posterior to each structure is different. Lymph nodes are homogeneous and thus transmit sound easily, whereas bowel presents a more complex pattern with dense central echoes representing its mucosal pattern. Often the duodenum will have some air within its walls, causing a shadow posteriorly. Enlarged lymph nodes should be reproducible on ultrasound. After the abdomen is completely

scanned, repeat sections over the enlarged nodes should demonstrate the same pattern as before.

The patient may be asked to return for a serial follow-up visit if there is uncertainty whether the pattern indicates enlarged lymph nodes or fluid-filled bowel.

Enlarged lymph nodes are more homogeneous than their surrounding organ structures, the pancreas, liver, kidneys, or spleen. With increased sensitivity, diffuse low-level echoes may be seen within the nodes. Proper adjustment of the enhance control on most equipment is necessary to record these fine echoes on the monitor. Their borders are generally smooth, but as they enlarge they may take on a more irregular appearance.

As described by Asher and Freimanis (1969), periaortic nodes are known to have specific characteristic patterns. They may drape, or mantle, the great vessels anteriorly. They may have a lobular, smooth, or scalloped appearance. As mesenteric involvement occurs, the adenopathy may fill most of the abdomen in an irregular complex pattern. (See Figs. 23-3 to 23-10.)

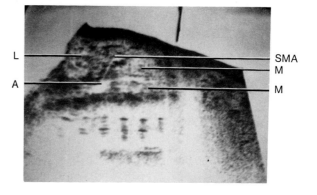

Fig. 23-6. Superior mesenteric artery is displaced by the tumor mass.

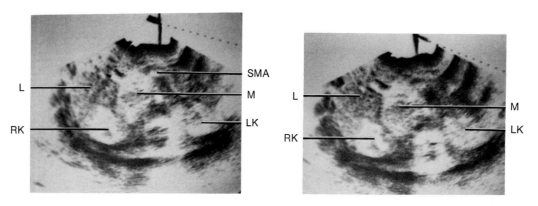

Fig. 23-7. Transverse scans of the retroperitoneal tumor in Fig. 23-6. Multiple internal echoes denote complexity of the mass.

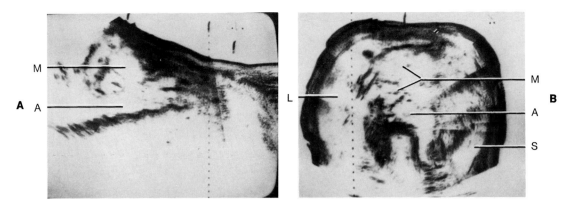

Fig. 23-8. A, Longitudinal scan of retroperitoneal nodes anterior to the aorta. B, Transverse scan at moderate gain shows an irregular clump of nodes anterior to the para-aortic area.

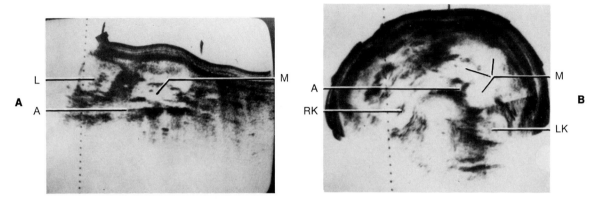

Fig. 23-9. A, Separate, well-defined enlarged nodes shown anterior to the aorta on a longitudinal scan. B, Mass of nodes extends mainly into the left upper quadrant.

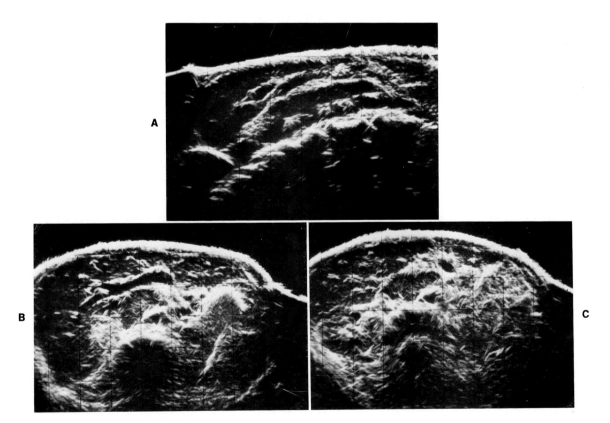

Fig. 23-10. A, Longitudinal scan of well-defined mass anterior to the abdominal aorta in a patient with lymphoma. B, Enlarged nodes are compressing the porta hepatis, causing dilatation of vascular structures on this transverse scan. C, Well-defined nodes laterally displacing the inferior vena cava and medially displacing the superior mesenteric vein.

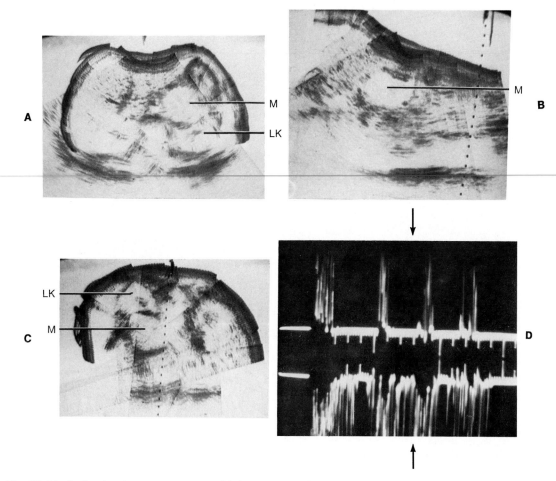

Fig. 23-11. A, Supine transverse scan of left upper quadrant mass. It could represent a pancreatic mass or cyst, adrenal mass, or retroperitoneal tumor. **B,** Supine longitudinal scan of left upper quadrant demonstrates a well-defined mass anterior to the left kidney, separate from the spleen. **C,** Prone transverse scan further defines the mass separate from the spleen and left kidney. **D,** A-mode study over a mass defines the characteristics of a solid tumor with low-gain (top) and high-gain (bottom) settings.

The localization of lymphadenopathy or a lymphomatous mass can be useful as a baseline study to the clinician. After treatment is administered, follow-up scans may be made to evaluate the shrinkage of the mass. If radiation therapy is used, it is helpful to mark the boundaries of the mass on the patient's skin for therapy planning.

If a retroperitoneal mass is seen separate from the lymph nodes, scans may be performed in the supine, prone, and decubitus positions to define its relationship to other organs. (See Fig. 23-11.)

24 □ Suprarenal glands

with assistance of
KEVIN KANE, C.X.T.

The suprarenal glands are yellowish retroperitoneal organs that lie on the upper pole of each kidney (Fig. 24-1). They weigh approximately 5 to 9 g. At birth the ratio of their weight to body weight is twenty times what it is in adulthood, but by one year of age their size is more proportional to the body. They are surrounded by perinephric fascia but are separated from the kidneys by the perinephric fat. Each gland has a yellow-colored cortex and a dark brown medulla. The right suprarenal gland is triangular or pyramidal in shape and caps the upper pole of the right kidney. It lies posterior to the right lobe of the liver and extends medially behind the inferior vena cava. It rests posteriorly on the diaphragm. The left suprarenal gland is semilunar in shape and extends along the medial border of the left kidney from the upper pole to the hilus. It lies posterior to the pancreas, the lesser sac, and the stomach. It also rests posteriorly on the diaphragm (Fig. 24-2).

There are three arteries supplying each gland: (1) the suprarenal branch of the inferior phrenic artery, (2) the suprarenal branch of the aorta, and (3) the suprarenal branch of the renal artery. A single vein arises from the hilus of each gland and drains into the inferior vena cava on the right and into the renal vein on the left.

FUNCTION

The adrenal cortex secretes hormones called corticosteroids. These are divided into mineral corticoids such as aldosterone (promotes sodium retention and potassium excretion) and glucocorticoids such as cortisol and corticosterone (relates the metabolism of carbohydrates, proteins, and fat). The cortex also secretes the gonadal hormones. The adrenal medulla secretes epinephrine (adrenaline) and norepinephrine (noradrenaline). Adrenaline affects all the structures innervated by the sympathetic nervous system, reinforcing its action.

ADRENAL CORTEX

Pathologic conditions of the adrenal cortex include congenital anomalies. Many of these are the basic causes of diseases that are manifested later in life. Two of these anomalies are congenital adrenal hypoplasia and ectopic adrenal glands.

There are two type of congenital adrenal hypoplasia. In the anencephalic type the two glands consist of only a provisional cortex with no adult zone. These are found in anencephalic fetuses, and the cause is either pituitary, hypothalamic, or cerebral. The cytomegalic type, in which a tiny adrenal with a cortex made up of large eosinophilic cells is found, has an unknown cause.

Ectopic adrenals consist mainly of accessory adrenal tissue that may be located anywhere from the diaphragm to the pelvis. This type of anomaly occurs only in the patient whose adrenal glands are removed as an aid in cancer therapy.

Hyperadrenalism assumes three main forms. They

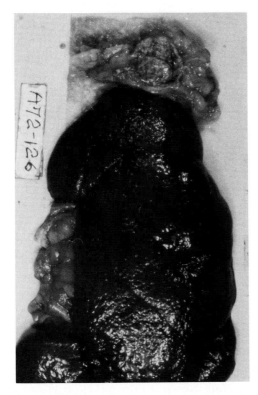

Fig. 24-1. Gross specimen of the kidney and adrenal gland on top of the renal capsule. Perinephric fascia and fat surround the adrenal gland.

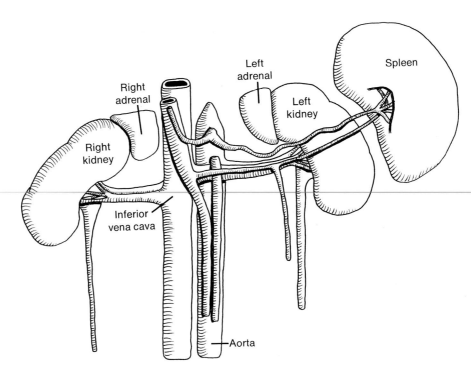

Fig. 24-2. Anteroposterior view of the medial location of both adrenal glands.

are adrenogenital (A/G) syndrome, Cushing's syndrome, and Conn's syndrome. They are all typified by an increase in secretion of one of the cortical steroids.

A/G syndrome is a term that indicates a variety of diseases. Each is caused by a deficiency in an enzyme that prevents normal hormone synthesis. Androgenic hormones are then manufactured, producing virilism. In infants and children the usual cause is a congenital lack of a specific enzyme, whereas in adults the cause is likely to be a hyperfunctioning adenoma or carcinoma. The virilism in A/G syndrome may be the only symptom or may be accompanied by hypertension or a salt loss.

Cushing's syndrome is a disease that has several causes: (1) excess production of cortisol by a benign or malignant tumor of the adrenal, (2) excess secretion of adrenocorticotrophic hormone (ACTH) by the pituitary (usually due to a pituitary tumor), and (3) the ectopic production of ACTH by a nonpituitary tumor. All three types of Cushing's syndrome are characterized by excess production of glucocorticoids. The disease can be recognized clinically by central obesity, moon face, diabetes mellitus, osteoporosis, hypertension, plethora, hirsutism, and weakness.

Conn's syndrome, which is also called primary hyperaldosteronism, is characterized by periodic muscle weakness, hypertension, polydipsia, and polyuria. These symptoms are accompanied by alkalosis, and renal potassium loss. The diagnosis is confirmed by increased serum aldosterone levels. About 90% of cases of Conn's syndrome are caused by solitary cortical adenomas, but the disease can also be caused by multiple adenomas, carcinoma, or cortical hypertrophy (hyperplasia).

Hypoadrenalism can be either acute or chronic. The chronic form is the most common and is called Addison's disease. The effects of Addison's disease include sodium loss, potassium retention, renal impairment, blood volume decrease, and blood sugar and lipid decrease. Fatigue, muscle weakness, weight loss, and gastrointestinal distress may also be present, along with hypotension and skin pigment increase.

Acute adrenal insufficiency is identified by low blood pressure, rapid pulse, vomiting, diarrhea, and sometimes abdominal pain. Without treatment, death follows in hours.

The causes of hypoadrenalism include disorders of the adrenal cortex, diminished ACTH production (due to pituitary or hypothalamic disease), or suppression of the hypothalamic-pituitary axis because of treatment with corticosteroids. Acute insufficiency can also be caused by necrotizing hemorrhage of the adrenals; Addison's disease causes include atrophy of the adrenals, tuberculosis, amyloidosis, carcinoma, or even fungal infections.

Hemorrhage of the adrenal gland is a common finding in newborns, especially following a difficult delivery in which fetal oxygen is cut off for varying periods of time. Hemorrhage, along with inflammation and necrosis of the adrenal, may also accompany severe infections such as diphtheria, pneumonia, and any meningococcal infection.

Atrophy of the adrenal gland, a main cause of Addison's disease, is the wasting away of the gland and has many causes. Some, such as chronic administration of glucocorticoid, are understood, but many others are not and are categorized as idiopathic atrophy.

Tumors of the adrenal cortex include both benign and malignant varieties. Most adrenal adenomas are nonsteroid producing. They are also poorly encapsulated cortical tissue usually ranging from 1 to 5 cm in diameter. As they get larger, they tend to degenerate and form areas of cystic deposits and hemorrhage. They also develop calcification.

Many of these tumors cannot be clearly classified. They contain elements of both benign and malignant cells. Nodular hyperplasia may look like a true adenoma, but in general if the nodules are multiple, bilateral, or loculated within the capsule or outside of it, they indicate hyperplasia; if there is a single lesion larger than 1 cm in diameter, it is an adenoma.

Most cortical carcinomas produce steroids and are associated with one of the hyperadrenal syndromes. Some do not produce steroids, however; such carcinomas are rare and highly malignant.

Adrenal cancers tend to invade the adrenal vein, the vena cava, and the lymphatics, metastasizing to regional and periaortic nodes, as well as to the lungs. Bone metastases are rare.

One other type of primary adrenal tumor is the myelolipoma, which is a mass consisting of bone marrow and fat often found in the adrenal glands.

It is not known whether metastases to the adrenal affect the medulla or cortex more commonly, but regardless of which part is affected, the adrenal is a common site for metastases from all types of cancer.

ADRENAL MEDULLA

The main pathologic processes that affect the adrenal medulla are tumors such as pheochromocytomas, neuroblastomas, and ganglioneuromas.

Pheochromocytoma is a tumor arising from the cells producing epinephrine or norepinephrine. Most pheochromocytomas are benign, but they can cause hypertension. This kind of tumor, found in both adults and children, is more likely to develop on the right side but is also commonly bilateral. In children it is more common in males, but in adults there is no sex link. It is also possible for multiple tumors to develop in one individual. Usual symptoms include hyperten-

sion, either chronic or episodal, headache, sweating, pallor, tachycardia, and a raised basal metabolism.

Since both benign and malignant pheochromocytomas have similar chemical and histologic characteristics, only distant metastases in the liver, lymph nodes, lungs, or bones establish a diagnosis of malignancy with certainty. Treatment is generally removal of the gland and substitution therapy. Radiotherapy or chemotherapy may be included.

Neuroblastoma is a highly malignant tumor generally found in children. It is one of the commonest childhood tumors and usually affects males. The lesion does not exclusively affect the adrenal gland, but 40% to 50% of all neuroblastomas are found there. The remainder are found principally in the abdominal and thoracic sympathetic chain.

These tumors are lobular and soft, with areas of necrosis and hemorrhage increasing with increase in tumor size. Calcification is also common. They metastasize quickly and widely to the liver, lungs, and bones. Some neuroblastomas spontaneously form a benign tumor called a ganglioneuroma. The reason for this is unknown, but a strong immunologic response to the tumor is suspected.

Treatment of a neuroblastoma is resection, if possible. This is combined with radiotherapy and chemotherapy. If resection is not possible, then radiotherapy and chemotherapy are used alone. The probability of cure is better if the tumor is discovered before 2 years of age and if the tumor is located outside the adrenals, but in general the prognosis is poor.

Apparently, true adrenal cysts are rare; most reported cases consist of pseudocysts and/or tumors with cystic degeneration. The only common feature of adrenal cysts is a tendency to form calcifications around their perimeters.

LABORATORY TESTS

The first group of tests are those which assess adrenocortical function. These tests can be divided into (1) determination of absolute values in serum and urine and (2) tests for the interdependency of various hormones.

The absolute value tests include the following:

1. Plasma cortisol level. These are obtained in the morning and evening, and the variations are tested. Extreme elevation of these levels without variation suggests carcinoma.

2. 24-hour urine steroids. This is the best test for adrenal function. The steroids tested include hydroxycorticosteroids (elevated levels indicate primary or secondary hyperadrenalism) and ketosteroids (ele-

vated levels may have the same meaning, but they may also indicate a tumor secreting androgenic steroids; the levels are increased in virilizing syndromes).

3. Aldosterone levels. These tests are ordered in hypertensive patients. Elevated levels indicate either hyperfunction of aldosterone-producing adrenal cells or the presence of aldosterone-producing adenomas.

4. Plasma ACTH. ACTH governs the production of some of the adrenal hormones. Its levels are increased with ectopic ACTH–producing tumors such as pituitary tumors.

The interdependency tests measure the true functioning of the hypothalamus, the pituitary, and the adrenal glands and include the following:

1. ACTH stimulation tests. These tests demonstrate the ability of the adrenal glands to produce steroids.

2. Aldosterone stimulation tests. These test aldosterone secretion.

3. Glucocorticoid suppression tests. If the levels of these hormones cannot be suppressed by chemical action, then a tumor is present.

4. Aldosterone suppression tests. If the patient has primary aldosteronism, the levels of this hormone cannot be suppressed chemically, but if he has essential hypertension, the levels are suppressed even more than normal.

The function of the adrenal medulla is not usually tested except in cases of hypertension or if pheochromocytoma is suspected. Elevated levels of catecholamines and/or VMA (vanillylmandelic acid) in the urine can indicate pheochromocytoma.

ULTRASONIC EVALUATION

Although ultrasonography has proved to be useful in the evaluation of most soft tissue structures within the abdomen, visualization of the adrenal gland has been very difficult because of its small size, its medial location, and the fact that its borders are outlined by perinephric fat. Recently, data have been presented by Sample (1976) concerning a successful technique in the localization and recognition of the adrenal gland. Of course, if the adrenal gland is enlarged due to disease, it is an easy task to separate the adrenal mass from that of the renal parenchyma and thus determine whether the mass is cystic, solid, or somewhat calcified. With current grey-scale equipment and a high-frequency transducer, visualization of the gland can be accomplished within the realm of 2 to 3 cm. If a normal frequency transducer of 2.25 MHz is used, the lateral resolution this transducer affords to the adrenal area makes it difficult to visualize the gland in a routine manner.

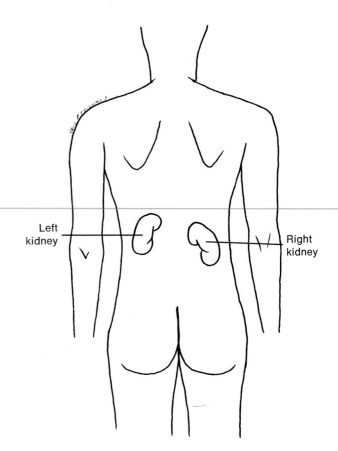

Fig. 24-3. Prone scans may initially be performed along the oblique margins of the renal area and psoas muscles in a search for the medial adrenal glands.

Scanning technique

Prone. The initial examination consists of prone longitudinal scans taken in deep inspiration. These scans are performed in an oblique path along the line of the renal area and psoas muscles (Fig. 24-3). It is important to outline the renal parenchyma well to demonstrate whether the mass may be a renal or adrenal lesion. Transverse views should also be used at 1 cm increments to demonstrate the full extent of the renal parenchyma and to note if there are extrarenal masses present. Generally, prone scanning is most beneficial for localization purposes. Better visualization of the adrenal area is afforded by decubitus, oblique, and lateral decubitus views.

Supine. Supine scanning is most effective if the lesion is in the right upper quadrant. The homogeneous liver provides an excellent sound transmitter to visualize the upper pole of the right kidney. If the upper pole is well seen, a mass superior to the upper pole would most likely represent an adrenal lesion. This technique is employed if the mass is at least 3 to 4 cm in size. (See Fig. 24-4.)

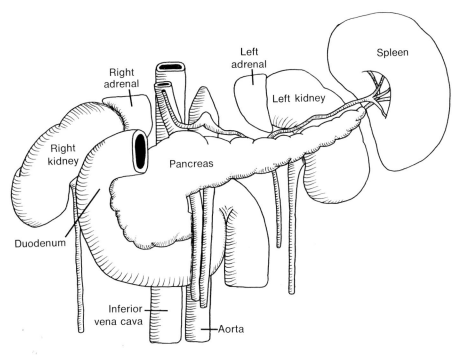

Fig. 24-4. Adrenals are often difficult to see because of their small size and the inability of the ultrasound beam to penetrate the duodenum, small bowel, and colon.

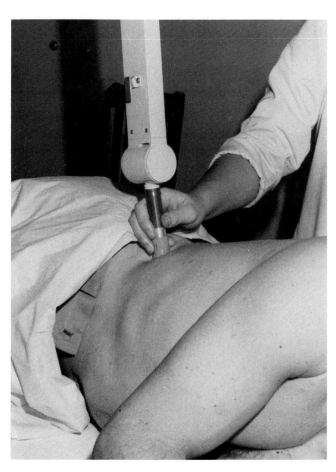

Fig. 24-5. Decubitus position for localization of the adrenal area.

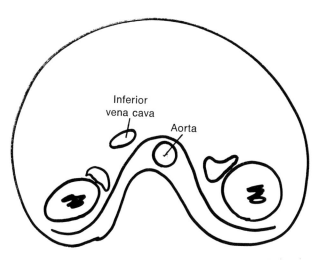

Fig. 24-6. Crux of the diaphragm can be seen to flow over the aorta and under the inferior vena cava. It serves as a landmark in the localization of the adrenal gland.

Decubitus. Since the left adrenal is more medial and anterior than the right adrenal, it is better demonstrated in the decubitus position (Fig. 24-5). Analysis of a cross section of the adrenal area will demonstrate the crux of the diaphragm as it lies posterior and medial to the right kidney, swinging over the abdominal aorta, then dipping medial to the adrenal gland, and then medial and posterior to the left kidney. With the patient in the left decubitus position, note the left kidney falling forward along with the adrenal

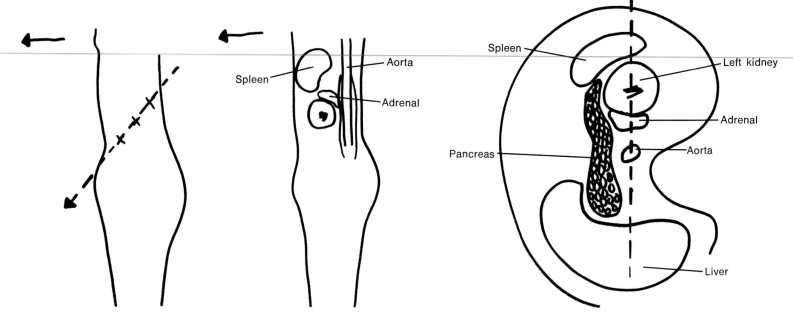

Fig. 24-7. Left decubitus position (see text).

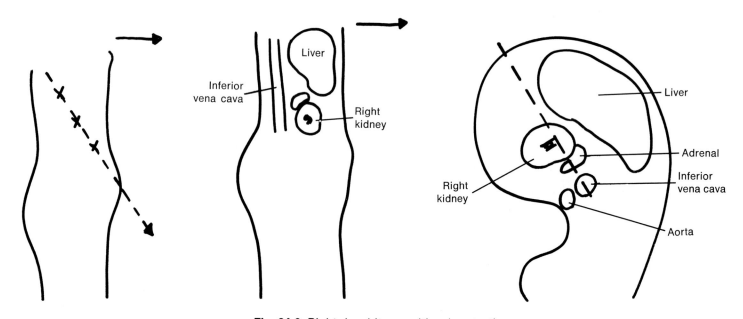

Fig. 24-8. Right decubitus position (see text).

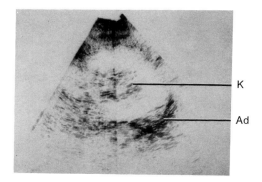

Fig. 24-9. Decubitus position of normal adrenal and kidney.

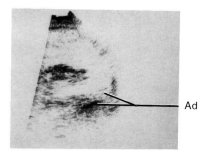

Fig. 24-10. Small capsular area medial to the kidney is the adrenal cortex area.

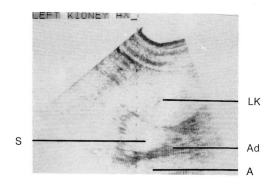

Fig. 24-11. Normal adrenal, aorta, spleen, and left kidney on a scan taken in the decubitus position.

gland. As the patient assumes the right decubitus position, the inferior vena cava moves forward and the aorta rolls over the crux of the diaphragm, thus offering good visualization of the right kidney and right adrenal area. (See Figs. 24-6 to 24-8.) To localize these structures in a correct fashion, most scans are performed in the prone position, with a grease pencil ready to mark the kidney, aorta, and inferior vena cava. Then, as the patient is rolled into the decubitus position, the transducer may be correctly placed in the oblique path to line up the structures for better localization of the adrenal gland. The pie sweep, or single sweep, technique should be utilized with the patient in midinspiration. If the patient is obese, it may be difficult to recognize the triangular or crescent-shaped adrenal gland. The adrenal gland should never appear as a rounded structure. This would most likely represent an abnormality. Because of the lateral resolution of the transducer it will always be difficult to outline one of the borders of the adrenal gland. The gland may vary in location from the top medial border of the kidney to the middle part of the kidney (Figs. 24-9 to 24-11). If kidney disease is involved, the adrenal gland should maintain its position. Children, of course, have larger adrenals than do adults, making it much easier to visualize these glands.

A study done at U.C.L.A. (Sample, 1977) to visualize the adrenal gland in normal patients revealed 85% positive visualization of adrenal glands over 2 cm in size. Obesity and para-adrenal fat were problems in some patients. The normal gland was usually triangular and thin.

Demonstration of pathologic conditions

Ultrasonically, adrenal cysts present a typical cystic pattern seen in other organs of the body—strong back wall, no internal echoes, and good sound transmis-

sion as seen on grey scale and A mode. It may be difficult to evaluate the consistency of the lesion if it is not a simple cyst. Adrenal cysts have the tendency to become calcified, which gives them an ultrasonic appearance of a somewhat solid mass with no internal echoes (sharp border but poor sound transmission). The cyst may have hemorrhaged and appear as a complex mass with multiple internal echoes but good through-transmission.

Pheochromocytomas, along with most lymphomas and sarcomas of the adrenal gland, present a homogeneous pattern which can be differentiated from that of cysts by the weak back walls caused by increased attenuation of the beam. As the gain is increased slightly, lymphomas and sarcomas tend to fill in with fine low-level echoes that distinguish them from cystic lesions. Metastatic adrenal tumors may appear as a homogeneous pattern due to necrosis and may give the appearance of a cystic mass. With higher sensitivity the complexity of these masses is generally brought out.

It is important to thoroughly examine both adrenal areas if metastasis is suspected, since there is incidence of metastases affecting both adrenals.

25 □ Kidneys

NORMAL ANATOMY

The kidneys lie in the retroperitoneal space under the cover of the costal margin. The right kidney lies slightly lower than the left because of the right lobe of the liver. During inspiration both kidneys move downward in a vertical direction by as much as 2.5 cm.

The normal adult kidney varies from 9 to 12 cm in length, 2.5 to 3 cm in thickness, and approximately 4 to 5 cm in width. Generally, both kidneys will attain approximately the same dimensions. A difference of more than 1.5 to 2 cm is significant.

Embryologically the kidneys develop in the pelvis and gradually ascend to their retroperitoneal position in the upper quadrants. They do not complete their ascension until the fifth to sixth year of life. Previous to this period the kidneys are large and extend below the iliac crest.

On the medial border of each kidney is a vertical slit, which is bounded by thick lips of the renal substance and is called the hilus. The hilus transmits from the front backward by means of the renal vein, two branches of the renal artery, the ureter, and the third branch of the renal artery. The kidneys are surrounded by a fibrous capsule that is closely applied to the cortex. Outside this capsule is a covering of perinephric fat. The perinephric fascia surrounds the perinephric fat and encloses the kidney and suprarenal glands.

The ureter is 25 cm long and resembles the esophagus in having three constrictions along its course: (1) where the pelvis of the ureter joins the ureter, (2) where it is kinked as it crosses the pelvic brim, and (3) where it pierces the bladder wall. The pelvis of the ureter is its funnel-shaped expanded upper end. It lies within the hilus of the kidney and receives the major calices. The ureter emerges from the hilus of the kidney and runs vertically downward along the psoas muscle, which separates it from the tips of the transverse processes of the lumbar vertebrae. It enters the pelvis by crossing the bifurcation of the common iliac artery in front of the sacroiliac joint. The ureter then runs down along the lateral wall of the pelvis to the region of the ischial spine and turns forward to enter the lateral angle of the bladder.

The kidney is composed of an internal medullary portion and an external cortical substance. The medullary substance consists of a series of striated conical masses called the renal pyramids. They vary from eight to eighteen in number and have their bases directed toward the outer circumference of the kidney. Their apices converge toward the renal sinus, where their prominent papillae project into the lumen of the minor calices.

The cortical substance is reddish brown in color and soft and granular in consistency. Microscopic examination of the cortex reveals a series of lighter colored conical areas termed the radiant part and a darker colored intervening part that, because of the complexity of its structure, is termed the convoluted part. The rays gradually taper toward the circumference of the kidney and consist of a series of outward prolongations from the base of each renal pyramid.

Within the kidney the upper expanded end, or pelvis, of the ureter divides into two or three major calices, each of which divides into two or three minor calices. The four to thirteen minor calices are cup-shaped tubes, each of which usually comes in contact with at least one but occasionally two or more of the renal papillae (the blunted apex of the renal pyramid). The minor calices unite to form two or three short tubes, the major calices, which in turn unite to form a funnel-shaped sac, the renal pelvis. Spirally arranged muscles surround the calices and may exert a milking action on these tubes, aiding in the flow of urine into the renal pelvis. As the pelvis leaves the renal sinus, it diminishes rapidly in size and ultimately merges with the ureter, the excretory duct of the kidney that ends in the urinary bladder.

The kidney, for the most part, is made up of renal tubules that commence in the cortical substance. After undergoing a tortuous journey through the cortical and medullary substances, they finally end at the apices of the renal pyramids near open "mouths," so that the fluid they contain is emptied through the calices into the pelvis of the kidney. The open mouths are actually small orifices of the renal tubules numbering anywhere from six to twenty, and if pressure were applied on a fresh kidney, urine would leak out through these openings.

The renal tubules arising from the cortical substance are also called malpighian bodies. They are small rounded masses, deep red in color, varying in size but averaging about 0.2 mm in diameter. Each of these bodies is composed of two parts—a central glomerulus of vessels and a double-walled membranous envelope, the glomerular capsule of Bowman, which is the pouchlike portion of the tubule. The glomerulus is a cluster of nonanastomosing capillaries. This capillary cluster is derived from an arteriole (the afferent vessel) that enters the capsule opposite to that at which the capsule joins the tubule. When it enters the capsule, the afferent arteriole divides into from two to ten primary branches, which in turn subdivide into fifty capillary loops that generally do not anastomose (communicate with other capillaries). Finally, the capillaries join to form the efferent arteriole, which leaves Bowman's capsule next to the afferent vessel. The efferent artery is usually larger than the afferent arteriole. The total surface area of the capillaries of all glomeruli is about 1 m². A renal tubule, which begins with the capsule of Bowman and ends where the tubule joins the excretory duct or collecting tubule, constitutes a nephron (the structural and functional unit of the kidney). There are about 1,250,000 of these units in each kidney.

The kidney is supplied with blood by the renal artery, a large branch of the abdominal aorta. Before entering the kidney substance, branches of the renal artery vary in number and direction. In most cases the renal artery divides into two primary branches, the larger anterior and a smaller posterior. The anterior branch supplies the anterior, or ventral, half of the organ, and the posterior branch supplies the posterior, or dorsal, part. Each renal artery usually divides into three branches, which enter the hilus of the kidney, two in front and one behind the ureter. These arteries break down finally to very minute arterioles. In the medullary portion these arterioles are called interlobar arteries. In the portion of the kidney between the cortex and medulla these arteries are called arcuate arteries. Of course, the veins of the kidney also break down into these categories. Five or six veins join to form the renal vein, which merges from the hilus in front of the renal artery. The renal vein drains into the inferior vena cava (Fig. 25-1). The arcuate arteries and veins break down further. The most important branches of these arteries and veins are the afferent and efferent glomerular vessels previously discussed.

CROSS-SECTIONAL AND SAGITTAL ANATOMY

Cross-sectional anatomy reveals that the right kidney is slightly lower (1 to 2 cm) than the left kidney because the right lobe of the liver prohibits the kidney's ascension. The superior borders of both kidneys are bounded by the suprarenal gland, perinephric fat,

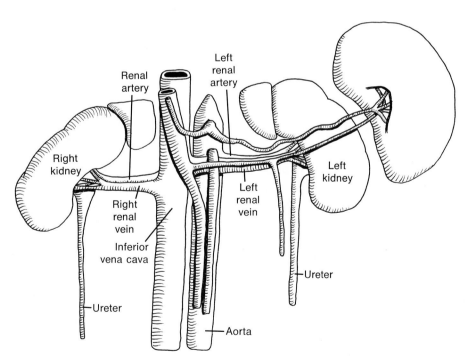

Fig. 25-1. Renal vascular relationships with other organs and great vessels. The right renal vein goes directly into the inferior vena cava. The right renal artery flows from the aorta under the IVC to enter the renal hilus. The left renal vein crosses anterior to the aorta and posterior to the superior mesenteric artery to enter the IVC. The left renal artery flows from the aorta directly to the renal hilus.

and fascia. The midportion of the kidneys contains the caliceal structures, renal vessels, and the beginning of the psoas muscle on the medial border of each kidney. The lower poles are surrounded by perinephric fat and fascia as well.

The sagittal plane demonstrates the renal capsule 4 to 6 cm to either side of the vertebral column. The upper pole of the kidney lies more posterior than the lower pole. In addition, the kidney lies along the lateral margin of the psoas muscles, which take an oblique course in the posterior retroperitoneal cavity, extending from the hilus of the kidney to the lateral walls of the pelvis.

PHYSIOLOGY

There are three processes the blood goes through to rid itself of unwanted material. The first is glomerular filtration. The initial step in the process of "making urine" takes place as the blood enters the glomeruli in the Bowman's capsule. Next is tubular resorption. Most of the substances in the blood (97% to 99%) are needed by the body. Resorption is accomplished by the cells that compose the walls of the convoluted tubules, loop of Henle, and collecting tubules. The final step is tubular secretion, which is the opposite of tubular resorption. The cells that resorb also secrete.

This is the movement of substances out of the blood into the filtrate in the kidney tubules.

Once the process of selection is completed, the remaining substances (urine) drain from the medulla into the ureters.

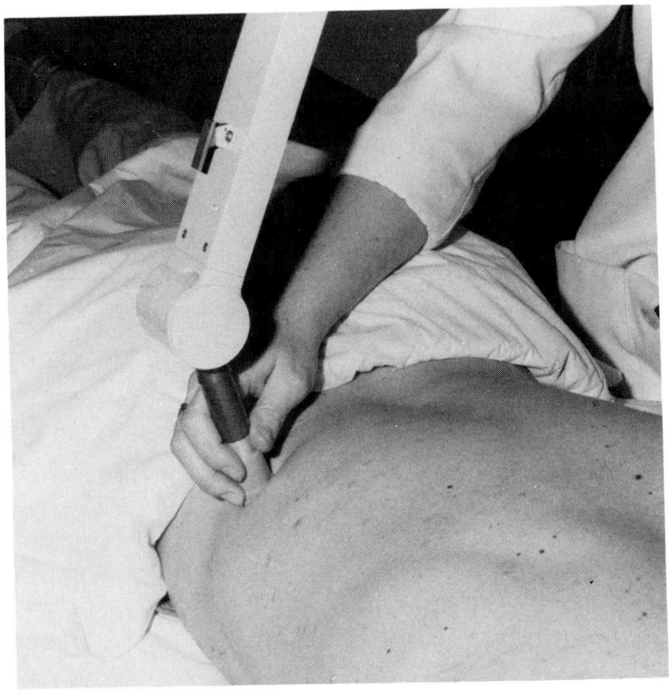

ULTRASONIC DETECTION OF RENAL PARENCHYMA

The patient should be positioned prone with a sandbag or small pillow placed under the abdomen. This allows more perpendicular contact of the renal area with the transducer (Figs. 25-2 and 25-3). The upper

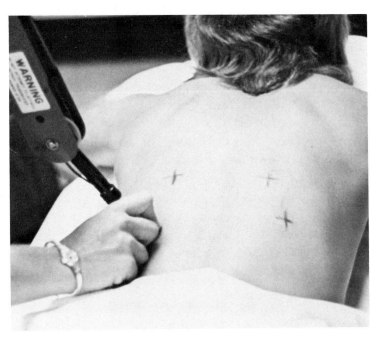

Fig. 25-3. Marks may be made on the skin surface at the upper, middle, and lower poles for correct longitudinal scans.

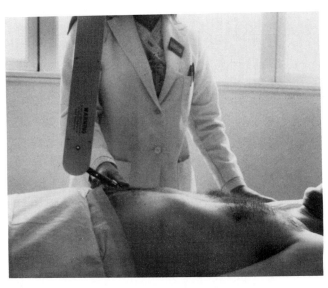

Fig. 25-4. Supine scans, especially of the right upper pole, are made in the longitudinal plane with deep inspiration.

Fig. 25-2. Transverse scans should begin at the level of the iliac crest. A slight angulation of the transducer allows perpendicular contact to the renal structures. Slight sector movement of the transducer allows one to scan between the rib cartilages.

poles of both kidneys are more difficult to visualize because of overlying lung tissue. Deep inspiration may aid in their visualization, or supine scans may allow more adequate demonstration of the upper pole (Figs. 25-4 and 25-5).

The patient should be well hydrated prior to the ultrasonic examination. The intravenous pyelogram permits precise localization of the renal mass and should be available at the time of the study.

Transverse scans begin at the level of the iliac crest and continue cephalad at 1 cm intervals until the entire renal parenchyma has been outlined. The exact

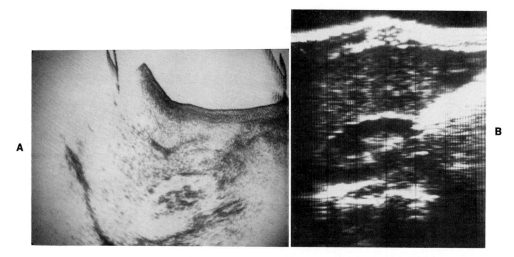

Fig. 25-5. A, Longitudinal supine scan of the liver and right kidney; the homogeneous liver permits adequate sound transmission to visualize the upper pole. **B,** Real-time longitudinal scan.

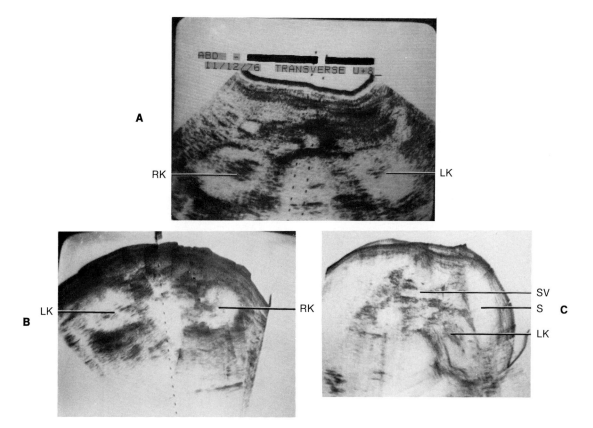

Fig. 25-6. A, Transverse supine scans usually do not permit adequate visualization of the renal area because of bowel gas interference. Very thin patients, however, may allow adequate visualization of both kidneys. **B,** Prone transverse scan across the midpole of both kidneys generally allows the best visualization of renal parenchyma. **C,** If there is an enlarged spleen, the left kidney will be well visualized from the supine plane.

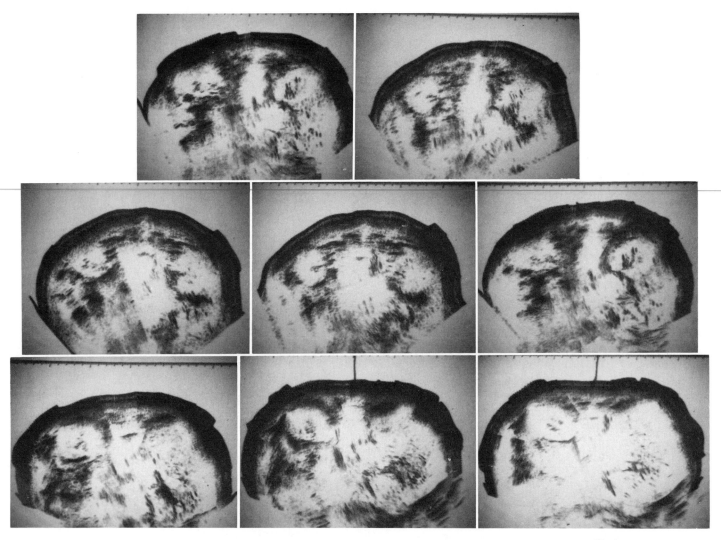

Fig. 25-7. Normal series of transverse scans. The spleen may be seen to the left of the scan and helps define the upper border of the kidney.

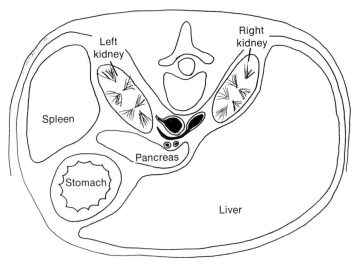

Fig. 25-8. Prone transverse scan demonstrates the relationship of the left kidney to the spleen, pancreas, and stomach and that of the right kidney to the liver.

location of the renal contour should be noted so the proper oblique longitudinal scans can be made. In the transverse plane the renal outline appears slightly round and measures approximately 4 cm in the antero-posterior diameter and 5 cm in the transverse diameter. The central strong echoes represent the caliceal system of the renal pelvis (Fig. 25-6).

The liver can be seen lateral and anterior to the right kidney. The left kidney is bounded laterally by the spleen and anteriorly by the pancreas and stomach (Figs. 25-7 and 25-8).

The longitudinal scans are made along the oblique mark to either side of the spine. The psoas muscle can be seen arising from the hilus of the kidney into the pelvis. The full contour of the kidney should be seen in this plane. Scans are made every 0.5 cm until the entire contour is demonstrated (Figs. 25-9 to 25-13).

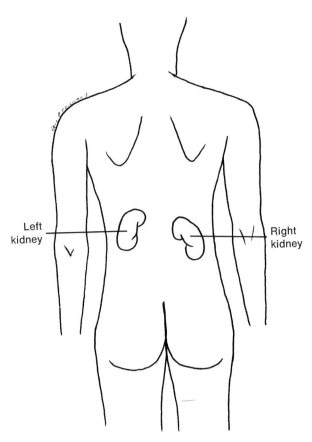

Fig. 25-9. Kidneys lie in an oblique path along the psoas muscles.

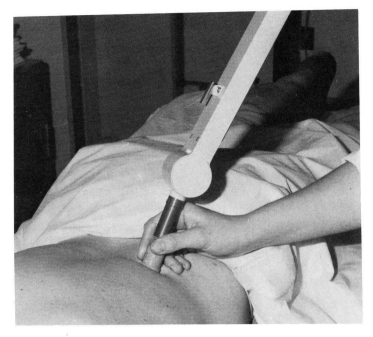

Fig. 25-11. Arm of the transducer should be angled slightly toward the midline of the spine.

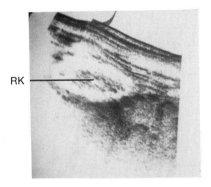

Fig. 25-12. Longitudinal scan of the right kidney.

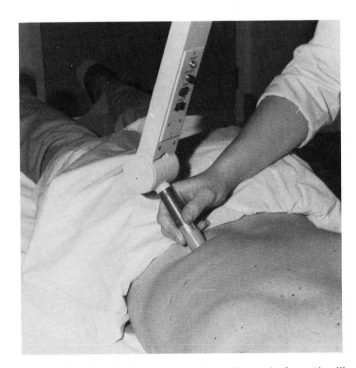

Fig. 25-10. Longitudinal scans are generally made from the iliac crest by sweeping the transducer slightly cephalad to obtain perpendicular information.

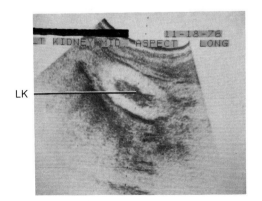

Fig. 25-13. Longitudinal scan of the left kidney.

ULTRASONIC IDENTIFICATION OF PATHOLOGIC CONDITIONS

Congenital agenesis

Congenital agenesis, absence of one kidney and ureter, may be difficult to assess clinically. Ultrasound can outline the normal kidney and tell with certainty whether one kidney is absent or pathologically afflicted.

Supernumerary kidney

Although rare, supernumerary kidney is a complete duplication of the renal system. It is generally found in the pelvis but occasionally may ascend with the other renal structures. Ultrasound may be able to outline two separate kidneys if they are within the normal renal area but may overlook the extra system if it is in the pelvis.

Horseshoe kidney

Horseshoe kidney occurs during fetal development with fusion of the upper or lower poles. It does not ascend to its normal position in the retroperitoneal cavity. Generally, the isthmus is found near the level of the iliac crest. It has separate ureters from either side of the kidney but is connected by tissue (the isthmus) draping across the midline.

Ultrasonically a horseshoe kidney should be evaluated from the supine position, since the kidneys generally appear lower in the abdomen and may be attenuated by the iliac crest in the prone position.

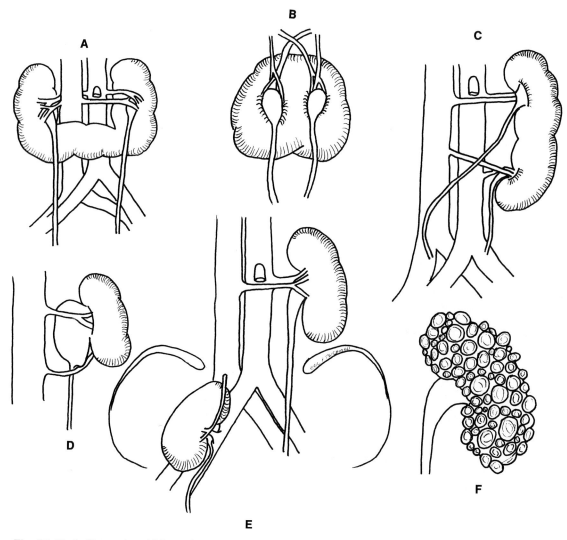

Fig. 25-14. A, Horseshoe kidney shown as two kidneys connected by an isthmus anterior to the great vessels and inferior to the inferior mesenteric artery. **B,** "Cake" kidney with double collecting system. **C,** Double collecting system in a single kidney. **D,** Obstruction of the renal pelvis resulting in hydronephrosis. **E,** Pelvic, or ectopic, kidney with one kidney in the normal retroperitoneal position. **F,** Polycystic disease.

The isthmus is best recorded with single sweep technique and is seen as a sonolucent band draping over the great vessels. It is difficult to diagnose lymphadenopathy in a patient with a horseshoe kidney, since the isthmus may mimic the lymph nodes. Real-time equipment should allow visualization of the renal parenchyma with the isthmus connecting the two capsules and thus may be an aid in distinguishing other disease from the isthmus (Fig. 25-14).

Hydronephrosis

Hydronephrosis is a dilatation of the renal collecting system that may be unilateral or bilateral. Ultrasonically it appears as a circular sonolucent ring on the transverse scans. The longitudinal scans show the entire caliceal system to be dilated, thus a tubular sonolucent pattern is seen (Figs. 25-15 and 25-16). This differs from a parapelvic cyst, which remains spherical in both planes.

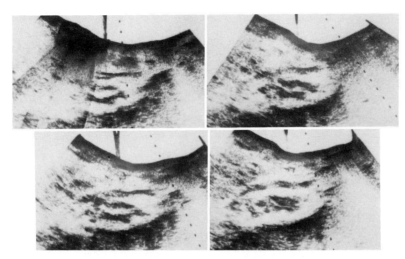

Fig. 25-15. Longitudinal scans of early hydronephrosis show dilation of the renal pelvis.

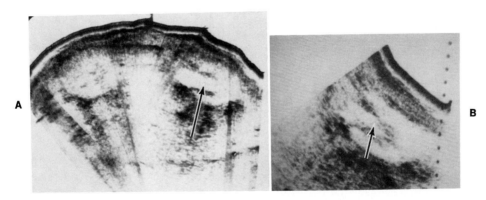

Fig. 25-16. Transverse **(A)** and longitudinal **(B)** scans of early hydronephrosis.

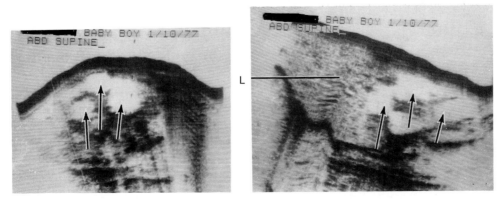

Fig. 25-17. Infant multicystic disease. Multiple small cysts are shown within the right kidney in the supine scans.

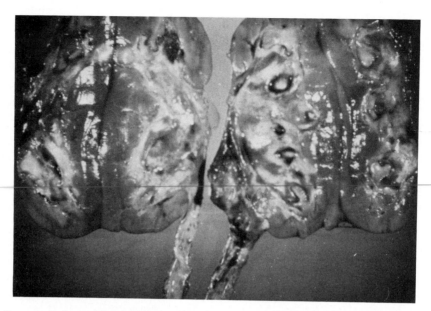

Fig. 25-18. Gross specimen of polycystic disease shows greatly enlarged kidneys with multiple cystic pockets.

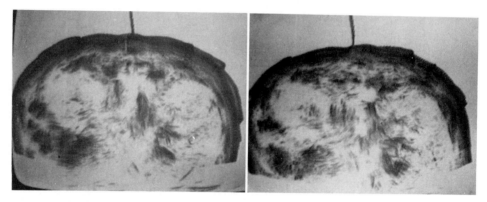

Fig. 25-19. Transverse scans of polycystic kidneys. The kidneys are enlarged with multiple interfaces within from the tiny cystic structures.

Multicystic kidneys

Multicystic kidneys are the most common childhood kidney disorder. Clinically there may be poor renal function or a palpable abdominal mass. Ultrasound can help screen these children in the search for renal cysts and renal dysfunction or obstruction (Fig. 25-17). Generally, only one kidney is affected by multicystic disease.

Polycystic kidneys

Polycystic kidneys are hereditary and may remain latent for years until cysts expand to obstruct normal renal function. If polycystic kidneys are suspected at birth, ultrasonic evaluation will demonstrate huge bilateral renal cysts throughout the parenchyma. These cysts vary in size but are always bilateral. It is much rarer to detect polycystic disease at birth, and this generally signifies imminent death. (See Figs. 25-18 to 25-22.)

Cystic renal masses

A cyst is the easiest abnormality to recognize in the kidney (Fig. 25-23). Most equipment limits the resolution of small masses, making it difficult to detect lesions smaller than 1 to 2 cm. Higher-frequency transducers, coupled with real-time equipment, enable the mass to be outlined with greater accuracy. The cyst should appear sonolucent with well-defined borders and good through-transmission. High gain allows the sonographer to fill in the renal area, with the cyst remaining echo free.

A simple cyst may cause partial obstruction of the collecting system. Clinically an abdominal mass may be palpated. It is usually cortical and will bulge

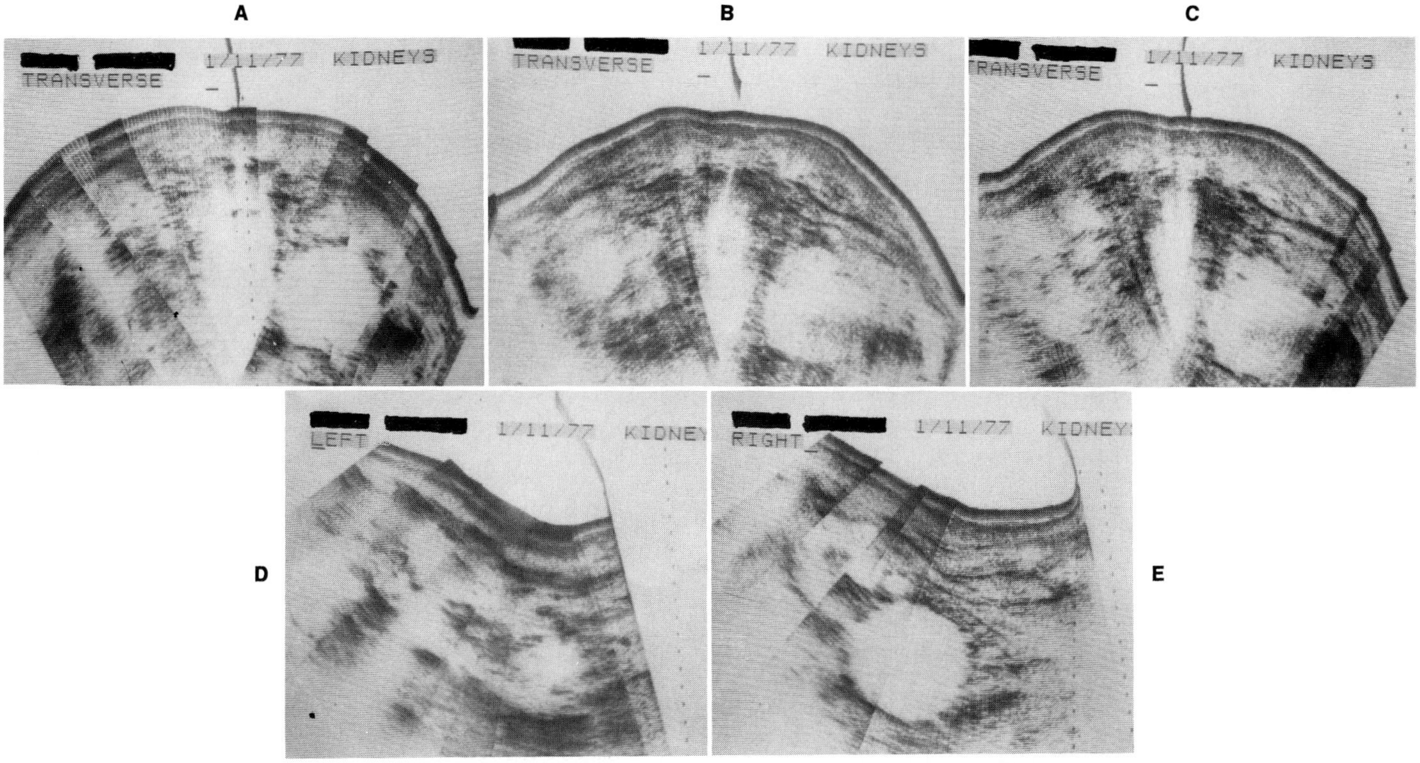

A   B   C

D   E

Fig. 25-20. A to **C,** Transverse scans of advanced polycystic disease showing large cysts throughout the kidneys. **D** and **E,** Longitudinal scans of the irregular shaped kidneys of the same patient.

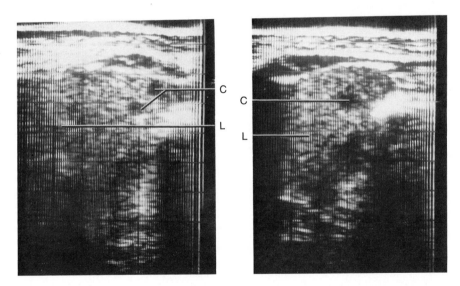

Fig. 25-21. Supine scans of the liver reveal small (1 cm) cysts within the parenchyma in a patient with polycystic renal disease. These small cysts may be difficult to visualize with contact scanners because of patient respiratory variability. Real-time evaluation is most effective.

through the renal capsule. Ultrasound will outline the cyst within the renal parenchyma and define whether it is single, multiple, trabeculated, or multilocular.

Most common is a simple serous cyst, which is ideal for aspiration. Multilocular cysts appear as simple cysts with many internal echo borders. Generally, these borders are sharp and well defined, which separates them from tumor echoes. It becomes diffi-

cult to aspirate these cysts, since there may be several different sacs within the lesion. (See Figs. 25-24 to 25-27.)

Adult polycystic disease is present at birth but may be asymptomatic until adulthood. Hypertension is one of the clinical signs, along with urinary tract infection. The polycystic disease is found in the multiple segments of dilated tubules. It is always bilateral, dis-

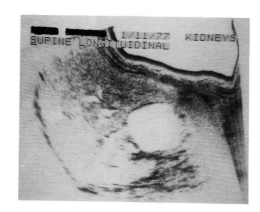

Fig. 25-22. Longitudinal supine scan of the right kidney of the patient in Fig. 25-21.

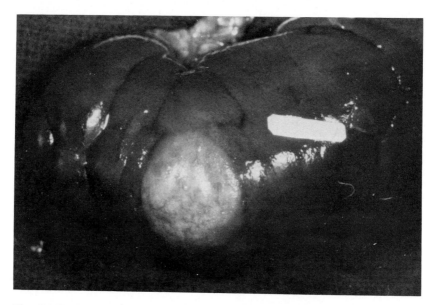

Fig. 25-23. Gross specimen of a renal cyst in the midpole of a right kidney.

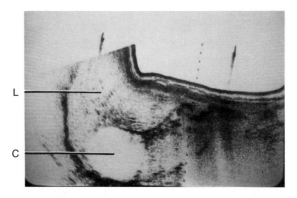

Fig. 25-24. Supine scan of a right upper pole renal cyst.

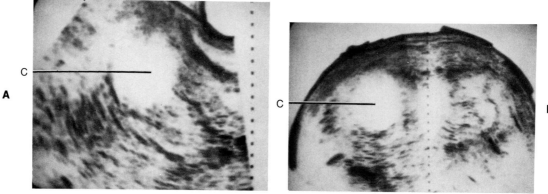

Fig. 25-25. Prone longitudinal (A) and transverse (B) scans of a right upper pole renal cyst.

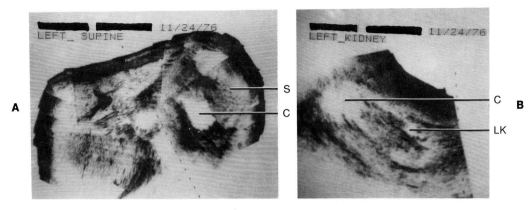

Fig. 25-26. A, Supine transverse scan of a left upper pole renal cyst. **B,** Prone longitudinal scan of a left upper pole renal cyst.

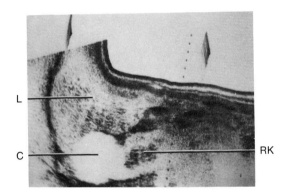

Fig. 25-27. Supine longitudinal scan of a right renal cyst.

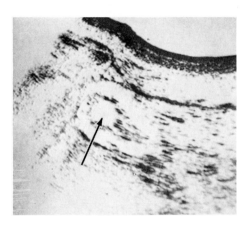

Fig. 25-28. Small parapelvic renal cyst within the renal parenchyma.

tinguishing it from multicystic disease, in which multiple cysts develop within the kidney. Attention should be directed to the liver parenchyma as well, since 30% to 40% of patients with renal polycystic disease have liver cysts.

Parapelvic cysts are generally very small and are found within the pelvic central core. They appear as a mild hydronephrosis in transverse scans but as a circle in longitudinal scans, which separates them from the tubular dilation of hydronephrosis (Fig. 25-28).

A renal carbuncle is an abscess in the renal cortex usually resulting from the union of smaller abscesses. Its rupture may cause a perirenal abscess surrounding the kidney (Figs. 25-29 and 25-30). The renal carbuncle, or perinephric abscess, may appear as a sonolucent pattern or as a complex pattern outside the renal capsule. Generally, clinical signs are flank pain, fever and chills, and increased white blood cell count. It may be secondary to an infection or postsurgical.

A subcapsular hematoma surrounding the renal capsule is secondary to trauma or surgical invasion or is spontaneously formed. It generally presents a ho-

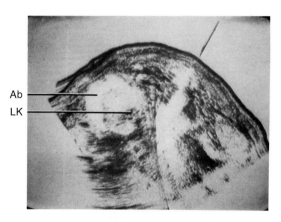

Fig. 25-29. Complex mass surrounding the left kidney represents a renal abscess.

mogeneous pattern, with some internal echoes representing clot formation.

Staghorn calculi within the renal capsule may be demonstrated as dense echo formations with shadowing posterior. Often it is difficult to visualize the renal parenchyma because of the sound attenuation of the calculi (Fig. 25-31).

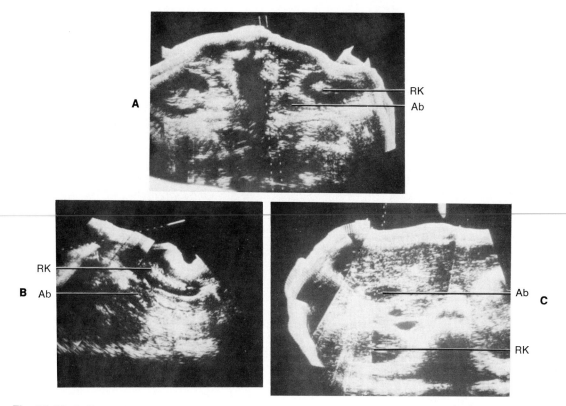

Fig. 25-30. A, Prone transverse scan of an abscess anterior to a right kidney. B, Prone longitudinal scan of the anterior complex mass. C, Supine transverse scan of an abscess anterior to the right kidney.

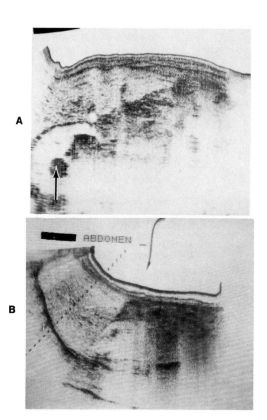

Fig. 25-31. Staghorn calculus is displayed as strong echoes within the renal parenchyma. Complete attenuation of sound may be due to the density of the calculi. A, Supine transverse scan demonstrating the anterior border of a kidney and dense internal echoes with shadowing posterior. B, Supine longitudinal scan of a right kidney demonstrates a shadowing effect from calculi within the renal parenchyma.

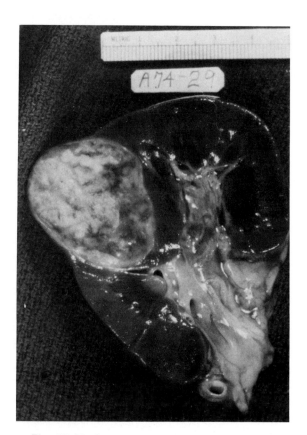

Fig. 25-32. Gross specimen of a renal tumor.

Benign renal tumors

Renal adenomas generally present no clinical symptoms and may be found on routine radiographs. The connective tissue tumors—fibroma, myoma, lipoma, hemangioma—indicate gross hematuria. Their pattern can present as complex to solid, depending on their growth and degenerative stage.

Malignant tumors

Possible symptoms of adenocarcinoma are flank pain, a palpable mass, fever, weight loss, and hematuria. It is the most common renal tumor. Its central core may undergo necrosis, but generally the tumor is well encapsulated, firm, and has a solid echo appearance. (See Figs. 25-32 to 25-36.)

In children nephroblastoma and Wilms' tumor are common renal lesions. They present complex patterns, generally so large that the kidney becomes difficult to distinguish from the mass.

Other tumors such as lymphoma and sarcoma are solid lesions with poor sound transmission and scattered fine internal echoes.

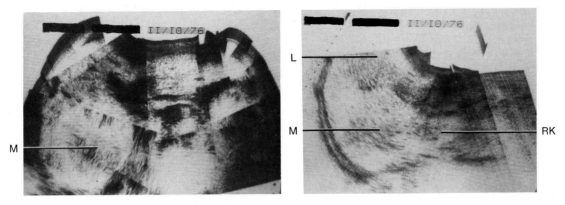

Fig. 25-33. Supine scans of a huge solid complex pattern of a right renal mass.

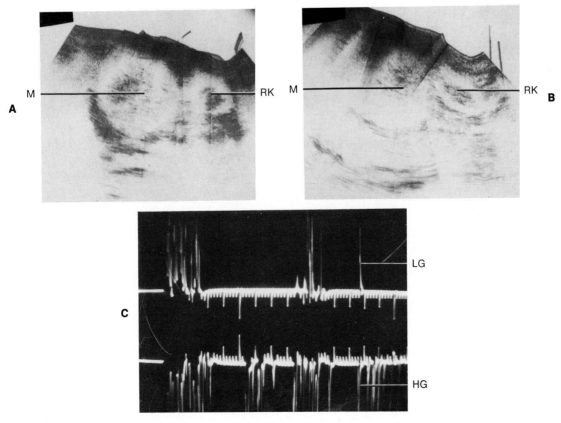

Fig. 25-34. A and **B,** Prone scans of a solid renal mass in the right upper pole renal mass with poor through-transmission and multiple internal echoes. **C,** A-mode scan of a mass demonstrates poor sound transmission at low gain and internal echoes within the borders at higher gain.

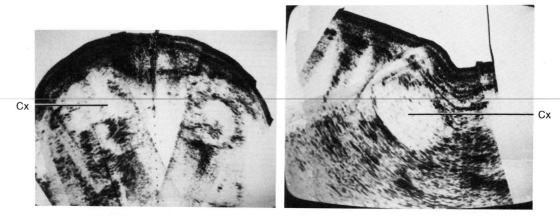

Cx   Cx

Fig. 25-35. Solid masses are more difficult to detect in the kidney because of the complex nature of the renal parenchyma. However, irregularities may be noted in the renal outline, which should lead to further investigation.

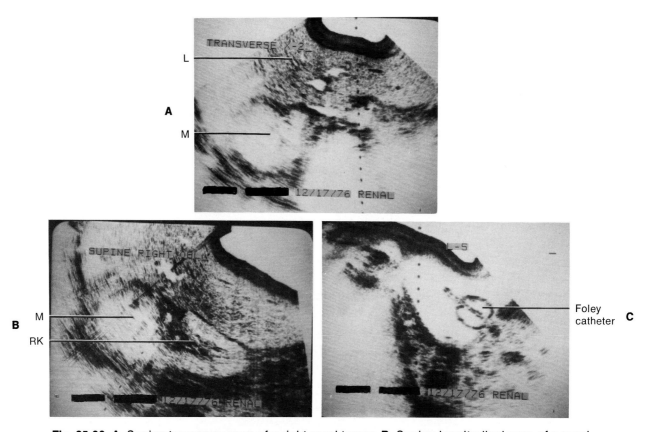

Fig. 25-36. A, Supine transverse scan of a right renal tumor. **B,** Supine longitudinal scan of a renal tumor on the upper pole of the kidney. **C,** Longitudinal scan of the lower pelvis reveals a distended bladder with a Foley catheter within.

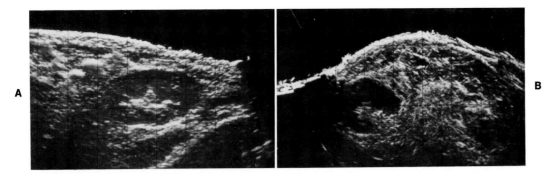

Fig. 25-37. Normal longitudinal **(A)** and transverse **(B)** scans of a renal transplant on top of the psoas muscle.

Renal transplant

Since the renal transplant is generally placed along the iliopsoas margin, the renal capsule may be well delineated in the supine position. Clinical signs of rejection are malaise, fever, leukocytosis, hypertension, abnormal urine output, pain, and tenderness over the renal area. Ultrasound should be performed as a baseline study postoperatively to determine caliceal pattern, renal size, and extrarenal fluid collections. Early signs of rejection may appear as hydronephrosis and increased renal size. Lymphocele collections or perirenal abscess may be seen surrounding the renal capsule. (See Figs. 25-37 to 25-40.)

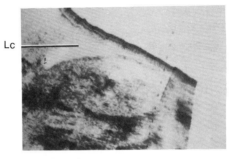

Fig. 25-38. Renal transplant with slight dilatation of the pelvis and lymphocele collection *(Lc)* anterior.

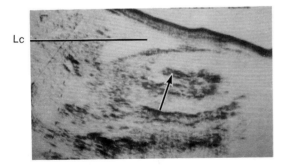

Fig. 25-39. Renal transplant with a lymphocele anterior to its border. Arrow points to the renal collecting system. Dilatation of these internal echoes indicates early rejection.

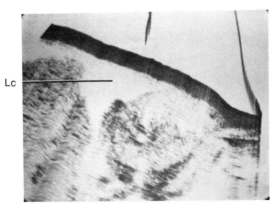

Fig. 25-40. Renal transplant with dilated tubules and surrounding lymphocyte collection, indicating rejection.

ULTRASONIC ASPIRATION TECHNIQUES

Once a renal mass has met the criteria for a cystic mass, most laboratories will recommend needle aspiration to obtain fluid from the lesion to further evaluate its internal composition.

The patient should be positioned with sandbags under the abdomen to help push the kidneys toward the posterior abdomen and to allow for a flat scanning surface. The cyst should be localized in the transverse and longitudinal planes with scans being performed at midinspiration. The depth of the mass should be noted from its anterior to posterior borders so the exact depth can be given to aid in the placement of the needle.

A special aspiration transducer with a hole in its central core will allow the sonographer to observe the A-mode trace of the cystic mass. If a metal needle is used, the tip will be shown as a sharp spike between the two walls on the A mode as the needle enters the cyst. This allows close monitoring of the mass as the fluid is withdrawn. Special B-mode aspiration transducers are now available that allow the scan to be made and the needle inserted in the same transducer, so the two-dimensional B scan and A mode allow for accurate puncture (Fig. 25-41).

A beveled needle will cause multiple echoes within the walls of the cyst. If the needle is slightly bent, many echoes will appear until the bent needle is completely out of the transducer's path. The larger the needle gauge, the stronger the reflection will be. Other needles, made of Teflon or other plastics, will not produce a strong echo within the cyst on A mode.

Most aspiration transducers are 2.25 MHz with higher frequencies used for superficial structures. The size of the lumen within the transducer should be close to the needle gauge to prevent wobbling or misdirection of the needle.

Sterile technique is used for aspiration and biopsy procedures. The transducer must be gas sterilized. The lumen of the transducer should be cleaned as well with a small brush and alcohol after each procedure. Sterile lubricant is used to couple the transducer to the patient's skin.

Once the area of aspiration is outlined on the patient's back, the distance is measured from the anterior

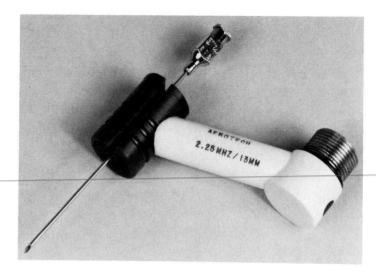

Fig. 25-41. B-mode aspiration transducer allows placement of the needle and slit within the transducer head to move the apparatus away once the needle is placed correctly.

surface to the middle of the cyst. This distance is added to the height of the transducer to give a total depth of the lesion. Special needle-stops act as a guide in preventing the needle from exceeding this precise distance.

The volume of the cyst may be determined by measuring the radius of the mass and using the following formula:

$$V = \frac{4}{3} \pi r^3$$

Or the diameter of the mass could be applied to this formula:

$$V = d^3 \div 2$$

The patient's skin should be painted with tincture of benzalkonium (Zephiran) and sterile drapes applied. A local anesthetic is administered over the area of interest, and the sterile transducer is then used to relocate the cyst. This may be done with A mode or B scan, depending on the type of transducer. The needle is inserted through the lumen of the transducer into the central core of the cyst. The needle stop will help in making sure the needle does not go through the cyst. The fluid is then withdrawn according to the volume calculations.

26 □ Spleen

with assistance of
PHYLLIS CAREY, R.D.M.S.

NORMAL ANATOMY

The spleen is reddish and lies in the left hypochondrium, with its long axis along the shaft of the tenth rib. The lower pole extends forward as far as the mid-axillary line. The spleen is roughly ovoid in shape and has a convex upper surface and a concave surface below, where vessels enter the organ. There is a notched anterior surface, and in an adult it weighs approximately 140 g. The spleen is the largest single mass of lymphoid tissue in the body, one of the so-called secondary lymphoid organs, in contrast to the thymus. It is active in blood formation during the initial part of fetal life. This function decreases, so that at the fifth or sixth month of gestation the spleen assumes its adult character and discontinues its hematopoietic activity.

RELATIONAL ANATOMY

Anterior to the spleen lies the stomach, the tail of the pancreas, and the left colic flexure. The left kidney lies along its medial border (Fig. 26-1). Posteriorly the diaphragm, the left pleura, left lung, and the ninth, tenth, and eleventh ribs are in contact with the spleen (Fig. 26-2).

The arterial blood supply is from the splenic artery, which travels along the superior border of the pancreas. On entering the spleen at the hilus, it immediately divides into about six branches. The splenic vein leaves the hilus and joins the superior mesenteric vein to form the portal vein. The lymph vessels emerge from the hilus and pass through a few lymph nodes along the course of the splenic artery and drain in the celiac nodes. The nerves to the spleen accompany the splenic artery and are derived from the celiac plexus.

PHYSIOLOGY

The red pulp of the spleen is composed of two principal elements—the splenic sinuses alternating with splenic cords. The sinuses are long irregular channels lined by endothelial cells or flattened reticular cells. A recent study indicated pores, or gaps, between the lining cells, implying that the circulation is open and

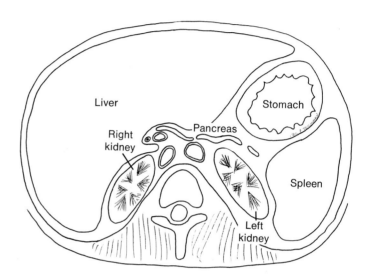

Fig. 26-1. Transverse diagram of the upper abdomen demonstrating the posterior position of the spleen behind the stomach and lateral to the left kidney.

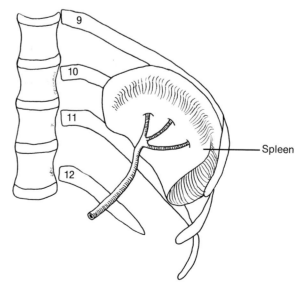

Fig. 26-2. Anteroposterior location of the spleen against the costal margin of the ninth, tenth, and eleventh ribs.

that blood cells can freely leave the sinuses to enter the intervening cords. The membrane shared by the cord and the adjacent splenic sinuses is also perforated. Reticular cells with delicate processes sometimes bridge the cords. Thus these highly phagocytic cells create an open meshwork of cords. The blood that leaves the splenic sinuses to enter the reticular cords passes through a complex filter.

The venous drainage of the sinuses and cords is not well defined, but it is assumed that tributaries of the splenic vein connect with the sinuses of the red pulp. From here the splenic vein follows the course of the artery, eventually joining the superior mesenteric vein to form the portal vein.

The white pulp is composed of the malpighian corpuscles, whereas the red pulp comprises the sinuses and the intervening spaces. Extending from the capsule inward are the trabeculae, containing blood vessels and lymphatics. The lymphoid tissue, or malpighian corpuscles, has the same structure as the follicles in the lymph nodes, but they differ in that the splenic follicles surround arteries, so that on cross section each contains a central artery. These follicles are scattered throughout the organ and are not confined to the peripheral layer or cortex, as are lymph nodes.

As part of the reticuloendothelial system, the spleen plays an important role in the defense mechanism of the body and is also implicated in pigment and lipid metabolism. The spleen is not essential to life, and it can be removed with no ill effects. The functions of the spleen can be classified under two general headings—those which reflect the functions of the reticuloendothelial system and the special functions characteristic of the organ. The functions of the spleen as an organ of the reticuloendothelial system are: (1) the production of lymphocytes and plasma cells, (2) the production of antibodies, (3) the storage of iron, and (4) the storage of other metabolites. The functions characteristic of the organ include those related to erythrocytes: (1) maturation of the surface of the erythrocytes, (2) reservoir function, (3) "culling" function, (4) "pitting" function, and (5) disposal of senescent or abnormal erythrocytes; also included are functions related to platelet life span and leukocyte life span.

The role of the spleen as an immunologic organ concerns the production of cells capable of making antibodies (lymphocytes and plasma cells); however, it should be understood that antibodies are produced at other sites.

Phagocytosis of erythrocytes and the breakdown of the hemoglobin occur throughout the entire reticuloendothelial system, but roughly half the catabolic activity is localized in the normal spleen. In splenomegaly the major portion of hemoglobin breakdown occurs in the spleen. The iron that is liberated is stored in the splenic phagocytes. In anomalies such as the hemolytic anemias, the splenic phagocytes become engorged with hemosiderin when erythrocyte obstruction is accelerated.

In addition to storing iron, the spleen is subject to the "storage diseases" such as Gaucher's disease and Niemann-Pick disease. Abnormal lipid metabolites accumulate in all phagocytic reticuloendothelial cells but may also involve the phagocytes in the spleen, producing gross splenomegaly.

The functions of the spleen that are characteristic of the organ relate primarily to the circulation of erythrocytes through it. In a normal individual the spleen contains only about 20 to 30 ml of erythrocytes. In splenomegaly the reservoir function is greatly increased, and the abnormally enlarged spleen contains many times this volume of red blood cells. The transit time is lengthened, and the erythrocytes are subject to destructive effects for a long time. In part, ptosis causes consumption of glucose, on which the erythrocyte is dependent for the maintenance of normal metabolism, and the erythrocyte is destroyed. Selective destruction of abnormal erythrocytes is also accelerated by the splenic pooling.

As erythrocytes pass through the spleen, the organ inspects them for imperfections and destroys those which it recognizes as abnormal or senescent. This is called the "culling" function. The "pitting" function is a process by which the spleen removes granular inclusions (Howell-Jolly bodies, siderotic granules, etc.) without destroying the erythrocytes. The normal function of the spleen keeps the number of circulating erythrocytes with inclusions at a minimum.

The spleen also pools platelets in large numbers. The entry of platelets into the splenic pool and their return to the circulation is extensive. In splenomegaly the splenic pool may be so large that it produces thrombocytopenia. Sequestration of leukocytes in the enlarged spleen may produce leukopenia.

PATHOLOGIC CONDITIONS
Congenital anomalies

Complete absence of the spleen (asplenia or agenesis of the spleen) is rare and, by itself, causes no difficulties. Often, however, asplenia is associated with congenital heart disease, such as defects in or the absence of the atrial or atrioventricular canal, pulmonary stenosis or atresia, transposition of the great vessels, and others. The abnormalities usually produce cyanotic disease in young patients and are seldom amenable to surgical correction.

Accessory spleen is a more common congenital anomaly. One of every six accessory spleens is located in the tail of the pancreas. Lesions affecting the main spleen usually affect the accessory spleen as well.

Regressive changes

Hyalinization. Hyaline degeneration of the arterial wall may be found in persons of any age and is non-specific in nature. In young patients hyalinization often accompanies hypertension.

Amyloidosis. In systemic diseases leading to amyloidosis the spleen is the organ most frequently involved. It may be normal in size or decidedly enlarged, depending on the amount and distribution of amyloid. Two types of involvement are seen—modular and diffuse. In the modular type, amyloid is found in the walls of the sheathed arteries and within the follicles but not in the red pulp. In the diffuse type the follicles are not involved, the red pulp is prominently involved, and the spleen is usually greatly enlarged and firm.

Atrophy. Atrophy of the spleen (50 to 70 g) is not uncommon in normal individuals. It may also occur in wasting diseases. In chronic hemolytic anemias, particularly sickle cell anemia, there is excessive loss of pulp, increasing fibrosis, scarring from multiple infarcts, and incrustation with iron and calcium deposits. In the final stages of atrophy the spleen may be so small that it is hardly recognizable. Advanced atrophy is sometimes referred to as autosplenectomy.

Pigmentation

The pigments found in the spleen are (1) hemosiderin and hematoidin, which are derived from hemoglobin, (2) malarial pigment, and (3) anthracotic pigments. Large amounts of hemosiderin are deposited in all phagocytic cells of the reticuloendothelial system when there is iron excess, as in chronic hemolytic anemia or after many blood transfusions. Deposits of hemosiderin iron in the spleen in abnormally large amounts is called siderosis. In moderate amounts it produces little effect on the tissue. In large amounts it stimulates proliferation of fibrous tissue. The nature of the pigment called hematoidin is largely unknown. It is formed in areas of hemorrhage or infarction.

In malaria the black pigment imparts a dark brown color to the pulp of the spleen. The pigment is of the hematin type and is found within phagocytes.

Anthracotic pigmentation of the spleen is rare.

Rupture

Rupture of the spleen is usually caused by a crushing injury or a severe blow. Much less often it is encountered in the apparent absence of trauma. This event is described as spontaneous rupture. Spontaneous rupture is encountered most often when the spleen is enlarged and soft in diseases such as infectious mononucleosis, leukemia, malaria, typhoid fever, and other types of acute splenitis.

Nonspecific acute splenitis

In nonspecific acute splenitis the spleen is enlarged by from 200 to 400 g, soft, and on section the pulp is often diffluent. The most common disease conditions producing acute splenitis are bacteremia, as in vegetative endocarditis, but any other severe systemic inflammatory disorder such as diphtheria, bacillary dysentery, or pneumonia, may effect similar splenic changes. Acute splenitis may be induced by noninfectious disease and is encountered in any extensive tissue destruction of chemical or physical nature, presumably because the spleen is active in resorption of necrotic cell products.

Nonspecific subacute or chronic splenitis

The organ with nonspecific subacute or chronic splenitis is enlarged, but rarely as much as 1000 g, and is firm in consistency. This condition is seen most commonly in certain specific diseases, which will be described later. The next most frequent cause is vegetative (bacterial) endocarditis.

Specific forms of splenitis

The specific infections that may affect the spleen are tuberculosis, syphilis, typhoid fever, brucellosis, malaria, sarcoid infectious mononucleosis, kala azar, histoplasmosis, torulosis, schistosomiasis, anthrax, actinomycosis, blastomycosis, echinococcosis, and cysticercosis. The more common infections will be discussed.

Tuberculosis. Although rare in adults, splenic involvement is common in children with pulmonary tuberculosis. The spleen is enlarged but usually does not exceed 500 or 600 g in weight. The tubercles are usually found in the malpighian corpuscles.

Syphilis. The spleen is often enlarged in congenital syphilis, but rarely more than twice its normal size. It is firm and microscopically shows an infiltration of lymphocytes and plasma cells and an increase in connective tissue. Here and in acquired syphilis, gummas occur rarely. Splenomegaly in the tertiary stage is usually secondary to the congestive changes induced by luetic cirrhosis of the liver.

Typhoid fever. The spleen is characteristically enlarged in the range of 250 to 500 g. The outstanding feature is the filling of the pulp with histiocytic cells containing numerous phagocytized red cells, although focal necrosis similar to that seen in other organs is present. The lining cells of the sinuses are hypertrophic and often display active phagocytosis of red cells and other cellular debris.

Malaria. In the acute stage of malaria the spleen is enlarged and soft. In the chronic stage the spleen is greatly swollen, usually in the range of 1000 g but possibly as much as 4000 g, and it is firm.

Sarcoid infectious mononucleosis. The spleen is enlarged in at least 50% of cases, usually two or three times its normal size. It is generally soft, fleshy, and hyperemic.

Vascular disease

Acute congestion. Active hyperemia accompanies the reaction in the spleen to acute systemic infections. The spleen is moderately enlarged, rarely over 250 g in weight.

Chronic congestion. Chronic venous congestion may cause enlargement of the spleen, a condition referred to as congestive splenomegaly. The venous congestion may be systemic in origin, caused by intrahepatic obstruction to portal venous drainage, or due to obstructive venous disorders in the portal or splenic veins. Systemic venous congestion is found in cardiac decompensation involving the right side of the heart. It is particularly severe in tricuspid or pulmonary valvular disease and in chronic cor pulmonale.

The most common causes of striking congestive splenomegaly are the various forms of cirrhosis of the liver. It is also caused by obstruction to the extrahepatic portal or splenic vein (e.g., spontaneous portal vein thrombosis).

Long-standing congestive splenomegaly results in severe swelling of the spleen (1000 g or more).

Hypersplenism. Hypersplenism is a term used to designate a symptom complex characterized by congestive splenomegaly, leukopenia, and anemia (McMichael, 1934). This condition was referred to as Bonti's disease and was considered a primary hematologic disorder with secondary involvement of the spleen. Currently it is believed that the spleen involvement is primary.

The hypersplenic syndrome has been divided into primary and secondary types. Primary hypersplenism refers to increased splenic activity and size in the absence of known underlying causes. Secondary hypersplenism may occur in patients whose splenomegaly has a known origin, such as leukemia, lymphoma, and others. In both forms the spleen is almost always enlarged.

Infarcts. Splenic infarcts are comparatively common lesions caused by occlusion of the major splenic artery or any of its branches. They are almost always due to emboli that arise in the heart, produced either from mural thrombi in the left auricle or ventricle or vegetation on the valves of the left side of the heart.

Hemolytic anemia

Hemolytic anemia is the general term applied to anemia referable to decreased life of the erythrocytes. When the rate of destruction is greater than can be compensated for by the bone marrow, then anemia results.

Disorders involving red cells

Hereditary spherocytosis (congenital spherocytic hemolytic anemia). In this disorder the spleen is enlarged and sometimes weighs over 1000 g. An intrinsic abnormality of the erythrocytes gives rise to erythrocytes that are small and spheroid rather than the normal, flattened biconcave disks. The two results of this disease are the production by the bone marrow of spherocytic erythrocytes and the increased destruction of these cells in the spleen. The spleen destroys spherocytes selectively.

Sickle cell anemia. In the earlier stages of the disease, as seen in infants and children, the spleen is enlarged with marked congestion of the red pulp. Later the spleen undergoes progressive infarction and fibrosis and decreases in size until, in adults, only a small mass of fibrous tissue may be found, weighing less than 1 g (autosplenectomy). It is generally believed that these changes result when sickled cells plug the vasculature of the splenic substance effectively, producing ischemic destruction of the spleen.

Polycythemia vera. The spleen is variably enlarged, rather firm, and blue-red. It usually weighs about 350 g, and infarcts and thrombosis are common.

Thalassemia. The spleen is severely involved. This hemoglobinopathy differs from the others in that an abnormal molecular form of hemoglobin is not present. Instead, there is a suppression of synthesis of beta or alpha polypeptide chains, resulting in deficient synthesis of normal hemoglobin. The erythrocytes are not only deficient in normal hemoglobin but are also abnormal in shape; many are target cells, whereas others vary considerably in size and shape. Their life span is short because they are destroyed by the spleen in large numbers.

The disease varies from mild to severe. The changes in the spleen are greatest in the severe form, called thalassemia major. The spleen is very large, often seeming to fill the entire abdominal cavity.

Autoimmune hemolytic anemia. This type of anemia can occur in its primary form without underlying disease, or it may be seen as a secondary disorder in patients already suffering from some disorder of the reticuloendothelial or hematopoietic systems, such as lymphoma, leukemia, infectious mononucleosis, and others. In the secondary form the splenic changes are dominated by the underlying disease; in the primary form the spleen is variably enlarged.

Disorders involving white cells

Leukemia. Chronic myelogenous leukemia may be responsible for more extreme splenomegaly than is any other disease. Depending on the duration of the disorder, the spleen may weigh anywhere from 1000 to 3000 g. Weights of 6000 to 8000 g are not rare. The organ is symmetrically enlarged and firm and has a thickened capsule.

Chronic lymphatic leukemia. This disorder produces less severe degrees of splenomegaly. The spleen rarely exceeds 2000 g in weight.

Monocytic leukemia. This kind of leukemia causes mild splenomegaly, rarely producing a spleen over 500 g.

Reticuloendotheliosis

Gaucher's disease. All age groups can be affected by Gaucher's disease. About 50% of patients are under the age of 8 years and 17% under 1 year. Clinical features follow a chronic course, with changes in skin pigmentation and bone pain. Usually, the first sign is splenomegaly, enlarging the spleen to as much as 8000 g.

Niemann-Pick disease. This rapidly fatal disease predominately affects female infants. The clinical features of the disease are hepatomegaly, digestive disturbances, and lymphadenopathy.

Letterer-Siwe disease. This is sometimes called nonlipid reticuloendotheliosis, and there is proliferation of reticuloendothelial cells in all tissues but particularly in the spleen lymph nodes and bone marrow. Usually, the spleen is only moderately enlarged, but the change may be more severe in affected older infants. This disease is generally found in children below the age of 2 years. Clinical features are hepatosplenomegaly, fever, and pulmonary involvement. It is rapidly fatal, as well.

Hand-Schüller-Christian disease. This disorder is benign and chronic in spite of many features similar to those of Letterer-Siwe disease. It usually affects children over 2 years of age. The clinical features are a chronic course, diabetes, and moderate hepatosplenomegaly.

Primary tumors of the spleen

In general, primary tumors of the spleen, either benign or malignant, are rare.

Benign. The cavernous hemangioma is the most common primary tumor of the spleen. Next in frequency is the lymphangioma. These may be very large, consisting of multicystic lesions. The other types of tumors that may arise in the spleen are fibromas, osteomas, and chondromas.

Malignant. Any of the types of lymphomas or Hodgkin's disease found in the lymph nodes may be primary in the spleen, and they have the same characteristics as in the lymph nodes. In addition to these lesions, hemangiosarcomas with metastases, especially in the liver, do occur.

The most common secondary tumors are sarcomas, principally the so-called malignant lymphoma group and Hodgkin's disease.

Metastases of other types of tumors, especially carcinomas, are rare and usually occur only when generalized carcinomatosis has developed. An exception is widely disseminated melanocarcinoma that involves the spleen in about half the cases.

Summary of splenic disorders

Disorders that usually cause massive enlargement of the spleen (over 1000 g) are chronic myelogenous leukemia, chronic lymphatic leukemia (less massive than the myelogenous form), lymphomas, primary or secondary, Gaucher's disease, myeloproliferative syndrome, primary tumors of the spleen (extremely uncommon, but both benign and malignant tumors may cause massive irregular splenomegaly), malaria, kala azar, and other parasitic infestations such as an echinococcus cyst. Congestive splenomegaly due to portal or splenic vein obstruction usually causes moderate enlargement (500 to 1000 g). Disorders brought about by this condition include chronic splenitis (particularly vegetative bacterial endocarditis), tuberculosis, sarcoid tumor, typhoid fever, chronic congestive splenomegaly, sickle cell anemia in early stages, hereditary spherocytosis, metastatic carcinoma or sarcoma, infectious mononucleosis, acute leukemias, Niemann-Pick disease, Hand-Schüller-Christian disease, thalassemia, autoimmune hemolytic anemia, idiopathic thrombocytopenia, and Hodgkin's disease. Condi-

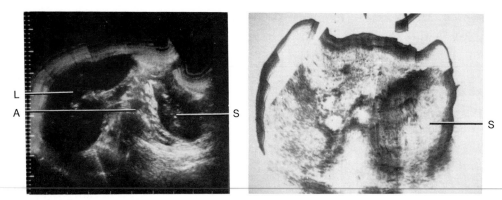

Fig. 26-3. Transverse supine scans of the upper abdomen demonstrate the splenic organ just posterior to the stomach.

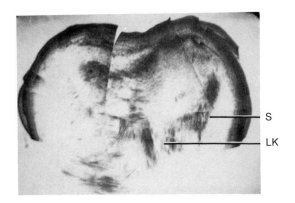

Fig. 26-4. Ribs may prevent the splenic parenchyma from filling in with fine echoes in the supine position.

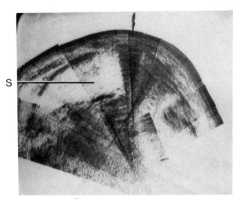

Fig. 26-5. Prone transverse scan of a slightly enlarged spleen with ascites lateral to the splenic margin.

tions causing minimal splenomegaly (usually under 500 g) are acute splenitis, acute splenic congestion, and miscellaneous acute febrile disorders such as bacteremic states, systemic toxemias, systemic lupus erythematosus, and intra-abdominal infections.

ULTRASONIC EVALUATION OF THE SPLEEN

Although the spleen is sometimes difficult to visualize when the patient is supine, this position often gives the examiner a clearer insight into splenic enlargement. One can compare the size of the spleen with that of the liver (Fig. 26-3). Usually, the spleen is not well visualized until 9 to 11 cm above the umbilicus. Generally, most of the liver is well visualized at the time of splenic visualization. In patients with enlarged spleens it may be seen as low as the umbilicus area.

The spleen should stipple in with fine snowflake echoes as is seen within the liver parenchyma. Generally, the stomach and ribs prohibit such visualization of the spleen, and only an outline can be noted from a scan along the left border (Fig. 26-4). If adequate visualization cannot be made from the supine

position, the patient should be rotated to the prone position to eliminate the stomach interference.

It has been reported by Leopold and Asher (1975) that one of the echo signs for splenic enlargement in the supine position is the visualization of the tip of the spleen exceeding the vertebral column in its transverse lateral projection. However, the examiner must be careful not to use this guide as the sole criterion for a diagnosis of enlargement. Like the liver, the spleen has various shapes and can be normal even when it exceeds the border of the vertebral column. Generally, the spleen lies posterior in the left upper quadrant, but occasionally it will lie fairly lateral along the left abdominal wall. In this instance, visualization of the left kidney and tail of the pancreas may be enhanced.

The prone scan is performed with a slight cephalic angulation of the transducer head. Transverse scans are probably the easiest in which to orient the transducer. Once the left kidney is well seen, serial scans are performed by moving the transducer gradually in a cephalic direction by 1 cm steps. As the scan moves superior from the caliceal area of the kidney, the spleen should be searched out along the left lateral

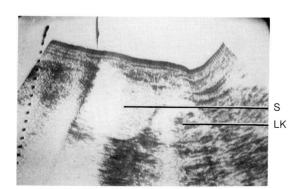

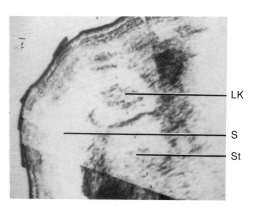

Fig. 26-6. Longitudinal prone scan of the spleen and upper pole of the left kidney.

Fig. 26-7. Transverse prone scan of the spleen and left kidney.

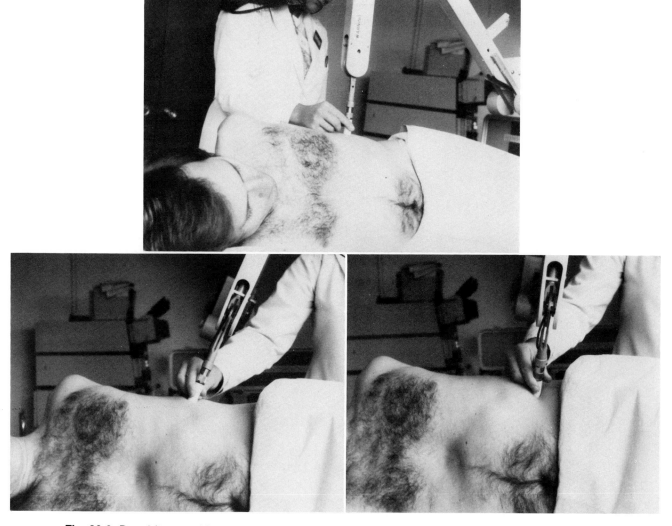

Fig. 26-8. Decubitus position permits scanning between the costal margin to record the maximum information from the splenic parenchyma.

border. Single scans are probably best to avoid rib artifacts. (See Figs. 26-5 to 26-7.) This view may give additional information about the splenic parenchyma, but the best information is probably obtained from the right decubitus position.

The decubitus, or axillary, position allows the examiner to scan in an oblique fashion in between the costal margins (Figs. 26-8 and 26-9). These scans should demonstrate the fine snowflake pattern within the spleen if gain settings are correct. Longitudinal decubitus scans can also be performed for an additional view. The ribs may be avoided by quickly skipping over them as the scan is being performed.

The automated scanners with a water bath delay are excellent machines to visualize the splenic parenchyma without rib artifact interference. These machines allow the scanner to glide over the splenic area without transducer "hang-up" over the ribs.

The determination of splenic enlargement is essential; once that has been established, the pathway to analyzing the cause for enlargement can be evaluated. It may be a general splenomegaly due to a blood disorder (leukemia), alcoholic cirrhosis, or other reasons or it may be splenomegaly secondary to a hemorrhage, tumor, or cyst. (See Figs. 26-10 to 26-18.)

If the patient has left upper quadrant pain secondary to trauma, a splenic hematoma or subcapsular hematoma should be considered. The patient should be scanned in the supine position first; then scans should be made in the prone and decubitus positions to define the hematoma. Increased gain settings should be used to define the extent of the hematoma. If the blood has organized, it may appear as an echo-free area within the spleen (Fig. 26-19). If it has clotted, it may appear as a complex mass. A subcapsular hematoma generally will appear as a complex mass partially surrounding the splenic capsule. If the patient has a slightly enlarged spleen without signs of organized hematoma, serial scans performed 6 hours apart may be helpful in the clinical diagnosis. The serial scans are especially helpful for the trauma patients who can afford to wait the 5 or 6 hours between scans to determine enlargement. A baseline scan must be done as soon as the patient arrives, with serial scans to follow up to a 24-hour period.

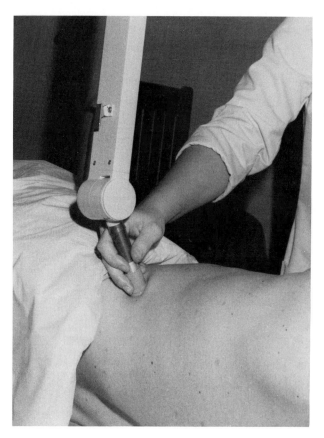

Fig. 26-9. Slight oblique path may be taken along the decubitus position to avoid the rib artifacts.

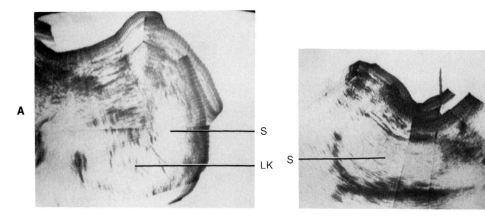

Fig. 26-10. Transverse **(A)** and longitudinal **(B)** supine scans demonstrate the splenic organ slightly enlarged.

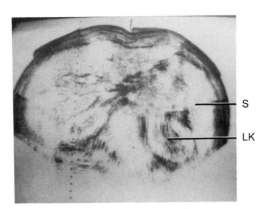

Fig. 26-11. Enlarged spleen secondary to Hodgkin's disease.

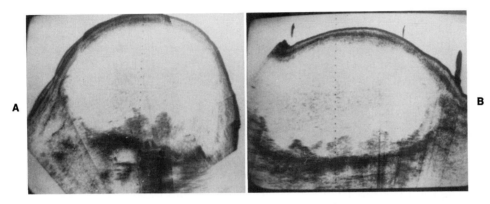

Fig. 26-12. Transverse **(A)** and longitudinal **(B)** scans demonstrate a huge dilated spleen secondary to an infarction.

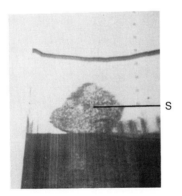

Fig. 26-13. Normal pattern of splenic parenchyma as shown in a water bath.

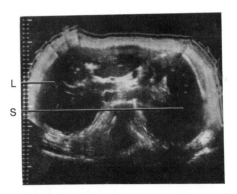

Fig. 26-14. Transverse supine scan demonstrates an enlarged spleen secondary to leukemia.

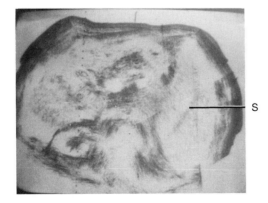

Fig. 26-15. Transverse scan of enlarged splenic organ.

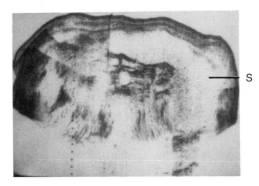

Fig. 26-16. Transverse supine scan of an enlarged spleen with ascites.

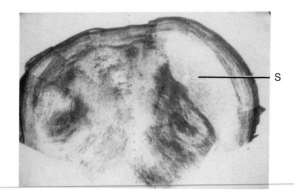

Fig. 26-17. Transverse supine scan of an enlarged spleen.

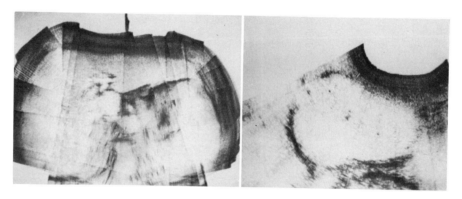

Fig. 26-18. Scans of a patient with cirrhosis and hepatosplenomegaly.

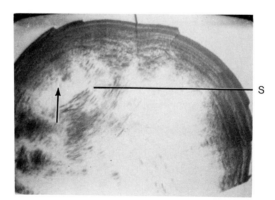

Fig. 26-19. Prone scan of an echo-free area within the periphery of the spleen represented in a splenic hematoma. The patient also had a filling defect on the nuclear medicine scan.

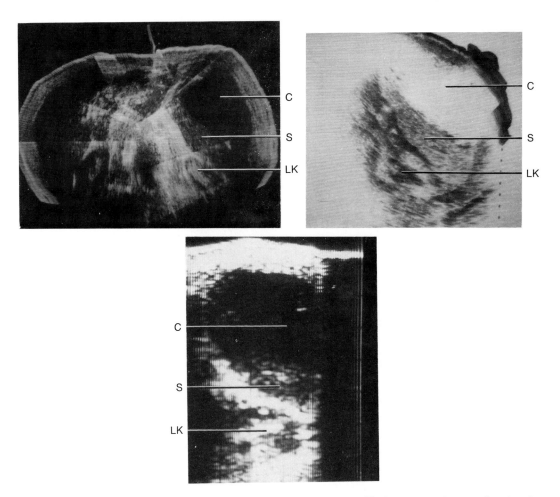

Fig. 26-20. Large echo-free area within the splenic capsule most likely represents a cystic structure within the spleen.

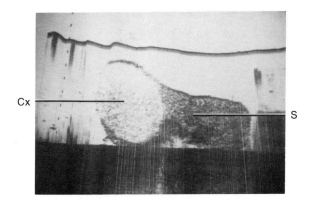

Fig. 26-21. Gross specimen was scanned, and the large echo-free area within the spleen had multiple fine stippled echoes within at high sensitivities. This was a benign tumor of the spleen.

An asplenic cyst shows up as an echo-free area within the spleen (Figs. 26-20 and 26-21). Sometimes it is difficult to discriminate a splenic cyst from a renal cyst or pseudocyst. Careful evaluation of these other organ systems should define their normal contour to rule out such a problem. Compression of normal structures sometimes is helpful in determining the origin of the mass. A splenic cyst may compress the renal parenchyma or even the tail of the pancreas. Of course, clinical evaluation of the patient is important in determining differential diagnosis.

Splenic tumors are not as common, and thus experience with them is limited in ultrasonic visualization. The tumors would probably resemble liver tumors—homogeneous, complex, solid, or denser than normal splenic parenchyma.

PART FOUR PELVIS

27 □ Anatomic and gynecologic considerations

ANATOMIC BOUNDARIES

The pelvic cavity is posterior and inferior to the abdominal cavity. The "false" pelvis is delineated by the ileum, whereas the "true" pelvis is delineated by the bow-shaped area within the iliac wings. Within the true pelvis are found the sacral promontory, the pubis, and the pelvic brim. The pelvis is tilted forward, so that the anterior iliac spine is more anterior than the pubic bone. This increases the lumbosacral curve in females and emphasizes the curvature of the buttocks.

The lower border of the pelvis has three bony structures—the ileum, ischium, and pubis. These meet to form the symphysis pubis, which generally serves as the external landmark of the lower pelvis.

The iliac crest holds the greater and lesser sciatic notches on its posterior surface. Blood vessels and nerves pass out of the sciatic region into the lower extremities.

The muscle groups relative to ultrasonic visualization are the psoas and iliacus, or iliopsoas, muscles. The psoas can be traced from the midpole of the kidney into the pelvic area where it becomes the iliacus. This generally marks the lateral landmark of the true pelvis. The muscular sling across the bottom of the pelvis is composed of the levator ani and the coccygeus. Together they form the pelvic diaphragm. Inferior to this diaphragm is the perineum.

The intraperitoneal structures within the pelvis are the cecum, small bowel, sigmoid colon, and rectum. The other structures are within what is more generally referred to as the retroperitoneal cavity and include urinary structures, vessels, and the reproductive system.

The common iliac artery bifurcates at the pelvic rim into the internal and external iliac arteries. The ureter crosses anterior to these vessels to enter the bladder posteriorly.

The uterus generally is found to lie at a 90° angle between the vagina and the bladder. The fallopian tubes extend to the lateral walls of the pelvis. The ureter comes very close to the cervix before it enters the bladder. The cervix is almost at a right angle to the vagina and extends into it.

PERITONEAL RELATIONS

From the anterior abdominal wall the parietal peritoneum passes over the superior surface of the bladder onto the anterior surface of the uterus as the vesicouterine reflection. The peritoneum then passes over the fundus of the uterus onto the posterior surface and extends inferiorly, covering the upper part of the vagina before reflecting on the rectum. This forms the rectouterine pouch of Douglas (Fig. 27-1).

The broad ligament is the fold of peritoneum related to the ovary, the uterine tubes, and the uterus. It is triangular in shape, extending from the lateral wall of the uterus to the lateral wall of the pelvis. Its free upper border encases the uterine tube and is directed anteriorly. Medially, the two layers envelope the uterus and are continuous with the layers of the opposite side. Inferiorly and laterally the two layers, anterior and posterior, extend over the floor of the true pelvis. The anterior surface is directed inferiorly as well as anteriorly, and the posterior surface, superiorly and posteriorly. The outer fifth of the upper free border contains the ovarian vessels and is termed the infundibulopelvic ligament of the ovary. The ovary projects from the posterior surface of the ligament sus-

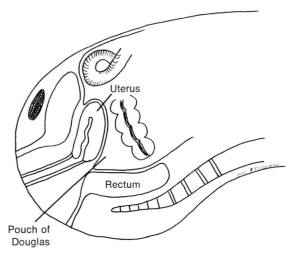

Fig. 27-1. Sagittal view of the lower pelvic cavity showing the uterus, rectum, and pouch of Douglas.

pended by a small peritoneal fold called the meso-varium. The portion of the ligament above this is termed the mesosalpinx and is related to the uterine tube. The portion of the broad ligament below the mesovarium is referred to as the mesometrium.

The support of the pelvic genital organs is further aided by several ligaments—the ovarian, round, lateral cervical, and uterosacral ligaments.

Ovaries

The ovaries develop from the germinal ridge and descend from their original position on the posterior abdominal wall into the pelvis. At this point they are found in an ovarian fossa, a depression bounded by the external iliac vessels above, obturator vessels below,

broad ligament anteriorly, and the ureter posteriorly. Their position varies and may occur in any part of the posterior portion of the pelvic cavity. The ovaries are suspended from the posterior layer by the meso-varium.

The infundibulopelvic ligament extends from the upper pole to the lateral pelvic wall and contains peri-vascular connective tissue surrounding the ovarian vessels. From the lower pole the ovarian ligament extends to the lateral uterine wall.

The lateral surface lies in relation to the ovarian fossa. The medial surface is related to the fimbriated end of the uterine tube and loops of small bowel. The posterior border lies free, but the anterior border is related to the mesovarium.

Uterine (fallopian) tubes

The fallopian tubes have two openings—the abdominal ostium and the uterine ostium. The four parts of each tube are (1) the infundibulum, a bulging extremity with a fimbriated mouth that overlies the ovary, to which one long fimbria adheres, (2) the ampulla, the largest portion of the tube, (3) the isthmus, a narrow, straight, thin-walled portion of the tube adjacent to the uterus, and (4) the intramural part, where the lumen narrows to 1 mm or less as it pierces the uterine wall.

Uterus

The uterus is a pear-shaped structure 7 to 8 cm in length (Fig. 27-2). It has three layers: (1) inner

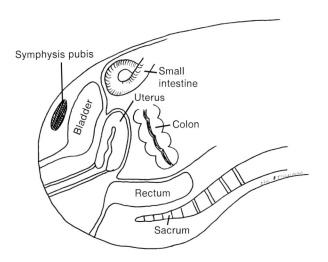

Fig. 27-2. Sagittal view of the female pelvis.

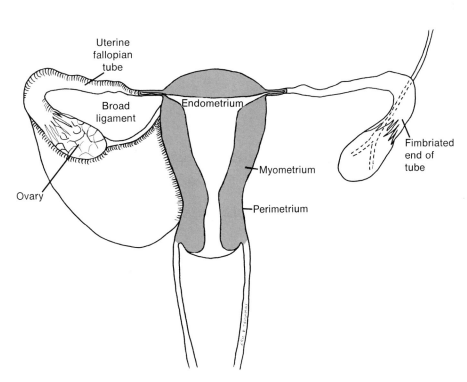

Fig. 27-3. Anteroposterior view of the female reproductive system.

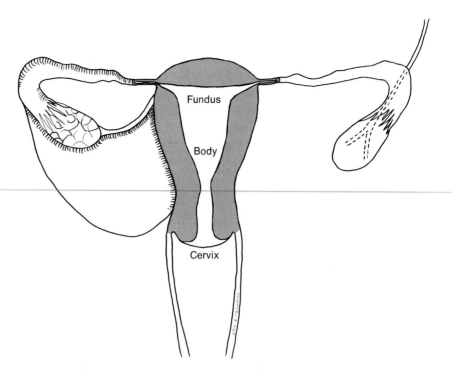

Fig. 27-4. Anteroposterior view of the uterine cavity.

mucosal, or endometrium; (2) thick muscular, or myometrium; and (3) serosal coat, or perimetrium. (See Fig. 27-3.) The parametrium is the loose connective tissue over the posterior surface of the anterior part of the body.

The uterine cavity is separated into three parts: (1) the fundus, the part lying above the entrance of the tubes; (2) the body, which is devoid of peritoneum along the lateral margin and is related to the parametrium; and (3) the cervix, where the body narrows to the area of the isthmus, which continues into the cervix. The cervix is 1.5 cm in length, and the lower portion protrudes into the vagina. (See Fig. 27-4.)

The uterine cavity is triangular, narrowing at the level of the isthmus. It communicates via the internal os with the cervical canal, which opens into the vagina by the external os.

The uterus normally is bent forward (anteflexed) in line with the horizontal axis at the level of the internal os. It also is bent forward in line with the vertical axis (anteverted). In contrast, the uterus may be bent backward at the horizontal and vertical axes (retroflexed and retroverted, respectively).

Vagina

The vagina is a flattened, but dilatable, canal. It pierces the pelvic floor and is directed down and forward. In the anteflexed position the cervix enters the wall of the vagina at a right angle.

GYNECOLOGIC COMPLAINTS

The female reproductive organs are the vagina, uterus, fallopian tubes, and ovaries. The external opening of the birth canal is the vagina; high in the vagina lies the neck of the uterus, called the cervix. The interior of the uterus joins the fallopian tubes, which open near the ovaries. The egg is released from the ovary and enters the fallopian tube, where fertilization normally occurs, then enters the uterus, where it attaches to the wall.

During a normal monthly cycle the lining cells of the uterus, influenced by the female hormones, grow to receive the fertilized egg. If fertilization does not occur, the lining cells of the womb are discharged through the vagina as the monthly menstrual flow.

Complaints related to the female reproductive organs may be caused by abnormalities of the menstrual flow or by pregnancy. Infection and tumor may cause pain, bleeding, or abnormal vaginal discharge; sexual problems and infertility are common sources of anxiety.

Cramps or pain

A pelvic infection may cause severe pain on one or both sides of the pelvis, becoming worse at the time of the menstrual period but persisting at other times. The pain of the pelvic infection is unremitting, punctuated by severe episodes from time and time. Fever as high as 103° F, or 39.5° C, accompanied by prostration may be noted. Nausea and vomiting may be seen in severe cases. Pelvic infections are treated with antibiotics.

Endometriosis

In endometriosis the lower abdomen and pelvis contain abnormally placed female hormones but are unable to release the discarded blood and cells, resulting in islands of old bloody discharge throughout the pelvis. The patient may complain of a dull, aching pelvic pain all month that becomes much worse at the time of the menstrual period. It is most common in women over 30 years of age who have not borne children. There is usually no nausea or vomiting, fever is not part of the disease, and the menstrual periods are regular except for the severe pain. Endometriosis responds well to pregnancy, but if pregnancy is not feasible, female hormones can be prescribed in a high enough dosage to simulate pregnancy, thereby allowing regression of the disease.

Uterine fibroids

Uterine fibroids are an overgrowth of the normal muscular wall of the uterus common after age 30. They may cause aching menstrual cramps, sometimes associated with bleeding periods. If the fibroid is very large, there may be a dull heavy feeling in the pelvis. Fibroids do not cause fever and there is no nausea or vomiting. The diagnosis of a fibroid uterus is made only after careful internal examination. If the fibroids are large and troublesome, they may be removed surgically with or without removal of the uterus.

GYNECOLOGIC ULTRASOUND

The pelvis must be evaluated with a full bladder. This serves four purposes: (1) it acts as a sonic window through which the ultrasound beam may travel; (2) it pushes the uterus cephalad and away from the symphysis pubis where it can be better evaluated; (3) it pushes the bowel cephalad and out of the pelvis; and (4) and fluid-filled bladder may be used as a comparison in evaluating the internal characteristics of a mass.

The female organs best visualized are the bladder, uterus, vagina, and cervix. Occasionally, the normal ovaries are visualized to either side of the uterine cavity. Midcycle ovulation permits slight dilation of the ovaries for better visualization. The transducer should be angled slightly toward the patient's head to slice through the bladder, uterus, and ovaries to either side.

The normal uterus is generally best seen in the longitudinal plane, where the cervix may be identified just beneath the triangle of the bladder. The body and fundus are shown posterior to the full bladder. The endometrial cavity presents an intense echo within the uterine cavity, and the myometrium generally fills in with fine low-level echoes. The normal uterus measures approximately 3 to 4 cm in the anteroposterior dimension and 6 to 7 cm in the longitudinal dimension.

The supine longitudinal scan is performed initially. This allows the sonographer to obtain the bladder-uterine relationship and to ascertain whether the bladder is sufficiently filled. The midline scan is centered midway between the symphysis and umbilicus, with subsequent scans made every 1 cm to both sides of the pelvic cavity. The iliacus muscle marks the lateral extent of the true pelvis and should be identified as a somewhat sonolucent band running along the posterior border of the pelvic cavity.

Transverse scans are then performed with a slight angulation of the transducer head to record the bladder and uterus simultaneously. Small increments are made in the cephalic direction until the transmission is attenuated by small bowel.

Intrauterine contraceptive device

There are several different types of IUCDs available, and the particular device should be known prior to ultrasound evaluation. The most common devices are the Lippes loop and the Cu-7. Each of these appears as a dense echo reflection within the fundus of the uterus. The Lippes loop generally appears as five separate echoes from each curvature in the device on the longitudinal scan. The Cu-7 does not appear as dense as the loop and is displayed as a fairly straight line with a slight bend at the upper end (Fig. 27-5). The Mazjlin spring and the Dalkon shield are more difficult to demonstrate; however, both can be recognized by a very dense echo within the uterine cavity as shown on transverse and longitudinal scans (Fig. 27-6).

Cyst

A cystic abnormality of the pelvic area should be evaluated in the following manner. Determination should be made as to whether a lesion is separate or part of the uterus. The scan should demonstrate the relationship of the mass to the uterus and bladder, and thus the consistency of the mass can be ascertained. If it is cystic, the same characteristics of the bladder should appear, that is, it should be echo free, show a strong posterior border, and exhibit good sound transmission. (See Figs. 27-7 to 27-12.)

An ovarian cyst may have interlocking cavities and

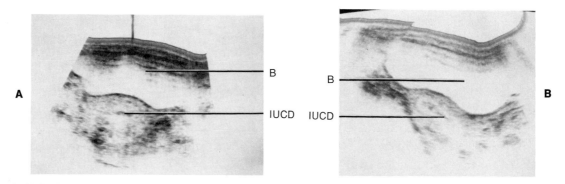

Fig. 27-5. A, Transverse view of the distended bladder and IUCD within the uterus. **B,** Longitudinal view of the Cu-7 device.

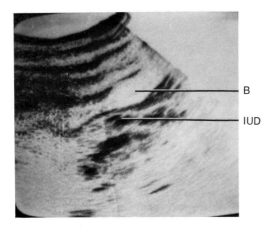

Fig. 27-6. Longitudinal view of the Mazjlin spring in a retroverted uterus.

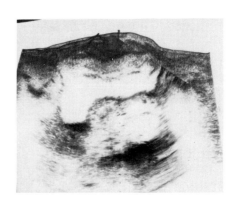

Fig. 27-7. Transverse view of the bladder with uterus deviated to the right by the cystic mass, most likely from the ovary.

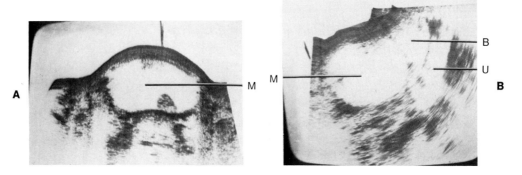

Fig. 27-8. A, Transverse scan of a large cystic mass in the pelvis. **B,** Longitudinal scan of the bladder, posterior uterus, and anterior cystic mass.

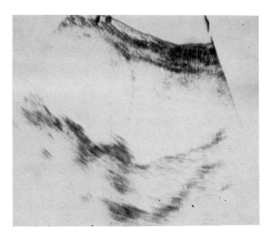

Fig. 27-9. Longitudinal scan of the bladder, posterior uterus, and anterior cystic mass.

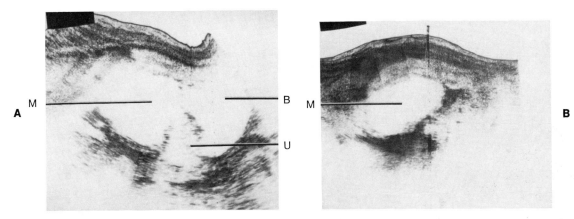

Fig. 27-10. A, Large cystic mass separate from the bladder and uterus. **B,** Transverse scan over the cystic mass. The echoes along the anterior wall represent reverberation artifacts.

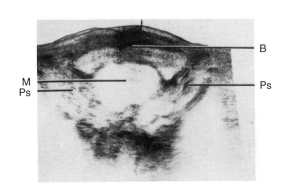

Fig. 27-11. Transverse scan of bladder, uterus, and cystic mass.

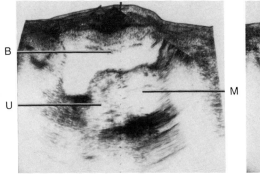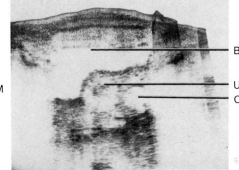

Fig. 27-12. Transverse scans show a small cystic structure indenting the uterine cavity posteriorly.

still be benign. The echo component is complex with good through-transmission and a sharp posterior border but with internal echoes from the interfaces of the cyst. If a cyst is over 5 cm in diameter, there is a chance of it twisting around itself. Thus the echo pattern may appear complex with irregular borders, depending on the nature of the twist and whether any rupture has occurred.

Infections within the fallopian tubes

Chronic cases of pelvic inflammatory disease appear ultrasonically as complex masses with irregular bor-

ders, usually in the cul-de-sac, or pouch of Douglas. A hydrosalpinx, as the result of an infection, is filled with serous fluid and is sometimes difficult to differentiate from an ovarian cyst. Endometriosis is a condition in which the blood from the uterus goes to the ovaries and tubes and appears echographically as a slightly enlarged uterus with multiple scattered internal echoes.

Leiomyoma

Leiomyoma is a benign tumor common in women. Black women have an eight to ten times greater chance

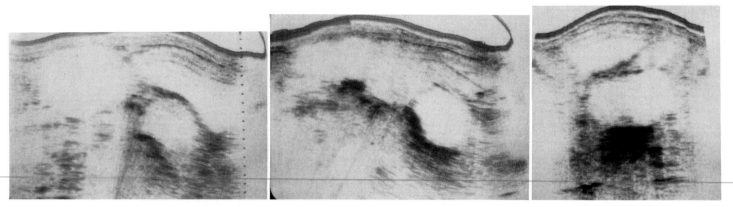

Fig. 27-13. Anterior fibroid with an ovarian cyst posterior to the bladder.

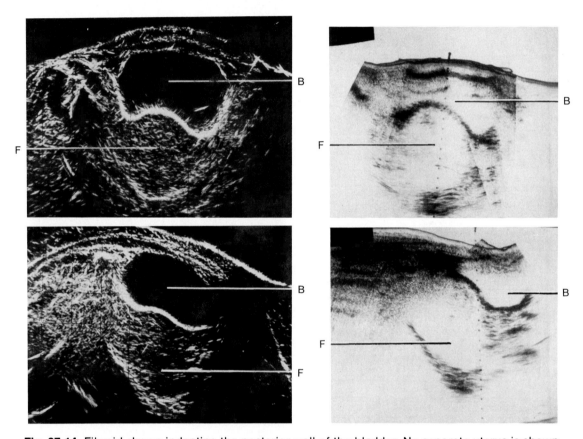

Fig. 27-14. Fibroid shown indenting the posterior wall of the bladder. No separate uterus is shown. Scans were done with high- and low-gain settings.

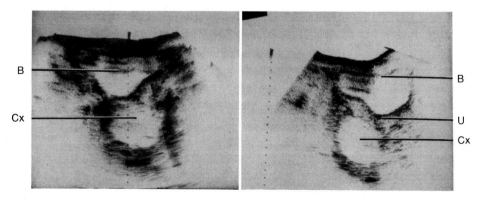

Fig. 27-15. Complex mass in the cul-de-sac may represent a fibroid of the posterior uterine wall.

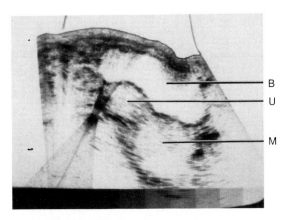

Fig. 27-16. Longitudinal scan of a fibroid in the cul-de-sac.

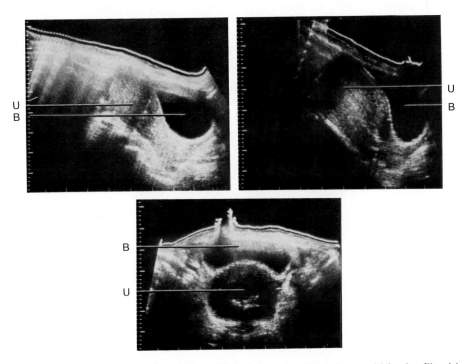

Fig. 27-17. Sensitivity denotes multiple internal echoes from within the fibroid.

of developing a myomatous tumor. Younger women show less incidence toward myomas than do postmenopausal women. Symptoms of bleeding, pain, and a feeling of pressure on the bladder are common. The ultrasound appearance is variable, from an echo-free area protruding from the uterine wall to a complex mass from the uterine wall. The amount of necrosis and degeneration the tumor undergoes is discerni le from the ultrasonic pattern. (See Figs. 27-13 to 27-17.)

Dermoid

The dermoid tumor generally shows calcification on a plain radiograph. It is known to grow quite large.

The patient is usually asymptomatic, sometimes with vague lower quadrant pain. Ultrasonically the pattern depends on the hair-fluid level within the dermoid. Generally, the hair-fluid sign is easily recognized as a dermoid tumor if the mass presses posteriorly on the bladder, separate from the uterus, or if the fluid level is sufficient to distinguish the mass from the bowel within the pelvis. Often the dermoid tumor will be so solid that it is difficult to separate the mass from the bowel patterns. Densities should be evaluated as well as deviation of the uterus to the right or an indentation of the posterior wall of the bladder, to indicate a mass compression sign. (See Figs. 27-18 to 27-20.)

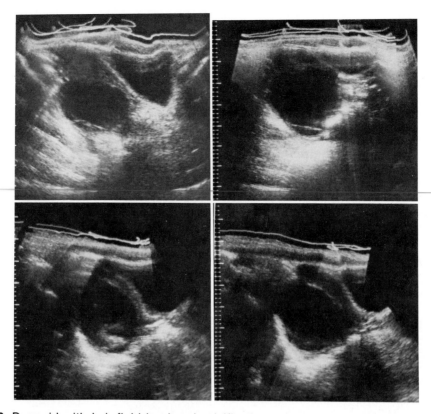

Fig. 27-18. Dermoid with hair-fluid level and calcification echoes within, shown posterior to the uterus.

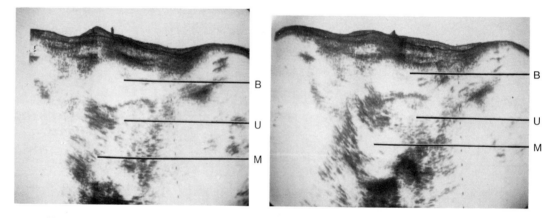

Fig. 27-19. Recurrent teratoma posterior to the uterus is seen as a complex mass.

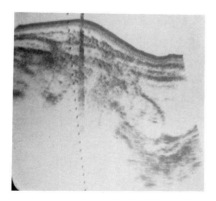

Fig. 27-20. Small dermoid tumor shown posterior to the bladder. The uterus is posterior to the bladder and inferior to the mass.

Complex masses

Most pelvic masses tend to be categorized as complex. It is often difficult to distinguish a pelvic abscess from a complex mass within the abscess by echo pattern recognition. It is important to be able to separate the mass from the bladder and uterus for further clinical evaluation. Often patients with intense pain are difficult to examine, but the ultrasound study can outline the abnormality, if present. Many endometrial tumors are complex masses within the uterine cavity, making it difficult to separate uterine parts from tumor echoes. The carcinomas often display complex patterns because of their necrosis and solid components. (See Figs. 27-21 to 27-23.) Ascites within the pelvis may be helpful in determining malignancy from obstructed bowel. With malignant ascites there is fluid in the flanks and matting of bowel with multiple echo-free areas in the pelvic cavity (Figs. 27-24 and 27-25).

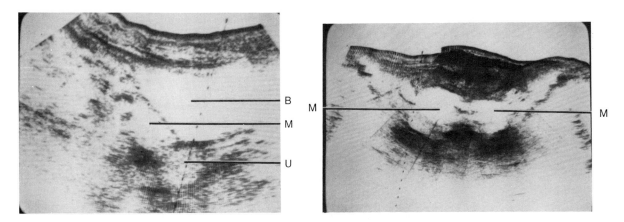

Fig. 27-21. Bilateral, complex adnexal mass separate from the uterus.

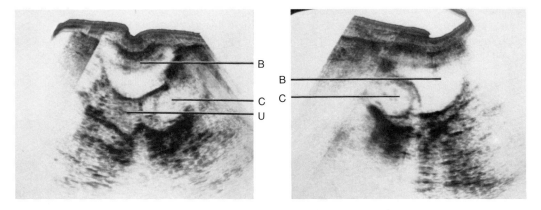

Fig. 27-22. Four to 5 cm complex adnexal mass could represent a cyst bled into an adnexal mass or dermoid.

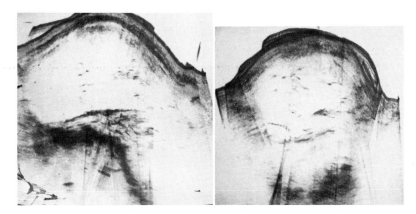

Fig. 27-23. Giant pelvic mass, most likely ovarian. Multiple internal echoes with echo-free areas denote a complex pattern, most likely cystadenoma or carcinoma.

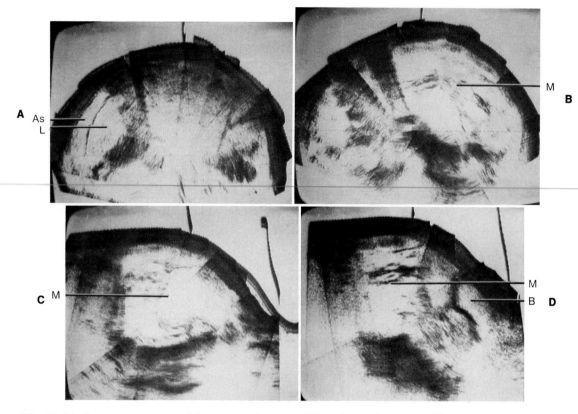

Fig. 27-24. Transverse scans of the upper abdomen **(A)** and umbilical area **(B)** showing ascites and separation of the liver from the abdominal wall. **C** and **D,** Longitudinal pelvic scans show massive ascites and a complex echo pattern with high-gain sensitivity. Most likely this indicates cystadeno-carcinoma with ascites.

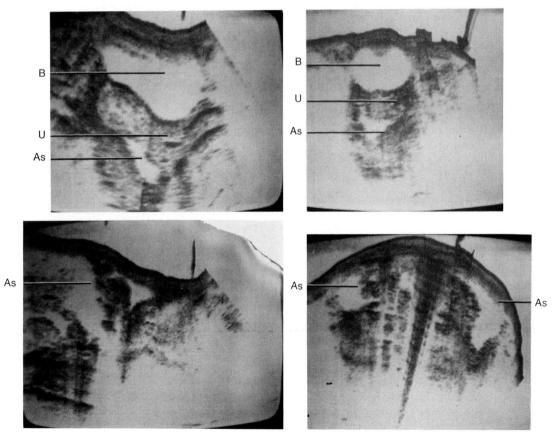

Fig. 27-25. Small amount of ascites just beneath the uterus and a large amount of ascites and bowel within the pelvic cavity are visible.

28 □ Normal gestation and obstetric complications

with assistance of
COLLEEN CARSON

NORMAL GESTATION

Normal human conception takes place at the fim-briated end of the fallopian tubes. After fertilization it takes three or four days for the egg to reach the uterus. Approximately three days after fertilization the egg has grown to a solid ball of about sixteen cells called a morula. On the fourth day the fluid from the uterus enters the morula, creating a cystic space; the morula is then called a blastocyst. This blastocyst has an outer cell mass of trophoblastic tissue and an inner cell mass destined to become the embryo.

From the sixth to the eleventh days the blastocyst goes through the process of attaching itself to the endometrium. After this implantation trophoblastic growth continues, and differentiation of the embryo germ cells into ectoderm, mesoderm, and endoderm layers occurs. The trophoblastic cells cause an erosion of the maternal vessels until veins and spiral arteries are reached. Thus a sluggish circulation is established on the maternal side of the placenta at about eleven and a half days.

During the first weeks after implantation, the embryo develops a neural plate soon to be a nervous system, a primitive heart, lung buds, and depression sites for the eyes. A growth of trophoblastic tissue covers the entire embryo, developing a structure called the chorion frondosum, which contains the amnion, amniotic fluid, and embryo. The base of the chorion frondosum is anchored to and communicates with the maternal vessels. This chorion frondosum continues to grow and become part of the fully developed placenta.

Up to this point the chorionic tissues contain no blood vessels, and the embryo does not have a circulatory system. The embryonic nutrition is carried out principally by osmosis from the amniotic fluid. By the end of the third week certain cells in the mesoderm layer differentiate into blood islands and then vessels, vascularizing the entire chorion. At the same time vessels are forming in the fetus, the circulatory system and the heart develop. By the end of the fourth week vessels from the fetus and the chorion connect and establish fetal-placental circulation through the umbilical cord.

The placenta absorbs nutrients and oxygen from the maternal blood, and these materials are transported to the fetus through the umbilical arteries. Waste products for excretion into the maternal blood are brought from the fetus through the large umbilical vein.

All this time the fetus continues to grow and specialize. During the fourth week it develops a primitive gallbladder and liver tubules, brain differentiation, facial parts, and a beating heart. With the sixth week the four chambers of the heart develop, cartilage for future bone is laid down, and arms and legs form.

By the seventh and eighth weeks the embryo is in recognizable human form with eyelids, genitals, thyroid gland, and buds for teeth. At the end of the first trimester the organ formation is almost complete. By the end of the seventh month or almost the second trimester, the fetus is often sufficiently well developed to survive outside the uterus.

Placenta

The maturation of the placenta is also crucial in a normal pregnancy. There seem to be three different phases of plancentation—a period of implantation, rapid placental growth, and maturation. The placenta matures in late gestation. This period is noted by a marked growth in the function of the organ without much change in its size. There is an increase in the total surface area but minimal changes in placental weight because the organ seems to have flattened and spread out.

The placenta at term is flat, cakelike, round or oval, with a diameter of approximately 15 to 20 cm and an approximate width of 2 to 3 cm at its thickest part. The normal placenta should weigh about one sixth the weight of the fetus. Oversized placentas (placentamegaly) are found in cases of erythroblastosis, syphilis, diabetes, or sometimes without apparent reason. Undersized placentas are often associated with fetal death. There can be conditions, such as multiple pregnancy, that would cause the placenta to be abnormally large for one fetus but smaller than would be functional for the two fetuses. Occasionally, two separate lobes with the same connecting vessels can also be found.

The normal placenta has a homogeneous spongy consistency. Sometimes at term a few subchorionic nodules of fibrin and flecks of calcification are found. These seem to have no clinical or pathologic significance.

Endocrine functions

Another essential factor of a normal pregnancy is endocrine function. The corpus luteum in the mother's ovaries produces increasing amounts of estrogen and progesterone to develop the endometrium layer in the uterus for early pregnancy. Blood levels in pregnancy roughly approximate the rise in progesterone production.

On about the sixth day of pregnancy the placenta begins producing estrogen and progesterone in progressive amounts until the end of gestation. After as little as thirty-six days sufficient progesterone production can be accomplished to allow a pregnancy to progress after the shriveling of the corpus luteum. Normally, the placenta does not take over production until the fourth month of gestation. By the third trimester it secretes about 250 mg of progesterone in 24 hours.

The placenta also takes over estrogen functions by synthesizing estrogens. The rising values of estrone, estradiol, and estriol in the mother's urine reflect the function and well-being of the fetus. Fetal distress or death can be predicted by the urinary estriol values. Estriol excretion depends on an intact fetal circulation.

Gonadotrophic hormone is also secreted by the placenta and excreted in the urine and serum. Excretion in pregnant women begins within the first two or three weeks of gestation and reaches its highest concentration between fifty and ninty days, following which is a decline to the low level that is maintained throughout the remainder of pregnancy. The function of this hormone is to maintain the corpus luteum until the placenta is capable of taking over the progesterone production. When it is no longer needed, it declines and the corpus luteum shrivels. This hormone is helpful in the evaluation of normal fetal growth and development in the first trimester of pregnancy. It also aids in the diagnosis of trophoblastic disease such as a hydatidiform mole or chorionepithelioma.

Pregnancy tests such as these are not always indicative of a normally progressing pregnancy; they only represent the presence of some functioning placental or trophoblastic tissue.

Respiration

Normal fetal respiration keeps the oxygen consumption per kilogram of body weight during fetal life approximately the same as that after the infant is born.

If the fetus in utero has an oxygen deficiency, a condition of asphyxia or anoxia develops. The fetus tries to compensate for its low P_{O_2} supply from placental veins by increasing its cardiac output. This increase of flow dilates the vascular beds in the placental and central nervous system and can cause increasing acidosis, growth retardation, central nervous system damage causing mental retardation, and finally, if the condition persists, fetal death.

Amniotic fluid

The volume of amniotic fluid is subject to considerable variation but is also an indication of fetal well-being. Normally, by the end of the first trimester of pregnancy there are approximately 50 ml of amniotic fluid. As pregnancy progresses so does the amniotic fluid level, up to about 1000 ml at thirty-seven to thirty-eight weeks. At term the amount of fluid decreases to about 800 ml. Thereafter the decrease can be dramatic, dropping to as little as 250 ml of fluid.

The fetus swallows about 210 to 760 ml of amniotic fluid a day. If there is some internal obstruction such as a thoracic tumor or esophageal atresia, the amount of fluid not swallowed will cause an increase in the total amount of amniotic fluid. About 2000 to 3000 ml or more is considered to be abnormal (Romney et al., 1975).

Polyhydramnios is a condition of excess amniotic fluid. It occurs in approximately 0.13% to 3.2% of known pregnancies. Acute polyhydramnios is associated with one amnion in a multiple pregnancy. It is also common in diabetes mellitus and anencephalic fetuses. Because of increased intrauterine pressures, congenital abnormalities and fetal distress conditions may occur. In about 50% of cases of polyhydramnios the fetus or newborn dies. Death is usually caused by abnormalities and premature labor.

Oligohydramnios is a condition wherein a smaller than normal volume of amniotic fluid is present. This condition is less common than polyhydramnios and tends to cause infants to be small for dates. Oligohydramnios is associated with the underdevelopment or obstruction of the fetal urinary tract, leaking of amniotic fluid, poor placental blood flow, or the death and retention of the fetus. An abnormal amount of fluid is considered to be below 400 ml.

Movement

Fetal movement or muscular activity usually begins after fourteen to twenty weeks of gestation and is most vigorous in the last trimester, but this varies according to the fetus. Some exhibit little activity yet are perfectly normal. One theory is that activity depends on the amount of REM sleep the fetus receives.

Cessation of fetal movement is usually associated with fetal death, but this is not always reliable. It has been proposed that the lack of fetal movement for 24 hours in the last trimester is indicative of fetal distress, and no movement for 72 hours means fetal death. (Romney, Gray, Little, Merrill, Quilligan, and Stander, 1975). This is only theory and should not be solely relied on.

Heart rate

Normal fetal heart rate is between 120 and 160 beats a minute (Romney et al., 1975). The more premature the infant, the faster the heart rate. This is a result of the increasing vaginal tone with fetal age and increased amniotic fluid, which tends to slow the heart rate.

Fetal tachycardia occurs above 160 beats a minute. Maternal fever tends to increase the heartbeat, causing tachycardia. Certain drugs, such as atropine, scopolamine, and isoxsuprine, also cause this condition of increased heartbeat.

Fetal bradycardia, which is considered to be a heart rate below 120 beats a minute, often results from severe hypoxia or conduction block. Prolonged fetal bradycardia due to hypoxia is often fatal.

Sometimes up and down changes in fetal heartbeat occur. Early deceleration of fetal heartbeat is often caused by the compression of the fetal heart from the umbilical cord. Late deceleration of the heart is due to fetal hypoxia, excessive uterine size, maternal hypotension, or placental insufficiency.

ABNORMAL DEVELOPMENT AND FETAL DEATH

Recognition of fetal distress or fetal demise is vital for the protection of the mother and the possible life of the fetus. Frequent evaluations of the progress of pregnancies could prevent many pending complications. The earlier fetal death is discovered, the safer it is for the mother.

Most fetuses deliver spontaneously soon after intrauterine demise. About 75% of mothers experience spontaneous labor by the end of the second week after fetal death, and by the end of the third week about 93% go into labor (Romney et al., 1975).

If the dead fetus is retained in utero longer than five weeks, the mother may develop disseminated intravascular coagulation. This is a situation in which the mother's clotting factor is not working properly, so she continues to bleed from the tear the placenta has made in the uterus. The blood cannot coagulate in this area, and a possible infection may also occur.

There is a fine line between abortion and premature labor. Some specialists contend that fetal death and expulsion up to the point of viability is abortion, and after that it is premature labor. It can also be broken down into stages: ovular abortion occurs during the first four weeks; embryonic abortion takes place after four to twelve weeks' gestation; and fetal abortion happens from twelve weeks to viability.

About 10% to 15% of all known pregnancies terminate in spontaneous abortions, most of them occurring in the first trimester. This period is the most important time in the development of the fetus.

Abortion may start after the death of the embryo or fetus, which is followed by the shriveling of the placenta and its separation from the uterine wall; or there is a possibility of initial placental separation followed by the death of the fetus. Fetal or placental death in the first two weeks of gestation is normally caused by noxious influences in the mother's body. During the three to eight weeks of gestation, death is usually caused by morphologic abnormalities of the fetus (Jones and Jones, 1975).

The clinical signs of abortion are lack of movement, no fetal heart sounds, abdominal colicky pain, vaginal bleeding with or without passage of parts of the uterine contents, elevation of temperature due to infection, and an enlarged soft uterus with tenderness and cervical dilation. If cervical dilation is not present and there is slight bleeding, there is the possibility of a threatened rather than an inevitable abortion.

In a missed abortion the fetus dies, but the placenta is still attached to the uterine wall. With the death of the fetus the cord and fetal membranes follow with postmortem changes, but the placenta does not. Postmortem changes cause the fetus to undergo dehydration and finally become mummified through a process of calcification.

Abruptio placentae is a premature separation of the normally implanted placenta and is one of the major causes of hemorrhage in the last trimester of pregnancy. The placenta may separate at varying degrees; thus the clinical results have a wide range of possibilities. The placenta may detach just a small corner that passes unnoticed, or the entire placenta may sever and cause serious bleeding and complications. It is possible that no bleeding would show if the presenting part of the fetus plugged the passage; all the bleeding would then be contained within the uterus. When the placenta does separate, in about 50% of patients the fetal heartbeat can still be heard.

Abruptio placentae seems to be caused by toxemia associated with pregnancy or other types of chronic hypertensive diseases. These diseases cause excessive amounts of thromboplastin and defibrination of the mother's blood. But there also seem to be numerous placental separations with no apparent cause.

DETECTION OF FETAL DISTRESS

There are several methods of detection of fetal death and fetal distress. In cases where there is a suspicion of fetal death, diagnostic interest is concentrated on fetal heart activity and movements as well as anatomic changes in the fetus.

Auscultation is one method of detection. The probability for error is great, however, and fetal heart sounds cannot be heard before the fifth month of pregnancy; thus auscultation is not a chosen method.

Radiology is another method that is not the most preferred. Changes in fetal anatomy can be detected, but the radiographs cannot be taken before the sixteenth week of gestation because of the lack of bone development. Also, there is a problem of radiation exposure hazard in cases where a pregnancy is developing normally.

Hormone studies with the analysis of serum, urine, or amniotic fluid are valuable in the assessment of fetal well-being. However, they do not always tell the whole story and so cannot be relied on exclusively. For example, a positive pregnancy test can be obtained in a case of a hydatidiform mole without any pregnancy at all.

At the present time the method of choice is diagnostic ultrasound. A-mode ultrasound can show fetal motion and anatomic changes. B scan can give a presentation of fetal parts, placenta, uterus, fetus head size, and shape showing anatomic changes as well as motion. Doppler ultrasound provides information about placental and fetal heart activity. A high-pitched blowing sound is indicative of the fetal heart, and a low-pitched roar is the maternal heart rate from the placental vessels. Doppler ultrasound is reliable from the twelfth week on and vaginal Doppler ultrasound from eight weeks on. Real-time ultrasound is also extremely valuable in showing fetal motion in utero, fetal breathing, and fetal heart motion.

Ultrasound has proved to be an excellent method of the detection of fetal death or progress. It is also helpful with amniocentesis in the localization of the placenta. The exact position can be marked and the best position for puncture site determined.

For ultrasound to detect fetal distress or demise there must be a record of normal ultrasonic findings for comparison.

ULTRASONOGRAPHY FOR THE NORMAL FETUS

At five weeks' gestation the embryonic sac can be recognized as a well-defined ring of echoes. From

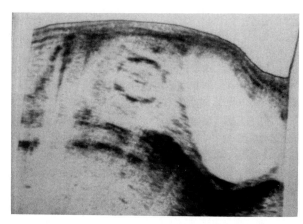

Fig. 28-1. Full bladder technique should be utilized in obstetric scans to serve as a window to the fetal structures and to push the uterus into the pelvic cavity.

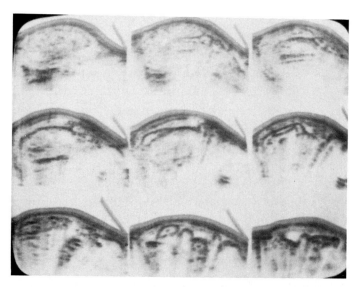

Fig. 28-2. Multi-image presentation demonstrates vertex presentation of a posterior placenta. Images are small for detail but present the basic information about fetal position.

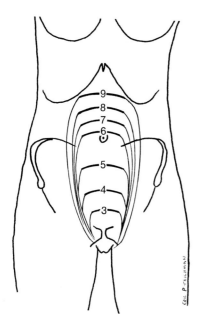

Fig. 28-3. Maternal uterine growth throughout pregnancy.

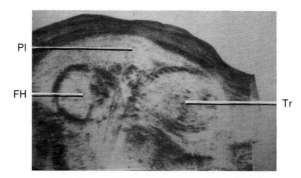

Fig. 28-4. Breech presentation with anterior fundal placenta.

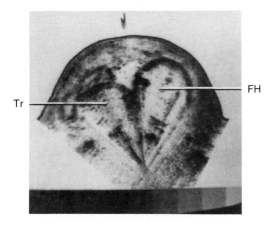

Fig. 28-5. Transverse lie showing fetal head and trunk.

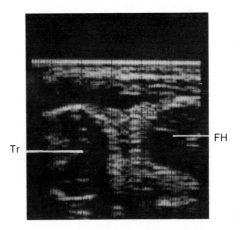

Fig. 28-6. Transverse lie shown on a real-time scan.

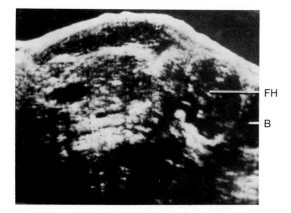

Fig. 28-7. Vertex presentation of a fetus with an anterior placenta.

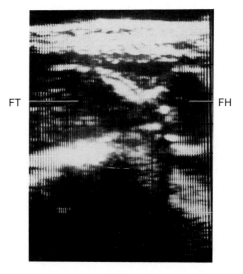

Fig. 28-8. Real-time scan showing vertex presentation.

seven to eight weeks the embryo can be detected as a small echo within the sac. An early placenta can sometimes be seen as a speckled area within the uterus after eight or nine weeks. At this period Doppler ultrasound can pick up fetal heart sounds, but it is not totally reliable until about ten weeks' gestation. Fetal movement can also be picked up at this time by real-time scanning.

At ten weeks the sac growth is so rapid it completely fills the uterine cavity with echoes. This period around ten to twelve weeks is considered the "blind spot." This is about the time that the gestational sac disintegrates, and the placental echoes are more noticeable. At this stage the intrauterine echoes are somewhat indefinite. Conditions other than intrauterine pregnancy might mistakenly be diagnosed, such as a fibroid or hydatidiform mole.

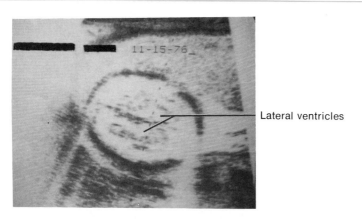

Fig. 28-9. Fetal skull with lateral ventricles and part of the falx.

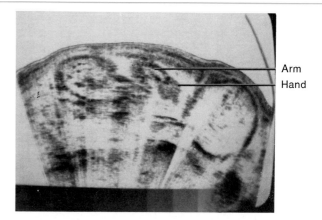

Fig. 28-10. Fetal hand, arm, and leg are distinguishable.

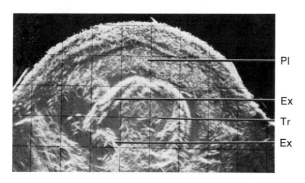

Fig. 28-11. Fetal shoulders, arms, and hands can be seen.

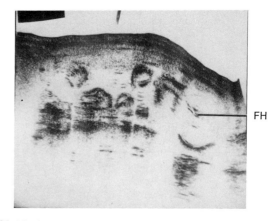

Fig. 28-12. Cross section showing fetal extremities and head.

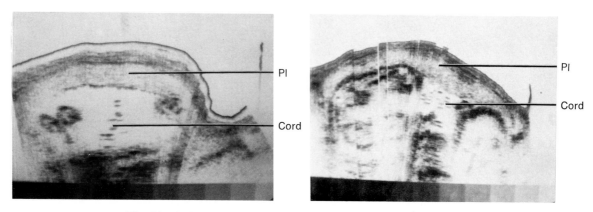

Fig. 28-13. Small horizontal lines represent the umbilical cord.

At eleven to twelve weeks the fetus has grown so much that the fetal head can be outlined separately. The placenta has a more speckled appearance with a well-defined line at the fetal surface—the chorionic plate. The placenta is mostly echo free at a low-gain setting, yet it becomes filled with fine echoes as the gain is increased.

The head outline is seen clearly with the midline echo. At this stage the skull is large enough to be measured. The trunk and limbs can be reliably distinguished. The fetal trunk and head size should have approximately the same diameter. (See Figs. 28-1 to 28-8.)

At twenty weeks the fetal spine becomes visible, and digits can be seen. Later the fetal aorta, kidneys, heart, bladder, and scrotum are visible. The best age for placental location is about thirty to thirty-two weeks. After this time the fetus is too large and partially covers the placenta. Ultrasonic accuracy of placental localization at this time is about 94% or 95% (Barnett and Morley, 1974). (See Figs. 28-9 to 28-27.)

Fetal breathing in utero can be detected using A-mode, B-scan, and real-time ultrasonic imaging. This is a potentially useful tool in the evaluation of the fetal condition, but at present it is not done routinely. Fetal chest wall movements are indicative of breathing in utero. Occasionally no fetal heartbeat or chest wall movements are observed, but with a good A-mode tracing they can often be picked up.

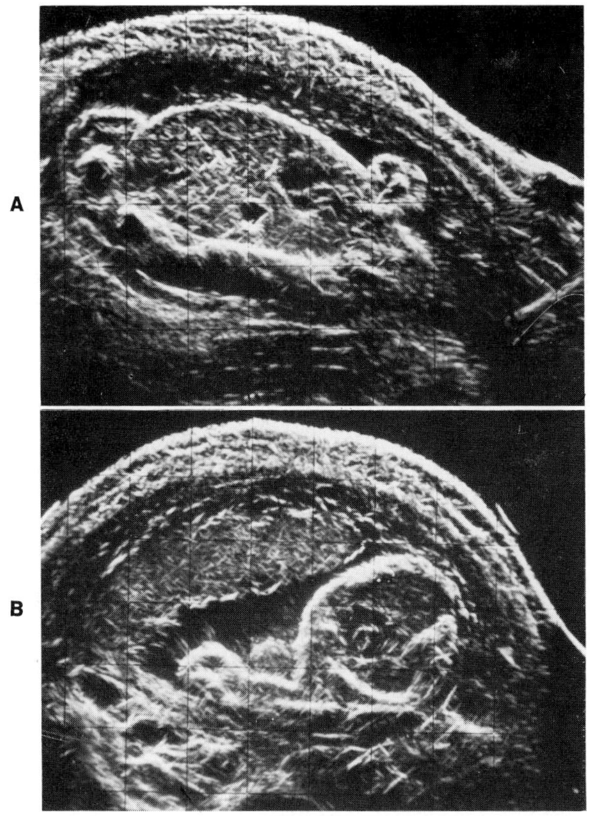

Fig. 28-14. A, Longitudinal section of a fetal trunk with a fetal heart. **B,** Transverse section of a fetal heart.

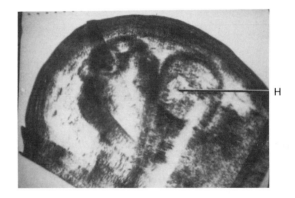

Fig. 28-15. Transverse sections of a fetal heart.

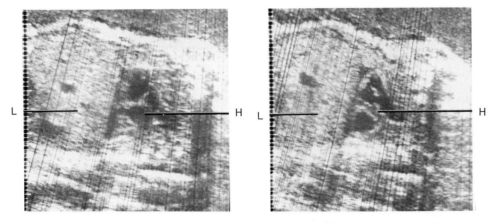

Fig. 28-16. Longitudinal sections of a fetal heart showing chambers and valve motion on various scans.

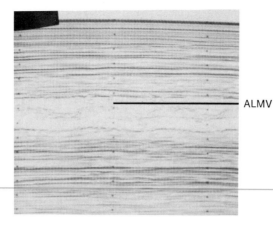

ALMV

Fig. 28-17. M-mode tracing can be done as the transducer is held over a fetal heart that has been localized by B-scan or real-time techniques.

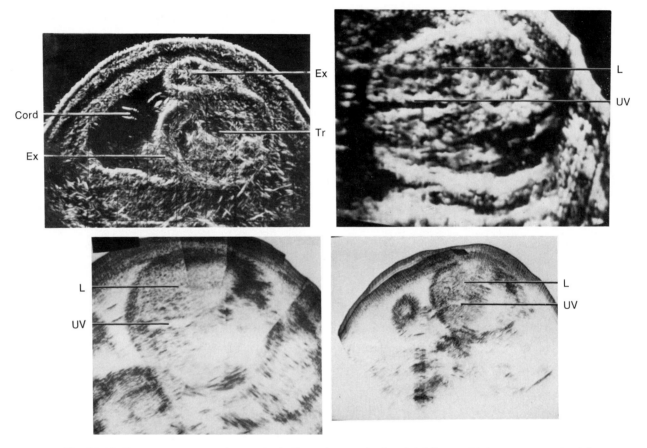

Fig. 28-18. Transverse scans demonstrate the echo-producing fetal liver, which covers much of the fetal trunk during development. The sonolucent tube shown in some scans represents the umbilical vein. It is at this section that accurate measurements can be made of the fetal thorax to compare with the fetal skull for growth determination.

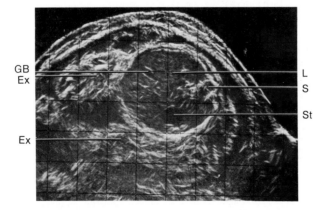

Fig. 28-19. Transverse scan of the fetal trunk to show liver, stomach (circular area), and fetal gallbladder (two horizontal lines within the fetal liver).

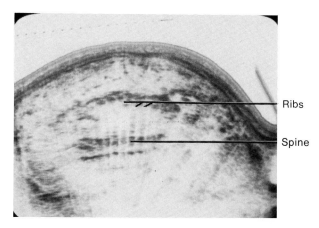

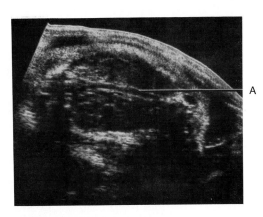

Fig. 28-20. Longitudinal scan demonstrates fetal ribs. As the transducer is passed along the fetal trunk, multiple echoes and shadows are produced by the fetal ribs.

Fig. 28-21. Two parallel lines represent the fetal aorta. Pulsations can be seen on a real-time scan.

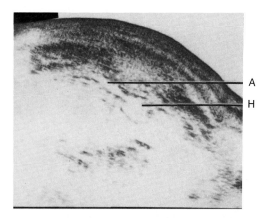

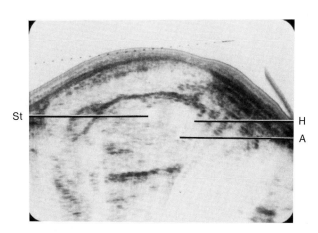

Fig. 28-22. Aorta can sometimes be seen to arise from the fetal heart.

Fig. 28-23. Irregular sonolucent structure within the fetal trunk is generally the stomach. The fetus swallows amniotic fluid, and this collects in the stomach.

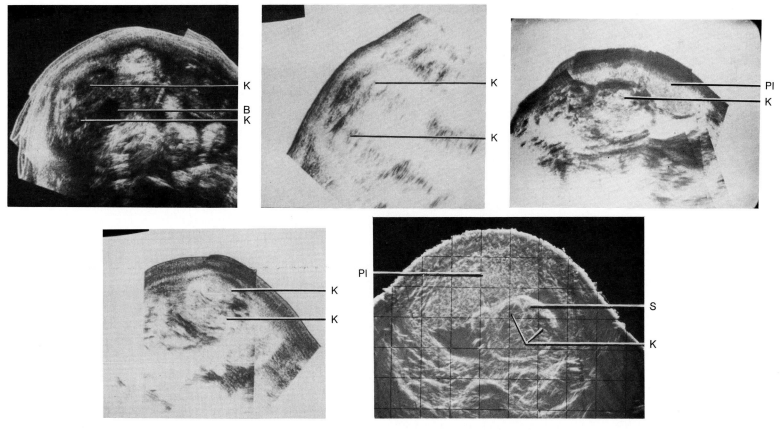

Fig. 28-24. Transverse scans best demonstrate the fetal kidneys along either side of the vertebral column. They should present as circular structures with small internal echoes representing the calyceal system.

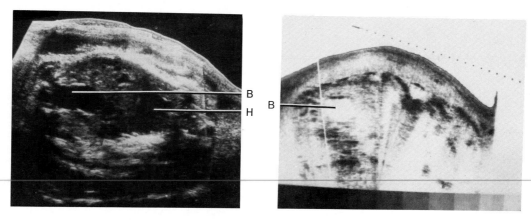

Fig. 28-25. Longitudinal views of the fetal bladder.

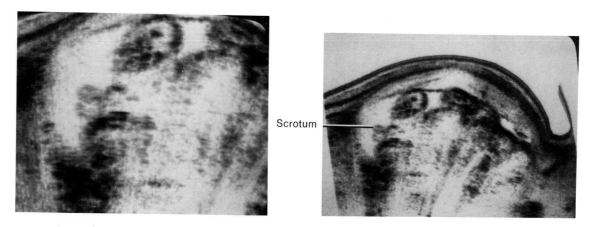

Fig. 28-26. It's a boy! If the fetus is lying in the correct position, the sex may be determined. The scrotum appears as a somewhat complex echo structure just adjacent to the area where the fetal bladder is shown. We have found it difficult to evaluate sex if the fetal bladder is not full.

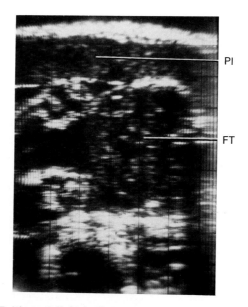

Fig. 28-27. It's a girl! Or is the transducer above the lower pelvic segment? Real-time equipment is probably the most efficient way to evaluate fetal sex.

FETAL DEATH DETERMINED WITH ULTRASOUND

In a determination of fetal death with B-scan ultrasound the degeneration of anatomic parts is the primary observation. The longer the interval following fetal death, the more pronounced the observations will be. The presentation of these results will depend on the length of time gestation had progressed.

In early pregnancy the gestational sac or fetal skull breaks up and is seen as strong scattered echoes within the uterus. After about eight weeks' gestation Doppler ultrasound is necessary to rule out fetal heartbeats.

In the later part of the second and third trimesters, deformities of the fetus are often indicative of demise. Approximately 24 to 48 hours after death there is development of a "fluffy" fetal contour and a double skull outline. The double outline is probably caused by edema of the scalp; it is not always a sign of death and may also be seen with distress, as in severely diabetic patients. Fetal movements can also create a double outline.

Another cause for suspicion of fetal death is a decrease in the biparietal diameter of about 4 mm. The midline echo becomes difficult to define within 12 hours of fetal death. The longer the interval following fetal death, the more frequent are scattered echoes within the skull. The fetal trunk should also be

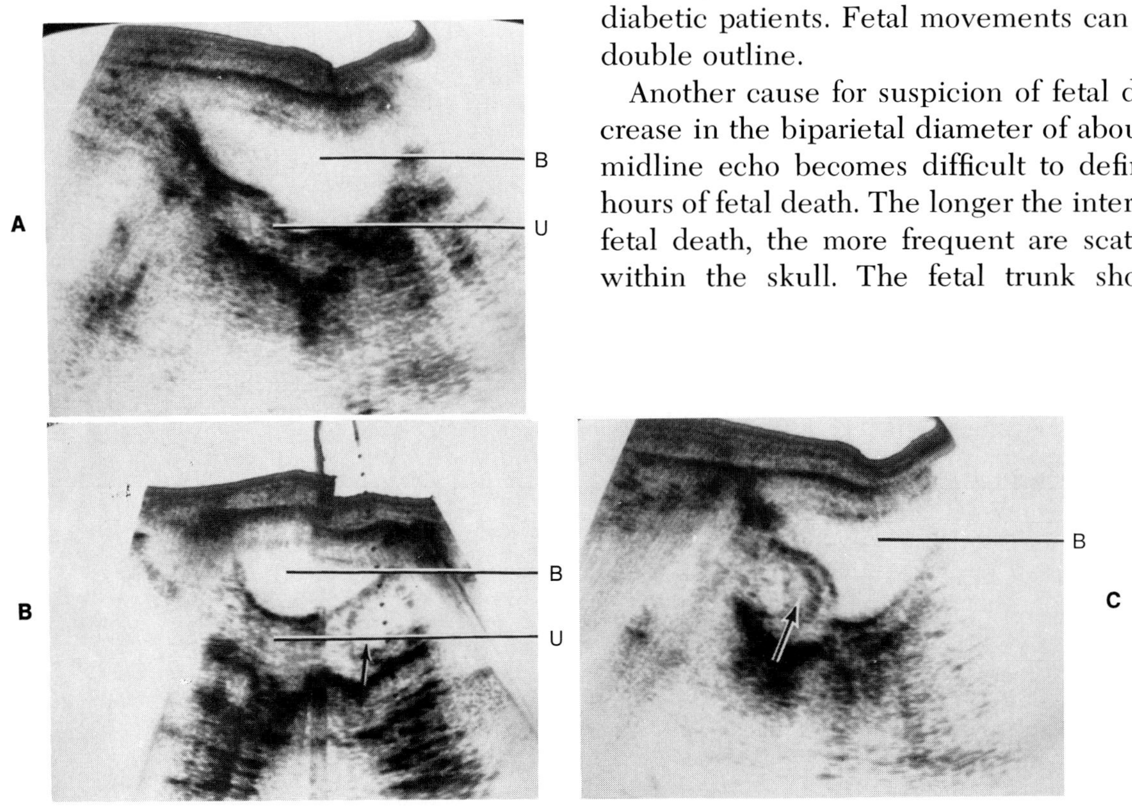

Fig. 28-28. A, Longitudinal view of the distended bladder and small uterus. **B,** Transverse scan of a uterus deviated to the right, with a tubal pregnancy shown to the left (a small gestational sac can be seen within the tube). **C,** Longitudinal scan over the tubal pregnancy.

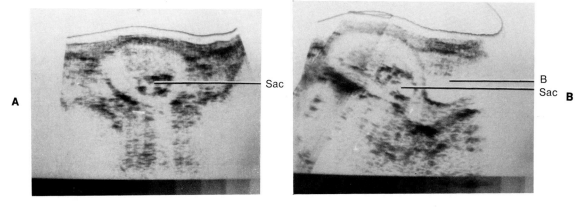

Fig. 28-29. Transverse **(A)** and longitudinal **(B)** scans of a uterus with a small-for-dates fetus. Poor fetal definition is shown with some stippling of placental tissue. A definite fetal skull should be shown with this uterine size (fourteen to fifteen weeks).

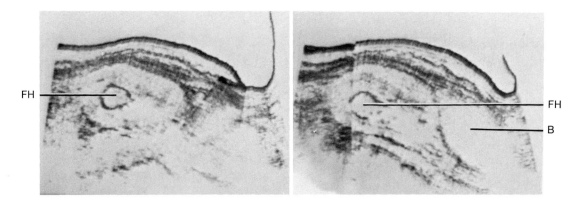

Fig. 28-30. Longitudinal scan of a second trimester pregnancy with a poorly defined fetal skull and no fetal motion shown on real time. These represent fetal demise.

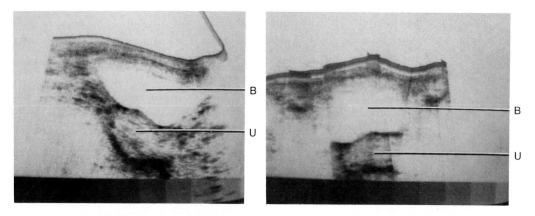

Fig. 28-31. Multiple scans of a pregnant uterus reveal that the fetus is small for dates. The uterus shows fine scattered echoes within. This most likely represents a missed abortion.

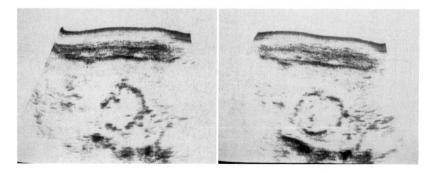

Fig. 28-32. Irregular, somewhat collapsed fetal skull may represent fetal demise or a very active fetus. In the latter case the fetus may move so much that it would be difficult to obtain a good biparietal diameter. Fetal heart motion would have to be evaluated to aid in the diagnosis.

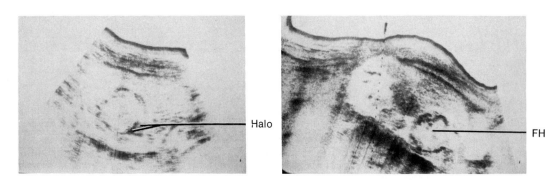

Fig. 28-33. Double outline sign *(halo)* may represent fetal motion, fetal diabetes, or fetal death. If fetal death, then no change would be made in the fetal skull throughout the study, whereas in fetal motion it would be difficult to repeat the same scan.

localized and considered with whatever fetal parts are depicted. Often the fetal spine on the transverse view is seen with a fuzzy outline. This is suspicious and is probably indicative of death. (See Figs. 28-28 to 28-33.)

The placenta should also be evaluated. An abnormally small placenta is noted in many cases of fetal demise. A thickened placenta with a change in echo pattern often occurs with anomalies such as diabetes mellitus or Rh incompatibility.

Ultrasound is an important method in determining whether an abortion has taken place and whether it is complete or incomplete. The lack of fetal structures is the criterion for fetal abortion. If the abortion is not complete, then scattered echoes are seen within the uterus. An infectious abortion causes an odd picture, which is similar to that of a mole and may be difficult to differentiate. The uterus tends to be rounded and filled with multiple diffuse echoes.

A blighted ovum leads to its death before the first trimester. About 12% of recognized pregnancies are defective, and the embryos die at this stage. Ultrasound shows a poorly defined gestational sac with fragmentation or a break in the sac outline. The maximum diameter of the intact gestational sac should be obtained at each diagnosis so the growth or shrinkage can be correctly diagnosed. The total absence of echoes is an indication of a true blighting.

ANOMALIES
Ectopic pregnancy

An ectopic pregnancy is defined as the implantation of the ovum anywhere outside the uterine cavity. Normally, there are considered to be four different categories—tubal (the most frequent), ovarian, abdominal or peritoneal, and cervical. Ectopic pregnancies develop about one out of every 270 to one in 400 pregnancies (Netter, 1974). They require immediate removal of the embryo and its attachments. Hemorrhaging is often uncontrollable, and maternal death rate is high.

Two kinds of factors that contribute to ectopic pregnancies are (1) those which cause a mechanical obstruction of the tube keeping the ovum from descending (some of these are adhesions, tumors, or angulation); (2) those which are functional (these are conditions of the ovum or tubal walls that cause an alteration in tubal contractions or early implantation of the ovum, and they are more difficult to pinpoint).

Early ectopic pregnancy is the same as a regular pregnancy in progression. The trophoblasts secrete the gonadotropin maintaining the corpus luteum. The estrogen and progesterone levels are maintained as in normal pregnancy, and the urine pregnancy test is positive. The symptoms of early ectopic pregnancy are bleeding accompanied by abdominal pain and a mass felt in an irregular area.

Tubal pregnancies rarely develop beyond the fourth or fifth month without discovery. Maternal mortality increases with the duration of the gestation. The tubal fetus usually has deformities of various kinds and seldom remains alive. The fetus is normally aborted through the tube into the peritoneal cavity. This occurs principally between the middle of the second and end of the third month or earlier. Degeneration of the ovum and blood clots then occur. In some cases the placental tissue ruptures the tubal wall. This causes extensive hemorrhage and acute shock to the mother. Occasionally, a tubal pregnancy is ended when the ovum dies in the tube and mummifies with dehydration. This missed tubal abortion is rare and often undetected.

Abdominal or peritoneal ectopic pregnancies are caused during a tubal abortion. Occasionally, the ovum will implant itself a second time somewhere in the peritoneum or broad ligament. Abdominal pregnancies curiously may continue to almost term before they are detected.

Ovarian ectopic pregnancies are the rarest of the group. They normally do not continue long and end with the death of the fetus and the degeneration of the fetal parts.

Interstitial pregnancies are also considered to be ectopic, even though they take place at the farthest end of the uterus next to the tubal opening. This area is called the interstitial segment of the uterus. These pregnancies continue longer without rupture than any other yet are most dangerous because of the massive hemorrhaging involved and possible death of the mother in a short period of time.

The appearance of an ectopic pregnancy ultrasonically depends on whether a rupture has occurred and what type it is. If an ectopic pregnancy is present, the uterus is normally bulky and a thick midcavity echo may be seen. An unruptured sac or tubal mole can be shown as a well-defined fluid mass beside the uterus. If there has been a rupture, then the hematocele can be seen as an extrauterine mass with poorly defined walls and a fluid appearance with small echoes within. Extrauterine pregnancies that are more advanced are harder to determine. The position of the fetus is usually abnormal, with the head and trunk extremely close together. The uterus and cervix should be separately identified.

Diabetes mellitus

Diabetes mellitus is a condition that occurs when the mother is a diabetic. With pregnancy the mother's tolerance for carbohydrates decreases, and more insulin is needed. This condition is more hazardous to the fetus than to the mother. There is a high rate of abortions, stillbirths, and neonatal deaths. Polyhydramnios is present in about 10% of these pregnancies. Toxemia due to ketosis and acidosis occurs in about 25% of these cases (Romney et al., 1975). Mortality is about 15% to 20%. The causes of death occur most frequently in the last month of pregnancy. These are usually placental insufficiency (although it is extremely large), cardiac arrest, respiratory distress syndrome, and congenital anomalies. One of these anomalies is macrosomia, an excessively large fetus of 10 pounds (4.5 kg) or more. The excessive birth weight is mainly from fetal obesity and organomegaly. This is caused by an overutilization of glucose in utero because of excessive amounts from the mother. The fetal pancreas hypertrophies and produces an excess of insulin; thus, if the infant does survive, it develops hypoglycemia after birth.

Ultrasonically diabetes mellitus shows the fetus and placenta as excessively large or thicker than normal. The fetal head is shown with a double contour, especially after thirty-four weeks.

Erythroblastosis fetalis

Erythroblastosis fetalis is an Rh disease in which the fetal blood is incompatible with the mother's blood. A fetus with Rh-positive blood is likely to develop hemolytic disease if carried by a mother with Rh-negative blood. If the mother is Rh positive and the fetus Rh negative, no problems should result. Usually, it is not the first child who is affected, since the mother's blood is given a chance to form antibodies to fight the Rh-positive blood of the next fetus. The fetal erythrocytes are destroyed by these antibodies. Three results of erythrocyte destruction are hemolytic anemia, icterus, and hydrops.

With fetal hydrops the fetus develops anemia and then edema of the subcutaneous tissues, ascites, and hepatomegaly and finally dies. This is the most severe of the three conditions. The fetus dies in utero and is often macerated, or soggy. Sometimes the infant is born with mild anemia and edema but dies within a few hours.

Icterus occurs when the red blood cells are destroyed, while delivering hemoglobin for transforma-

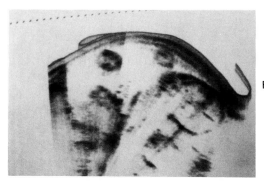
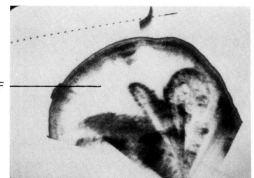

F

Fig. 28-34. Polyhydramnios may lead to another diagnosis in pregnancy. See text for explanation.

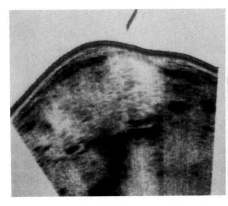
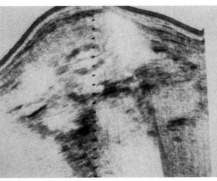
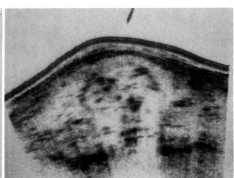

Fig. 28-35. In contrast, the loss of amniotic fluid, or oligohydramnios, may represent ruptured membranes or a congenital renal abnormality. Fetal viability should be evaluated or renal outlines determined to aid in the diagnosis.

tion into bilirubin, faster than they can be eliminated by the liver. Hepatomegaly occurs, and death is possible within a few days.

In hemolytic anemia the nucleated red cells completely outnumber the white cells. Blood vessels in the lungs are engorged with erythroblasts. The outcome depends on the severity of the condition.

Ultrasound defines erythroblastosis fetalis as a double outline of the fetal trunk and skull (a result of edema) occurs. The placenta is shown abnormally large, and later in the disease the fetal trunk shows ascites and hepatomegaly.

Polyhydramnios

Polyhydramnios is a condition of excessive amniotic fluid. By ultrasound the fetus and placenta appear much more sharply etched than normal. Often the placenta will appear compressed by the excessive fluid. The fetal limbs seem to be floating and separated. Minimal increases of fluid will not be detected by ultrasound and will not distress the fetus. (See Figs. 28-34 and 28-35.)

Anencephalic fetus

Anencephalic fetus is the failure of the fetus to develop a fetal head. The central nervous system stumps at the neck. Often this condition is accompanied by polyhydramnios.

Ultrasound facilitates the diagnosis of this condition with the failure to demonstrate a fetal head after the fourteenth week of gestation.

Syphilis

Syphilis is the most common cause of fetal death in the later months of gestation. The fetus is infected from the mother through the placenta. Most of these fetuses are born dead. If the fetus remains in utero after death, maceration occurs. Inflammatory and degenerative changes are present in the liver, lungs, spleen, kidneys, and pancreas. There is disturbed ossification in the fetal bones, which is most prominent. The placenta is enlarged, lobulated, and swollen with fluid, yet pale and bloodless.

Ultrasonically, this disease is shown with the normal degenerative process following death, along with an enlarged sonolucent placenta.

Small for gestational age

For the reduction of mortality, early diagnosis of the abnormally small fetus is important. Small-for-dates infants have over eight times the mortality of all other babies of similar gestational age. When fetal growth ceases, it cannot be determined how long the preg-

nancy can continue before fetal death occurs. When the growth rate is below normal in two successive weeks, this puts the fetus in the borderline category. Early diagnosis of such cases helps in the anticipation of early birth and delivery problems.

Some of the causes of a small-for-dates condition are fetal malnutrition, dysmaturity, intrauterine growth retardation, placental insufficiency syndrome, toxemia, multiple pregnancies, congenital infections, and congenital anomalies. There is an increase in the number of small-for-dates babies in the maternal age group over 38 years and in teenage pregnancies.

Amniocentesis is helpful in the diagnosis with tests such as creatinine concentrations, lecithin/sphingomyelin ratios, and the fetal fat cell test.

Ultrasound diagnoses the small-for-gestational age fetus through the measurement of the biparietal diameter obtained and compared with the chart of normal growth. Taking sources of error into consideration, it is normally accepted that three weeks off the normal growth rate is clinically abnormal (Barnett and Morley, 1974).

Large for gestational age

Large-for-dates babies are usually a more difficult group to define than are the small-for-dates. Their mortality is also higher because they develop more serious complications. Three general problems tend to arise: (1) a transposition of the aorta, which is a congenital cardiovascular oddity; (2) Beckwith's syndrome, the signs of which are large body weight and length, umbilical problems, renal enlargement, severe hypoglycemia, and microcephaly; and (3) maternal diabetes or diabetes mellitus, in which hypoglycemia usually occurs, along with the increased body and head size caused by edema.

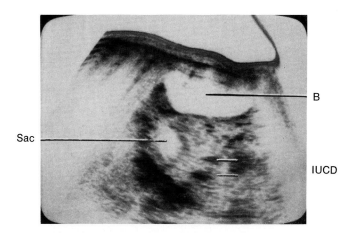

Fig. 28-36. Pregnancy can still result with an IUCD in place. The uterus should be evaluated to see if the IUD can be separated from the other echoes and to see if it has perforated and formed an abscess collection outside the uterus.

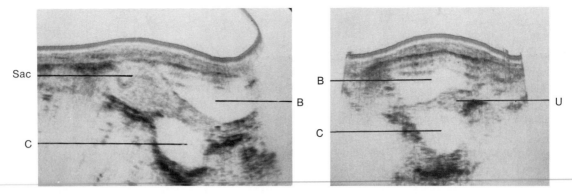

Sac

B

C

B

U

C

Fig. 28-37. Early pregnancy with a corpus luteum cyst in the cul-de-sac. This can cause pain in the lower pelvic segment; fullness in the uterine cavity would be palpated. The cyst generally disappears in early pregnancy, and it is abnormal for it to persist beyond twenty to twenty-four weeks.

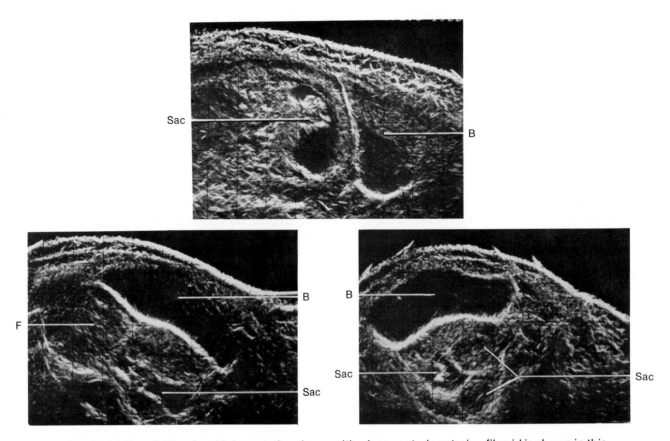

Sac

B

F

B

B

Sac

Sac

Sac

Fig. 28-38. Possibility of multiple gestational sacs with a large anterior uterine fibroid is shown in this scan of early gestation. Repeat scan in four weeks would define the possibility of multiple gestation.

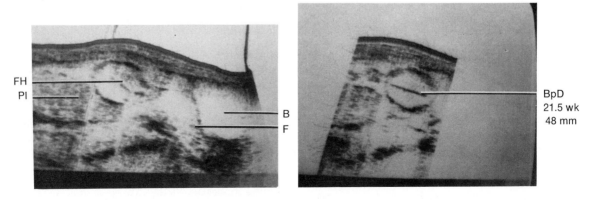

FH
Pl

B
F

BpD
21.5 wk
48 mm

Fig. 28-39. Large fibroid in the cul-de-sac of the lower uterine segment.

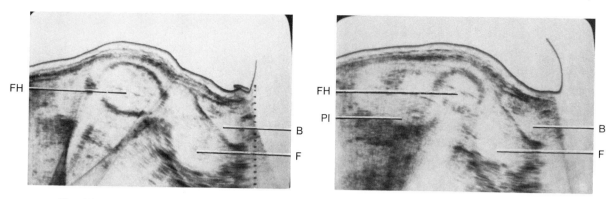

Fig. 28-40. Longitudinal scan of a second trimester pregnancy with a lower uterine fibroid.

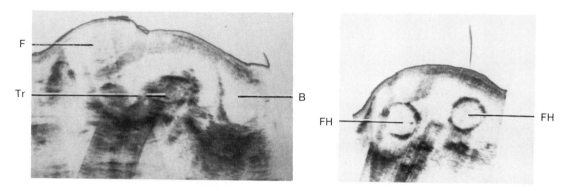

Fig. 28-41. Twin pregnancy with an anterior uterine mass, most likely a fibroid.

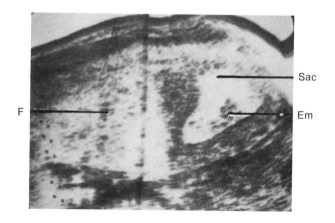

Fig. 28-42. Ten-week gestation with a fibroid to the right.

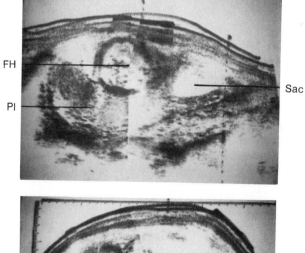

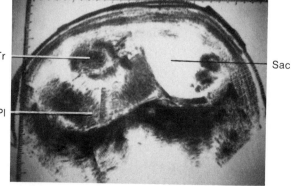

Ultrasound can easily determine if the baby is large for dates, but it cannot do much specifically to define the pathologic cause. There tend to be large placentas along with the large bodies and heads. Death is recognized with the body and head fuzziness along with increased echoes.

No one finding should be solely relied on for the diagnosis of fetal death. There are so many things to consider in the diagnosis that as much information as can be easily obtained should be reviewed. (See Figs. 28-36 to 28-43.)

Fig. 28-43. Bicornuate uterus with one horn empty and the other with a normal fetus and posterior placenta.

29 □ Fetal cephalometry

with assistance of
NANCY WRIGHT, B.S., R.D.M.S.

Modern prenatal care demands an accurate assessment of fetal maturity. Traditionally this was based on a prediction of the estimated date of confinement calculated by Nägele's rule from the first day of the last menstrual period. (Underhill, 1971). However, it is impossible to detect the estimated date of confinement of some patients using Nägele's rule for several reasons, the most obvious being that some women have no knowledge of the date of their last menstrual period. Clinical examination of the uterine fundus during pregnancy has also been shown to be an inaccurate method of estimating fetal maturity (Beazley and Underhill, 1970). This is based on the accepted fact that at certain times during gestation the fundus of the uterus will be at a known height above the symphysis pubis. Although this may act as a guideline, there is no consideration of conditions such as polyhydramnios, multiple pregnancy, or small-for-dates fetuses. The use of radiologic techniques is dependent on the recognition of ossification centers (Brown, 1975). Radiology is the most accurate of all these methods; however, repeated x-ray examinations involve a risk of irradiation to be avoided if possible. Therefore, until ultrasonic techniques became available, accurate measurement of the fetal head size in utero was not obtainable.

In 1961 Donald and Brown published an article on the use of ultrasound for measuring the size of the fetal head. Following their report several other authors used ultrasound for the determination of the biparietal diameter (BpD) in utero and recorded results within 3 mm of the actual postnatal caliper measurements (Goldberg et al., 1966).

The proved accuracy of the ultrasonic technique of cephalometry has served as a stimulus for other workers to adopt the procedure and use it as a replacement or supplement to diagnostic x-ray studies. At present the safety of ultrasonography has never been disproved. Extensive clinical use has failed to indicate any injurious effects or discomfort to the fetus or the mother.

The primary importance of knowledge of the size and shape of the fetal head to understand the mechanism of labor was recognized by Smellie in 1752. Cephalometry today has been used for two principal reasons: (1) to assess the growth and maturity of the fetus and (2) to assess disproportion (Willocks, Ian, et al., 1964).

The original method of performing fetal cephalometry, developed by Donald and associates, was the A-mode technique. (Donald and Brown, 1961). It called for obtaining equal spikes of approximately equal amplitude from each wall of the fetal skull as evidence that the biparietal diameter was being measured. The basis on which the measurement was made follows.

The fetal head in the horizontal plane view is ovoid with only two pairs of parallel surfaces—between the brow and the occipital lobe and between the two parietal lobes. The head is first located by palpation. Then the transducer is placed over the head and moved over the area of interest. A beam of ultrasound passing through the fetal head is partially reflected by the skull margins and by discontinuities in density within the brain. A given echo will return along the path of the ultrasonic beam to the originating probe only when its axis is at right angles to the reflecting surface. Opposing skull margins will therefore produce simultaneous echoes of maximum amplitude only when the beam axis lies along either the occipitofrontal or the biparietal diameter.

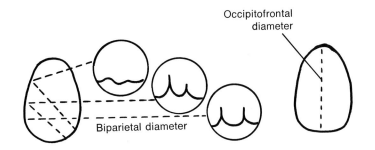

The fetal biparietal diameter is usually more or less at right angles to the anterior surface of the maternal abdomen. Therefore it is readily accessible to a searching ultrasonic beam generated by a transducer probe placed on the abdominal wall. The occipito-frontal diameter is less accessible because of its lateral position, and it is so much larger than the biparietal diameter that it is unlikely to be confused with it (Willocks, Ian, et al., 1964).

The biparietal diameter of the fetal head, as measured by the A-mode technique, is slightly smaller than the true diameter. The ultrasound records the distance between the anterior surface of the head and the anterior surface of the posterior parietal bone. For the true biparietal diameter of the head the thickness of the posterior parietal bone and the scalp should be added to that measurement (Pystynen, 1967).

When this uncorrected diameter is compared with the control measurement obtained postnatally by ultrasound from the fetal head, it is useful to remember that there are sources of error. First, the diameter recorded prenatally may not be identical with the corresponding postnatal diameter because of technical reasons involved in measurement. Second, the probable change in the shape of the head during delivery can effect a difference in measurements (Pystynen, 1967). If these two sources of error are kept in mind, the results may be considered satisfactory.

To simplify the A-mode technique and improve the accuracy, Campbell (1968) devised a system that involved both the A-scan instrument and a two-dimensional scanner. The patient is scanned longitudinally using a two-dimensional scanner, and the plane of the scan is adjusted until a sector scan showing the skull outline and the falx is obtained. The angle of the transducer is measured when the greatest diameter is being traversed. A transverse scan is taken at this angle and a search is made for a larger diameter, and the examiner tries at the same time to maintain a clear image of and be at right angles to the falx. When the largest diameter is located, the transducer is switched to the A-mode instrument so that an accurate measurement can be taken. This method, with its facility for the positive determination of the position of the skull, has greatly improved the accuracy and reliability of the technique (Hall et al., 1970).

More recently the performance of the equipment has been improved, and a considerable amount of previously unseen fetal detail has been visualized (Kossoff and Garrett, 1972).

B-scan techniques can be carried out for fetal head identification as early as the fourteenth week of gestation. This allows measurement of the fetal head and continued assessment of the rate of fetal growth during pregnancy. In early pregnancy the head usually can best be assessed in a longitudinal scan at the midline.

If the fetus is in a vertex presentation, a coronal section of the head is usually identified. It is then important to determine a transverse plane drawn at right angles to the midsagittal plane. This is called the angle of ascynclitism (Brown, 1974). By determining this variation from the vertical plane, the necessary rotation of the transducer for the transverse scan can be derived.

In early pregnancy a midline echo is noted to extend from the front to the back of the skull. This is related to either the interhemispheric sulcus or to the falx cerebri. In later pregnancy it is preferable to identify the transverse section of the skull showing the falx echo and then move the scanning plane toward the base of the skull until the central portion of the falx echo is lost. Either at that point or slightly below, when a midline echo complex is noted, will be a satisfactory point for measurement of a biparietal diameter.

Available information suggests that fetal biparietal diameter is an accurate index of fetal maturity, unless growth retardation or one of several other malfunctions occurs.

Campbell and Dewhurst (1971) performed a study on the diagnosis of small-for-dates fetuses by serial ultrasonic cephalometry. They assessed the prenatal fetal growth of 406 patients whose fetuses were considered to be at risk from placental failure. To facilitate comparisons with the growth rate catagories, the fetuses were placed in one of three weight categories for gestation groups, that is, above the 10th percentile (normal), between the 5th and 10th percentiles (borderline), and below the 5th percentile (small for dates). They found that when the growth rate of the fetal biparietal diameter was below the 5th percentile, 82% of the fetuses were below the 10th percentile of weight for gestation and 68% were below the 5th percentile. This study shows how instrumental serial ultrasonic cephalometry can be in the diagnosis of fetal maturity. If any of these patients had been scanned only once for fetal age, the chances are good that the results would have shown miscalculation by several weeks.

Ultrasonic fetal cephalometry is also helpful in cases of suspected disproportion and in malpresentations. Observation of the growth of the fetal head by repeated measurements has been found to be worthwhile in both normal and abnormal pregnancies.

Hibbard and associates (1967) performed several studies with fetal cephalometry in various clinical conditions, the first of which was toxemia. Severe toxemia usually requires termination of the pregnancy without regard to fetal survival. With lesser degrees of toxemia the length of pregnancy and fetal maturation are factors to be considered in deciding the optimum time for termination. Because toxemia is such an unpredictably dangerous complication, there is no justification for procrastination once fetal maturity has been established.

Another study (Hibbard et al., 1967) was performed on the use of ultrasonic fetal cephalometry in cases of third trimester hemorrhage caused by placenta previa, ruptured marginal sinus, and minor degrees of premature separation of a normally implanted placenta. Diagnostic ultrasound is valuable in selecting the optimum time of delivery.

A biparietal measurement was also obtained in a group of patients in whom an uncertain expected date of delivery was associated with premature rupture of membranes. All the infants with biparietal diameters greater than 8.8 cm were delivered spontaneously or by induced labor within 24 hours after admission, and all of them survived. If the biparietal diameter was 8.6 cm or less, the decision was to wait for the spontaneous onset of labor. It was believed that this delay contributed to the survival of two, and possibly three, of these infants (Hibbard et al., 1967).

Elective cesarean section is a convenience for both the patient and the physician, but it is justified only when there is certainty that the fetus has matured. Ultrasonic biparietal diameter measurement can give this additional assurance of maturity.

Lee and associates (1971) presented their results on a series of seventy-five patients who had elective repeat cesarean sections preceded by serial ultrasonography to determine the optimum time for operation. When the fetal biparietal diameter had reached 8.7 cm or more before the surgery, the incidence of prematurity was zero based on 2500 g birth weight. This study indicates that serial sonographic measurement of fetal biparietal diameters before all repeat cesarean sections is an effective way to decrease the rate of prematurity associated with the procedure.

As stated earlier, in addition to the assessment of fetal growth and maturity, ultrasonic cephalometry can be used to determine position and disproportion of the fetus. In breech presentation ultrasonic measurement has helped to evaluate the size of the head and to predict a successful vaginal delivery. Often the head measurement is too large for the vagina to accommodate it. Many complications can be avoided if this information is known prior to delivery.

Cephalopelvic relationships can also be evaluated to determine any disproportions of the fetus. Before the advent of ultrasound, routine radiographic evaluation for possible cephalopelvic disproportion had always included anteroposterior and lateral views of the pelvis using the interspinous diameter on the anteroposterior film. The results of the ultrasonic determination have been sufficiently impressive to discourage the lateral view in the absence of any gross pelvic deformity, thereby greatly reducing the exposure to x rays (Goldberg, 1966).

Hydrocephaly, anencephaly, and microcephaly have also been determined by ultrasonic fetal cephalometry. The technician must be careful in such cases not to simply obtain a biparietal diameter and disregard the remainder of the uterine contents. It is a good practice to scan the entire uterus in both dimensions and make a comparison of the fetal trunk in relation to the fetal head. If there is any discrepancy between the two, a follow-up study is advisable.

Several attempts have been made at correlating fetal weight with biparietal diameters. Ianniruberto and colleagues (1971) performed a study of a hundred normal pregnancies to estimate fetal biparietal diameter and thereby predict neonatal weight. Fetal weight estimates were determined with an absolute mean error of 368 g. This was found to be too great a variance for clinical use.

In another study, by Goldberg and co-workers (1966), the birth weights of approximately 300 newborn infants and their respective biparietal diameters, as obtained with calipers, were charted. It was apparent that fetal weight could be predicted from the biparietal diameters within an accuracy of about one-half pound in over 80% of cases. Serial determinations of the biparietal diameter serve as an index of progressive increase in weight and can thereby be used to determine the optimum time for intervention in patients scheduled for elective termination of pregnancy. Willocks and associates (1964) state what they consider a simple rule: If the ultrasonic measurement of the biparietal diameter is 8.5 cm or more, the baby is unlikely to weigh less than 4 pounds (1.8 kg); if the diameter is 9 cm more, the expected weight of the baby is 5 pounds (2.25 kg) or over.

Numerous graphs and charts have been compiled in an attempt to correlate the fetal biparietal diameter with the actual gestational age. Which chart is the most accurate depends on several factors. First, the area where the chart is being used may have a major influence on its accuracy. Individuals vary in size from one area of the world to another. Also, in some areas the gestational periods may be longer or shorter than in others. Thus one chart may be adequate for one region and off by several weeks somewhere else. It is the responsibility of the individual department to determine which chart is best suited for each patient. Ideally, "each institute must establish its own curve for reliable estimates" (Perkins, 1974). It would probably take a new laboratory at least two or three years to begin to evolve meaningful data. The greatest task is ensuring the reproducibility of the results. Lunt and co-workers (1974) found that measurements are most reproducible when the size of the head is between 59 and 83 mm, which corresponds to twenty-three to thirty-one weeks. It is also important to scan a

Table 29-1. Ultrasonic estimation of fetal weight and maturity

BpD (cm)	Grams	Pounds	Ounces	Weeks of gestation	BpD (cm)	Grams	Pounds	Ounces	Weeks of gestation
1.0	NA	NA		9	6.0	660.4	1	8	25.5
1.1	NA	NA		9	6.1	737.6	1	10	26.0
1.2	NA	NA		9.5	6.2	814.8	1	13	26.0
1.3	NA	NA		10.0	6.3	892.1	2		26.5
1.4	NA	NA		10.0	6.4	969.3	2	2	27.0
1.5	NA	NA		10.5	6.5	1046.5	2	5	27.0
1.6	NA	NA		11.0	6.6	1123.7	2	8	27.5
1.7	NA	NA		11.0	6.7	1200.9	2	10	28.0
1.8	NA	NA		11.5	6.8	1278.2	2	13	28.0
1.9	NA	NA		12.0	6.9	1355.4	3		28.5
2.0	NA	NA		12.0	7.0	1432.6	3	3	29.0
2.1	NA	NA		12.5	7.1	1509.8	3	5	29.0
2.2	NA	NA		13.0	7.2	1587.0	3	8	29.5
2.3	NA	NA		13.0	7.3	1664.3	3	11	29.5
2.4	NA	NA		13.5	7.4	1741.5	3	14	30.0
2.5	NA	NA		14.0	7.5	1818.7	4		30.5
2.6	NA	NA		14.0	7.6	1895.9	4	3	30.8
2.7	NA	NA		14.5	7.7	1973.1	4	5	31.0
2.8	NA	NA		15.0	7.8	2050.4	4	8	31.7
2.9	NA	NA		15.0	7.9	2127.6	4	11	32.0
3.0	NA	NA		15.5	8.0	2204.8	4	14	32.7
3.1	NA	NA		16.0	8.1	2282.0	5		33.0
3.2	NA	NA		16.0	8.2	2359.2	5	3	33.6
3.3	NA	NA		16.5	8.3	2436.5	5	6	34.0
3.4	NA	NA		17.0	8.4	2513.7	5	8	34.6
3.5	NA	NA		17.0	8.5	2590.9	5	11	35.0
3.6	NA	NA		17.5	8.6	2668.1	5	14	35.5
3.7	NA	NA		18.0	8.7	2745.3	6		36.0
3.8	NA	NA		18.0	8.8	2822.6	6	3	36.5
3.9	NA	NA		18.5	8.9	2899.8	6	6	37.0
4.0	NA	NA		19.0	9.0	2977.0	6	8	37.4
4.1	NA	NA		19.0	9.1	3054.2	6	11	38.0
4.2	NA	NA		19.5	9.2	3131.4	6	14	38.4
4.3	NA	NA		20.0	9.3	3208.7	7	2	39.0
4.4	NA	NA		20.0	9.4	3285.9	7	3	39.0
4.5	NA	NA		20.5	9.5	3363.1	7	6	39.8
4.6	NA	NA		21.0	9.6	3440.3	7	10	40.0
4.7	NA	NA		21.0	9.7	3517.5	7	11	40.8
4.8	NA	NA		21.5	9.8	3594.8	7	14	41.0
4.9	NA	NA		22.0	9.9	3672.0	8	2	41.7
5.0	NA	NA		22.0	10.0	3749.2	8	3	NA
5.1	NA	NA		22.5	10.1	3826.4	8	6	NA
5.2	42.6		2	23.0	10.2	3903.6	8	10	NA
5.3	119.9		5	23.0	10.3	3980.9	8	13	NA
5.4	197.1		6	23.5	10.4	4058.1	8	14	NA
5.5	274.3		10	24.0	10.5	4135.3	9	2	NA
5.6	351.5		13	24.0	10.6	4212.5	9	5	NA
5.7	428.7		14	24.5					
5.8	514.9	1	2	25.0					
5.9	583.2	1	5	25.0					

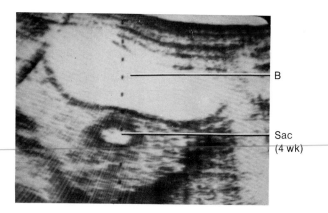

Fig. 29-1. Magnified transverse scan of a full bladder with the pregnant uterus posterior. The small gestational sac represents four weeks by measurements.

sufficient number of individuals to establish a curve. The examiner should be aware of possible hydrocephalic and microcephalic fetuses.

Dewhurst and Campbell (1971) have recently claimed that B-mode ultrasound scanning can provide about a 95% accuracy rate in predicting the estimated date of confinement through serial biparietal diameters if the patient is first scanned in the twenty- to thirty-week range.

The standard deviation begins to increase in the third trimester; therefore early scanning is essential to accuracy. Linear increases in the biparietal diameter are to be expected during this period, and in the absence of such an increase placental insufficiency may be presumed. A decrease of several millimeters during an interval of one week is a strong suggestion of fetal

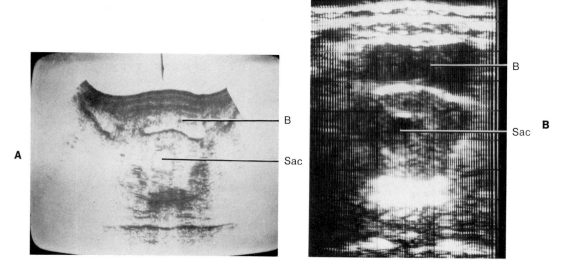

Fig. 29-2. Transverse scan of a four-to-five-week gestational sac as seen on grey scale **(A)** and real time **(B)**.

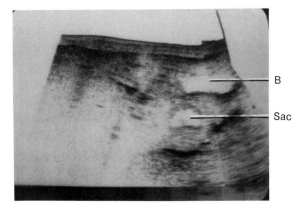

Fig. 29-3. Longitudinal scan of a semifull bladder with a five-week gestational sac within the uterus.

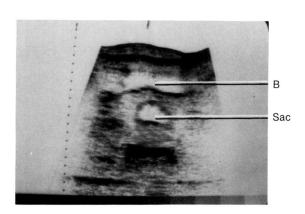

Fig. 29-4. Transverse scan of a five-week gestational sac within the uterus.

death (Goldberg et al., 1966). According to some authors, the biparietal diameter of the fetal head increases by an average of 1.6 mm (Willocks, 1964) to 1.8 mm (Thompson, 1965) weekly. Although measurements can lead to diagnostic error, in such cases ultrasound is an accurate means of determining growth rate in the late second and early third trimesters of pregnancy.

Table 29-1 presents data on ultrasonic estimation of fetal weight and maturity. Figs. 29-1 to 29-32 illustrate examples of the use of ultrasonic scans in determining this same information.

Text continued on p. 425.

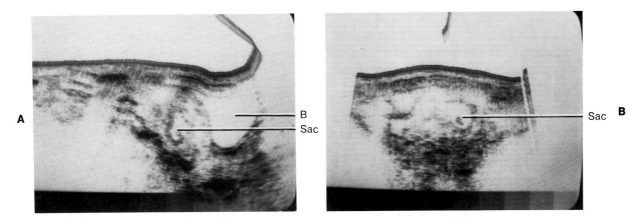

Fig. 29-5. A, Longitudinal scan of a six-week gestational sac. **B,** Transverse scan of a six-week gestational sac with an embryo within.

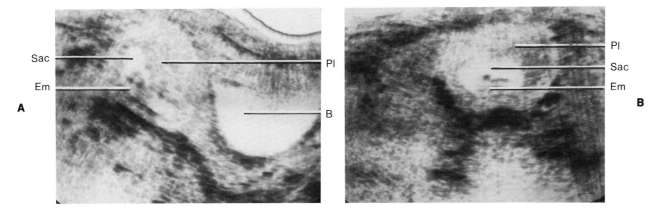

Fig. 29-6. A, Longitudinal scan of an eight-week gestational sac with fetal echoes representing the embryo. **B,** Transverse scan of embryo and sac.

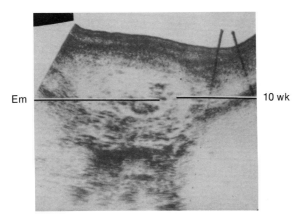

Fig. 29-7. Magnified view of an embryo within the gestational sac.

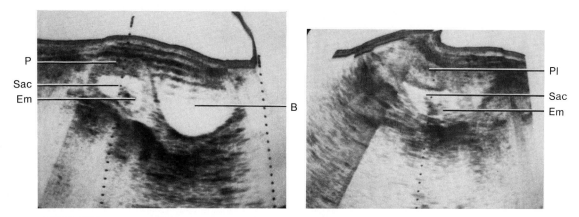

Fig. 29-8. Longitudinal scan of nine-to-ten-week gestational sac with embryo. The magnified view demonstrates part of the embryo within the uterus.

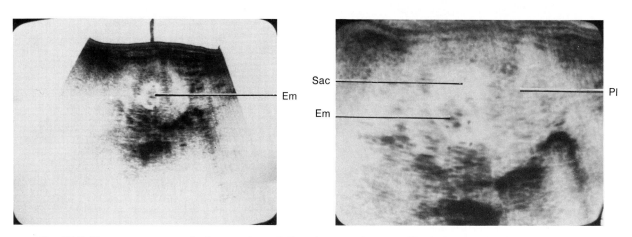

Fig. 29-9. Transverse scan of a ten-week gestational sac and a magnified view of the embryo within the sac. The increased echoes to the left represent placental tissue.

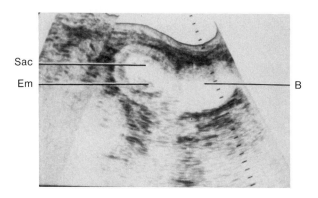

Fig. 29-10. At ten to eleven weeks the gestational sac nearly fills the entire uterine cavity.

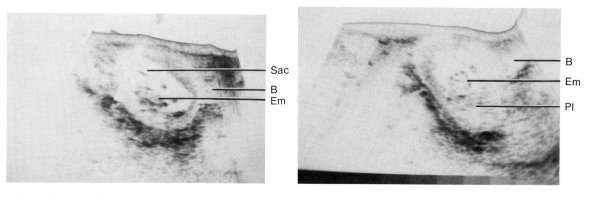

Fig. 29-11. Scattered echoes are seen within the eleven- to twelve-week gestational period as the sac breaks and fetal parts take more definite form. Organized echo formation in this period represents the site of the placental tissue.

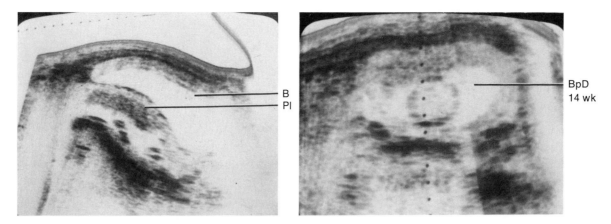

Fig. 29-12. Longitudinal scan of a fourteen-week gestation with an anterior placenta. The fetal skull correlates with fourteen weeks. The biparietal diameter can be very difficult to record in this early period of gestation because the fetus continually swims in the amniotic fluid.

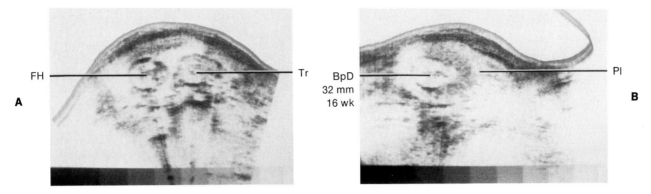

Fig. 29-13. A, Transverse lie of a sixteen-week gestation. **B,** Biparietal diameter of the fetal skull measures 32 mm.

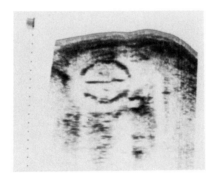

Fig. 29-14. Fetal skull of twenty and a half weeks' gestation.

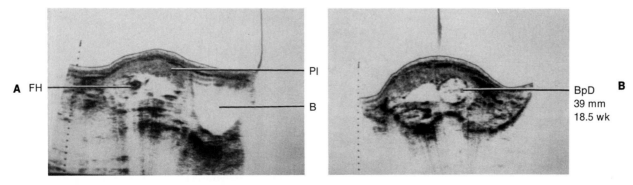

Fig. 29-15. A, Longitudinal scan of an eighteen and a half–week fetus in breech presentation. **B,** Small biparietal diameter measures 39 mm.

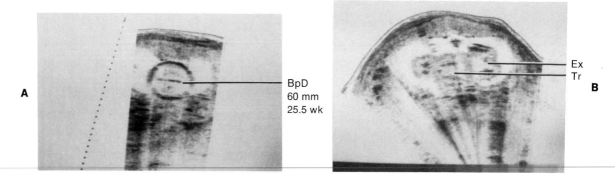

Fig. 29-16. A, Biparietal diameter measures 60 mm at twenty-five and a half weeks' gestation. **B,** Transverse scan of thorax and fetal extremities.

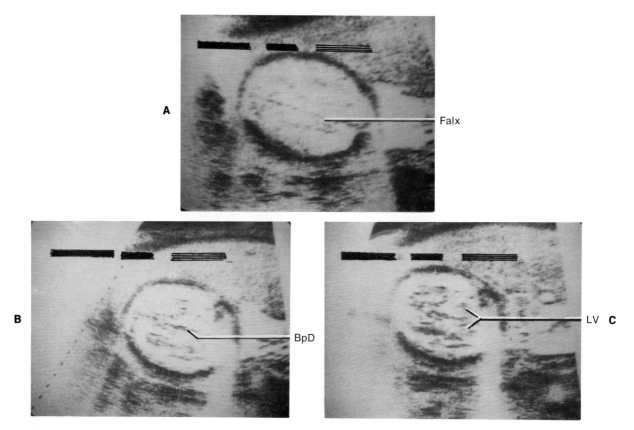

Fig. 29-17. A, Fetal skull with falx and pieces of lateral ventricles. **B,** Biparietal diameter at twenty-nine and a half weeks' gestation. **C,** Better visualization of the lateral ventricles is provided as the transducer is moved cephalad to the falx.

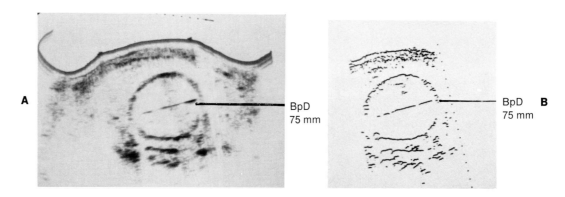

Fig. 29-18. A, Biparietal diameter at thirty weeks' gestation measuring 75 mm. **B,** Leading edge technique used with bistable equipment provides the same measurement as does grey-scale equipment.

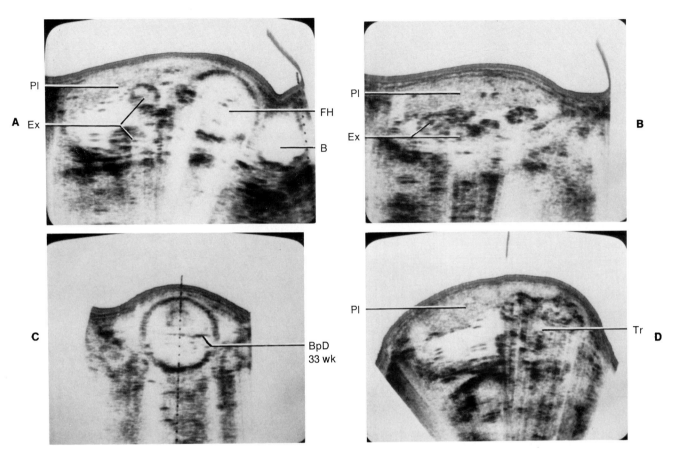

Fig. 29-19. A, Vertex fetus of thirty-one and a half weeks' gestation with an anterior placenta. **B,** Longitudinal scan of an anterior placenta and fetal extremities. **C,** Biparietal diameter at thirty-three weeks' gestation. **D,** Transverse section of the fetal trunk, cord, and placenta.

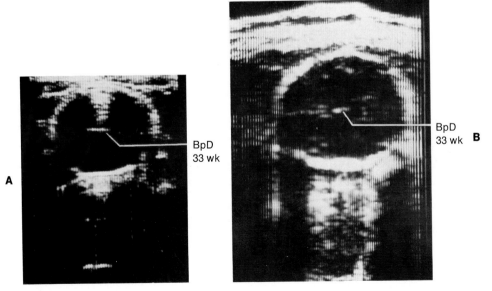

Fig. 29-20. A, Real-time scan at thirty-three weeks' gestation. **B,** Real-time scan with water bath at thirty-three weeks' gestation.

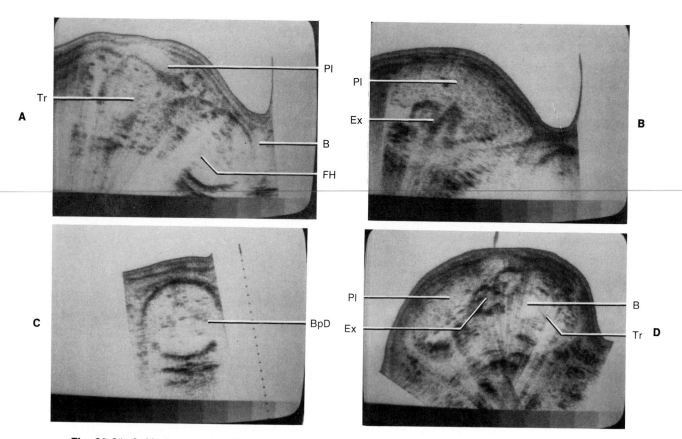

Fig. 29-21. A, Vertex presentation at thirty-six weeks' gestation. **B,** Longitudinal view of an anterior placenta and fetal extremities. **C,** Biparietal diameter of 88 mm. **D,** Transverse section of the fetal trunk with bladder.

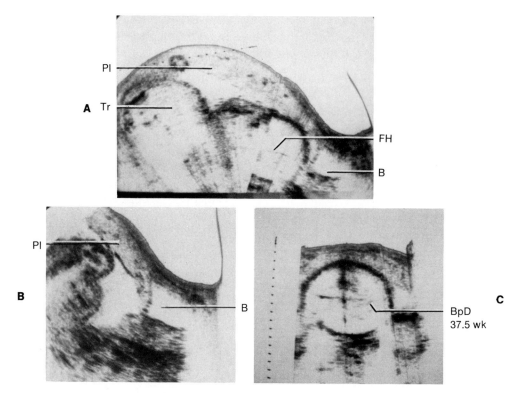

Fig. 29-22. A, Questionable low-lying placenta. **B,** Repeat scan after the fetus has moved from a vertex presentation demonstrates the placental edge extending to the lower uterine segment but not covering the cervical os. **C,** Biparietal diameter of thirty-seven and a half weeks' gestation.

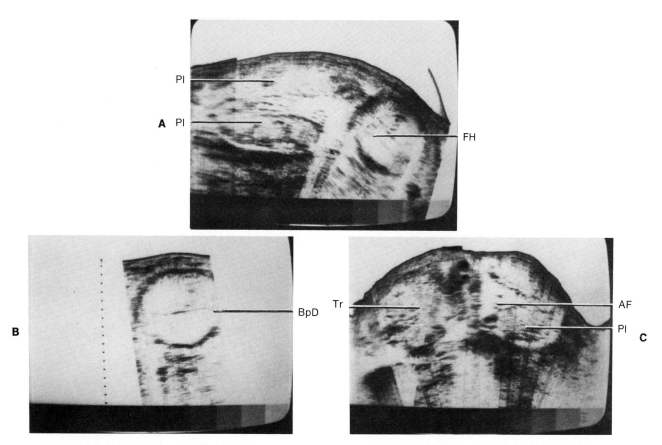

Fig. 29-23. A, Vertex presentation at thirty-nine weeks' gestation with anterior and posterior placentas. **B,** Biparietal diameter measures 94 mm. **C,** Transverse section of the fetal trunk, tangential placenta, and amniotic fluid.

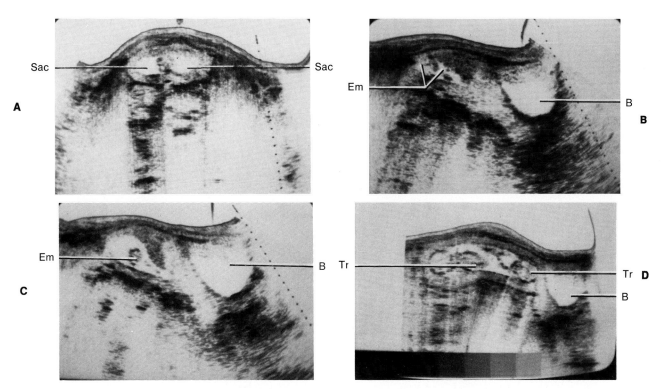

Fig. 29-24. A, Early five- to six-week gestation shows two distinctly separate sacs. **B,** Longitudinal scan over one of the gestational sacs. **C,** Longitudinal scan shows the embryo of one of the twins. **D,** Two distinct fetal bodies are shown with pieces of the fetal skull. Since twins are usually smaller than a single fetus, special charts must be utilized in computing gestational age. Care must be taken to record biparietal diameters from each skull, since one is usually smaller.

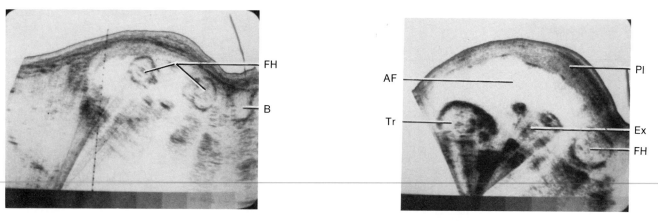

Fig. 29-25. Two distinct fetal skulls are shown on the same scan, indicating twin gestation.

Fig. 29-26. One fetal skull and a separate fetal trunk are shown in this uterus with massive polyhydramnios.

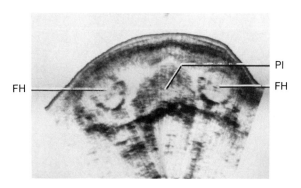

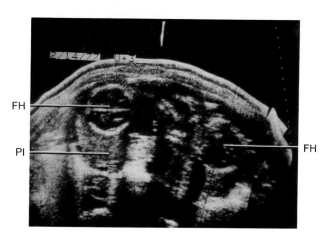

Fig. 29-27. Two distinct fetal heads are shown in this twenty-five–week gestation.

Fig. 29-28. Twins at twenty-six to twenty-seven weeks' gestation with a posterior placenta.

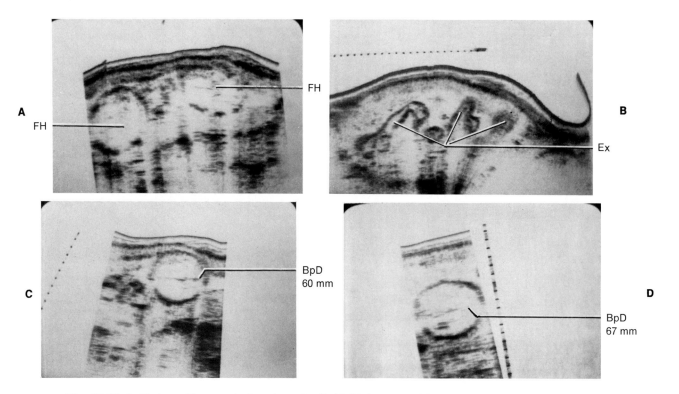

Fig. 29-29. **A,** Twins with a posterior placenta. **B,** Multiple extremities may also be a clue that more than one fetus is present. **C,** One biparietal diameter measures 60 mm. **D,** The other biparietal diameter measures 67 mm.

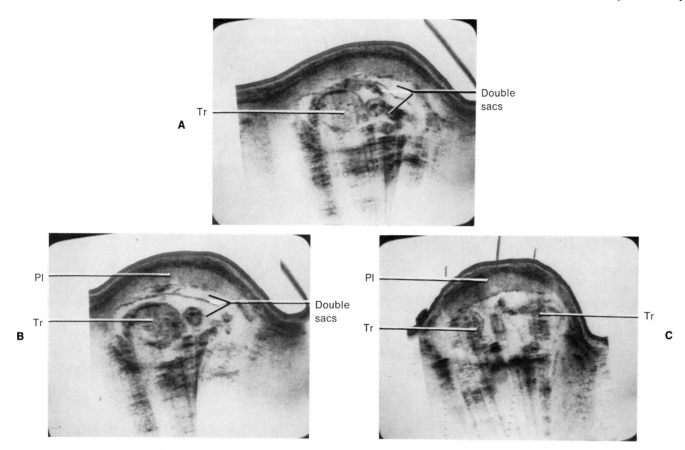

Fig. 29-30. **A,** Sometimes the actual echo reflection from the double sac may be seen on the sonogram. One fetal trunk is seen to the right of the sac. **B,** Double sac is shown posterior to the anterior placenta. **C,** Two fetal trunks shown on one transverse scan.

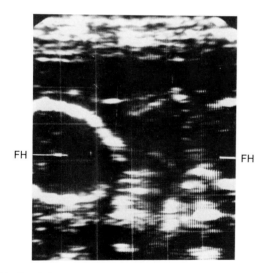

Fig. 29-31. Real-time demonstration of twins at thirty weeks' gestation.

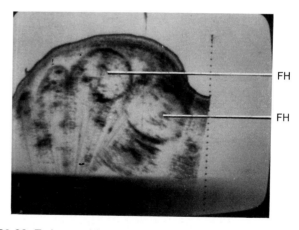

Fig. 29-32. Twins at thirty-two weeks' gestation with a posterior placenta.

Ultrasonic fetal cephalometry is a painless, safe, and reliable method of measuring the biparietal diameter of the fetal skull in utero. The technical aspects of the procedure are uncomplicated and can be learned quickly. The correlation between the ultrasonic biparietal diameter and the postpartum caliper measurement is excellent. There is also a high degree of correlation between the biparietal diameter and fetal weight. Fetal age, maturity, cephalopelvic relationships, and disproportion can all be adequately assessed using this method. Finally, ultrasonography can accurately locate the fetal head in the occasional situation when clinical examination is unsatisfactory, and it is rapidly becoming the procedure of choice in the field of obstetrics.

30 □ Placenta

with assistance of
MICHAEL LUTZ, R.T., *and* **JANET SCHEETS, R.T.**

Placental localization and analysis by diagnostic ultrasound may be the safest, easiest, and least painful way of examining this life-sustaining organ currently available.

The pregnant abdomen has proved particularly ideal for pulse-echo ultrasonic techniques because of its anatomic configuration; also, the pregnant uterus is filled with amniotic fluid, which provides good sonic transmission for outlining intrauterine structures.

Gottesfeld described placental localization by ultrasonic technique in 1966 and reported an accuracy of about 97%. Since that time, the accuracy has been maintained while additional applications for and information through ultrasound are being found to help obstetricians with their diagnosis.

The reasons for doing an ultrasonic examination of the placenta are varied. Localization of the placenta and its relationship to the fetus and cervical os are the most common, and ultrasound can detect any previa that may exist. Other instances include antepartum hemorrhage (dysfunctional bleeding from the uterus during pregnancy), unstable presentation of placenta or fetus, before selective cesarean section, and always as a guiding tool for amniocentesis (Kohorn, Walker, Morrison, and Campbell, 1969).

ANATOMY AND DEVELOPMENT

The placenta is a highly specialized organ through which the fetus makes its functional contact with the uterine wall. It has a fetal and a maternal portion.

The fetal surface consists of the villi of the chorion frondosum. The greatly branched and interwoven villi are suspended in the intervillous space and are bathed in maternal blood. The branches of the umbilical arteries enter the villi and ramify into capillary branches, which are drained by capillary branches of the umbilical vein.

The fetal blood currents pass through the blood vessels of the placental villi, and the maternal blood passes through the intervillous space. The two currents do not intermingle, being separated from each other by the delicate walls of the villi. Nevertheless,

the fetal blood is able to absorb oxygen and nutritional materials from the maternal blood through the walls of the villi and give up its waste products in the same manner.

The placenta is usually attached near the fundus of the uterus and more frequently on the posterior than on the anterior wall (about 60% of the time).

The maternal portion of the placenta is formed by the stratum spongiosum (a type of tissue) and placental deciduae (mucosal lining). It contains a placental septum and a basal plate, which is the boundary between the fetal and maternal portions of the placenta.

Following birth the placenta and membranes are expelled from the uterus as the afterbirth. The separation of the placenta from the uterine wall takes place through the stratum spongiosum and causes rupture of the uterine vessels. The vessels are tightly compressed and closed by the firm contraction of the uterine muscular fibers, and thus postpartum hemorrhage is controlled.

The expelled placenta is a discoid mass weighing about 450 g and has a diameter of 15 to 20 cm. Its average thickness is about 3 cm. Table 30-1 presents data concerning how the placenta, from the fifteenth week to term, increases in size, volume, surface area, and weight accordingly.

Table 30-1. Placental dimensions

Duration (weeks)	Diameter (cm²)	Volume (ml)	Surface (cm²)	Weight (g)
15 to 19	10	115	62	120
19 to 23	12	235	167	245
23 to 28	14	239	169	245
28 to 32	15	349	199	365
32 to 34	16	394	219	407
34 to 42	18	430	243	464

TYPES OF PLACENTAS

A listing of the possible kinds of placentas follows.

abruptio Premature separation of the placenta.
annular Placenta that extends like a belt around the interior of the uterus.
anterior Placenta attached to anterior portion of uterus.

bipartite Placenta divided into two separate parts.

circinate Cup-shaped placenta.

double Placental mass of the two placentas of a twin gestation.

fundal Placenta attached to the uterine wall within the fundal zone.

horseshoe Formation in which the two placentas of a twin gestation are united.

lateral Placenta attached to the lateral wall of the uterus.

membranous Thinning of the placenta from atrophy.

posterior Placenta attached to the posterior portion of the uterus.

previa Placenta implanted in the lower uterine segment. The three types are (1) central, in which the placenta implants in the lower uterine segment and grows to completely cover the internal cervical os; (2) lateral, in which the placenta lies just within the lower uterine segment; and (3) marginal, in which the placenta partially covers the internal cervical os.

reniformis Kidney-shaped placenta.

succenturiate Accessory placenta.

tripartita Three-lobed placenta.

triple Placental mass of the three placentas of a triple gestation.

ULTRASONIC LOCALIZATION

The need for precise placental localization concerns the evaluation of bleeding and/or the performance of atraumatic amniocentesis.

The placenta may be reliably identified from the thirteenth week through term. The chorionic plate, or fetal surface, of the placenta is seen as a sharply etched line paralleling the internal contour of the uterus. Between the plate and the wall of the uterus, multiple small speckles representing the placental villi are usually apparent. The precise margins of the placenta may be accurately determined and related to any desired external landmark. Although it is not an inviolate rule, anterior placentas tend to be chiefly right-sided,

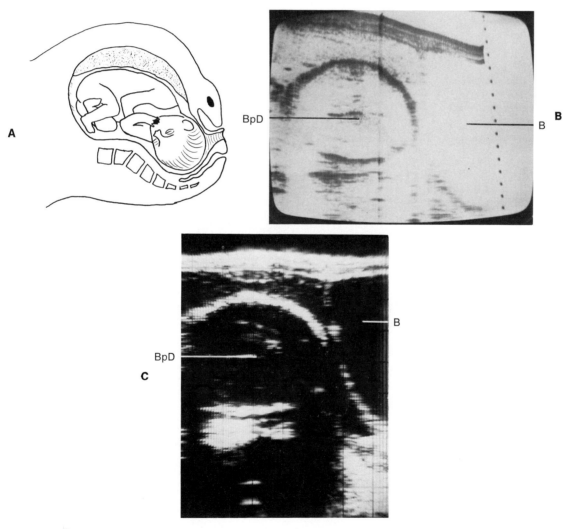

Fig. 30-1. A, Depiction of a full bladder to demonstrate the lower uterine segment. The fetal skull is shown flush against the bladder and next to the mother's sacrum. The anterior placenta is shown to extend just to the upper border of the bladder. **B,** Longitudinal scan of a vertex fetal head flush against the full bladder. **C,** Real-time scan of the same area.

whereas posterior placentas are more often left-sided. This phenomenon probably occurs because of uterine rotation as it rises out of the pelvis.

The new methodology of ultrasonography has demonstrated a striking feature of placentation. Many patients studied in the first trimester appear to have very low–lying placentas. In general, the internal cervical os is positioned halfway between the base of the distended bladder and the sacral promontory. When the placenta is adjacent to or covers the os, placenta previa is present. Surprisingly, the placenta of many of these patients, when restudied, occupies a much higher position and may actually end up in the fundus of the uterus at term. This phenomenon has been termed placental migration, but it is believed by most specialists to reflect a differential growth rate of the upper and lower uterine segments. We have therefore been reluctant to make the diagnosis of placenta previa before thirty weeks' gestation and have recommended repeat studies at that time in all patients who appear to have this finding in early pregnancy. Many observers believe that this particular circumstance may be re-sponsible for what otherwise is inexplicable first trimester bleeding.

It is sometimes possible to record the presence of abruptio placentae, which is the separation of a portion of the placenta due to hemorrhage. A minimal separation cannot usually be identified; however, moderate-to-massive hemorrhage is recorded as an outward bulging of the placenta with an echo-free zone located between the placenta and uterine wall.

Ultrasound is used in amniocentesis to localize the position of the fetal head and body as well as the placenta. Once this has been accomplished using a B-scan ultrasonic technique, the site for placement of the needle can be easily determined. Guidance of the amniocentesis needle into place can be successfully accomplished using this ultrasonic approach.

ULTRASONIC EVALUATION

The patient should have a full bladder prior to ultrasonic evaluation of the fetus and placental localization. This allows good visualization of the lower uterine segment and permits a distinct margin between the

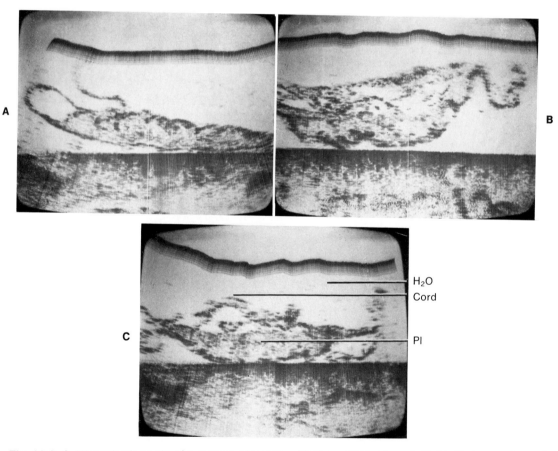

H₂O
Cord

Pl

Fig. 30-2. A, Water bath study of a mature placenta with the umbilical cord. **B,** Multiple sonolucent structures within the placenta are the signs of a mature placenta. These represent organized blood pools within the placenta. **C,** The umbilical cord can be seen to extend from the placenta as it weaves in and out of the water bath.

bladder, placenta (if lying low), and fetal structures (Fig. 30-1). Often a fetal extremity may be in the lower uterine segment, especially if the fetus is in a breech presentation. If the placenta is lying low, it may be difficult to separate the fetal limb from placental tissue, and the examiner will have to note movement in that area or manipulate the fetus in an attempt to define the lower uterine segment better. Real-time equipment allows visualization of this segment without difficulty, since the fetal parts can be seen to move throughout the procedure.

Longitudinal scans are made first, beginning at the midline and moving at 1 or 2 cm increments to cover the entire uterine cavity. Transverse scans are then performed at 2 cm increments from the symphysis pubis in a cephalad direction.

The placenta is seen as a finely mottled grey area through which run short white strands. It is also described as having a speckling effect that represents the substance of the placenta (Fig. 30-2). This speckling appears more sharply at high-sensitivity settings and gradually disappears as lower-sensitivity settings are used. During the scanning procedure an attempt should be made at outlining the cervix and adjacent uterine wall through the full urinary bladder, since this will demonstrate the distance of the lower edge of the placenta from the cervix and aid in determining placenta previa (Campbell and Kohorn, 1968). One of the most important structures to locate is the fetal surface of the placenta, also referred to as the chorionic plate.

Anterior placenta is easily identified by the presence of a clearly defined chorionic plate and multiple internal echoes. (See Figs. 30-3 to 30-13.) Fundal pla-

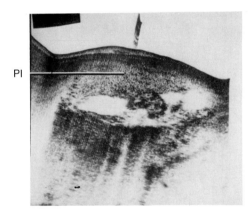

Fig. 30-3. Anterior placentas are the easiest to outline by ultrasound, since there is no attenuation by the fetal parts. The placenta should stipple in with fine echoes throughout with a dense linear formation along the fetal surface representing the chorionic plate.

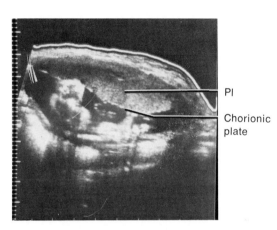

Fig. 30-4. Longitudinal scan of an anterior placenta stippled in with fine echoes. Chorionic plate is seen on the fetal side of the placenta.

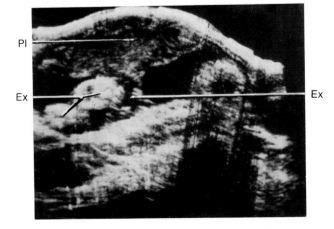

Fig. 30-5. Longitudinal scan of an anterior placenta. Circular echoes represent fetal parts.

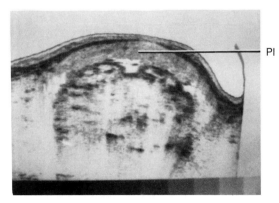

Fig. 30-6. Longitudinal scan of an anterior placenta with the fetal trunk and extremities shown posterior to its border.

centas may be seen in the anterior, fundal, and posterior positions as they wrap around the upper uterine segment (Figs. 30-14 to 30-16). Posterior placentas, whether previa or not, are more difficult to clearly identify because of the longer distance between the transducer and the placenta as well as attenuation caused by the fetal parts lying over the chorionic plate (Kobayashi, 1972). When a posterior placenta is suspected, a high-sensitivity setting should be used, even though it still may only be demonstrated by a few internal echoes and a chorionic plate seen only in certain portions, wherever fetal parts are not obscuring it. (See Figs. 30-17 to 30-31.)

When interpreting a placental sonogram, the examiner should always have a clear idea of the position and tilt of the transducer in relation to the placental size. The size and thickness of the placenta may vary with the scanning location and angle (Fig. 30-32). After having obtained recordings of all the desired areas, the sonographer should consider both longitudinal and transverse scans for a three-dimensional relationship (Kobayashi, 1972).

Text continued on p. 436.

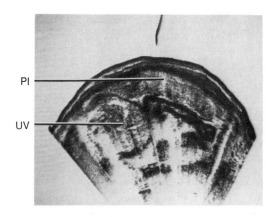

Fig. 30-7. Transverse scan of an anterior placenta. The fetal trunk and lower extremities are shown posterior to the placenta.

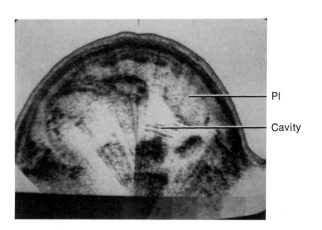

Fig. 30-8. Transverse scan of an anterior placenta shown more to the right of the uterine cavity.

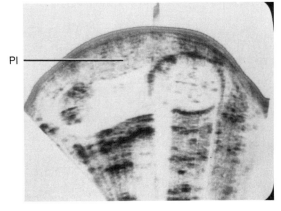

Fig. 30-9. Transverse scan of a placenta anterior to the fetal skull.

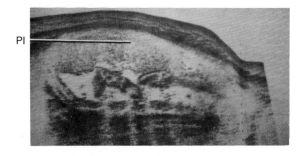

Fig. 30-10. Mature anterior placenta is shown on this longitudinal scan. Multiple sonolucent areas are seen within its borders.

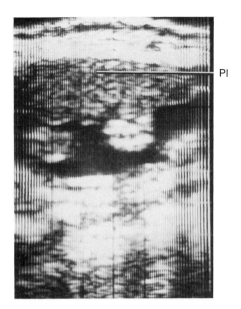

Fig. 30-11. Real-time evaluation of an anterior placenta is easily attained with good definition of placental borders.

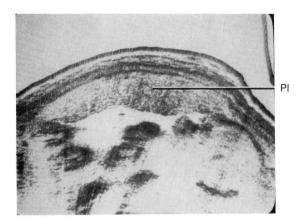

Fig. 30-12. Longitudinal view of an anterior placenta. The fetal skull and extremities are shown posterior.

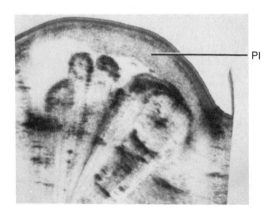

Fig. 30-13. Longitudinal anterior placenta with the fetal skull flush against the bladder wall. This rules out previa.

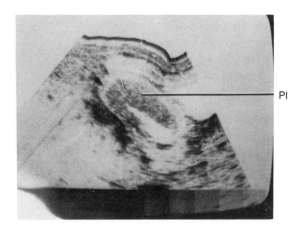

Fig. 30-14. Fundal placenta is easily shown as it stretches along the anterior wall of the uterus on the fundal edge to the posterior wall. Care must be taken to record the placenta in several areas to note its size and lateral extension. It can be mistaken for an enlarged placenta or a hydatidiform mole if not fully evaluated.

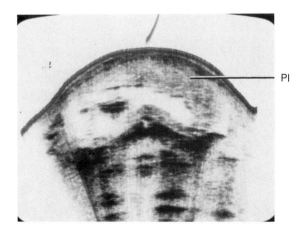

Fig. 30-15. Transverse scan shows fundal placenta to wrap around the anterior and posterior walls of the uterine cavity.

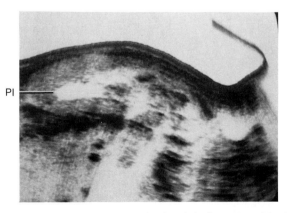

Fig. 30-16. Longitudinal scan of a fundal placenta with the fetal extremities shown in the lower uterine segments.

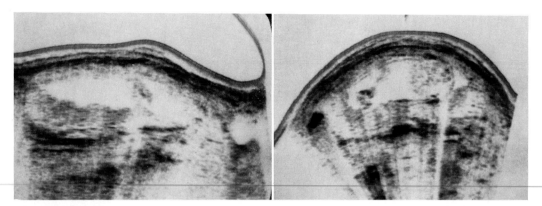

Fig. 30-17. Easiest way to identify the posterior placenta is to identify the fetal trunk. Since the normal placenta is approximately 3 cm thick, the fetal trunk will be closer to the wall on which the placenta is not attached. Therefore a posterior placenta may be more difficult to visualize initially, but the fetal trunk will be seen close to the anterior uterine wall. The placenta may be identified with the typical stippled pattern as the sensitivity is increased.

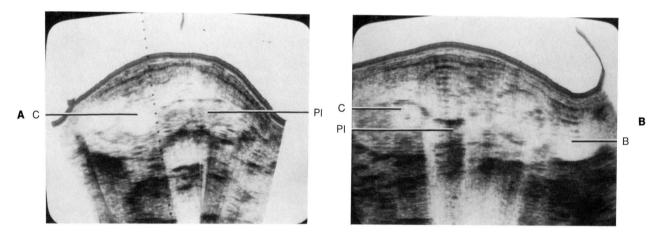

Fig. 30-18. A, Transverse scan of a posterior placenta shows a small cyst within its anterior border. The mature placenta is more likely to show this type of pattern. The "cyst" may be a homogeneous pocket of blood that has walled itself off from the placental tissue. **B,** Longitudinal scan of a posterior placenta with a small cyst.

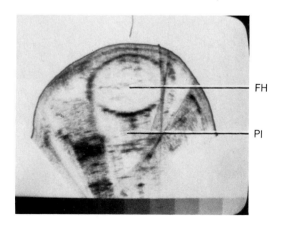

Fig. 30-19. Transverse scan of a fetal skull attenuating sound from posterior placental tissue.

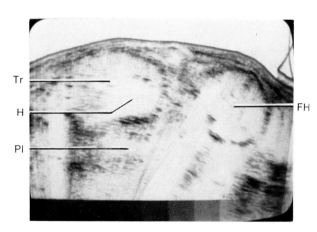

Fig. 30-20. Often it is difficult to stipple the posterior placenta because of attenuation from the fetal skull and trunk.

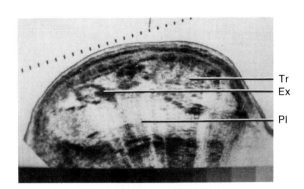

Fig. 30-21. Transverse scan of a posterior placenta. The fetal trunk is seen anterior to the placenta.

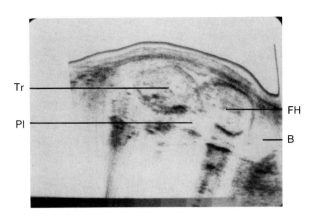

Fig. 30-22. Longitudinal scan of a posterior placenta. The fetal skull is separated from the posterior uterine wall. The placenta would be considered low-lying to marginal previa.

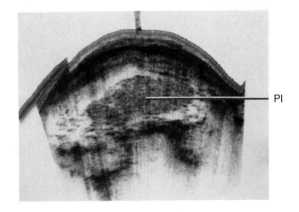

Fig. 30-23. Posterior placenta can be distinguished in this transverse scan.

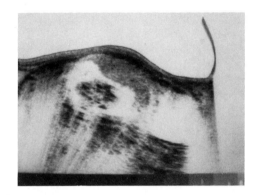

Fig. 30-24. Longitudinal scan of an early gestation with a low-lying placenta.

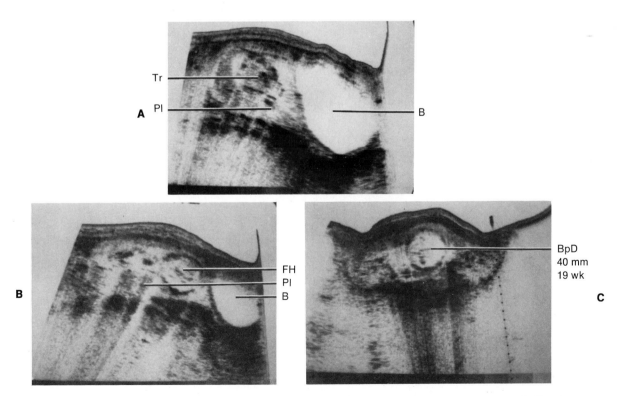

Fig. 30-25. A, Longitudinal scan at nineteen weeks' gestation with marginal placenta previa. **B,** Fetal skull is very close to the sacrum, which does not allow placental tissue to cover the cervical os. **C,** Transverse scan over the lower uterine segment shows the fetal skull with little placental tissue posterior.

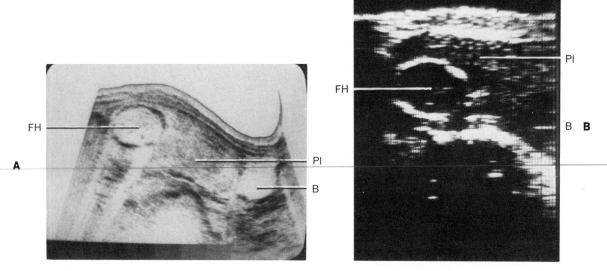

Fig. 30-26. A, Longitudinal scan of complete placenta previa with the fetus in the breech presentation. **B,** Real-time demonstration of placenta previa.

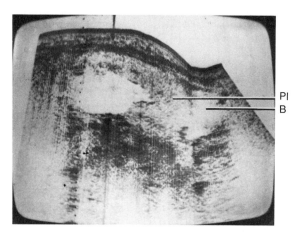

Fig. 30-27. Placenta previa is usually shown when the fetus presents in a breech position. If the fetal skull is in the vertex presentation and the placenta is posterior, there must be at least 1.5 cm distance between the fetal parts and the mother's spine for placental tissue to be seen.

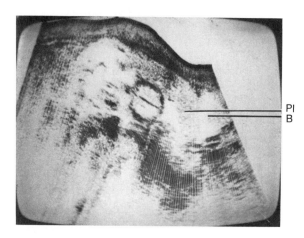

Fig. 30-28. Longitudinal scan of posterior placenta previa shown covering the entire lower uterine segment. The fetal skull is shown in the miduterine cavity. The maternal bladder is shown to the right of the scan.

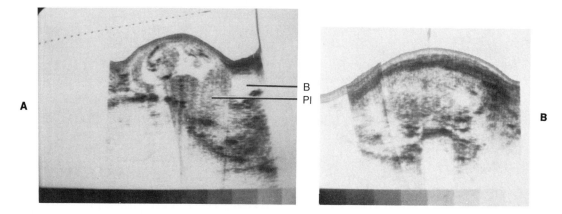

Fig. 30-29. Longitudinal **(A)** and transverse **(B)** scans of placenta previa. In the second trimester the placenta may migrate as the uterine cavity grows and thus may require follow-up scans to determine its position within the uterus.

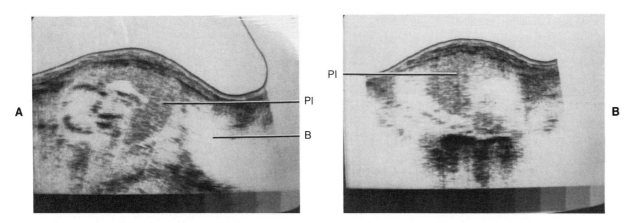

Fig. 30-30. A, Longitudinal scan of placenta previa with a distended bladder to the right of the scan. **B,** Transverse scan of placenta previa.

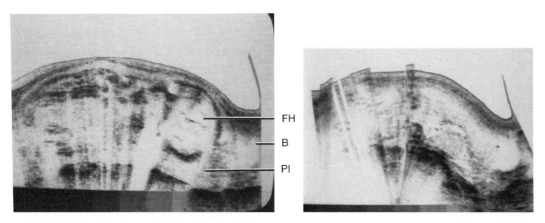

Fig. 30-31. Longitudinal scans of posterior placenta separating the fetal skull from the posterior uterine wall by more than 1.5 cm. The placenta extends to the cervical os.

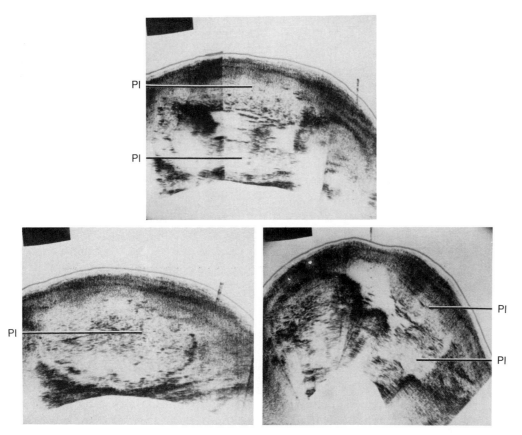

Fig. 30-32. Tangential placenta that appears to be abnormally thickened.

DIFFICULTIES IN LOCALIZATION
AND DIAGNOSIS

As with any new field in medical diagnosis, ultrasound has posed some problems or limitations in the diagnosis of uncommon pathologic conditions.

Underestimations, or false negatives, of previa, hydatidiform mole, and other abnormalities must be evaluated. False negatives regarding previa are more likely to occur with a posterior placental implantation than with an anterior one. Overestimations, or false positives, may be caused by inexperience or placental migration.

One of the most difficult combinations of all placental scanning is the posterior placenta with a large fetus without any amniotic space between the fetal head, the placenta, and the bladder. The placenta appears to be directly behind the head, but the chorionic plate seems to be obscured by the position of the fetus. Gain settings must be increased to penetrate through the fetus, which is why there are so many confusing anterior echoes in the uterus. Perhaps by manipulating the head (externally) a space containing amniotic fluid can be seen and the chorionic plate better defined.

Follow-up studies are always recommended for patients that have low-lying posterior placentas on their first ultrasound examination. These are done at three- or four-week intervals. It should be noted that what may seem to be previa or borderline previa at an early date may change in the weeks to follow. This migration, or change in position, of the placenta is the result of the elongation of the lower uterine segment that occurs as gestation progresses or because of episodes of placental bleeding (Gottesfeld, 1975).

Difficulties in the diagnosis of hydatidiform mole are few when the presenting symptoms are classic. However, a substantial number of cases fail to meet a textbook description, and special procedures become necessary. B-mode ultrasonography is foremost because of its diagnostic accuracy.

PATHOLOGIC CONDITIONS
Placenta previa

Previa is defined as a condition that results whenever the placenta covers all or part of the internal os of the cervix. It usually occurs when the placenta is implanted too low in the uterine segment. Whenever previa exists, normal delivery of the fetus is impossible. This abnormality of the placenta occurs at a ratio of 1:200 deliveries (Peery and Miller, 1972) and is more common in posterior placental implantations than in anterior ones.

In a study by Kobayashi (1973), he stated that with posterior placenta previa and the fetus in cephalic presentation, the degree of difficulty of locating the chorionic plate was easy, determining the presence of internal echoes within the placenta was moderately difficult, and the overall technical difficulties experienced were from easy to very difficult. With the fetus in breech presentation, locating the chorionic plate was easy, internal echoes (speckling) were easy to demonstrate, and the overall degree of technical difficulties was negligible. Finally, in a transverse presentation of the fetus, identifying the chorionic plate was easy, producing the speckling effect was easy, and overall technical difficulties were minimal. In general, the technical difficulty in demonstrating placenta previa is inversely related to its severity. Thus the total placenta previa is the easiest to identify.

Degrees of placenta previa are categorized according to how much of the internal os is covered by the placenta:

1. Total placenta previa. The internal os is totally covered.
2. Partial placenta previa. The internal os is only partially covered and could possibly change position, if diagnosed early in pregnancy.
3. Low-lying placenta (marginal). The region of the internal os is encroached on by the placenta, and the placental edge can be palpated by examining through the cervix; the placenta does not extend beyond the margin of the os.

Little is known about the causes of previa, but advancing age and multiparity are most likely contributory. One other factor may be the lack of adequate blood supply to the placenta. This condition can cause the placenta to spread out over a larger area to compensate for the lack of blood, and as a result its lower portion may approach the area of the internal os, thus causing previa.

Abruptio placentae

Abruptio placentae is the term given to a condition in which the normally located placenta undergoes a separation from its uterine attachment. This usually occurs between the twentieth week of pregnancy and birth (Hellman and Pritchard, 1972). Other names given to this condition are premature separation of the normally implanted placenta, ablatio placentae, and accidental hemorrhage. Detachment of the placenta before the twentieth week is a frequent cause of abortion. The reason for regarding placental separations early and late in pregnancy as different problems is that the clinical and pathologic features of the accidents at these two times are quite different. The earlier in pregnancy abruptio placentae occurs, the more it may resemble abortion and frequently be treated as such. This accident in the middle trimester, however, may have serious consequences.

The bleeding brought on by placental separation usually escapes through the cervix and appears externally. Less often the blood does not escape and is retained between the detached placenta and the uterus, leading to concealed hemorrhage. Abruptio placentae with concealed hemorrhage may be more serious than placental abruption with external hemorrhage, and it carries with it much greater maternal hazards, probably because the extent of the hemorrhage is not appreciated. With external hemorrhage, detachment of the placenta is generally incomplete, whereas with concealed hemorrhage it is usually more extensive. Concealed hemorrhage, furthermore, is associated with hypertension in a substantial proportion of cases. This association is less common in cases with external bleeding. In about 80% of cases of abruptio placentae the bleeding is predominantly external, but in about 20% it is concealed.

All degrees of premature separation of the placenta may occur, from an area only a few millimeters in diameter to the entire placenta, with intermediate signs and symptoms. As a consequence abruptio placentae is not a sharply defined condition. The placenta separating at its margin may disrupt the marginal sinus. It should be noted that of all cases of antepartum hemorrhage in the latter half of pregnancy, about half can be ascribed positively to placenta previa and abruptio placentae (Kobayashi, 1973). The frequency of occurrence of abruptio placentae ranges between 1:55 to 1:150 (Kobayashi, 1972; Hellman and Pritchard, 1972).

Abruptio placentae is diagnosed by the following ultrasonic findings:

1. Presence of an echo-free space behind the placenta (this represents retroplacental hematoma)
2. Thick appearance of placenta (longitudinal and transverse scans should be combined to interpret the thickness of the placenta)
3. Bulging chorionic plate (it may appear to bulge into the amniotic cavity)

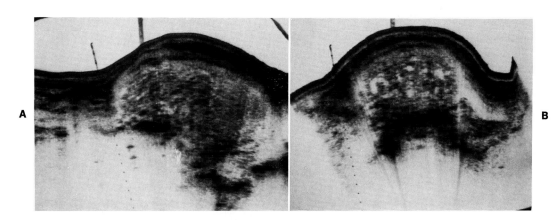

Fig. 30-33. A, Hydatidiform mole is shown throughout the uterus as placental tissue grown wild. It should completely fill the uterine cavity with fine stippled echoes. **B,** In some cases sonolucent areas represent an organized blood clot or hematoma formation within the mole. An additional finding would be the lutein cysts in either or both ovaries, which would appear as multicystic structures.

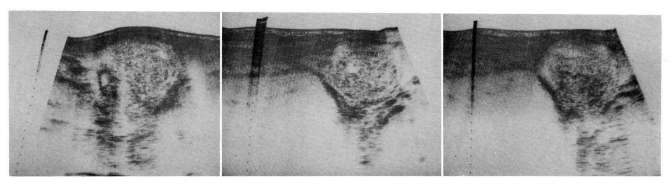

Fig. 30-34. Multiple scans of the uterine cavity reveal placenta-like tissue throughout the hydatidiform mole.

Hydatidiform mole

Hydatidiform mole is a developmental anomaly of the placenta that is often regarded as a benign neoplasm. Some or all of the chorionic villi are converted into a mass of clear vesicles. Usually, no embryo is present, although in occasional cases a mole arises in part of the placenta in association with a normal fetus. The vesicles vary in size from less than a millimeter to more than a centimeter in diameter and hang in grapelike clusters from thin pedicles. The mass may grow large enough to fill the uterus to the size occupied by a six or seven months' normal pregnancy. In rare instances a small fetus may be present in addition to the mole. This condition is called partial hydatidiform mole, but the life of the fetus may be sustained only a short time (Hellman and Pritchard, 1972) (Figs. 30-33 and 30-34).

In early stages of development of the mole there are no characteristics distinguishing it from normal pregnancy. The only clue may be the rapidity of growth of the abdomen and the supposed gestational age of the fetus. This rapid growth can cause pain and some bleeding. Uterine bleeding is probably the most outstanding sign and may vary from spotting to profuse hemorrhage. Hydatidiform mole is often diagnosed by expulsion of the specimen, but since the initiation of ultrasound, its diagnosis can be made before that point. Hydatidiform mole may also be the forerunner of choriocarcinoma. The frequency is 1:2000 in the United States and Europe but is much more frequent in parts of Asia and the South Pacific (Hellman and Pritchard, 1972).

Hydramnios

Hydramnios, sometimes called polyhydramnios, is an excessive amount of amniotic fluid. The normal volume of amniotic fluid near term is about 1000 ml. In general, more than 2000 ml may be considered excessive.

Little is known about the reasons for hydramnios, but it is assumed to be more frequent in cases of anencephaly. In normal cases the fetus swallows amniotic fluid, but when atresia of the esophagus is present in the fetus and swallowing is inhibited, an excessive amount of fluid collects. Again, this is only a theory. But it has been indicated that fetal swallowing is by no means the only mechanism for preventing hydramnios and should not be considered so.

The weight of the placenta tends to be high in hydramnios as does the rate of premature birth. Some other symptoms include dyspnea, edema of the lower extremities, vulva, and the abdominal wall, and generalized pain in the uterus as a result of overstretching of the myometrium. The effect on maternal breathing is a result of pressure exerted by the overdistended uterus on adjacent organs. When accumulation of fluid takes place gradually, the patient may tolerate excessive abdominal distention with relatively little discomfort. In acute hydramnios, however, the distention may lead to disturbances sufficiently serious to threaten the life of the patient. Acute hydramnios tends to occur earlier in pregnancy than does the chronic form, often as early as the fourth or fifth month, and it rapidly expands the uterus to enormous size. The dyspnea experienced by the patient may be so severe that she is unable to breathe while lying flat.

Hydramnios can be diagnosed by ultrasound through identification of a disproportionately large amniotic cavity (appears as a black area on the sonogram) in relation to the size of the fetus or fetal volume. When hydramnios is diagnosed, the examiner should look further for any evidence of gross malformations of the fetal head, comparing the size of the head with the fetal body (Hellman and Pritchard, 1972).

The incidence of hydramnios of a minor degree is common, but more marked grades are not frequent.

PART FIVE OTHER CLINICAL APPLICATIONS

31 □ Thyroid gland

THOMAS SZEWEZYK, R.T., R.N.M.

ANATOMY

During embryonic development the thyroid gland is derived from the ventral wall of the primitive pharynx. This median outgrowth migrates downward, and at its lower end it bifurcates to form the isthmus and lateral lobes of the thyroid. In some cases the thyroid gland does not progress down into the neck but remains at the base of the tongue. Thyroid tissue may continue down into the mediastinum and thus become substernal. However, the thyroid is usually found between the thyroid cartilage and the suprasternal notch. The isthmus is astride the trachea with one lobe on either side. In many cases there is a slight extension of the thyroid tissue from the lobes, from the isthmus, or from both. This is normal thyroid tissue that lines the tract the thyroid follows down into the neck. It is called the pyramidal lobe.

Thyroid tissue is composed of cuboidal epithelial (acinar) cells arranged in single layers around spherical spaces called follicles. In these follicles colloid is found. In the human fetus the thyroid becomes functional during the third month of gestation.

Normally, control of thyroid activity is exerted by the thyroid thyrotropic hormone (TSH), which is secreted by the anterior pituitary gland. The normal weight of the human thyroid is from 20 to 35 g, and the normal adult thyroid gland is barely palpable, if at all. The thyroid's primary function is to synthesize, store, and secrete the thyroid hormones.

The arterial blood supply of the thyroid is derived from each common carotid artery lying directly behind the lateral half of the respective lobes of the thyroid. The gland receives the principal part of its blood supply superiorly from the external carotid artery and inferiorly from the subclavian artery and arch of the aorta. For each gram of tissue the blood flow to the thyroid well exceeds that of the kidneys. Venous drainage is through the facial and internal jugular veins superiorly and the innominate veins inferiorly.

The lymphatic drainage of the thyroid gland corresponds to the superior and inferior thyroid arteries. These are medial and lateral channels for both the superior and inferior parts of the thyroid. The medial and lateral lymphatics from the upper portion of the thyroid drain into the deep cervical lymph nodes. The lower medial drainage is to the pretracheal and paratracheal nodes, and the lateral inferior drainage is to the supraclavicular nodes.

PHYSIOLOGY

The thyroid gland is an endocrine organ, and thyroid hormones have a direct effect on the body's metabolism. The thyroid's function is under the direct control of the anterior pituitary gland, which secretes thyroid-stimulating hormone (TSH). The output of TSH is directly related to the secretion of thyroid factor (thyrotropin-releasing factor) by the hypothalamus. This relationship between thyroid factor, TSH, and thyroxine is called the hypothalamic pituitary thyroid axis.

The negative feedback system controls the amount of thyroid hormone present in the body at any time. If the thyroid hormones are not needed in the body, they are stored in the colloid portion of the follicle. If they are needed, they are secreted into the bloodstream where they bind with thyroid-binding globulin and are carried to the specific site where it is needed. Here the hormone diffuses into the interstitial spaces and is released from the thyroid-binding globulin. In the body cells the T_3 and T_4 complexes are broken down to form I^- and elemental iodine (I_2). This breakdown creates energy that is used by the cells to carry out their specific function. Eventually, the I^- and elemental iodine (I_2) get back into the bloodstream where the complete cycle starts all over again. If this mechanism is affected by trauma or disease, the result is a gradual change in normal metabolic activities.

PATHOLOGIC CONDITIONS
Colloid nodules

Adenomatous goiters are the most common cause of single and multiple thyroid nodules. The incidence of nodular goiters increases with the age of the patient. Formerly endemic in parts of the United States, these goiters are still seen even though iodine deficiency has been eliminated. Increased dietary iodine has made these goiters smaller and their multinodularity less obvious to palpation; they are the only cause of autonomous nodules.

Thyroiditis

Chronic and subacute thyroiditis generally involve most of the thyroid gland, producing a diffuse enlargement. However, some thyroid glands contain discrete areas of thyroiditis, which give the examiner the impression of palpating a true nodule. When subacute thyroiditis has subsided, the gland may become irregular and nodules may be felt.

Adenomas

Thyroid pathologic subclassification of adenomas is of little clinical importance. Prior irradiation may be a cause of adenoma formation. Adenomas are not precancerous, and autonomous nodules are not adenomas.

Cancer

Thyroid neoplasia appears in five general forms. The well-differentiated types (papillary and/or follicular adenocarcinomas) are the least malignant. Medullary carcinoma arises in the thyroid gland but not from thyroxine-producing cells. This cancer secretes thyrocalcitonin and histaminase. The presence of such tumors is proved and even predicated by finding detectable serum levels of thyrocalcitonin. They produce amyloid and are usually asymptomatic. Medullary carcinomas are slow growing and yet are many more times malignant than papillary follicular carcinomas. Cure is not common. These cancers are often familial, being part of the multiple endocrine syndromes, with bilateral pheochromocytomas the most common. Metastatic cancer in the thyroid is rarely noted. Lymphosarcoma can develop primarily in the thyroid gland. It is associated with similar disease of the stomach. Undifferentiated thyroid carcinomas, both large and small cell types, probably arise from and are a retrogressive change in papillary follicular carcinomas. When undifferentiated cancer appears, there is no effective therapy.

Congenital abnormalities

Thyroglossal duct cysts. Commonly thin walled, these cysts are 1 to 2 cm in diameter and contain sticky yellow fluid. The cyst wall is formed either by mature thyroid epithelium or by ciliated columnar or metaplastic stratified squamous epithelium. Because of its propinquity, the hyoid bone is often removed surgically to prevent recurrent cyst formation. Except for occasional small thyroid follicles in the wall, only the midline location distinguishes most thyroglossal duct cysts from laterally placed brachial cleft cysts.

Substernal thyroid tissue. This condition is a result of embryologic descent into the anterior mediastinum. Substernal goiters may rise with respiration into the suprasternal notch or become incarcerated there. Lingual and subhyoid thyroid tissues sometimes also form goiters. When larger lateral thyroid masses are removed, practically all prove to be prominent metastases of an unrecognized intrathyroid carcinoma.

Cretinism. Cretinism (hypothyroidism) centers around congenital thyroid deficiency. Cretins typically have a large head, broad nose, wide-set eyes, low forehead, large thick tongue, and dry skin. The most serious clinical aspect is failure of central nervous system development. If infantile hypothyroidism is not discovered and treated within six months of birth, irreversible mental retardation may result. Cretins show stunted growth, enamel dysplasia, umbilical hernia, and sexual infantilism, and they may have other defects of the central nervous system, such as hearing and speech loss.

Goiter and altered hormonal biosynthesis

Goiter refers to persistent thyroid enlargement. Most goiters weigh over 40 g, but some are as small as 25 g. Simple goiter is called diffuse or colloid-storage goiter. Adolescent girls and pregnant women and other women exposed to increased estrogens may develop the symmetrical thyroid enlargement and swanlike neck.

Nodular goiter is the most familiar thyroid disease. It is called adenomatous, endemic nodular colloid and nontoxic multinodular goiter. The last term implies a correlation of function and structure.

Iodine deficiency is the ordinary cause of nodular goiter. Before the widespread use of iodized salt, iodine-poor diets predisposed goiter. Women are affected more than men in a ratio of about 6:1. With iodine deficiency thyroid extraction of blood iodine is increased, and relatively more triiodothyronine is secreted. At first the entire thyroid gland becomes enlarged and more vascular. Follicles shrink, and their epithelium proliferates. An opportunity to see this early diffuse hyperplastic reaction is uncommon except experimentally.

Typical nodular goiters are large, weighing from 60 to over 1000 g. Grossly and microscopically they have four characteristics: nodules, hemorrhage, fibrous structure, and calcification. The nodules vary in size and colloid content, and some are red or brown from recent or old hemorrhage.

In established nodular goiters the major processes are irregular degeneration and regeneration, hypertrophy, and colloid storage. The characteristic nodules are benign and have no known precancerous significance. Nodular goiters are usually removed for diagnosis or cosmetic reasons when the individuals are euthyroid. Two important complications are local hemorrhage with sudden enlargement of the goiter and secondary hyperthyroidism.

Genetically mutant humans or animals may lack an enzyme involved in one of the major biosynthetic reactions necessary for the secretion of thyroxine. The metabolic blocks are generally believed to be caused by autosomal recessive genes. Familial goiter may result, either with euthyroidism or hypothyroidism. Familial goiters are grossly indistinguishable from other nodular goiters.

Primary hyperplasia

Clinically Graves', or Basedow's, disease is a hypermetabolic state associated with a fine tremor, a vascular bruit over the thyroid lobes, and often exophthalmos. An exophthalmic goiter removed surgically usually weighs 35 to 60 g. The thyroid gland is diffusely enlarged, firm, red-brown, opaque, and nongelatinous.

Thyroid storm, or crisis, is a life-threatening exacerbated thyrotoxicosis. Psychosis, shock, and death from cardiopulmonary complications may occur. Severe primary thyroid hyperplasia is usually responsible, but thyroiditis with hyperplasia rarely is.

Secondary hyperplasia

Nodular goiter complicated by hyperthyroidism chiefly affects older individuals, in whom the clinical signs are often atypical. Grossly, red-tan granular thyroid tissue is found either in or between the nodules. Microscopically, nodular goiter with secondary hyperplasia is characterized by some follicles containing peripherally scalloped colloid and columnar epithelial cells.

The clinical term "hot nodule" usually refers to a focus of secondary hyperplasia in nodular goiter that concentrates ^{131}I with or without demonstrable hyperthyroidism. Until surgical removal it may not be evident whether the entire gland is nodular and whether it is enlarged or of normal weight.

Acute thyroiditis

Acute thyroiditis often appears to be a complication of bacterial or viral infection of the oropharynx or salivary glands. The thyroid gland becomes temporarily enlarged and tender but rarely requires operation except for drainage of suppuration.

Chronic thyroiditis

Chronic thyroiditis represents a more difficult problem, since there is no agreement on its classification or pathogenesis. The distinctive clinicopathologic features of five recognized noninfective types follow.

Hashimoto's struma. Hashimoto's struma, or struma lymphomatosa, is characterized by a firm, rubbery, enlarged gland that weighs from 60 to 225 g and is covered by an unaltered thin capsule. On section the thyroid tissue has a uniform, faintly lobulated, opaque yellow-tan surface unlike the grayish pink granularity indicative of cancer. It is often difficult microscopically to recognize thyroid follicles because of a notable lymphocytic infiltrate in sheets and follicles with germinal centers.

Lymphocytic thyroiditis. Lymphocytic thyroiditis, also called juvenile or adolescent thyroiditis, was recognized relatively recently. The gland is larger than in Hashimoto's struma.

Nonspecific chronic thyroiditis. Nonspecific chronic thyroiditis, also called chronic sclerosing thyroiditis, is the most common type of thyroiditis and is often confused with Hashimoto's struma. However, it differs from the latter in three ways. The gland is smaller, weighing 35 to 60 g. Microscopically the thyroid parenchyma is easily recognized despite some follicular disruption, mild fibrosis, and infrequent lymph follicles. The most distinctive feature is an abundance of interstitial plasma cells. There also may be focal squamous metaplasia.

Granulomatous thyroiditis. Granulomatous thyroiditis is synonymous with giant cell, pseudotuberculous, de Quervain's, or so-called subacute thyroiditis. Neither clinically nor pathologically is it subacute. Grossly the thyroid gland is moderately enlarged, but the tissue is pale and hard, like a raw turnip.

Riedel's struma. Riedel's struma is the rarest type of thyroiditis. It produces a localized hard cervical mass that on resection proves to be a dense fibrous scar involving the thyroid and contiguous tissues.

Age changes, degeneration, and atrophy

Beyond 50 years about half of normal-sized thyroid glands contain single or multiple nodules with increased colloid storage, mostly clinically impalpable. Irregular colloid repletion and depletion appear responsible. The nodular thyroid gland has no known clinical significance. Mild interstitial fibrosis, calcium oxalate crystals, and medial calcification of the thyroid arteries also are common in elderly persons.

Hyaline interstitial fibrosis and follicle shrinkage represent the most familiar thyroid degeneration. When the hyalin is abundant and partly involves vessel walls, special staining may demonstrate amyloid. Amyloid goiter is a massive deposit predominantly restricted to the thyroid gland.

Mild thyroid atrophy with small follicles may accompany aging or chronic systemic diseases. Moderate atrophy reduces the gland weights to 10 to 12 g. In severe atrophy the thyroid gland weighs only 3.5 to 6 g, representing mostly capsule, vessels, and infiltrative nonadipose connective tissue.

Myxedema results from subtotal or total thyroid inactivity. The characteristic features of myxedema comprise a puffy, pasty complexion, sparse eyebrows, coarse hair, and large tongue. Menorrhagia and increased sensitivity to cold are common. Mental activity is sluggish, frequently with irritability. Deep tendon reflexes are slow. Coma may complicate myxedema, associated with hypothermia, carbon dioxide retention, and hyponatremia. Bradycardia, low-voltage ECGs, cardiac hypertrophy with basophilic myocardial degeneration, and circulating thyroid antibodies are common in myxedema.

Usually, myxedema appears due to idiopathic thyroid failure. Fewer cases are secondary to TSH insufficiency or panhypopituitarism, whereas hypothalamic myxedema is rare. In all three situations the thyroid gland is moderately or severely atrophied. Chronic thyroiditis also causes hypothyroidism.

Benign neoplasms

Thyroid adenomas are true neoplasms, usually solitary and predominating in women, with a sex ratio of about 5 or 6:1. Thyroid nodules outnumber adenomas at least 10:1, but adenomas require special scrutiny because they are sometimes precancerous. About 10% show invasive characteristics. Five diagnostic criteria of thyroid adenoma are (1) complete fibrous encapsulation, (2) a different architecture inside and outside the capsule, (3) a uniform internal growth pattern, (4) compression of follicles outside the capsule into crescent shapes, and (5) singleness.

Adenomas

Adenomas are divided into follicular, papillary, and atypical types.

Follicular adenomas. In the center of larger adenomas may be a dense white fibrous scar. Fetal adenoma is by far the most common. The miniature fetal follicles contain small colloid masses and lie closely packed or loosely arranged in an edematous fibrovascular stroma. In embryonal adenoma the epithelium grows in branching cords with little or no follicle formation. Simple adenomas have follicles of normal adult size. This is the type that, on rare occasions, develops hyperplasia and constitutes the genuine toxic adenoma. In colloid adenoma the follicles are unusually large. Hürthle cell adenoma is characterized by large granular oxyphil cells that form cords and follicles containing scanty colloid.

Follicular adenomas require careful study of the capsule and the vessels within and outside to determine the presence of invasion. Tumor that penetrates a vessel wall and also occupies its lumen can most clearly be considered invasive.

Papillary adenoma. Papillary adenoma is grossly distinctive, since on sectioning it typically contains wine-red fluid and a capsule lined by granular gray tissue nodules. Microscopically, few papillary adenomas are completely encapsulated. Expert opinion differs on what designation should be applied to papillary adenomas with capsular invasion. In the absence of any significamt cytologic dysplasia and other evidence of invasive activity, it is not clear that incomplete encapsulation of a papillary adenoma indicates cancer.

Atypical adenoma. Atypical adenoma is rare, making up about 2% to 5% of the adenomas. A few atypical adenomas are composed of clear cells or pale follicles resembling parathyroid tissue. Others possess bizarre giant nuclei without indications of carcinoma. Despite the peculiar and somewhat ominous cytologic findings, their course is benign.

Teratoma

Teratoma of the thyroid gland is a disorder that usually affects newborn infants. Grossly teratomas are partly cystic with mesodermal components including muscle, glia, and glandular or other epithelial elements of ectodermal and endodermal origin. The benign thyroid teratoma is dangerous chiefly because of its strategic cervical location.

Malignant neoplasms

Papillary carcinoma. The most common thyroid cancer, papillary carcinoma comprises over 60% of thyroid carcinomas in large series. Generally, it has a long, sluggish natural history, corresponding to carcinomas elsewhere. Grossly, papillary carcinomas may not be discernible. Larger carcinomas are either partly encapsulated or unencapsulated, or the tumor may massively involve the thyroid and adjacent tissues.

Massive papillary carcinoma spreading into the extrathyroid tissues and lymph nodes is lethal in about a third of patients within twenty years. Peculiar to papillary carcinomas are its notable tendency to lymphatic invasion with metastasis to regional cervical lymph nodes and the calcospherites found in the stroma. Calcospherites may remain in areas of local tumor regression, and their presence suggests nearby papillary carcinoma.

Papillary carcinoma may grow purely in this pattern, or papillary and follicular carcinoma may be found together in the original site, in metastases, or in both. Occasionally, an apparently pure papillary carcinoma has lymph node metastasis with predominant follicular carcinoma. Squamous foci are also sometimes present.

Follicular carcinoma. A follicular carcinoma is ordinarily a hard, gritty, grayish pink unencapsulated mass 2 cm or more in diameter, not unlike a breast carcinoma in appearance. Sometimes the best differentiated follicular carcinomas metastasize to lymph nodes, bones, or elsewhere and focally are of a practically normal thyroid appearance. However, a careful study usually reveals some neoplastic qualities. Benign metastasizing thyroid is largely a myth. Blood vessel invasion, which is not uncommon in follicular carcinoma, contributes to the likelihood of pulmonary and osseous metastases.

Medullary carcinoma with amyloid stroma. Medullary carcinoma of the thyroid gland with amyloid stroma is also called solid carcinoma. Medullary carcinoma varies from less than 1.5 cm to a massive size. It has a rounded demarcated outline without encapsulation, and the tumor tissue is gray or white with focal hemorrhages. Amyloid occurs also in the metastases. Despite the rather undifferentiated appearance of medullary thyroid carcinomas and a tendency to bilaterality, these tumors behave like moderately malignant neoplasms. Recently, cases of diarrhea and the carcinoid, or Cushing's, syndrome attributable to medullary thyroid carcinoma have been recognized. In its aberrant endocrine activities medullary carcinoma now rivals oat cell lung carcinomas and pancreatic islet tumors, all of which are derived from foregut endoderm.

Undifferentiated carcinoma. Undifferentiated carcinomas also are termed anaplastic. Ordinarily, their hard consistency and rapid growth renders them clinically, grossly, and microscopically malignant. Older individuals are more often affected. Occa-sionally, a long history begins with an invasive adenoma, progresses to follicular carcinoma, and ends with death from undifferentiated carcinoma twenty-five years or more thereafter.

Small cell, compact undifferentiated carcinoma in some series is the most common variety. Giant cell carcinoma, also called spindle and giant cell carcinoma or carcinosarcoma, is the other relatively well-known undifferentiated carcinoma. Some arise from adenomas. The bizarre and disorderly neoplastic cells are unrecognizable as thyroid, and tumor giant cells striking variability are present.

Small cell diffuse carcinoma is uncommon and not easily distinguished from malignant lymphoma, even in well-prepared sections. Both in the thyroid and nodal metastases the small cells retain some epithelial characteristics, such as cordlike growth and compression of the preexisting reticulin.

Rarer and ordinarily lethal carcinomas include adenoacanthoma, squamous cell carcinoma, and mixed carcinoma. Hürthle cell carcinoma is now regarded as a metaplastic alteration of some other neoplasm and not as an entity.

Stromal tumors. Sarcoma of the thyroid gland most often is malignant lymphoma, lymphosarcoma, reticulum cell sarcoma, or Hodgkin's disease. Elderly women usually are the victims of either primary or secondary thyroid lymphomas. The features used to distinguish thyroid lymphoma from carcinoma or thyroiditis are essentially the same as those employed in lymph nodes. Plasmacytoma restricted to the thyroid gland is belived to have the same benign course observed in certain other extramedullary sites.

Metastatic cancer. Metastatic cancer of the thyroid gland is fairly common at autopsy, with widely disseminated malignant melanoma the most common source of thyroid metastasis.

ULTRASOUND EVALUATION

Ultrasonographic evaluation of the thyroid gland provides a simple and reproducible method of differentiating between solid and cystic thyroid nodules and accurately measuring the thyroid gland and nodular size. In addition to these capabilities, the introduction of grey scale with high-frequency transducers may allow differentiation between benign and malignant thyroid lesions.

Radionuclide scans provide valuable data on the functional status of the thyroid gland. "Cold" areas represent glandular tissue with malignancy or cystic changes. "Hot" areas represent possible benign conditions. With ultrasonic examinations, low-level

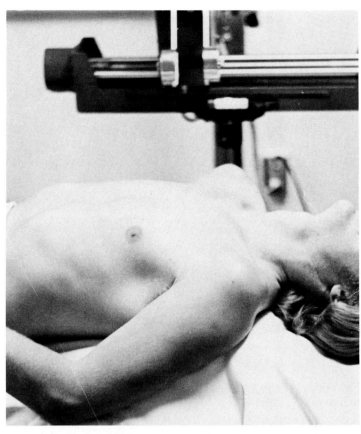

Fig. 31-1. Normal patient setup for a thyroid examination. The neck should be hyperextended with a pillow under the shoulder area for support. This allows the thyroid area to be in better contact with the transducer.

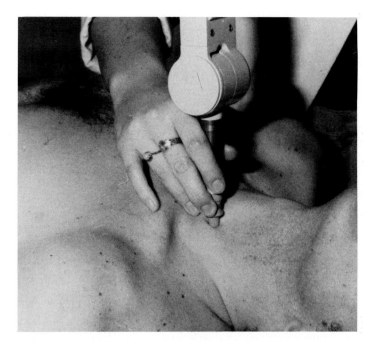

Fig. 31-2. High-frequency transducer with a small diameter should be used to avoid near-field ring down and better resolution of the superficial structures.

echoes from normal glandular tissue add considerably to the differential diagnosis of thyroid conditions, making it a valuable complementary tool for visualizing the anatomic and pathologic structures of the involved areas.

Techniques vary according to the institution, but basic methods of localization should be followed for good statistical results. The patient is positioned supine with a slight hyperflexion of the cervical spine (Fig. 31-1). Begin scanning at the sternal notch for transverse cuts and move cephalad at 0.5 cm intervals. Scans at 0.5 cm intervals are also obtained in the longitudinal sections to outline the thyroid tissue with the carotid artery or jugular vein posterior.

In a case of a superficial structure such as the thyroid, sound attenuation is not a problem. A 5 MHz transducer with a 6 mm diameter beam width is used for optimal resolution (Figs. 31-2 and 31-3). The 2.25 MHz transducer offers better penetrating power but with a considerable loss of resolution. Scans should be performed with both low- and high-gain settings to differentiate the tissue patterns.

The complex contour of the neck and the rapid scanning action may create a problem. Therefore it is advantageous to use a transducer with an intervening water bath. The bath is filled with degassed warm water, and the plastic is coupled to the skin with a layer of mineral oil. The transducer is placed so that the thyroid lies within the focal plane of the transducer (Fig. 31-4). One pass of the transducer completes the scan (Fig. 31-5). The transducer is then stepped 5 cm and the process repeated. Longitudinal and transverse scans are required for a complete examination.

A-mode thyroid echography is useful for differentiating cystic and solid masses of the thyroid that fail to concentrate radioactive iodine. This is accomplished by placing the transducer over the area of interest and observing the A-mode oscilloscope.

In this mode a sound pulse is emitted and travels into the tissue, attenuating with greater depth because of interfacing surfaces. On reaching a fluid-filled cyst, the sound travels through the medium with minimal reflection, therefore displaying a pattern of spikes separated by an area of free spikes. In a solid component many interfaces are encountered and reflected back to the transducer causing repetitive attenuating spikes without a clear space.

B-mode ultrasonography adds another dimension of depth and is especially useful in the resolution of supposedly warm nodules, which could in fact be cold nodules surrounded by normal functioning tissue on the nuclear medicine scans. It is also useful in the differentiation of hypofunctioning and nonfunctioning nodules.

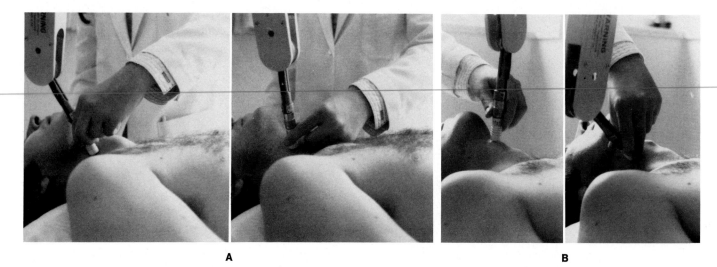

A   **B**

Fig. 31-3. A, Longitudinal scans made directly on the patient's neck should be done with a single
sweep technique with the patient in full inspiration. This will dilate the jugular vein posterior to the
thyroid and delineate the gland more fully. **B,** Transverse scans directly over the thyroid area should
also be made with a single sweep technique. It may be difficult to keep contact with the patient's skin.
The sonographer may start at the midline to scan one side of the neck and then return to the midline
to scan the other side of the thyroid area.

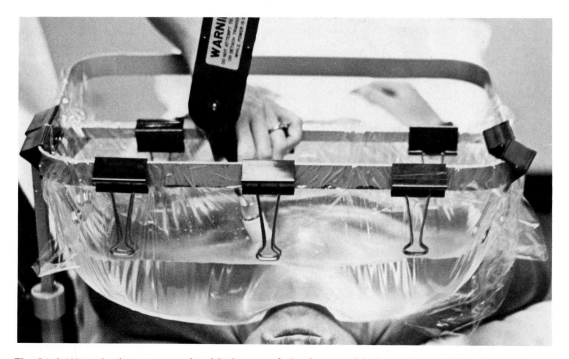

Fig. 31-4. Water bath system made with the use of plastic material clipped onto a Mayo stand allows
excellent coupling with the anterior skin surface. A generous supply of mineral oil is applied to the
water bath and skin surface to avoid air interference. The transducer is placed in the water approximately 2 to 3 cm deep. A single sweep or a slight sector sweep may be used to obtain perpendicular angles from the thyroid structure. Longitudinal scans may be performed without moving
the water bath.

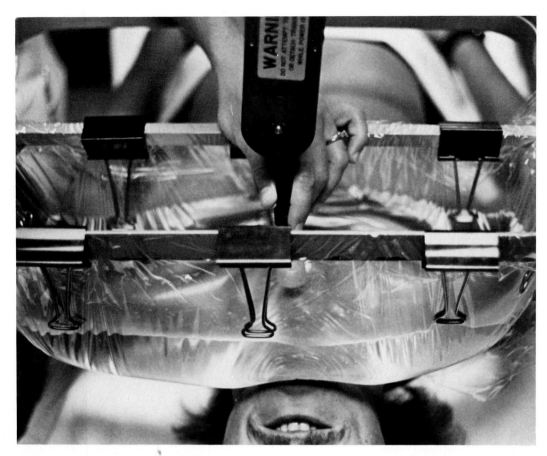

Fig. 31-5. Patient feels no discomfort during this water bath procedure. We have found it advantageous to use warm water (body temperature) to allow the sound to travel at the same speed the equipment is calculated for.

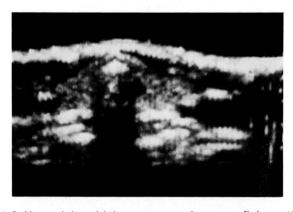

Fig. 31-6. Normal thyroid tissue appears in a snowflake pattern of uniform echoes draping over the trachea and esophagus and lying anterior to the carotid and jugular vascular structures. The strap muscles are sometimes seen lateral and posterior to the vascular structures.

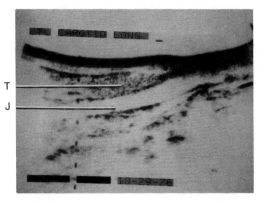

Fig. 31-7. Longitudinal scan of the normal thyroid with the dilated jugular posterior.

In a normal thyroid the distribution of echoes should be uniform throughout the gland (Fig. 31-6). The boundaries of the lobes are usually not clearly displayed over the whole surface. However, the size of the lobe is apparent by the uniform echo pattern of the lobe as distinguished from the surrounding structures (Fig. 31-7).

The trachea is visualized lying behind the isthmus. The anterior surface of the trachea is always displayed by a strong echo because of the large tissue-air impedance mismatch. The side walls are usually displayed by weaker echoes because of the unfavorable angle to the ultrasonic beam. Shadowing caused by its air content prevents the posterior surface of the trachea from being visualized. On either side are seen the common carotid arteries and the internal jugular veins. Structures such as the muscles and some of the

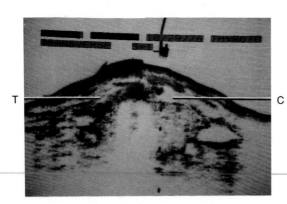

Fig. 31-8. Small cystic mass shown displacing the normal thyroid tissue on the left neck. The jugular vein and carotid artery can be seen posterior.

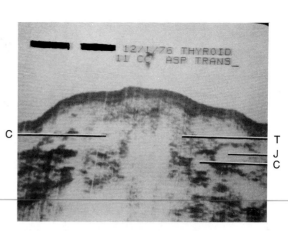

Fig. 31-9. Two to 3 cm cystic structure with internal echoes on the left side of the neck. The normal right thyroid can be seen on the right anterior to the carotid artery. The jugular vein is shown on the lateral margin of the carotid artery.

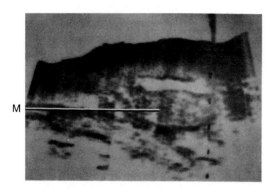

Fig. 31-10. Complex mass on the left thyroid. This may represent a solid tumor with central necrosis or an adenoma with hemorrhage.

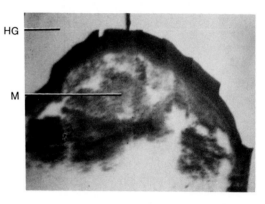

Fig. 31-11. Complex structure on the left neck displacing normal thyroid tissue. Multiple cystic areas within the solid mass may represent necrosis, hemorrhage, or degenerating tissue.

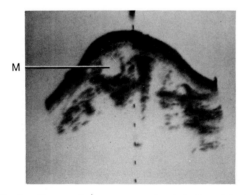

Fig. 31-12. Small complex mass on the left thyroid with a large, central, echo-free area, follicular adenoma, and degeneration.

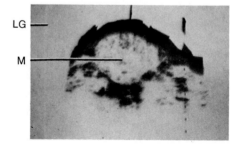

Fig. 31-13. Four to 5 cm nodule on the right thyroid with multiple internal echoes. This represents a large solitary hyperfunctioning nontoxic autonomous thyroid nodule.

larger nerves are also often visualized. The esophagus, on the other hand, is not generally seen, since it is shadowed by the trachea.

A cystic pattern is typically seen with a colloid cyst. Other cystic masses, such as a thyroglossal duct cyst, can present a similar echo pattern but are recognized by their locations. A hemorrhage without clot can present a cystic pattern as well. The pattern of simple cysts in B mode is characterized by persistent sonolucency with high-gain settings. Echoes that may appear at high-gain settings tend to occur in the more superficial part of the cyst, but, the discrete, thin, deep wall of the cyst remains discernible. In A-mode scans, as the sensitivity is increased, the cystic pattern tends to fill with echoes (ring down) from the periphery. (See Figs. 31-8 and 31-9.)

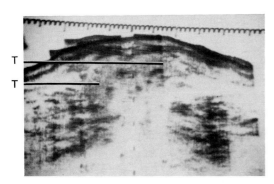

Fig. 31-14. Dense echoes within the normal thyroid tissue representing calcification.

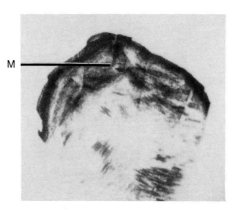

Fig. 31-15. Solid mass in the right lobe of the thyroid, a diffuse toxic goiter.

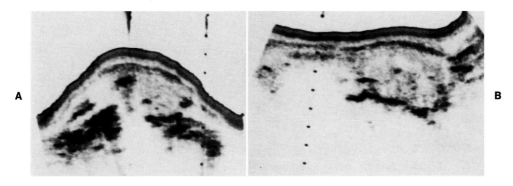

Fig. 31-16. A, Solid mass shown in the left lobe of the thyroid. Jugular vein is shown on the right. **B,** Longitudinal scan of the solid nodule shown in **A.**

A complex pattern is commonly seen in multinodular goiter, with a relative proportion of cystic and solid components corresponding with the morphology of the mass. A tumor with central necrosis and an adenoma with patchy areas of central hemorrhage can both present similar patterns (Figs. 31-10 to 31-14).

A solid pattern can be seen in malignancy, benign adenomas, hyperplasia, thyroiditis, Hashimoto's disease, goiter, and normal thyroid. With grey-scale, malignancies appear to contain echoes of slightly lesser intensity than the normal gland or an adenoma. A solid nodule is represented by (1) internal echoes appearing in the middle and deeper portions at intermediate-to-high–gain settings; (2) obliteration of the sonolucency of the nodule by echoes as the sensitivity is increased, and (3) the inability to demonstrate a discrete, thin, deep wall at higher gain settings. With A mode the echoes tend to appear first in the center of the lesion. (See Figs. 31-15 to 31-17.)

The ultrasonic appearance of various anomalies follows:

1. Cyst—liquid-filled area surrounded by normal tissue and a strong back wall

2. Degenerating adenoma—abnormal tissue containing interspread liquid-filled areas
3. Adenoma—evenly distributed low-level echoes
4. Thyrotoxicosis—varying-level echoes, evenly distributed; symmetrical enlargement of both lobes
5. Multinodular goiter—complex echo pattern with uneven echo distribution
6. Anaplastic carcinoma—even distribution of very low–level echoes
7. Follicular carcinoma—recorded as a predominately cystic mass
8. Lymphoma—usually produces a complex pattern
9. Thyroglossal duct cyst—cystic pattern superior to the thyroid gland

Certain pitfalls are apparent in ultrasonic assessment of the thyroid gland. Nodules less than 1 cm might not be clearly defined. If the nodule is flat and broad, it is also difficult to define. Nodules that bulge prominently, and the diameter of which is the same or smaller than the area of the transducer surface, may be difficult to determine because of the problem in keeping the transducer flat on the skin. A water bath might be useful in these situations.

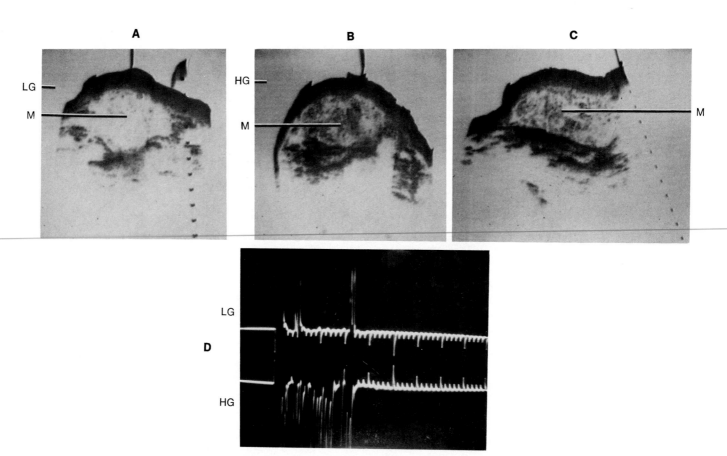

Fig. 31-17. **A,** Low-gain study of a multinodular thyroid. Diffuse internal echoes are shown through-out the mass. **B,** Increased gain settings demonstrate complete fill-in of the multinodular thyroid. **C,** Longitudinal high-gain settings of a multinodular thyroid. Note sonolucent areas within the central core. **D,** A-mode study of above lesion at low-gain and high-gain settings. Additional information is obtained when high gain is used with higher-frequency transducers. A solid mass will not penetrate with higher frequencies, whereas a cystic mass would.

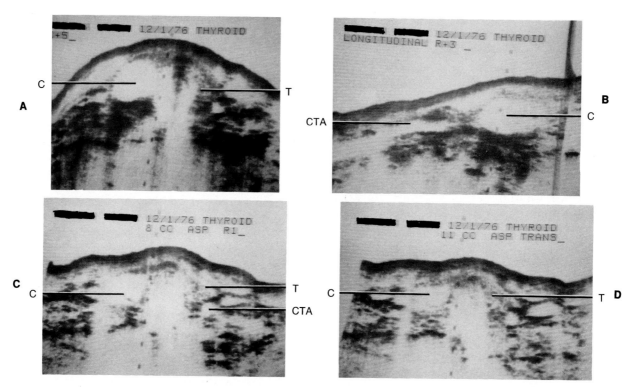

Fig. 31-18. **A,** Large cyst on the left lobe of the thyroid before aspiration. **B,** Longitudinal view of the cystic structure prior to aspiration. **C,** Repeat scan after 8 ml of fluid was withdrawn. **D,** Final scan after 11 ml of fluid was withdrawn.

Multiloculated cystic nodules may appear solid on echogram because of the many reflecting interfaces within. Nodules that are initially solid may undergo necrosis or hemorrhage internally with clots and appear solid on ultrasonography, whereas their contents are actually liquid. Lesions that extend behind the sternum are obscured from ultrasonographic view because of the absorption by the bone. Extrathyroidal cystic lesions (branchial cleft cysts, cystic degeneration in a lymph node) or extrathyroidal solid lesions (glomus tumor, parathyroid tumors, lymph nodes) cannot routinely be distinguished by echography from intrathyroidal lesions.

ASPIRATION BY A-MODE ECHOGRAPHY

If a nodule appears suddenly and is large enough to be visible in the neck, it is almost certainly a cyst or the result of a hemorrhage developing into an adenoma. No malignant tumors of the thyroid, except the easily recognized lymphomas and anaplastic cancers, grow rapidly. This condition is best treated by aspiration. Aspiration of a cyst, whether it contains fluid or old blood, not only establishes the diagnosis but also avoids the necessity of operation in about 90% of patients (Fig. 31-18).

The three situations for which aspiration or needle biopsy is commonly used are (1) diffuse enlargement of the thyroid thought to be the result of struma lymphomatosa, (2) nodules of the thyroid thought to be benign, and (3) cysts of the thyroid or hemorrhage into adenomas in which the diagnosis is suspected because of the sudden appearance or rapid growth of the nodule (a history that rules out the presence of differentiated or operable carcinoma).

If a cyst is suspected, an aspiration is performed to examine the fluid for the possible presence of abnormal cells. (These cells often are not seen unless special care is taken to aspirate them with a large-gauge needle.) This in turn may cause recurrence of the cyst because of hemorrhage. For this reason, cysts of the thyroid usually are aspirated with a 20-gauge needle.

If there is a persistent mass after a cyst is aspirated, aspiration biopsy should be taken with a 15-gauge needle to rule out the possibility of cancer. Occasionally, a papillary carcinoma may be cystic and could be missed if cellular material is not obtained.

The routine use of needle biopsy in patients with thyroid nodules that have none of the characteristics of malignancy could diminish the need for thyroidectomy by a factor of about 10:1.

• • •

Ultrasound examination has proved helpful in the assessment of the thyroid gland and in particular of solitary hypofunctioning thyroid nodules. It also provides an accurate method of differentiating between solid and cystic abnormalities. This information aids the clinician in deciding on the course of treatment. The ability to accurately measure the size of the thyroid gland and the individual nodules and to follow these with serial measurements during therapy is also useful.

With the development of newer and better equipment and the elaboration of highly resolving real-time scanners and mechanical scanners, the approach to thyroid evaluation by means of ultrasonography can only be improved in the diagnosis of thyroid gland abnormalities.

32 □ Doppler techniques

DARLENE BIBERDORF, R.T., R.N.M.

The circulatory system has always been difficult to examine in a noninvasive manner. The development of the transcutaneous Doppler ultrasound flow detection method now permits this assessment. Prior to this, radiographic contrast studies were about the only means for evaluation. Angiography has many disadvantages, which have prevented its widespread use as a screening method.

Ultrasonic Doppler evaluation of the peripheral vessels has proved to be an effective and useful diagnostic tool. This discussion will include the basic principles of the Doppler effect and, in greater detail, the techniques used in specific examination of the vascular system.

First an understanding of the Doppler effect and its use in this examination must be established. This effect has been known for over 130 years. The change in pitch (frequency) of the sound of the whistle on a passing train is a familiar phenomenon. The frequency is higher as the train approaches and lower as the train moves away. This change is explained by the fact that, as the train approaches, the sound waves are compressed, thereby producing more waves per unit of time and thus a higher frequency. As the train passes, there is an instantaneous decrease in the whistle sound frequency and the waves are stretched out, traveling back toward the listener. This change in frequency is related to the velocity of the moving source and is termed the Doppler effect, in honor of Christian Doppler, its discoverer. Use of the Doppler effect in the detection of blood flow began in about 1957. Since that time further research has improved the technique.

INSTRUMENTATION

The basic Doppler flowmeter consists of an electronic oscillator, a transducer probe, a signal processor, and an output device for presenting the information received.

The electronic oscillator applies a high frequency to the transducer, which contains the transmitting piezoelectric crystal. This signal is a continuous wave type. The same probe also contains the receiving crystal. Although many Doppler flowmeters are available, those equipped with a pencil probe are the easiest to maneuver in vascular examination. The frequencies used in the diagnosis of vascular disease range from 2.5 to 10 MHz. The lower frequencies tend to penetrate more and are useful in examining slow-moving structures such as arterial walls. Higher frequencies are used to detect the flow of blood in more superficial arteries and veins.

The frequencies transmitted into the blood vessels are in the ultrasonic range; however, the frequency change caused by the Doppler effect is within the audible range. This change in frequency results because the flowing blood reflects the sound transmitted. This reflected backscatter is of a different frequency than the transmitted wave, causing a Doppler shift. The difference is directly proportional to the velocity of the blood flow. Therefore, because it is within the audible range, with appropriate amplification or with a speaker or headphones the examiner can hear the blood flow.

This output is not quantitative. Since the procedure is done transcutaneously, the volume of flow cannot be estimated because the cross-sectional area of the blood vessel is not known and the true velocity cannot be measured. The directional Doppler flowmeter presents frequency shifts of flow toward the probe in one channel and those of flow away from the probe in a second channel. Stereophonic headphones can be used to hear the flow moving toward the probe in one ear and away from the probe in the other ear.

For permanent records the Doppler audio signal may also be displayed on an oscilloscope and then photographed. The signal can also be printed on a strip-chart recorder.

DOPPLER OPHTHALMIC TEST

Strokes are the third most common cause of death in the United States. Although there are many controversial aspects about management of stroke victims, there is agreement that efforts should be directed toward the detection of patients, symptomatic and asymptomatic, with surgically correctable lesions. This brings about a need for an effective screening method for potential stroke victims. Although cerebral angiography is available, this test carries with it a high mortality, thereby making its use as a screening tool limited. Introduction of the Doppler ophthalmic test as a noninvasive means of evaluation has opened up this field for investigation of cerebrovascular occlusive disease.

Association of extracranial vascular occlusions with cerebral infarction was described as early as 1914. However, it was not until the late 1930s and the introduction of cerebral arteriography that interest was focused on its importance in the investigation of cerebrovascular insufficiency. It was soon learned that arteriography carried with it a high risk. A search began for a means of diagnosing, with relative reliability and ease, extracranial vascular lesions.

The introduction of the Doppler flowmeter for blood flow evaluation opened up new doors in the search for a noninvasive screening method. Early investigators confined their studies to direct monitoring of the common or internal carotid artery in the neck. This, however, proved unreliable because of the difficulty in separating the internal and external carotid arteries, which are situated close together. This anatomic proximity made examination of the vessels impossible, thus, Doppler evaluation was limited to the common trunk.

The next stage was the realization that there was a change in pressure relationships between the internal and external carotid arteries, via their collateral anastomoses, with the occlusion of the internal carotid artery. Thus, as perfusion pressure decreased in the branches of the internal carotid artery, particularly the ophthalmic artery, a point was reached when the flow was channeled into the ophthalmic artery from the external carotid collaterals.

Studies indicate that the stenosing carotid lesion must exceed 63% of the luminal diameter before a pressure drop can be expected. With the Doppler flowmeter this reversal of flow can be detected in the supraorbital artery, which is a terminal branch of the ophthalmic artery.

The important point in this examination is its anatomic basis. The carotid artery originates at the sternoclavicular joint and terminates midway between the angle of the mandible and the mastoid process of the temporal bone. The common caroid arteries are not of equal length. The right common carotid artery arises from the bifurcation of the brachiocephalic artery behind the right sternoclavicular joint. The left common carotid artery is a direct branch of the aortic arch. Therefore the left common carotid artery exceeds the superior mediastinum of the thorax by about 2 cm before it enters the neck. The common carotid arteries have no collateral branches but divide terminally into the internal and external carotid arteries.

The internal carotid artery has no branches in the neck but continues up into the cranium to become the principal artery of the brain and of the structures of the orbit. The first branch of the internal carotid artery is the ophthalmic artery, which then terminates in the supraorbital artery. It exits from the orbit via the supraorbital notch and anastomoses with the temporal frontal branches of the superficial temporal artery, which is also part of the carotid system. Under normal circumstances flow in the supraorbital artery is antegrade, outward from the orbit toward the superficial temporal anastomosis.

The external carotid artery is equal in diameter to the internal artery. It extends from the upper thyroid to the neck of the mandible, where it divides into the superficial temporal and maxillary arteries. There are other branches of the external carotid artery, but they are not directly related to this test.

The Doppler ophthalmic test examines the pathway between the external carotid artery and the ophthalmic artery. This serves as a loop to restore pressure and flow to the internal carotid artery distal to its extracranial point of occlusion or stenosis (Fig. 32-1).

The test is performed with the patient in the supine position and the examiner positioned at the head of the table. The supraorbital notch is palpated at the rim of the orbit, and the coupling gel is applied to this area. It is best to have the patient's eyes closed. The transducer is placed over the supraorbital notch, which houses the supraorbital artery. The probe should be angled slightly upward toward the vertex of the skull, not into the orbit. Proper angulation allows the ultrasound beam to be directed against the normal flow of blood. It is important to adjust the probe until maximum audio signal is heard. Remember, under normal circumstances the flow in the supraorbital artery is antegrade. Any significant lesion in the internal carotid artery system proximal to and including the ophthalmic branch may cause reversal of the normal pressure and therefore result in retrograde flow in the supraorbital artery.

After determining the direction of flow in the supraorbital artery, the examiner should then compress the superficial temporal artery just anterior to the homolateral auditory canal. The change that occurs in the supraorbital signal with compression forms the basis for interpretation of the Doppler ophthalmic test.

In normal circulation, compression of the superficial temporal artery causes augmentation of the antegrade supraorbital artery signal. However, with internal

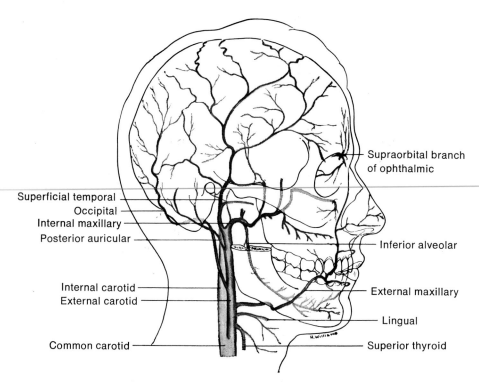

Fig. 32-1. Normal anatomy of the supraorbital and superficial arteries as terminal branches of the internal and external carotid arteries. (From Anthony, C. P., and Kolthoff, N. J.: Textbook of anatomy and physiology, ed. 9, St. Louis, 1971, The C. V. Mosby Co.)

carotid artery stenosis the flow is decreased through the superficial temporal artery, and therefore with compression the signal may cease totally. Occasionally, supraorbital artery flow may change from retrograde to antegrade with superficial temporal compression. This also implies significant internal carotid artery stenosis.

As with all methods of diagnostic testing there is the possibility of technical errors, which lead to false readings. The exact placement of the transducer is important. If placed too far laterally it may be over the orbital branch of the superficial temporal artery. If this occurs, it is obvious that during compression anterior to the auditory canal (of the superficial temporal artery) there will be a decrease in the supraorbital signal, indicating disease of the internal carotid artery when none is present.

It is also important not to move the probe from the correct position once it has been established. Movement of the probe causes the ultrasound beam to either sound other vessels in the area or to completely lose all signals. Probe immobility is especially important during the time of superficial temporal artery compression. Also at the time of compression, care should be taken to not press the probe against the skin, which would obliterate the supraorbital artery signal completely.

Unfortunately, false negative test results do occur. This can happen whenever antegrade flow in the supraorbital artery occurs in the presence of significantly altered internal carotid artery hemodynamics. This situation occurs whenever equally severe internal and external carotid stenoses coexist. Negative results are also found when a single stenosis is located in the common carotid artery. Supraorbital artery flow remains antegrade because the net pressure is not changed. False negative readings also occur in cases of unusually efficient intracranial collateral flow via the circle of Willis.

Also found are false positive results. As stated earlier, these are most often caused by technical error, usually in connection with probe placement and movement during testing.

It has been reported that a false positive test result has occurred in patients having transient ischemia attacks due to extracranial cerebrovascular disease. It is possible that emboli obstruct the ophthalmic artery or its branches in the absence of an obstructive lesion of the internal carotid artery. However, in carotid arteriography the ophthalmic artery and its branches are usually not visualized well enough to verify this.

The safety of the Doppler ophthalmic test has been established. There has been a failure to demonstrate retinal or ophthalmic lesions on pathologic examination of experimental animals. The remote possibility of this occurring is obviated by correct positioning of the transducer. There also have been no reported instances of transient ischemia attacks during the brief time of superficial temporal artery compression.

It is therefore believed that the diagnostic Doppler ophthalmic test has a definite place in the evaluation of patients with cerebrovascular disease or with a family history of stroke. The necessary equipment is relatively inexpensive, and the test is harmless and easy to accomplish. Results show a close correlation with subsequent arteriographic and surgical results.

DOPPLER EVALUATION OF VENOUS DISEASE OF THE LOWER EXTREMITY

Deep venous disease is usually harder to diagnose clinically than is peripheral arterial disease. Clinical evidence is based solely on indirect evidence. There is no venous pulse that can be palpated in the periphery. Physical symptoms such as tenderness, swelling, dilated and varicosed superficial veins, and skin changes become the basis for diagnosis of deep venous disease. Furthermore, venous thrombosis of the lower extremity may go undetected until a complication such as pulmonary emboli has developed.

Venography may be used to diagnose venous disease. However, it is generally employed to better define the problem after it is clinically suspected on the basis of the physical symptoms. Venography is not suitable or practical to use as a screening procedure; therefore the Doppler ultrasound blood flow detector provides a device to detect venous abnormalities in a simple, rapid, and safe manner.

It is important to understand and know the venous anatomy of the lower extremity. There are two sets of veins. The superficial are immediately under the skin and the deepset veins accompany the arteries. Both sets have valves; however, there are more in the deep venous system. (See Figs. 32-2 and 32-3.)

The superficial set of veins contains two major vessels, the great and small saphenous. The great saphenous is the longest vein in the body. It begins at the medial margin of the foot and runs along the medial aspect of the leg until it ends in the femoral vein about 3 cm below the inguinal ligament. The small saphenous begins behind the lateral malleolus as a continuation of the lateral marginal vein of the foot and runs along the middle of the back of the leg, ending in the popliteal vein about 3 to 7 cm above the knee joint. It communicates with the deep veins of the dorsum of the foot and sends several branches superior and medial to join the great saphenous vein.

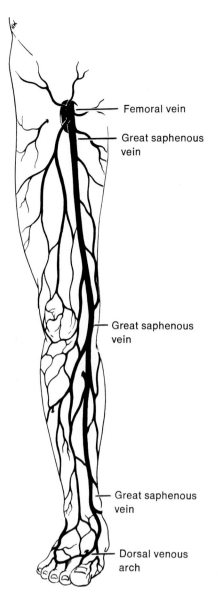

Fig. 32-2. Main superficial veins of the lower extremity. (From Anthony, C. P., and Kolthoff, N. J.: Textbook of anatomy and physiology, ed. 9, St. Louis, 1971, The C. V. Mosby Co.)

The deep venous system accompanies the arteries. Therefore the femoral vein follows the femoral artery, and the popliteal, anterior tibial, and posterior tibial veins all follow their respective arteries.

The patient is examined in the supine position with the head slightly elevated to maintain a larger pool of venous blood in the lower extremity. To evaluate the deep venous system multiple sites must be studied. Three customary sites are the common femoral vein at the inguinal ligament, the popliteal vein in the popliteal fossa, and the posterior tibial vein behind the medial malleolus. These are sites where the veins of the deep system can be readily identified. External anatomic landmarks and the presence of the accompanying arterial flow signal both aid in localization.

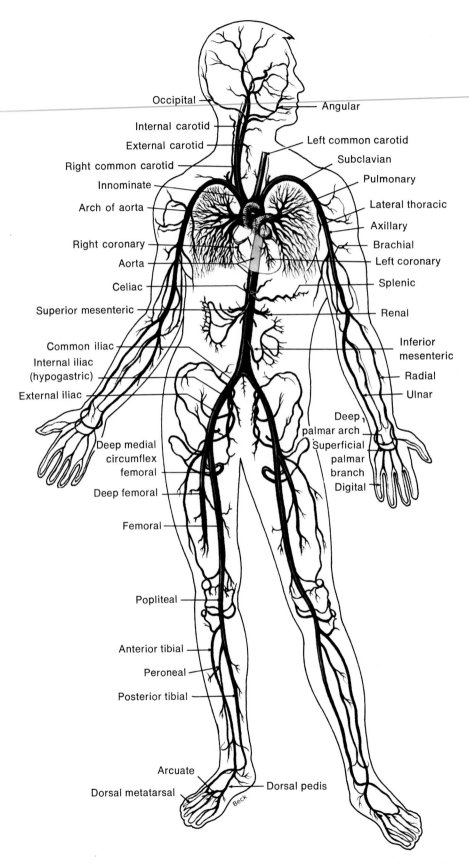

Occipital — — Angular

Internal carotid — — Left common carotid

External carotid — Subclavian

Right common carotid — Pulmonary

Innominate — Lateral thoracic

Arch of aorta — Axillary

Right coronary — Brachial

Aorta — Left coronary

Celiac — Splenic

Superior mesenteric — Renal

Common iliac — Inferior mesenteric

Internal iliac (hypogastric) — Radial

External iliac — Ulnar

Deep palmar arch
Superficial palmar branch
Digital

Deep medial circumflex femoral

Deep femoral —

Femoral —

Popliteal —

Anterior tibial —

Peroneal —

Posterior tibial —

Arcuate

Dorsal metatarsal — — Dorsal pedis

Beck

Fig. 32-3. Principal arteries of the body. (From Anthony, C. P., and Kolthoff, N. J.: Textbook of anatomy and physiology, ed. 9, St. Louis, 1971, The C. V. Mosby Co.)

If the transducer is placed over a large vein, an audible signal is heard as a result of the Doppler effect. This signal resembles a wind storm. It is cyclic in phase with respiration. During inspiration the signal decreases in amplitude and pitch and usually disappears completely. During expiration this sound, termed the S sound, for spontaneous flow sound, returns. The S sound may be continuous and high-pitched in the presence of velocity flow. In normal venous flow the S sound is always heard over the common femoral vein, usually over the popliteal, and only occasionally over the posterior tibial vein.

By manually compressing the extremity for a second or two, blood flow in the deep veins is accelerated. As a flow wave of greater velocity is detected by the Doppler transducer, a new distinct and relatively high-pitched signal is heard. This signal is termed the augmented flow sound, or the A sound. The A sound is brief and is superimposed on the S sound, but it is readily perceived. The A sound may also be heard over veins that do not have an audible S sound. In these circumstances spontaneous flow velocity is below the threshold of detection by ultrasound, and therefore only the faster flow caused by compression may be heard.

With a normal venous system an A sound produced by compression propagates toward the heart. Compression distal to the transducer will elicit an augmented sound, whereas release of compression does not. If an occlusion is present in the vein between the probe and the site of the distal compression, an A sound will not be heard, since the propagated wave of accelerated flow will be damped by the occlusion. If the vein is open but the valves incompetent, distal compression will also produce an A sound. However, after release of compression another A sound will be heard. Because of valve incompetence some blood flows in a retrograde direction toward the site where the compression has been released. As this retrograde flow passes the transducer, an A sound is produced. Distal compression may therefore cause two types of A sounds—positive and negative. Positive refers to flow motion initiated by compression and negative the sound on release of compression.

Proximal compression also produces two types of A sound—positive on compression and negative on release of compression. The proximal positive A sound is not heard if there are functional valves between the site of compression and the probe. With compression the valve will close, and flow will be toward the heart. If no valves are in the intervening segment or if the valves are incompetent, proximal compression will

produce an A sound. A proximal negative A sound is normally heard. During compression blood is held back by closed valves. On release this blood flows past the probe, and an A sound is heard. The negative A sound after the release of proximal compression may be diminished or absent in the presence of occlusion or incompetent valves; therefore four possible A sounds may be detected. The sound reveals whether flow is present in the vein being examined. If flow is present, it may also be determined whether retrograde flow is possible.

For examination of the femoral vein the patient is placed in the supine position. Palpation and sounding of the common femoral artery help locate the common femoral vein. After proper location of the femoral vein, the S sound should be heard. The arterial signal is often present in the background.

There are four common abnormalities. The first is the continuous S sound. This indicates a lack of cycle variation with respiration. The second abnormality is a high-pitched S sound. A greater than normal pitch is difficult to ascertain, and experience is most often required to make this judgment. The third is a decreased S sound. Not only is there a decrease in volume and pitch, but the length of the signal is shortened during the respiratory cycle. The fourth and final abnormality is a totally absent S sound.

The next part of the examination is to make an assessment of the common femoral vein A sound. Without moving the probe from its previous position, compression of the lower thigh is done for several seconds. This produces a distinct, loud, new sound superimposed on the background S sound. This new sound is transient, lasting for one or several seconds. The examiner should release compression after the distal positive A sound has totally disappeared. During and after release, attention should be directed to the presence of a distal negative A sound. Distal positive A sounds should be heard as distinct signals that are comparable to those on the opposite extremity. Two types of abnormalities are distinguished in eliciting the distal positive A sound. The first is diminished distal positive A sounds. If on repeated testing a low-intensity signal is produced by compression, interpretation of a possible abnormality may be made. The second is absent distal positive A sounds. If the transducer is positioned properly and no A sound is heard, a definite abnormality is indicated.

Distal negative A sounds are not normally heard; therefore release of thigh compression should not be followed by an A sound. If a distal negative A sound is heard, an abnormality is considered.

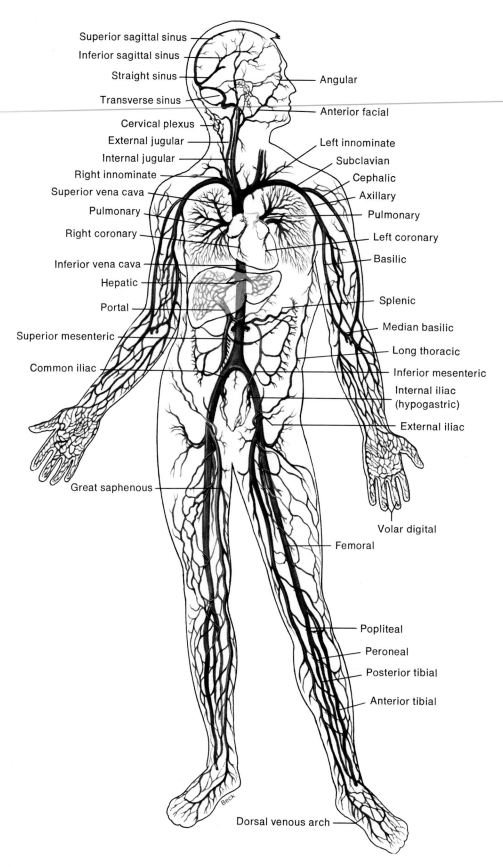

Superior sagittal sinus
Inferior sagittal sinus
Straight sinus
Transverse sinus
Cervical plexus
External jugular
Internal jugular
Right innominate
Superior vena cava
Pulmonary
Right coronary
Inferior vena cava
Hepatic
Portal
Superior mesenteric
Common iliac
Great saphenous

Angular
Anterior facial
Left innominate
Subclavian
Cephalic
Axillary
Pulmonary
Left coronary
Basilic
Splenic
Median basilic
Long thoracic
Inferior mesenteric
Internal iliac (hypogastric)
External iliac
Volar digital
Femoral
Popliteal
Peroneal
Posterior tibial
Anterior tibial
Dorsal venous arch

Beck

Fig. 32-4. Principal veins of the body. (From Anthony, C. P., and Kolthoff, N. J.: Textbook of anatomy and physiology, ed. 9, St. Louis, The C. V. Mosby Co.)

Next, compression of the calf should be done at its midpoint. Grasping is done from the anterior. Usually, the A sound at the femoral vein is heard. The discernment of diminished and absent distal positive A sounds and negative A sounds is similar to that found in the thigh.

The examiner should dorsiflex the patient's foot. Normally, an A sound is heard following this. It is important not to move the leg during this maneuver, since this may simulate an abnormality. Most examiners do not attempt to discern a negative A sound.

The posterior tibial vein is usually examined next with the patient still in the supine position. The vein is found by palpation next to the medial malleolus. Usually, an S sound is not heard. The foot is grasped and the sole compressed. A distal positive A sound should be heard. On release of the foot the examiner should listen for the presence of a distal negative A sound. Compression is also applied on the posterior medial aspect of the calf at the upper third. A proximal A sound is normally heard on release.

With the patient in the prone position the popliteal vein is examined. The leg should be flexed about 30° and supported on a pillow. Full extension of the leg interferes with the venous return. An S sound is normally heard over the popliteal vein. The calf is again compressed. After the complete subsidence of the distal A sound the grip is released, and the presence of a distal negative A sound is noted. Proximal compression of the lower third of the thigh is done, which normally gives a proximal positive A sound. On release a proximal negative A sound is heard. Compression of the middle third of the thigh usually does not elicit a proximal positive A sound. However, the presence of a proximal positive A sound from the upper third is regarded as an abnormality.

To diagnose any venous abnormality all the findings of the Doppler evaluation must be considered. The Doppler method has proved to be a safe and effective tool for this purpose.

DOPPLER EVALUATION OF ARTERIAL DISEASE IN THE LOWER LEG

The earliest use of Doppler technique was the assessment of arterial blood flow. Clinical evidence of arterial disease is derived from direct and indirect physical findings. The presence or absence of a pulse is considered. Color and temperature of skin and the presence of muscle and skin atrophy is noted. Special arteriography can further aid in the diagnosis.

The arterial anatomy of the leg is fairly simple and

straightforward. The femoral artery is a branch of the common iliac artery. As the femoral artery reaches the area of the knee, it becomes the popliteal artery. In the upper third of the lower leg the popliteal artery divides into the anterior tibial artery and the posterior tibial artery. These vessels then go on to the foot, and the dorsalis pedis is derived from them (Fig. 32-4).

Stenosis of the femoral artery has been detected by noting an increased frequency signal in the Doppler shift. Because of the changes in the depth of the femoral artery as it passes in the tissue of the leg, as well as the difficulty in maintaining a constant transducer angle, it has not proved to be a useful technique. However, in the lower extremity, diagnosis and approximate location of an arterial lesion can be assessed by the quality of the sounds of the blood flow present. Normal arterial flow has a high-frequency first sound of short duration followed by a lower-frequency longer second sound. There is always a pause before the next high-frequency first sound. Arterial abnormalities proximal to the monitoring site produce changes in the sounds. (See Table 32-1.)

Information gained from this examination has proved helpful in a number of situations. Doppler evaluation can indicate whether leg pain is a result of arterial disease and provide information about a pulseless limb. If arterial disease is present in one limb, this method can help evaluate the asymptomatic limb to determine if it should also be studied further. Doppler assessment is also helpful in postoperative follow-up cases. It is employed for the evaluation of limbs with minimal symptoms, since the limb can be serially examined to determine if there is progression of arterial disease.

Table 32-1. Diagnosis of arterial occlusion by quality of Doppler signals*

Quality of signal	Interpretation
High-pitched first sound, lower-pitched second sound, followed by a pause	Normal
Low-pitched first sound, no second sound	Partial occlusion proximally
Prolonged low-frequency first sound, undulating, continous	Complete occlusion proximally; flow is via collaterals
No Doppler signal	Complete occlusion proximally with no collaterals

*From Felix, W. R., Jr., Siegel, B., and Popky, G. L.: Doppler ultrasound in the diagnosis of peripheral vascular disease, Semin. Roentgenol. **10:**315, 1975. Used by permission.

APPENDIXES **EDUCATIONAL REQUIREMENTS AND GUIDELINES**

Appendix A □ The diagnostic ultrasonographer and guidelines for establishing an educational program

DIAGNOSTIC ULTRASONOGRAPHER

The diagnostic ultrasonographer is a skilled person qualified by academic and clinical training to provide patient services using diagnostic ultrasound under the supervision of a physician or osteopath responsible for the use and interpretation of ultrasound procedures. The sonographer may be involved with the patients of the physician in any medical setting for which the physician is responsible.

Education

Individuals admitted for training should have completed high school or the equivalent and should have post–secondary education in the following areas: medical ethics, medical terminology, clinical anatomy and physiology, medical orientation and administration, nursing procedures, general human anatomy, and elementary physics. Individuals in the allied health field of nuclear medicine or radiologic technology are good applicants for diagnostic ultrasound, since they already possess imaging capabilities. Cardiopulmonary technologists and cardiac catheterization technologists have proved to be capable candidates for the echocardiology section of diagnostic ultrasound.

Personal qualifications

Individuals should be mature, responsible, and able to use initiative and independent judgment when necessary. They should have a high standard of medical ethics and empathy with the patient.

Sonographers must have the ability to establish and maintain effective working relationships with patients, employees, physicians, and the general public. They should be capable of working without supervision within the guidelines set by department heads.

Self-motivation to maintain an increasing level of understanding and knowledge of the field and new procedures is necessary for the development of the sonographer.

Skills

The sonographer should have a high degree of technical aptitude with an in-depth knowledge of anatomy and physiology. An ability to improvise the standard of procedure when necessary is essential. The sonographer must be able to supervise the work activities of the backup technologist and ancillary personnel.

Knowledge of ultrasound techniques should be thorough. The number of procedures known will depend on the sonographer's particular interests, background, and training. The general sonographer should have current knowledge of neurology, cardiology, and abdominal and gynecologic applications. In addition, the sonographer must have the ability to deal effectively with patients and to act quickly in an emergency.

A complete knowledge and understanding of the complex instrumentation used to extract the finest quality performance from the equipment is necessary.

The ability to deviate from the normal techniques when necessary and to develop new and better techniques to keep the department up to date is also the responsibility of the sonographer and the physician.

Duties

There are numerous duties the sonographer performs daily. The following duties have been proposed by the American Society of Ultrasound Technical Specialists (A.S.U.T.S.):

1. Prepare the patient for examinations and explain procedures to the patients prior to the examination.

2. Correlate the clinical history with the examination to be performed and obtain the result from other pertinent diagnostic tests to correlate with the ultrasound study.

3. Consult with the referring physician regarding the patient's previous history and the appropriate ultrasonic procedures required.

462

4. Recognize the significance of all structures that are visualized on the oscilloscope.

5. Differentiate artifacts from the normal or pathologic process and recognize electronic equipment limitations.

6. Recognize a diagnostic scan and interpret it but not necessarily give an official reading.

7. Properly label, coat, and mount permanent recordings of the scans for filing.

8. Evaluate new products and equipment for possible future purposes.

9. Research, develop, and formulate new techniques and procedures to be done in the ultrasound department.

10. Maintain a library of ultrasound books and journals for reference by the sonographers and students of the department.

11. Read journals to keep abreast of new techniques and procedures in the field of diagnostic ultrasound.

12. Attend annual conventions and symposiums for the same purpose.

13. Maintain a log to document proof of the sonographic diagnosis with surgical biopsy or autopsy.

Supervision

The sonographer is under the supervision of the director of diagnostic ultrasound. Working under personal initiative to achieve quality work after initial assignments are received, the sonographer may also supervise other staff sonographers with less experience, students of ultrasound, visiting sonographers and physicians, or visiting house staff, medical students, and fellows.

Line of promotion

The larger medical centers with diagnostic ultrasound programs have a more extensive staff than do community hospital laboratories. The former program may have a staff consisting of an educational coordinator, a clinical coordinator, staff instructors, and staff sonographers specializing in neurology, cardiology, and B-scan techniques. The smaller departments may have one to three sonographers sharing the duties of the department.

Performance

The number of cases a sonographer can perform in a day depends on the type of examination ordered; for example, abdominal and cardiac cases may take longer than an obstetric case. Although there is usually a protocol established for each examination, the sonographer may take additional views of the area of interest for a more accurate diagnostic interpretation by the physician. It is difficult to place a rigid time factor for each examination performed because of the anatomic and acoustic properties of each patient. The experienced sonographer, in most cases, should be able to perform an average of ten to twelve cases a day. The approximate time to complete each ultrasound study is as follows:

Echoencephalography, complete: 30 minutes
Echocardiography, complete: 15 to 30 minutes
Doppler: 5 to 10 minutes
Abdominal: 20 to 40 minutes
Renal: 15 to 30 minutes
Gynecologic: 15 to 30 minutes
Obstetric: 10 to 15 minutes
Thyroid: 15 to 20 minutes
Real time: 5 to 10 minutes

Of course, the number of patients a sonographer can examine depends on ancillary personnel to aid in the function of the ultrasound department. Escort service for the patient, secretarial assistance for the mounting, labeling, and sorting the scans, and telephone assistance for appointments and reports are necessary to increase the number of patients the sonographer can examine daily.

Availability

The ultrasound laboratory should determine if 24-hour service is necessary for quality patient care. If it is deemed necessary, the sonographer and physician should provide adequate technical and interpretive skills.

Curriculum

The structure of the curriculum for individuals meeting the entrance requirements should be based on a minimum of a calendar year (twelve months) of full-time study. This is to provide didactic content of appropriate scope and depth as well as clinical experiences of sufficient variety and quantity to ensure adequate opportunity to acquire the needed knowledge and skills.

The subject matter for a one-year program would include introduction to basic physics, ultrasound applications of physics and biologic safety, laboratory experiments, instrumentation, biometrics, cross-sectional anatomy, pathology, physiology, cardiology, clinical medicine, differential diagnosis, comparison of other diagnostic modalities, ultrasonic techniques, interpretation, and journal review, research, and clinical experience.

The number of students selected for each program

should be proportional to the ultrasound staff and should not exceed a ratio of 3:1. The instructors should be qualified in their respective areas of ultrasound. Additional nonultrasound instructors are valuable in areas of anatomy, physics, and pathology for correlation with the ultrasound presentation.

Continuing education

The sonographer should maintain an active interest in the field of ultrasound. A current library of ultrasound textbooks, videotapes, slide series, and journals should be maintained in the laboratory as a reference for updating current techniques and interpretations. The sonographer should be encouraged to attend local and regional ultrasound seminars. Attendance at the national ultrasound and echocardiography meetings is important for the sonographer to keep abreast of current developments in the field. Visiting experts in ultrasound should be encouraged to visit particular laboratories if special techniques are newly employed.

GUIDELINES FOR THE ESTABLISHMENT OF A DIAGNOSTIC ULTRASOUND EDUCATIONAL PROGRAM

Since the 1970s, interest in ultrasound has risen geometrically, causing an acute shortage of educated sonographers and physicians. This demand has been the impetus for the extensive development of training facilities.

The A.S.U.T.S. and several of the leading medical schools have developed extensive programs in diagnostic ultrasound. These programs have evolved through the cooperative efforts of physicians and sonographers dedicated to quality education in ultrasound. Much of the material has been revised through the experience of the program directors. It is through these revisions that the following guidelines are presented to institutions interested in establishing such an educational program.

Admission requirements

The diagnostic sonographer is a unique member of the allied health field, working closely with the physician to reach a diagnosis through the use of ultrasound. Qualifications and duties of the sonographer have already been discussed; therefore it will suffice to re-emphasize the responsibility and clinical exposure the sonographer must have to be an asset to the clinician. Thus it was decided not to admit students directly from high school but to admit instead those students who have completed a two-year allied health program or two years of undergraduate work.

Persons admitted for training into diagnostic medical sonography programs should have completed high school or the equivalent and should have post–secondary education in the following areas:
1. Anatomy and physiology
2. Basic physics
3. Basic mathematics
4. Medical terminology
5. Oral and written communications
6. General chemistry
7. Psychology/sociology
8. Basic patient care
9. Medical ethics and jurisprudence

Institutions

The ideal location for such programs has been within the confines of the medical center, hospital, clinic, or busy physician's office. Junior and senior colleges and universities have had success establishing ultrasound programs when working in conjunction with an active medical center. Some institutions will work cooperatively to offer a total program to the students. Thus specialized hospitals performing echocardiograms, obstetric care, and so on could be attended on a rotating basis for the student's learning experience. If carefully structured and monitored, this rotating program could be effective in providing the student with several technical outlooks during the training period.

Number of students

The number of students selected for each program should be proportional to the ultrasound staff and should not exceed a ratio of 3:1. Ideally, two students to each sonographer allows a more in-depth clinical exposure.

Length of the program

Because ultrasound encompasses so many aspects, a general program involving all aspects of diagnostic ultrasound should be a minimum of one year. Shorter programs have been attempted without success. The six-month program does not allow sufficient didactic and clinical exposure to the field. A sample curriculum is provided on p. 465.

Instructors

Instructors should be qualified in their respective areas of ultrasound. It is recommended that the instructors complete a formal training program in ultrasound and have clinical experience beyond training. The Registry for Diagnostic Medical Sonographers

DIAGNOSTIC ULTRASOUND CURRICULUM: ONE-YEAR PROGRAM

	Hours			Hours
Quarter 1			**Quarter 2—cont'd**	
Hours 480			**Hours 480—cont'd**	
Anatomy			Clinical medicine	24
Introductory gross anatomy	5		Ultrasound techniques	
Physics			Neurology	5
Introductory physics	12		Cardiology	12
Cardiology			Abdominal	12
Clinical conference	12		Obstetrics	8
Interpretation	15		Gynecology	4
Technique	12		Doppler	4
Neurology			Superficial	3
Technique	12		Interpretation	30
Interpretation	8		Journal club	12
Abdomen			Clinical experience	67
Technique	12		Holiday (1)	8
Interpretation	12			
Obstetrics/gynecology			**Quarters 3 and 4**	
Technique	12		**Hours 960**	
Interpretation	10			
Research	48		Anatomy	
Journal club	12		Research project	24
Clinical experience	274		Clinical rotations	
Holidays (3)	24		Neurology	45
			Cardiology (includes conference)	144
Quarter 2			Abdominal	120
Hours 480			Superficial	45
			Obstetrics/gynecology	90
Anatomy			Doppler	42
Gross anatomy	8		Elective	90
Cross-sectional	8		Review session	64
Sagittal	8		Journal club	32
Review	6		Teaching file	32
Physics			Interpretation	120
Lecture	36		Holidays (6)	48
Laboratory	48		Vacation	64
Pathology	12			
Cardiology				
Didactic	24			
Clinical	12			
Auscultation and				
physical examination	5			

should be taken by the instructors to measure their competence on a national level. The physicians involved in the program likewise should have formal training either through short courses or in their residency or fellowship program. It is generally agreed that physicians should spend a minimum of three months to an ideal of one year in ultrasound prior to entering the teaching profession.

If the program has at least six students, the staff may be composed of a director of ultrasound and staff physicians with specialty areas in anatomy, neurology, cardiology, abdominal and renal studies, and obstetrics and gynecology. A physicist who specializes in

acoustic energy or ultrasound is highly recommended. The sonographers should comprise an educational coordinator, chief sonographer, and staff sonographers with specialty areas in neurology, cardiology, abdominal and renal studies, and obstetrics and gynecology. These staff members may overlap in some areas, but as the program expands, so should the staff specialty areas develop.

Tuition

Fees should be kept at a minimum to support the program. Outside speakers and additional teaching equipment such as audiovisual aids, library facilities, organ models, and so on may have to be financed through the students' tuition. It is recommended that most institutions charge $100 or less a month to support such a program. Grants or stipends are offered in a few educational centers.

Recommended program for diagnostic sonographers

Physics is an important part of ultrasound, and care should be taken to chose a physicist with experience in acoustic properties or ultrasound modalities. The course should consist of an introduction to the basic laws of physics, followed by a concentrated approach in ultrasound physics, including biologic safety. Laboratory experiments should be used to further emphasize lecture material, with concentration on transducer construction, testing and evaluation, frequency change effects, and so on. A thorough understanding of ultrasonic equipment is necessary to facilitate quality operation of such machinery. An understanding of biometrics and statistical analysis may be beneficial in the research-directed program.

Anatomic relationships are the core of the ultrasound examination; therefore this subject cannot be overemphasized. We have found it particularly useful to begin with gross anatomy and then proceed to cross-sectional and sagittal relationships of anatomy. Our anatomist has sectioned two cadavers, one in the sagittal plane and the other in the transverse plane, and has had these sections mounted in plastic containers for use in the classroom. Additional instruction in embryology would give the students a better understanding of anatomic anomalies, defects, and variations that appear in the developmental process.

Pathology provides the sonographer with an insight into the ultrasonic visualization of disease. Gross pathology is probably the most helpful to the sonographer. This class could be held in the surgical pathology classroom or could be illustrated by slides of gross pathologic specimens and their sections. The consistency of cystic masses versus solid tumors enables the sonographer to gain a better understanding of the scans to be performed.

Physiology should be a prerequisite to the program so that the subject may be presented in more depth in specialized areas of neurology, cardiology, and specific organ function.

The sonographer needs to have an understanding of various aspects of clinical medicine as related to ultrasound. We have found it useful to be able to evaluate the patients' clinical symptoms and history prior to performing the examination. This eliminates unnecessary scanning time if an initial differential diagnosis is made prior to the study. After the study is completed, the sonographer should be able to present an initial preliminary reading with differentials to be presented to the physician. The other diagnostic modalities should be presented to provide the sonographer with a better understanding of the final diagnosis.

Cardiology lectures may be provided in electrocardiography, phonocardiography, vector cardiography, carotid and jugular pulse tracings, cardiac catheterization, cardiac disease processes, and congenital anomalies. Attendance at joint conferences between cardiology and ultrasound personnel should be encouraged to evaluate echocardiograms. In addition, the clinical cardiology conference presents the total history, diagnostic evaluation, interpretation, and discussion of the cardiac patient.

Ultrasonic techniques include scanning protocol and procedures necessary to perform an adequate examination. This should be combined with clinical experience and ultrasonic interpretation.

Journal review of current articles enables the student to keep abreast of current developments and to gain an insight into investigative research and data collection for use in the student's own particular research project.

Ultrasonic equipment

Sufficient equipment should be available for the students to gain clinical competence in the ultrasonic examination. Each student should be able to spend at least 25% to 30% of the daily allotted time physically learning the "art" of scanning. The state-of-the-art equipment should be available for the training center. Ideally it would include commercially different greyscale, real-time, A-mode, M-mode, and Doppler equipment. Optional equipment would include the pulsed Doppler, ophthalmologic instruments, a computerized real-time scanner, and the Octoson.

Teaching aids

Attendance at weekly cardiac conferences is beneficial to the students involved in echocardiography. These conferences are generally of two types. A clinical cardiac conference involves clinical case presentations of two or more patients. Patient symptoms, history, and results of ECG, vector, phonocardiography, treadmill, echocardiography, cardiac catheterization, and surgical evaluation are presented. The other type of cardiac conference is more didactic, involving specific cardiac subjects including invasive and noninvasive cardiac procedures.

Additional teaching aids should be used throughout

the program. Attendance at outside courses and seminars provides the individual with exposure to current new developments in ultrasound. Visiting physicians and sonographers often add to the educational program by relating personal experience with ultrasonic techniques and problems. Review of problem cases with these visitors is sometimes a beneficial exercise. New techniques can also be adopted or experimented with as the result of such visits.

Local society meetings may be educationally stimulating to the training programs. Guest speakers and case presentations provide the sonographer with continued challenge in this field. Many regions now have specialized local meetings, and thus echocardiography may be discussed exclusively or in combination with other ultrasound modalities.

Currently there are video slide sets, videotapes, and cassette tapes available from the known experts in ultrasound. These should be a supplementary part of the ultrasound program.

Library facilities should include all current books, journals, and reprints on diagnostic ultrasound. Students should be encouraged to read as much material as they can during their educational exposure. Journals can routinely be assigned to certain students. Each student should be required to copy the pertinent ultrasound articles for reference and discussion in the weekly or bimonthly journal club review. This exposes students to current literature in a uniform manner and encourages them to read and selectively interpret the available information.

Research assignments are an important part of the student's training. The first project should be a review of literature and/or cases on a particular subject of the student's choice. This paper will be critiqued by and discussed among the other students. The second project should consist of research in which the student actually evaluates one particular aspect of ultrasound. Thus scanning techniques, artifacts, patient data, and evaluation, as well as a review of the pertinent literature are included in this paper.

Some laboratories may find field trips to other laboratories useful. This exposes the student to new or different techniques available to the ultrasonographer. Trips to manufacturers of equipment or transducers may promote understanding and appreciation of ultrasonic equipment.

Of course, interdepartmental exposure to other diagnostic modalities should be incorporated if the student has limited exposure in this area. Thus exposure to cardiac catheterization, phonocardiography, treadmill, electrocardiography, cardiac clinic, radiology, and nuclear medicine will add to the student's understanding of the echographic procedure.

Appendix B □ Specialized echocardiographic training

Diagnostic ultrasound has been widely established as a valuable clinical tool over the past two decades. Within the realm of diagnostic ultrasound is echocardiography, which has proved to be the fastest growing specialty within this noninvasive field. "It is a well-known fact that, in skilled hands, echocardiography provides reliable and valuable information on the structure and function of the heart. The basis for diagnosis is evaluation of the size, position, configuration, and motion of structures, and the assessment of anatomical and functional relationships within the heart."*

The purpose of this discussion is to provide echocardiographers with guidelines for developing quality training programs. The growth of echocardiography will only be as efficient as the echocardiographer's growth. Thus education plays a primary role in the development of this nontraumatic technique.

ECHOCARDIOGRAPHIC EXAMINATION

Echocardiography is a unique field in medicine in that it requires a tremendous amount of experience and knowledge on the operator's part. Unlike other diagnostic tests that have eliminated the operator error, echocardiograms are only as good as the operator can produce.

Currently the mode of ultrasound used most frequently in the echocardiographic examination is the time-motion pulse-echo. This mode allows the echocardiographer to graphically display the dynamic motion and function of the heart. The anatomy and hemodynamics existing within the heart cause the intracardiac structures to move in patterns that have been identified as indicative of specific diseases (Feigenbaum, 1972). It has proved itself a superior diagnostic tool in the evaluation of pericardial effusion. Increasingly it has been used in the detection of vegetations on the mitral and aortic apparatus, and the

evaluation of atrial myxomas has proved advantageous as a noninvasive technique in echocardiography. The determination of enlarged left ventricular dimensions versus increased left ventricular mass is especially helpful in patients who display an enlarged cardiac silhouette on chest x-ray examination. Increased left ventricular mass is generally due to hypertensive cardiac disease, which appears echographically as a symmetrical increase in interventricular septum and posterior left ventricular wall dimensions. Cardiomyopathy has now been established by the demonstration of particular echographic patterns, such as thinning of the interventricular septum and posterior left ventricular wall, increased echoes in systole on the ALMV, increased distance from e point of the mitral valve to the interventricular septum, and generalized cardiac enlargement. Evaluation of the degree of aortic insufficiency can be made by examining the ALMV with a decrease in the E-F slope, the amount of flutter, and premature closure of the ALMV. The evaluation of mitral and aortic stenosis has been widely accepted through echocardiography. Pulmonary and tricuspid valves are generally more difficult to record, but when shown they can also be evaluated for stenosis or regurgitant patterns.

Research is currently being done to determine the effects of drugs on cardiac function. Through echocardiography the amount of increase or decrease in both the E-F slope of the ALMV and the endocardial velocity of the left ventricular wall can be measured. Echocardiology is also useful as a follow-up technique in postoperative cardiac patients, in renal patients to detect pericardial effusion, and in patients on cardiac drug therapy (propranolol [Inderal]) to measure changes in cardiac function.

GUIDELINES FOR EDUCATIONAL PROGRAMS

Guidelines for educational programs have been established by the American Society for Echocardiography (A.S.E.), the American Society for Ultrasound Technical Specialists (A.S.U.T.S.), and the American Institute of Ultrasound in Medicine (A.I.U.M.). Al-

---

*From Gramiak, R., et al.: Report of the Inter-Society Commission for Heart Disease Resources: optimal resources for ultrasonic examination of the heart, Circulation **51**:A1-A7, June, 1975. By permission of the American Heart Association, Inc.

though there is controversy among these societies regarding the length of training, the basic requirements for a quality echocardiographic program are similar. Each viewpoint will be discussed in regard to physician and technology programs.

Physician training

Echocardiography is an operator-dependent examination that demands instantaneous and continuous interpretive evaluation as well as a high level of technical skill (Gramiak et al., 1975). Unless the nature and significance of various echo patterns are immediately recognized, they will not usually be adequately recorded, and an examination of diagnostic quality will not be obtained. Thus a *physician* responsible for obtaining and interpreting the echocardiogram should have the following qualifications as determined by the Inter-Society Commission for Heart Disease Resources:

1. A thorough background in cardiac anatomy, physiology, hemodynamics, and pathology and the ability to conceptualize three-dimensional spatial relationships in functioning cardiac structures
2. The ability to recognize and interpret variations of normal and pathologic patterns on the echocardiographic tracing
3. A thorough understanding of the physical and technical principles of ultrasound instrumentation and its proper and safe use
4. A working knowledge of the electrocardiogram and phonocardiogram to facilitate their correlation with the echocardiographic tracing
5. A knowledge and understanding of each patient's clinical problem*

Many programs are now incorporated within the cardiology fellowship rotation, in which three or more months are spent actively involved in echocardiology, and the physician's echocardiographic ability is verified by the echocardiographer in charge. These laboratories should perform at least twenty cases a week under the supervision of qualified personnel. Active participation should be included in the training program, which involves echocardiographic correlation with the patient's phonocardiogram, vector, treadmill, cardiac catheterization, and surgery results. Participation in cardiac conferences is highly recommended, not only for the echocardiographer's sake but also to instruct the hospital staff on the uses of echocardiography.

*From Gramiak, R., et al.: Report of the Inter-Society Commission for Heart Disease Resources: optimal resources for ultrasonic examination of the heart, Circulation **51**:A1-A7, June, 1975. By permission of the American Heart Association, Inc.

Noncardiologist physicians believe that a specialty in echocardiography should be at least one year in length beyond residency. Instruction in cardiac anatomy, physiology, hemodynamics, pathology, electrocardiology, phonocardiology, and basic ultrasound physics should be included in the program. Minimum case load should be between twenty-five and forty cases a week. If the student is involved in a general ultrasound program, 20% to 30% of the time should be spent in echocardiology.

Echocardiographers must keep up with new developments through available literature. Since many journals now include echocardiography articles, it is necessary to be aware of all sources. *Current Contents* may be useful in this respect. Many articles appear monthly in *Circulation, The American Journal of Cardiology, Annals of Internal Medicine*, and *Chest.*

Numerous short-term courses in echocardiology are offered to keep the echocardiographers informed of current information. The national cardiology meetings now devote a considerable amount of attention to the most significant developments in echocardiography. Several postgraduate courses are being planned through medical schools in cooperation with the American Heart Association to keep physicians abreast of the current concepts in cardiac care with echocardiography. In addition, several laboratories conduct one-week courses specifically in echocardiography, which serves as a good introduction for the novice echocardiographer. In a field as operator-dependent as echocardiography, it is impossible to master the technique in a short period of time. Care must be taken to correlate data with cardiac catheterization and clinical symptoms of each patient. Misinterpretations are made by the inexperienced and those with limited training, and this leads to poor quality echocardiography.

Technologist training

"Technicians should examine patients only under supervision of a physician competent in echocardiography who, if at all possible, should be available to assist with difficult studies. Close supervision is necessary because information selected or rejected for inclusion in the echocardiographic tracing requires repeated medical judgements to assure its diagnostic content and accuracy. The ultimate responsibility for these judgements must remain with the physician."*

*From Gramiak, R., et al.: Report of the Inter-Society Commission for Heart Disease Resources: optimal resources for ultrasonic examination of the heart, Circulation **51**:A1-A7, June, 1975. By permission of the American Heart Association, Inc.

The technologist, if properly motivated and trained, has the capacity to function as a true physician's assistant, playing a dynamic and intelligent role in the diagnosis and management of the cardiac patient (Chang, 1975).

The exact training of the technologist is probably under more controversy with A.S.E. and A.S.U.T.S. than is the physician's training, although each group maintains that the program should be at least three months of full-time study. The merits of each approach will be discussed.

The first viewpoint maintains that technicians usually learn echocardiography best if they have already had exposure to cardiac anatomy and physiology. Understanding of electrocardiography, phonocardiography, and hemodynamics involved with cardiac catheterization are extremely helpful. The best technicians seem to come from cardiac catheterization or phonocardiographic laboratories (Feigenbaum, 1974). Many of these technicians are trained by the physician who employs them (Chang, 1975), and many have had at least some college, a degree in a science-related field, or previous nursing experience (Chang, 1974). All have prior experience with multiple diagnostic laboratories (Chang, 1975). On-the-job training with a physician experienced in echocardiography is emphasized. The technologists are exposed to new techniques by attending short-term courses, national meetings, or obtaining information from the available cardiac journals. Periodic visits to other active echocardiographic laboratories also promotes continued growth. Of course, the daily feedback obtained by other noninvasive cardiac examinations, cardiac catheterization, and surgery and/or autopsy is included routinely.

The second viewpoint maintains that there should be a multidisciplinary ultrasound program available with echocardiography as one of its disciplines. The technologist may be qualified in more than one area and may specify competence in a particular area. The degree of responsibility a technologist may assume requires that the knowledge, skills, and abilities necessary to provide those services appropriate to the diagnostic ultrasound sonographer be assimilated by the conclusion of the formal education.

These programs may be established in junior or senior colleges and universities, medical schools, hospitals and clinics, or vocational/technical schools and institutions. Most of these programs are affiliated with medical schools or hospitals. Prerequisites for persons entering such programs are two years of allied health background or two years of college with an emphasis on biologic sciences.

The number of students selected for each program should be proportional to the ultrasound staff and should not exceed a ratio of 3:1. The general consensus is that the length of this program should be one year (Hagen, 1974). However, the curriculum may be structured to allow students to progress at an individual pace, thus enabling students to finish in less than the normal required time.

Instructors should be qualified in their respective area of ultrasound. Within the general ultrasound program a cardiologist, preferably with experience in echocardiography, is a necessity for a good program. The clinical correlation, auscultatory findings, and cardiac diagnosis lend to a well-coordinated program that which only the cardiologist can employ. There must also be sonographic technical competence in echocardiography to classify as a quality program.

Echocardiographic equipment

Echocardiographic equipment necessary to execute this examination is becoming specialized to the point whereby it will be virtually useless for other ultrasound examination procedures (Chang, 1975). Former storage scope monitors have been supplanted by continuous low-persistence sweeping monitors. Many echocardiography machines have specific modifications to make their equipment more compatible for echocardiography. Gain adjustments, damping effects, and transducer megahertz controls are all specific for echocardiography. An additional characteristic of echocardiographic equipment is portability. It becomes imperative to be able to examine many critically ill cardiac patients at their bedside or in the emergency room before further evaluation. Thus the equipment should be mobile, as compact as possible, and available on an emergency basis.

Current strip-chart recorders with multichannel options are now routinely used with echographic equipment.

New advances in cardiac imaging may deem it necessary to share equipment with other departments or may support the concept of a generalized ultrasound laboratory. Real-time two-dimensional imaging is currently available as a recognized diagnostic modality. Its usefulness has been shown in the detection of small pericardial effusion, calcified mitral valve apparatus, prolapse of the mitral valve, asymmetrical septal hypertrophy, and detection of ventricular aneurysms. As a result, many echocardiographic examinations are incomplete without real-time equipment.

The pulsed Doppler technique is another method with multiple capabilities. The increase or decrease in blood flow has proved to be clinically useful, especially with regurgitation and septal defects.

Echocardiographic program

Besides including other diagnostic ultrasound modalities, the recommended program for sonographers is so extensive that it covers many areas pertinent to the echocardiographer. The program would present material in an organized, well-developed format. Instructors in ultrasonography, physics, anatomy, physiology, pathology, and clinical medicine would conduct the majority of the didactic training. All clinical experience would be performed under the guidance of highly qualified ultrasonographers.

Specific requirements for an echocardiographic program include gross anatomy, cross-sectional anatomy, cardiac physiology, hemodynamics, disease process, pathology, clinical signs and symptoms, differential diagnosis, auscultation, and noninvasive and invasive techniques.

Teaching aids

Attendance at weekly cardiac conferences is beneficial to students involved in echocardiography. These conferences are generally of two types—clinical and theoretical. A clinical cardiac conference involves clinical case presentations of two or more patients, including patient symptoms, history, ECG, vector, phonocardiography, treadmill, echocardiography, cardiac catheterization, and surgical evaluation; the other type of conference is more didactic, involving specific cardiac subjects including invasive and noninvasive cardiac procedures.

Additional teaching aids should be utilized throughout the program. Attendance at outside courses and seminars provides the individual with exposure to new developments in ultrasound. Visiting physicians and sonographers often add to the educational program by relating personal experience to ultrasonic techniques and problems. Review of problem cases is sometimes a rewarding exercise with these visitors. New techniques can also be adopted or experimented with as the result of such visits.

Local society meetings may be educationally stimulating to the training programs. Guest speakers and case presentations provide the sonographer with continued challenge in this field. Many regions now have specialized local meetings; thus echocardiography may be discussed exclusively or in combination with other ultrasound modalities.

Currently there are numerous video slide sets, videotapes, and cassette tapes made available by the experts in ultrasound. These should be a supplementary part of the ultrasound program.

Library facilities should include all current books, journals, and reprints on diagnostic ultrasound. Students should be encouraged to read as much material as possible during their educational exposure. Journals can routinely be assigned to certain students. Each student should be required to copy the pertinent ultrasound articles for personal reference and for discussion in the weekly or bimonthly journal club review. Students are thus exposed to current literature and encouraged to read and selectively interpret a wealth of information.

Research assignments are an important part of the student's training. The first project should be a review of literature and/or cases on a particular subject of the student's choice. This paper will be discussed among the other students, who in turn will critique the paper. The second project should consist of a research project in which the student actually evaluated one particular aspect of ultrasound. Thus scanning techniques, artifacts, patient data and evaluation, as well as a review of the pertinent literature are included in this paper.

Some laboratories may find field trips to other laboratories valuable. These expose the students to new or different techniques available to the ultrasonographer. Trips to manufacturers of equipment or transducers may prove useful to the understanding and appreciation of ultrasonic equipment.

Of course, interdepartmental exposure to other diagnostic modalities should be incorporated if the student has limited exposure in this area. Thus exposure to cardiac catheterization, phonocardiography, treadmill, electrocardiography, cardiac clinic, radiology, and nuclear medicine will add to the student's understanding of the echographic procedure.

Bibliography

Physics (Chapters 1 and 2)

Brown, B., and Gordon, D.: Ultrasonic techniques in biology and medicine, Springfield, Ill., 1967, Charles C Thomas, Publisher.

Brown, R.: Ultrasonography, St. Louis, 1975, Warren H. Green, Inc.

Carlin, B.: Ultrasonics, New York, 1960, McGraw-Hill Book Co.

Condon, B., and Oddishaw, H.: Handbook of physics, New York, 1967, McGraw-Hill Book Co.

Freeman, I.: Sound and ultrasonics, New York, 1968, Random House, Inc.

General Dynamics Convair Division: Nondestructive testing: basic principles. Volume I. 1967.

Goldberg, B. B., Kotler, M., Ziskin, M., and Waxham, R.: Diagnostic uses of ultrasound, New York, 1975, Grune & Stratton, Inc.

Hagen, S. L., et al.: Body scanning, Cleveland, 1975, Picker Corporation.

Halliday, D., and Resnick, R.: Physics for students of science and engineering, New York, 1963, John Wiley & Sons, Inc.

Heuter, T., and Bolt, R.: Sonics, New York, 1955, John Wiley & Sons, Inc.

Hussey, M.: Diagnostic ultrasound, London, 1975, Blackie & Sons, Ltd.

Kazner, E., Ceulieger, M., Muller, H. R., and McCready, V. R.: Ultrasonics in medicine, Amsterdam, Excerpta Medica.

Kelly, E.: Ultrasonic energy, Urbana, Ill., 1965, University of Illinois Press.

King, D.: Diagnostic ultrasound, St. Louis, 1974, The C. V. Mosby Co.

McDicken, W. N.: Diagnostic ultrasonics: principles and use of instruments, New York, 1976, John Wiley & Sons, Inc.

Miller, F.: College physics, New York, 1972, Harcourt Brace Jovanovich, Inc.

Wells, P. N. T.: Physical principles of ultrasonic diagnosis, New York, 1969, Academic Press, Inc.

Wells, P. N. T.: Ultrasonics in clinical diagnosis, Edinburgh, 1972, Churchill Livingstone.

Echocardiography (Chapters 3-16)
General

Allen, H., Goldberg, S., Sahn, D., Ovitt, T., and Goldberg, B.: Suprasternal notch echocardiography: assessment of its clinical utility in pediatric cardiology, Circulation 55:605, 1977.

Borer, J. S., Henry, W. L., and Epstein, S. E.: Echocardiographic observations in patients with systemic infiltrative disease involving the heart, Am. J. Card. 39:184, 1977.

Cooper, R., and Leopold, G.: Diagnostic ultrasound in cardiology, Med. Ann. D.C. 41:748, 1972.

Cortina, A., and Lopez-Bescos, L.: Ultrasonics in cardiology, Rev. Esp. Cardiol. 26:15, 1973.

Dillon, J., and Feigenbaum, H.: Echocardiography, J. Indiana State Med. Assoc. 67:104, 1974.

Feigenbaum, H.: Clinical applications of echocardiography, Prog. Cardiovasc. Dis. 14:531, 1972.

Feigenbaum, H.: Echocardiography, Philadelphia, 1972, Lea & Febiger.

Feigenbaum, H.: Echocardiography, Cardiovascular Review, World Medical News, 1973.

Feigenbaum, H.: Newer aspects of echocardiography, Circulation 47:833, 1973.

Feigenbaum, H.: Ultrasound as a clinical tool in valvular heart disease, Cardiovasc. Clin. 5:219, 1973.

Feigenbaum, H.: Educational problems in echocardiography (editorial), Am. J. Cardiol. 34:741, 1974.

Feigenbaum, H.: Hazards of echocardiographic interpretation (editorial), N. Engl. J. Med. 289:1311, 1974.

Feigenbaum, H., Dillon, J., and Chang, S.: Recent developments in echocardiography. In Russek, H. I., editor: New horizons in cardiovascular practice, Baltimore, 1975, University Park Press.

Friedman, W. F., et al.: A review: newer, noninvasive cardiac diagnostic methods, 1977, International Pediatric Research Foundation.

Goldberg, B. B.: Suprasternal ultrasonography, J.A.M.A. 215:245, 1972.

Goldberg, S., Allen, H., and Sahn, D.: Pediatric and adolescent echocardiography: a handbook, Chicago, 1975, Year Book Medical Publishers, Inc.

Goldschoager, S., et al.: Right atrial myxoma with right to left shunt and polycythemia presenting as congenital heart disease, Am. J. Cardiol. 30:82, 1972.

Gramiak, R.: Cardiac ultrasonography. A review of current applications, Radiol. Clin. North Am. 9:469, 1971.

Gramiak, R.: Echocardiography, J.A.M.A. 229:1009, 1974.

Gramiak, R., Shah, P., and Kramer, D.: Ultrasound cardiography: contrast studies in anatomy and function, Radiology 92:939, 1969.

Gramiak, R., et al.: Report of the inter-society commission for heart disease resources. Optimal resources for ultrasonic examination of the heart, J. Clin. Ultrasound 3:2, 1975.

Harbold, N., Jr., and Gau, G.: Echocardiographic diagnosis of right atrial myxoma, Mayo Clin. Proc. 48:284, 1973.

Kerber, R.: Errors in performance and interpretation of echocardiograms, J. Clin. Ultrasound 1:330, 1973.

Kerber, R., Kioschos, J., and Lauer, R.: Use of an ultrasonic contrast method in the diagnosis of valvular regurgitation and intracardiac shunts, Am. J. Cardiol. 34:722, 1974.

Pai, A. L., Cahill, N. S., Dubroff, R. J., et al.: Digital computer analysis of M-scan echocardiograms, J. Clin. Ultrasound 4:173, 1976.

Schieken, R. M., and Kerber, R. E.: Echocardiographic abnormalities in acute rheumatic fever, Am. J. Cardiol. 38:458, 1976.

Mitral valve

Abbasi, A. S., MacAlpin, R. N., Eber, L. M., et al.: Echocardiographic diagnosis of idiopathic hypertrophic cardiomyopathy without outflow obstruction, Circulation 46:897, 1972.

Barlow, J. B., Pocock, W. A., Marchand, P., and Denny, M.: The significance of late systolic murmurs, Am. Heart J. 66:443, 1963.

Bolton, M. R., Jr., King, J. F., Polumbo, R. A., et al.: The effects of operation on the echocardiographic features of idiopathic subaortic stenosis, Circulation 50:897, 1974.

Botvinick, E. H., Schiller, N. B., Wickramasekaren, R., et al.: Echocardiographic demonstration of early mitral valve closure in severe aortic insufficiency. Its clinical implications, Circulation 51:836, 1975.

Burgess, J., Clark, R., Kamigaki, M., et al.: Echocardiographic findings in different types of mitral regurgitation, Circulation **48:**97, 1973.

Chung, K., Manning, J., and Gramiak, R.: Echocardiography in coexisting hypertrophic subaortic stenosis and fixed left ventricular outflow obstruction, Circulation **49:**673, 1974.

Craige, E., and Fortuin, J.: Studies on mitral valve motion in the presence of the Austin-Flint murmur, Trans. Am. Clin. Climatol. Assoc. **83:**209, 1972.

DeMaria, A. N., King, J. F., Bogren, H. G., et al.: The variable spectrum of echocardiographic manifestations of the mitral valve prolapse syndrome, Circulation **50:**33, 1974.

DeMaria, A., Lies, J. E., King, J. F., et al.: Echographic assessment of atrial transport, mitral movement, and ventricular performance following electroversion of supraventricular arrhythmias, Circulation **51:**273, 1975.

Dillon, J. C., Feigenbaum, H., Konecke, L. L., Davis, R. H., and Chang, S.: Echocardiographic manifestations of valvular vegetations, Am. Heart J. **86:**698, 1973.

Dillon, J. C., Haine, C. L., Chang, S., et al.: Use of echocardiography in patients with prolapsed mitral valve, Circulation **43:**503, 1971.

Dodd, M., and Wilcken, D.: Echocardiography in left atrial myxoma: relation to the findings in mitral stenosis, Aust. N.Z. J. Med. **2:**124, 1972.

Duchak, J. M., Jr., Chang, S., and Feigenbaum, H.: The posterior mitral valve echo and the echocardiographic diagnosis of mitral stenosis, Am. J. Cardiol. **29:**628, 1972.

Finegan, R., and Harrison, D.: Diagnosis of left atrial myxoma by echocardiography, N. Engl. J. Med. **282:**1022, 1970.

Flaherty, J., Livengood, S., and Fortuin, N.: Atypical posterior leaflet motion in echocardiogram in mitral stenosis, Am. J. Cardiol. **35:**675, 1975.

Fortuin, N., and Craige, E.: Echocardiographic studies of genesis of mitral diastolic murmurs, Br. Heart J. **35:**75, 1973.

Goodman, D., Harrison, D., and Popp, R.: Echocardiographic features of primary pulmonary hypertension, Am. Heart J. **86:**847, 1973.

Goodman, D., Harrison, D., and Popp, R.: Echocardiographic features of primary pulmonary hypertension, Am. J. Cardiol. **33:**438, 1974.

Gramiak, R., and Waag, R. C.: Cardiac ultrasound, St. Louis, 1975, The C. V. Mosby Co.

Henry, W., Clark, C., and Epstein, S.: Asymmetric septal hypertrophy: the unifying link in the IHSS disease spectrum. Observations regarding its pathogenesis, pathophysiology and course, Circulation **47:**827, 1973.

Henry, W. L., Clark, C. E., Glancy, D. L., et al.: Echocardiographic measurement of the left ventricular outflow gradient in idiopathic hypertrophic subaortic stenosis, N. Engl. J. Med. **288:**989, 1973.

Hernberg, J., Weiss, B., and Keegan, A.: The ultrasonic recording of aortic valve motion, Radiology **94:**361, 1970.

Johnson, A., Lonky, S., and Carleton, R.: Combined hypertrophic subaortic stenosis and calcific aortic valvular stenosis, Am. J. Cardiol. **35:**706, 1975.

Johnson, M. L., Holmes, J. H., Spangler, R. D., et al.: Usefulness of echocardiography in patients undergoing mitral valve surgery, J. Thorac. Cardiovasc. Surg. **64:**922, 1972.

Johnson, M. L., et al.: Echocardiographic diagnosis of a left atrial myxoma found attached to the free left atrial wall, J. Clin. Ultrasound **1:**75, 1973.

Kamigaki, M., and Goldschlager, N.: Echocardiographic analysis of mitral valve motion in atrial septal defect, Am. J. Cardiol. **30:**343, 1972.

Kerber, R., Kelly, D., Jr., and Gutenkauf, C.: Left atrial myxoma.

Demonstrated by stop-action cardiac ultrasonography, Am. J. Cardiol. **34:**838, 1974.

King, J. F., De Maria, A. N., Miller, R. R., et al.: Markedly abnormal mitral valve motion without simultaneous interventricular pressure gradient due to uneven mitral-septum contact in idiopathic hypertrophic subaortic stenosis, Am. J. Cardiol. **34:**360, 1974.

Konecke, L. L., Feigenbaum, H., Chang, S., et al.: Abnormal mitral valve motion in patients with elevated left ventricular diastolic pressures, Circulation **47:**989, 1973.

Levisman, J. A., and Abbasi, A. S.: Abnormal motion of the mitral valve with pericardial effusion: pseudo-prolapse of the mitral valve, Am. Heart J. **91:**18, 1976.

Lortscher, R. H., Toews, W. H., Nora, J. J., et al.: Left atrial myxoma presenting as rheumatic fever, Chest **66:**302, 1974.

Markiewicz, W., Stoner, J., London, E., Hunt, S., and Popp, R. L.: Effect of transducer placement on echocardiographic mitral valve systolic motion, Eur. J. Cardiol. **4:**359, 1976.

Meyer, J. F., Frank, M. J., Goldberg, S., and Cheng, T. O.: Systolic mitral flutter, an echocardiographic clue to the diagnosis of ruptured chordae tendineae, Am. Heart J. **93:**3, 1977.

Nanda, N. C., Gramiak, R., Shah, P. M., et al.: Echocardiography in the diagnosis of idiopathic hypertrophic subaortic stenosis coexisting with aortic valve disease, Circulation **50:**752, 1974.

Nanda, N. C., Gramiak, R., Shah, P. M., et al.: Mitral commissurotomy versus replacement: preoperative evaluation by echocardiography, Circulation **51:**263, 1975.

Nasser, W. K., Davis, R. H., Dillon, J. C., Tavel, M. E., Helmen, C. H., Feigenbaum, H., and Fisch, C.: Atrial myxoma. Part I. Clinical and pathologic features in nine cases, Am. Heart J. **83:**694, 1972.

Nasser, W., et al.: Atrial myxoma. Part II. Phonocardiographic, echocardiographic, hemodynamic and angiographic features in nine cases, Am. Heart J. **83:**810, 1972.

Nichol. P. M., Gilbert, B. W., and Kisslo, J. A.: Two-dimensional echocardiographic assessment of mitral stenosis, Circulation **55:**120, 1977.

Parisi, A., and Milton, B.: Relation of mitral valve closure to the first heart sound in man: echocardiographic and phonocardiographic assessment, Am. J. Cardiol. **32:**779, 1973.

Popp, R., and Levine, R.: Left atrial mass simulating cardiomyopathy, J. Clin. Ultrasound **1:**96, 1973.

Popp, R., et al.: Echocardiographic abnormalities in the mitral valve prolapse syndrome, Circulation **49:**428, 1974.

Pridie, R. B., Beham, R., and Oakley, C. M.: Echocardiography of the mitral valve in aortic valve disease, Br. Heart J. **33:**296, 1971.

Quinones, M., et al.: Reduction in the rate of diastolic descent of the mitral valve echogram in patients with altered left ventricular diastolic pressure-volume relations, Circulation **49:**246, 1974.

Rubenstein, J., et al.: The echocardiographic determination of mitral valve opening and closure: correlation with hemodynamic studies in man, Circulation **51:**98, 1975.

Shah, P., et al.: Role of echocardiography in diagnostic and hemodynamic assessment of hypertrophic subaortic stenosis, Circulation **44:**891, 1971.

Shah, P., et al.: Echocardiographic assessment of the effects of surgery and propranolol on the dynamics of outflow obstruction and hypertrophic subaortic stenosis, Circulation **45:**516, 1972.

Spangler, R., D., Johnson, M. L., Holmes, J. H., et al.: Echocardiographic demonstration of bacterial vegetations in active infective endocarditis, J. Clin. Ultrasound **1:**126, 1973.

Spangler, R., and Okin, T.: Echocardiographic demonstration of left atrial thrombus, Chest **67:**716, 1975.

Sweatman, T., et al.: Echocardiographic diagnosis of mitral regurgitation due to ruptured chordae tendineae, Circulation **46:**580, 1972.

Weaver, W. F., et al.: Mid-diastolic aortic valve opening in severe acute aortic regurgitation, Circulation **55**:145, 1977.

Winkle, R., Goodman, D., and Popp, R.: Simultaneous echocardiographic-phonocardiographic recordings at rest and during amyl nitrite administration in patients with mitral valve prolapse, Circulation **51**:522, 1975.

Winsberg, F., and Mercer, E.: Echocardiography in combined valve disease, Radiology **105**:405, 1972.

Aorta and left atrium

Brown, O., Harrison, D., and Popp, R.: An improved method for echographic detection of left atrial enlargement, Circulation **50**:58, 1974.

Chang, S., Clements, S., and Chang, J.: Aortic stenosis: echocardiographic cuspi separation and surgical description of aortic valve in 22 patients, Am. J. Cardiol. **39**:499, 1977.

Cooperberg, P., Mercer, E. N., Mulder, D. S., et al.: Rupture of a sinus Valsalva aneurysm. Report of a case diagnosed preoperatively by echocardiography, Radiology **113**:171, 1974.

DeMaria, A. N., King, J. F., Salel, A. F., et al.: Echography and phonography of acute aortic regurgitation in bacterial endocarditis, Ann. Intern. Med. **82**:329, 1975.

Feizi, O., Symons, C., and Yacoub, M.: Echocardiography of the aortic valve. Studies of normal aortic valve, aortic stenosis, aortic regurgitation and mixed aortic valve disease, Br. Heart J. **36**:341, 1974.

Francis, G. S., et al.: Echocardiographic criteria of normal left atrial size in adults, Cath. Cardiovas. Diagnosis **2**:69, 1976.

Glasser, S.: Late mitral valve opening in aortic regurgitation, Chest **70**:70, 1976.

Goldberg, B.: Suprasternal ultrasonography, J.A.M.A. **215**:245, 1971.

Gottlieb, S., Khuddus, S. A., Balooki, H., et al.: Echocardiographic diagnosis of aortic valve vegetations in candida endocarditis, Circulation **50**:826, 1974.

Gramiak, R., and Shah, P.: Echocardiography of the aortic root, Invest. Radiol. **3**:356, 1968.

Gramiak, R., and Shah, P.: Echocardiography of the normal and diseased aortic valve, Radiology **96**:1, 1970.

Henry, W. L., Morganroth, J., Pearlman, A. S., et al.: Relation between echocardiographically determined left atrial size and atrial fibrillation, Circulation **53**:273, 1976.

Hirata, T., Wolfe, S. B., Popp, R. L., Helmen, C. H., and Feigenbaum, H.: Estimation of left atrial size using ultrasound, Am. Heart J. **78**:43, 1969.

Hirschfeld, D. S., and Schiller, N.: Localization of aortic valve vegetations by echocardiography, Circulation **53**:280, 1976.

Johnson, A. D., Alpert, J. S., Francis, G. S., Vieweg, V. R., Ockene, I., and Hagan, A. D.: Assessment of left ventricular function in severe aortic regurgitation, Circulation **54**:975, 1976.

Johnson, M. L., Warren, S. G., Waugh, R. A., et al.: Echocardiography of the aortic valve in non-rheumatic left ventricular outflow tract lesions, Radiology **112**:677, 1974.

Kelly, D., Wulfsberg, E., and Rowe, R.: Discrete subaortic stenosis, Circulation **46**:309, 1972.

Kronzon, I., and Mehta, S.: Giant left atrium, Chest **65**:677, 1974.

Martinez, E., Burch, G., and Giles, T.: Echocardiographic diagnosis of vegetative aortic bacterial endocarditis, Am. J. Cardiol. **34**:845, 1974.

Millward, D., Robinson, N., and Craige, E.: Dissecting aortic aneurysm diagnosed by echocardiography in a patient with rupture of the aneurysm into the right atrium, Am. J. Cardiol. **30**:427, 1972.

Nanda, N. C., Gramiak, R., Manning, J., et al.: Echocardiographic recognition of the congenital bicuspid aortic valve, Circulation **49**:870, 1974.

Nanda, N., Gramiak, R., and Shah, P.: Diagnosis of aortic root dissection by echocardiography, Circulation **48**:506, 1973.

Nanda, N. C., Gramiak, R., Shah, P. M., et al.: Echocardiography in the diagnosis of idiopathic hypertrophic subaortic stenosis coexisting with aortic valve disease, Circulation **50**:752, 1974.

Petsas, A. A., Gottlieb, S., Kingsley, B., et al.: Echocardiographic diagnosis of left atrial myxoma, Br. Heart J. **37**:627, 1976.

Popp, R. L., Silverman, J. F., French, J. W., et al: Echocardiographic findings in discrete subvalvular aortic stenosis, Circulation **49**:226, 1974.

Pratt, R. C., Parisi, A. F., Harrington, J. J., et al.: The influence of left ventricular stroke volume on aortic root motion: an enchocardiographic study, Circulation **53**:947, 1976.

Rothbaum, D. A., Dillon, J. C., Chang, S., et al: Echocardiographic manifestations of right sinus of Valsalva aneurysm, Circulation **49**:768, 1974.

Spangler, R. D., Johnson, M. L., Holmes, J. H., et al.: Echocardiographic demonstration of bacterial vegetations in active infective endocarditis, J. Clin. Ultrasound **1**:126, 1973.

Strunk, B. L., Fitzgerald, J. W., Lipton, M., Popp, R. L., and Barry, W. H.: The posterior aortic wall echocardiogram, its relationship to left atrial volume change, Circulation **54**:744, 1976.

TenCate, F., et al.: Dimensions and volumes of left atrium and ventricle determined by single beam echocardiography, Br. Heart J. **36**:737, 1974.

Vredevoe, L., Creekmore, S., and Schiller, N.: The measurement of systolic time intervals by echocardiography, J. Clin. Ultrasound **2**:99, 1974.

Weyman, A. E., Feigenbaum, H., Dillon, J. C., et al.: Noninvasive visualization of the left main coronary artery by cross-sectional echocardiography, Circulation **54**:179, 1976.

Winsberg, F., and Goldman, H.: Echo pattern of cardiac posterior wall, Invest. Radiol. **4**:173, 1969.

Tricuspid valve

Ainsworth, R. P., Hartmann, A. F., Aker, U., and Schad, N.: Tricuspid valve prolapse with late systolic tricuspid insufficiency, Radiology **107**:309, 1973.

Chandraratna, P., et al.: Echocardiographic detection of tricuspid valve prolapse, Circulation **51**:823, 1975.

Gooch, A. S., Maranhao, V., Scampardones, G., Cha, S. D., and Yang, S. S.: Prolapse of both mitral and tricuspid leaflets in systolic murmur-click syndrome, N. Engl. J. Med. **287**:1218, 1972.

Green, E., Agruss, N., and Adolph, R.: Right-sided Austin-Flint murmur: documentation of intracardiac phonocardiography, echocardiography and postmortem findings, Am. J. Cardiol. **32**:370, 1973.

Hagan, A., Sahn, D. J., and Friedman, W. F.: Cross-sectional echocardiographic features of Ebstein's malformation (abstr.), Circulation **50** (suppl. III): 17, 1974.

Lundstrom, N.: Echocardiography in the diagnosis of Ebstein's anomaly of the tricuspid valve, Circulation **47**:597, 1973.

Nanda, N., Gramiak, R., and Manning, J.: Echocardiography of the tricuspid valve in congenital left ventricular-right atrial communication, Circulation **51**:268, 1975.

Seides, S. F., DeJoseph, R. I., Brown, A. E., and Damato, A. N.: Echocardiographic findings in isolated, surgically created tricuspid insufficiency, Am. J. Cardiol. **35**:679, 1975.

Tavel, M. E., Baugh, D., Fisch, C., and Feigenbaum, H.: Opening snap of the tricuspid valve in atrial septal defect: a phonocardiographic and reflected ultrasound study of sounds in relationship to movements of the tricuspid valve, Am. Heart J. **80**:550, 1970.

Waxler, E. B., Kawai, N., and Kasparian, H.: Right atrial myxoma: echocardiographic, phonocardiographic and hemodynamic signs, Am. Heart. J. **83**:251, 1972.

Wolfe, S. B., Popp, R. L., and Feigenbaum, H.: Diagnosis of atrial tumors by ultrasound, Circulation 39:615, 1969.

Pulmonary valves

Chung, K. J., Alexson, C. G., Manning, J. A., and Gramiak, R.: Echocardiography in truncus arteriosus: the value of pulmonic valve detection, Circulation 48:281, 1973.

Goldberg, S., Allen, H., and Sahn, D.: Pediatric echocardiography, Chicago, 1974, Year Book Medical Publishers, Inc.

Goodman, D., Harrison, D., and Popp, R.: Echocardiographic features of primary pulmonary hypertension, Am. J. Cardiol. 33:438, 1974.

Gramiak, R., Nanda, N. C., and Shah, P. M.: Echocardiographic detection of the pulmonary valve, Radiology 102:153, 1972.

Nanda, N., et al.: Evaluation of pulmonary hypertension by echocardiography, J. Clin. Ultrasound 1:225, 1973.

Nanda, N. C., Gramiak, R., Robinson, T. I., and Shah, P. M.: Echocardiographic evaluation of pulmonary hypertension, Circulation 50:575, 1974.

Nanda, N., et al.: Echocardiographic evaluation of pulmonary hypertension, Circulation 50:575, 1974.

Wann, L. S., et al.: Premature pulmonary valve opening, Circulation 55:128, 1977.

Weyman, A. E., Dillon, J. C., Feigenbaum, H., and Chang, S.: Echocardiographic patterns of pulmonary valve motion in valvular pulmonary stenosis, Am. J. Cardiol. 34:644, 1974.

Weyman, A. E., Dillon, J. C., Feigenbaum, H., and Chang, S.: Echocardiographic patterns of pulmonic valve motion with pulmonary hypertension, Circulation 50:905, 1974.

Weyman, A., et al.: Echocardiographic patterns of pulmonary valve motion with pulmonary hypertension, Circulation 50:905, 1974.

Weyman, A., et al.: Echocardiographic patterns of pulmonic valve motion in pulmonic stenosis, Am. J. Cardiol. 34:644, 1974.

Weyman, A., et al.: Premature pulmonic valve opening following sinus of Valsalva aneurysm rupture into the right atrium, Circulation 51:556, 1975.

Prosthetic valves

Alderman, E. L., Rytand, D. A., Crow, R. S., Finegan, R. E., and Harrison, D. C.: Normal and prosthetic atrioventricular valve motion in atrial flutter, Circulation 45:1206, 1972.

Assad-Morell, J., et al.: Malfunctioning tricuspid valve prosthesis. Clinical, phonocardiographic, echocardiographic and surgical findings, Mayo Clin. Proc. 42:443, 1974.

Belenkie, I., Carr, M., Schlant, R. C., Nutter, D. O., and Symbas, P. N.: Malfunction of a Cutter-Smeloff mitral ball valve prosthesis: diagnosis by phonocardiography and echocardiography, Am. Heart J. 86:399, 1973.

Brodie, B. R., Grossman, W., McLaurin, L., Starek, P. J. K., and Craige, E.: Diagnosis of prosthetic mitral valve malfunction with combined echo-phonocardiography, Circulation 53:93, 1976.

Burgraff, G. W., and Craige, E.: Echocardiographic studies of left ventricular wall motion and dimensions after valvular heart surgery, Am. J. Cardiol. 35:473, 1975.

Douglas, J., and Williams, G.: Echocardiographic evaluation of the Bjork-Shiley prosthetic valve, Circulation 50:52, 1974.

Gold, H., and Hertz, L.: Death caused by fracture of Beall mitral prosthesis, Am. J. Cardiol. 34:371, 1974.

Horowitz, M., Goodman, D., and Popp, R.: Echocardiographic diagnosis of calcific stenosis of a stented aortic homograft in the mitral position, J. Clin. Ultrasound 2:179, 1974.

Johnson, M. L.: Echocardiographic evaluation of prosthetic heart valves. In Gramiak, R., and Waag, R. C., editors: Cardiac ultrasound, St. Louis, 1975, The C. V. Mosby Co.

Johnson, M. L., Paton, B. C., and Holmes, J. H.: Ultrasonic evaluation of prosthetic valve motion, Circulation 41, 42 (suppl. II): 3, 1970.

Johnson, M. L., Holmes, J. H., and Paton, B. C.: Echocardiographic determination of mitral disc valve excursion, Circulation 47:1274, 1973.

Miller, H., Gibson, D., and Stephens, J.: Role of echocardiography and phonocardiography in the diagnosis of mitral paraprosthetic regurgitation with Starr-Edwards prostheses, Br. Heart J. 35:1217, 1973.

Miller, H., Stephens, J., and Gibson, D.: Echocardiographic features of mitral Starr-Edwards paraprosthetic regurgitation, Br. Heart J. 35:560, 1973.

Nanda, N. C., Gramiak, R., Shah, P. M., and DeWeese, J. A.: Mitral commissurotomy versus replacement: preoperative evaluation by echocardiography, Circulation 51:263, 1975.

Nanda, N. C., Gramiak, R., Shah, P. M., DeWeese, J. A., and Mahoney E. B.: Echocardiographic assessment of left ventricular outflow width in the selection of mitral valve prosthesis, Circulation 48:1208, 1973.

Nanda, N., et al.: Echocardiographic assessment of left ventricular outflow width in the selection of mitral valve prosthesis, Ciculation 48:1208, 1973.

Popp, R., and Carmichael, B.: Cardiac echography in the diagnosis of prosthetic mitral valve malfunction, Circulation 44:33, 1971.

Siggers, D. C., Srivongse, S. A., and Deuchar, D.: Analysis of dynamics of mitral Starr-Edwards valve prosthesis using reflected ultrasound, Br. Heart J. 33:401, 1971.

Smith, R. A., et al.: Non-invasive diagnostic evaluation of the normal Beall mitral prosthesis, Cath. Cardiovasc. Diagnosis 2:289, 1976.

Srivastava, T. N., et al.: Echocardiographic diagnosis of a stuck Bjork-Shiley aortic valve prosthesis, Chest 70:94, 1976.

Willerson, J. T., Kastor, J. A., Dinsmore, R. E., Mundth, E., Buckley, M. J., Austen, W. G., and Saunders, C. A.: Non-invasive assessment of prosthetic mitral paravalvular and intravalvular regurgitation, Br. Heart J. 34:561, 1972.

Yoshikawa, J., Owaki, T., Kato, H., and Tanaka, K.: Abnormal motion of interventricular septum of patients with prosthetic valve. In White, D., editor: Ultrasound in medicine, New York, 1975, Plenum Publishing Corporation.

Right ventricle

Brown, O. R., Harrison, D. C., and Popp, R. I.: Echocardiography study of right ventricular hypertension producing asymmetrical septal hypertrophy (abstr.), Circulation 48 (suppl. IV):47, 1973.

DeMaria, A. N., Vismara, I. A., Miller, R. R., Neumann, A., and Mason, D. T.: Unusual echocardiographic manifestations of right and left heart myxomas, Am. J. Med. 59:713, 1975.

Diamond, M. A., Dillon, J. C., Haine, C. L., Chang, S., and Feigenbaum, H.: Echocardiographic features of atrial septal defect, Circulation 43:129, 1971.

Henry, W. L., Clark, C. E., and Epstein, S. E.: Asymmetric septal hypertrophy (ASH): the unifying link in the IHSS disease spectrum, Circulation 47:827, 1973.

Popp, R. L., Wolfe, S. B., Hirata, T., and Feigenbaum, H.: Estimation of right and left ventricular size by ultrasound. A study of the echoes from the interventricular septum, Am. J. Cardiol. 24:523, 1969.

Interventricular septum and interatrial septum

Abbasi, A., et al.: Echocardiographic diagnosis of idiopathic hypertrophic cardiomyopathy without outflow obstruction, Circulation 46:897, 1972.

Cohen, M. V., et al.: B-scan ultrasonography in idiopathic hypertrophic subaortic stenosis, Br. Heart J. 37:1976.

Devereux, R. B., and Reichek, N.: Echocardiographic determination of left ventricular mass in man. Anatomic validation of the method, Circulation 55:613, 1977.

Dillon, J., et al.: Cross-sectional echocardiographic examination of the interatrial septum, Circulation **55**:115, 1977.

Epstein, S. E., Henry, W. L., Clark, C. E., Roberts, W. C., Maron, B. J., Ferrans, V. J., Redwood, D. R., and Morrow, A. G.: Asymmetric septal hypertrophy, Ann. Intern. Med. **81**:650, 1974.

Henry, W. L., Clark, C. E., and Epstein, S. E.: Asymmetric septal hypertrophy (ASH): the unifying link in the IHSS disease spectrum, Circulation **47**:827, 1973.

Henry, W. L., Clark, C. E., and Epstein, S. E.: Asymmetric septal hypertrophy: echocardiographic identification of the pathognomonic anatomic abnormality of IHSS, Circulation **47**:225, 1973.

Henry, W. L., Clark, C. E., Roberts, W. C., Morrow, A. G., and Epstein, S. E.: Difference in distribution of myocardial abnormalities in patients with obstructive and nonobstructive asymmetric septal hypertrophy (ASH): echocardiographic and gross anatomic findings, Circulation **50**:447, 1974.

Kerber, R., et al.: Effects of acute coronary occlusion on the motion and perfusion of the normal and ischemic interventricular septum, an experimental echocardiographic study, Circulation **54**:1976.

Kerin, N., et al.: Ventricular septal defect complicating acute myocardial infarction, Chest **70**:560, 1976.

King, J. F., DeMaria, A. N., Miller, R. R., Hilliard, G. K., Zelis, R., and Mason, D. T.: Markedly abnormal mitral valve motion without simultaneous intraventricular pressure gradient due to uneven mitral-septal contact in idiopathic hypertrophic subaortic stenosis, Am. J. Cardiol. **34**:360, 1974.

Nanda, N. C., Gramiak, R., Shah, P. M., Stewart, S., and DeWeese, J. A.: Echocardiography in the diagnosis of idiopathic hypertrophic subaortic stenosis co-existing with aortic valve disease, Circulation **50**:752, 1974.

Popp, R. L., and Harrison, D. C.: Ultrasound in the diagnosis and evaluation of therapy of idiopathic hypertrophic subaortic stenosis, Circulation **40**:905, 1969.

Pridie, R., and Oakley, C.: Mechanism of mitral regurgitation in hypertrophic obstructive cardiomyopathy, Br. Heart J. **32**:203, 1970.

Roberts, W. C.: Valvular, subvalvular, and supravalvular aortic stenosis: morphologic features, Cardiovasc. Clin. **5**:98, 1973.

Rossen, R. M., Goodman, D. J., Ingham, R. E., and Popp, R. L.: Ventricular systolic septal thickening and excursion in idiopathic hypertrophic subaortic stenosis, N. Engl. J. Med. **291**:1317, 1974.

Shah, P.: IHSS—HOCM—MSS—ASH? (editorial), Circulation **51**:577, 1975.

Shah, P., et al.: Role of echocardiography in diagnostic and hemodynamic assessment of hypertrophic subaortic stenosis, Circulation **44**:891, 1971.

Shah, P., et al.: Echocardiographic assessment of the effects of surgery and propranolol on the dynamics of outflow obstruction and hyperpranolol on the dynamics of outflow obstruction and hypertrophic subaortic stenosis, Circulation **45**:516, 1972.

Weyman, A., et al.: Cross-sectional echocardiography in evaluating patients with discrete subaortic stenosis, Am. J. Cardiol. **37**:358, 1976.

Weyman, A., et al.: Mechanism of abnormal septal motion in patients with right ventricular volume overload, a cross-sectional echocardiographic study, Circulation **54**:179, 1976.

Left ventricle

Abbasi, A., et al.: Paradoxical motion of interventricular septum in LBBB, Circulation **49**:423, 1974.

Bergeron, G. A., Cohen, M. V., Teichholz, L. F., and Gorlin, R.: Echocardiographic analysis of mitral valve motion after acute myocardial infarction, Circulation **51**:82, 1975.

Burch, G. E., Giles, T. D., and Martinez, E.: Echocardiographic detection of abnormal motion of the interventricular septum in ischemic cardiomyopathy, Am. J. Med. **57**:293, 1974.

Chang, S., and Feigenbaum, H.: Subxiphoid echocardiography, J. Clin. Ultrasound **1**:14, 1973.

Chang, S., Feigenbaum, H., and Dillon, J.: Condensed M-mode echocardiographic scan of the asymmetrical left ventricle, Chest **68**:93, 1975.

Chang, S., Feigenbaum, H., and Dillon, J.: Subxiphoid echocardiography: a review, Chest **68**:233, 1975.

Corya, B. C., Feigenbaum, H., Rasmussen, S., and Black, M. J.: Anterior left ventricle wall echoes in coronary artery disease: linear scarring with a single element transducer, Am. J. Cardiol. **34**:652, 1974.

Diamond, M., et al.: Echocardiographic features of atrial septal defect, Circulation **43**:129, 1974.

Dillon, J., Chang, S., and Feigenbaum, H.: Echocardiographic manifestations of left bundle branch block, Circulation **49**:876, 1974.

Fortuin, N., et al.: Determinations of left ventricular volumes by ultrasound, Circulation **44**:575, 1971.

Goldstein, S., and Willem de Jong, J.: Changes in left ventricular wall dimension during regional myocardial ischemia, Am. J. Cardiol. **34**:56, 1974.

Gramiak, R., and Nanda, N.: Echocardiographic diagnosis of ostium primum septal defect, Circulation **45** (suppl. II):46, 1972.

Hagan, A., et al.: Ultrasound evaluation of systolic anterior septal motion in patients with and without right ventricular volume overload, Circulation **50**:248, 1974.

Henning, H., Schelbert, H., Crawford, M. H., Karliner, J. S., Ashburn, W., and O'Rourke, R. A.: Left ventricular performance assessed by radionuclide angiocardiography and echocardiography in patients with previous myocardial infarction, Circulation **52**:1069, 1975.

Karliner, J., et al.: Mean velocity of fiber shortening: a simplified measure of left ventricular myocardial contractility, Circulation **44**:323, 1971.

Kerber, R. E., and Abboud, F. M.: Echocardiographic detection of regional myocardial infarction: an experimental study, Circulation **48**:997, 1973.

Kraunz, R., and Kennedy, J.: Ultrasonic determination of left ventricular wall motion in normal man. Studies at rest and after exercise, Am. Heart J. **79**:36, 1970.

Kraunz, R., and Ryan, T.: Ultrasound measurements of ventricular wall motion following administration of vasoactivity drugs, Am. J. Cardiol. **27**:464, 1971.

Kreamer, R., Kerber, R., and Abbound, F.: Ventricular aneurysm: use of echocardiography, J. Clin. Ultrasound **1**:60, 1973.

Layton, C., et al.: Assessment of left ventricular filling and compliance using an ultrasound technique, Br. Heart J. **35**:559, 1973.

Levitsky, S., and Merchani, F.: Non-invasive methods of measuring myocardial contractility, Surg. Annu. **5**:205, 1973.

Ludbrook, P., et al.: Comparison of ultrasound and cineangiographic measurements of left ventricular performance in patients with and without wall motion abnormalities, Br. Heart J. **35**:1026, 1973.

Ludbrook, P., et al.: Posterior wall velocity: an unreliable index of total left ventricular performance in patients with coronary artery disease, Am. J. Cardiol. **33**:475, 1974.

Ludbrook, P., Karliner, J. S., London, A., Peterson, K. L., Leopold, G. R., and O'Rourke, R. A.: Posterior wall velocity: an unreliable index of total left ventricular performance in patients with coronary artery disease, Am. J. Cardiol. **33**:475, 1974.

McDonald, I.: Assessment of myocardial function by echocardiography, Adv. Cardiol. **12**:221, 1974.

McLaurin, I., et al.: A new technique for the study of left ventricular pressure-volume relations in man, Circulation **48:**56, 1973.

Morganroth, J., et al.: Comparative left ventricular dimensions in trained athletes, Ann. Intern. Med. **82:**521, 1975.

Payvandi, M., et al.: Echocardiography in congenital and acquired absence of the pericardium. An echocardiographic mimic of right ventricular volume overload, Circulation **53:**86, 1976.

Pombo, J., et al.: Comparison of stroke volume and cardiac output determination by ultrasound and dye dilution in acute myocardial infarction, Am. J. Cardiol. **27:**630, 1971.

Pombo, J., Troy, B., and Russell, R., Jr.: Left ventricular volumes and ejection fraction by echocardiography, Circulation **43:**480, 1971.

Popp, R., et al.: Ultrasonic cardiac echography for determining stroke volume and valvular regurgitation, Circulation **41:**493, 1970.

Popp, R., et al.: Sources of error in calculation of left ventricular volumes by echography, Am. J. Cardiol. **31:**152, 1973.

Popp, R., et al.: Effect of transducer placement on echocardiographic measurement of left ventricular dimensions, Am. J. Cardiol. **35:**537, 1975.

Ratshin, R., Rackley, C., and Russell, R.: Serial evaluation of left ventricular volumes and posterior wall movement in the acute phase of myocardial infarction using diagnostic ultrasound, Am. J. Cardiol. **29:**286, 1972.

Ratshin, R., Rackley, C., and Russell, R. L.: Determination of left ventricular preload and afterload by quantitative echocardiography in man, Circ. Res. **34:**711, 1974.

Ratshin, R., et al.: Quantitative echocardiography: correlations with ventricular volumes by angiography in patients with coronary artery disease with and without wall motion abnormalities, Circulation **48** (suppl. IV): 48, 1973.

Ratshin, R., et al.: The accuracy of ventricular volume analysis by quantitative echocardiography in patients with coronary artery disease with and without wall motion abnormalities, Am. J. Cardiol. **33:**164, 1974.

Redwood, D., Henry, W., and Epstein, S.: Evaluation of the ability of echocardiography to measure acute alterations in left ventricular volume, Circulation **50:**901, 1974.

Stack, R., et al.: Left ventricular performance in coronary artery disease evaluated with systolic time intervals and echocardiography, Am. J. Cardiol. **37:**331, 1976.

Weyman, S., et al.: Localization of left ventricular outflow obstruction by cross-sectional echocardiography, Am. J. Med. **60:** 33, 1976.

Pericardium

Abbasi, A., Ellis, N., and Flynn, J.: Echocardiographic M-scan technique in the diagnosis of pericardial effusion, J. Clin. Ultrasound **1:**300, 1973.

Casarella, W., and Schneider, B.: Pitfalls in the ultrasonic diagnosis of pericardial effusion, Am. J. Roentgenol. **110:**760, 1970.

D'Cruz, I. A., Cohen, H. C., Prabhu, R., and Glick, G.: Diagnosis of cardiac tamponade by echocardiography: changes in mitral valve motion and ventricular dimensions, with special reference to paradoxical pulse, Circulation **52:**460, 1975.

Ellis, K., and King, D.: Pericarditis and pericardial effusion. Radiologic and echocardiographic diagnosis, Radiol. Clin. North Am. **11:**393, 1973.

Feigenbaum, H.: Echocardiographic diagnosis of pericardial effusion, Am. J. Cardiol. **26:**475, 1970.

Goldberg, B., and Pollack, H.: Ultrasonically guided pericardiocentesis, Am. J. Cardiol. **31:**490, 1973.

Horowitz, M. S., Schultz, C. S., Stinson, E. B., Harrison, D. C., and Popp, R. L.: Sensitivity and specificity of echocardiographic diagnosis of pericardial effusion, Circulation **50:**239, 1974.

Levisman, J. A., and Abbasi, A. S.: Abnormal motion of the mitral valve with pericardial effusion: pseudo-prolapse of the mitral valve, Am. Heart J. **91:**18, 1976.

Ratshin, R., Smith, M., and Hood, W., Jr.: Possible false-positive diagnosis of pericardial effusion by echocardiography in presence of large left atrium, Chest **65:**112, 1974.

Rothman, L., et al.: Ultrasonic diagnosis of pericardial effusion, Circulation **35:**358, 1967.

Sakamoto, T., et al.: Unusual diastolic heart beat in pericardial effusion, Jpn. Heart J. **13:**379, 1972.

Abdomen (Chapters 17-26)
General

Asher, W., and Freimanis, A. K.: Echographic diagnosis of retroperitoneal lymph node enlargement, Am. J. Roentgenol. Radium Ther. Nucl. Med. **105:**438, 1969.

Cunningham, J.: False-positive gray-scale ultrasonography for intra-abdominal abscesses, Arch. Surg. **111:**810, 1976.

Doust, B., et al.: Ultrasonic diagnosis of abdominal abscess, forums in gastrointestinal roentgenology, Dig. Dis. **21:** 1976.

Gosink, B. B., and Leopold, G. R.: Abdominal echography, Semin. Roentgenol. **10:**299, 1975.

Holm, H. H.: Ultrasonic scanning in the diagnosis of space occupying lesions of the upper abdomen, Br. J. Radiol. **44:**24, 1971.

Leopold, G. R., and Asher, W.: Fundamentals of abdominal and pelvic ultrasonography, Philadelphia, 1975, W. B. Saunders Co.

Lomonaco, A., et al.: Nuclear medicine and ultrasound; correlation in diagnosis of disease of liver and biliary tract, Semin. Nucl. Med. **5:**307, 1975.

Maklad, N., et al.: Ultrasonic diagnosis of postoperative intra-abdominal abscess, Radiology **113:**417, 1974.

Sample, W. F.: A new technique for the evaluation of the adrenal gland with gray-scale ultrasonography, Radiology **124:**463, 1977.

Sample, W. F.: Techniques for improved delineation of normal anatomy of the upper abdomen and high retroperitoneum with gray-scale ultrasound, Radiology **124:**197, 1977.

Walls, W. J.: The evaluation of malignant gastric neoplasms by ultrasonic B-scanning, Radiology **118:**159, 1976.

Liver

Garrett, W., et al.: Gray scale compound scan echography of the normal upper abdomen, J. Clin. Ultrasound **3:**3, 1975.

Hebert, G., and Gelinas, C.: Hepatic echography, Radiology **125:**4, 1975.

Rasmussen, N. S., et al.: Three-dimensional imaging of abdominal organs with ultrasound, Radiology **121:**4, 1974.

Taylor, K. J. W., et al.: Gray scale echography in the diagnosis of intrahepatic disease, J. Clin. Ultrasound **1:**284, 1973.

Taylor, K. J. W., et al.: The anatomy and pathology of the porta hepatis demonstrated by gray scale ultrasonography, J. Clin. Ultrasound **3:**117, 1975.

Gallbladder

Bartrum, R. J., et al.: Ultrasound examination of the gallbladder. An alternative to "double-dose" oral cholecystography, J.A.M.A. **236:**1147, 1976.

Doust, B., et al.: Ultrasonic B-mode examination of the gallbladder, Radiology **110:**643, 1974.

Filly, R., and Carlsen, E. N.: Choledochal cyst: report of a case with specific ultrasonographic findings, J. Clin. Ultrasound **4:**7, 1976.

Goldberg, B.: Ultrasonic cholangiography, Radiology **118:**401, 1976.

Leopold, G. R., and Sokoloff, J.: Ultrasonic scanning for the diagnosis of biliary disease, Surg. Clin. North Am. **53:**1043, 1973.

Leopold, G. R., et al.: Gray scale ultrasonic cholecystography: a comparison with conventional radiographic techniques, Radiology 121:445, 1976.

Malini, S., et al.: Ultrasonography in obstructive jaundice, Radiology 123:429, 1977.

Perlmutter, G., and Goldberg, B. B.: Ultrasonic evaluation of the common bile duct, J. Clin. Ultrasound 4:107, 1976.

Stone, L. B., et al.: Gray scale ultrasound diagnosis of obstructive biliary disease, Am. J. Roentgenol. Radium Ther. Nucl. Med. 125:47, 1975.

Taylor, K. J. W., et al.: Gray scale echography in the diagnosis of intrahepatic disease, J. Clin. Ultrasound 1:284, 1973.

Taylor, K., et al.: Grey-scale ultrasonography in the differential diagnosis of jaundice, Arch. Surg. 112:820, 1977.

Weill, F., et al.: Ultrasound study of the venous patterns in the hypochondrium: an anatomical approach to differential diagnosis of obstructive jaundice, J. Clin. Ultrasound 3:23, 1975.

Vessels

Birnholz, J. C.: A noninvasive approach to the derivation of quantitative pathophysiological data concerning the diseased aortic wall, Radiology 107:675, 1973.

Birnholz, J. C.: Alternatives in the diagnosis of abdominal aortic aneurysm: combined use of isotope aortography and ultrasonography, Radiology 118:809, 1973.

Filldy, R. A., and Carlsen, E. N.: Newer ultrasonographic anatomy in the upper abdomen. II. The major systemic veins and arteries with a special note on localization of the pancreas, J. Clin. Ultrasound 4:91, 1976.

Goldberg, B. B., et al.: Aortosonography: ultrasound measurement of the abdominal and thoracic aorta, Arch. Surg. 100:652, 1970.

Gore, I., et al.: Arteriosclerotic aneurysms of the abdominal aorta: a review, Prog. Cardiovasc. Dis. 16:113, 1973.

Holm, H. H., et al.: Ultrasonic diagnostic of arterial aneurysms, Scand. J. Thorac. Cardiovasc. Surg. 2:140, 1968.

Kristensen, J. K., et al.: Ultrasonic diagnosis of aortic aneurysms, J. Cardiovasc. Surg. (Torino) 13:168, 1972.

Lee, T., et al.: Ultrasonic aortography: unexpected findings, Am. J. Roentgenol. 128:273, 1977.

Leopold, G. R.: Ultrasonic abdominal aortography, Radiology 96:9, 1970.

Leopold, G. R., et al.: Ultrasonic detection and evaluation of abdominal aortic aneurysms, Surgery 72:939, 1972.

Sarti, D., et al.: Correlation of the ultrasonic appearance of the portal vein with abdominal arteriography, J. Clin. Ultrasound 3:263, 1975.

Winsberg, F., et al.: Continuous ultrasound visualization of the pulsating abdominal aorta, Radiology 103:455, 1972.

Pancreas

Beck, I., et al.: The exocrine pancreas, Baltimore, 1971, The Williams & Wilkins Co.

Carey, L. C.: The pancreas, St. Louis, 1973, The C. V. Mosby Co.

Doust, B., et al.: Gray-scale ultrasonic properties of the normal and inflamed pancreas, Radiology 120:653, 1976.

Dreilung, D. A., et al.: Pancreatic inflammatory disease, New York, 1964, Harper & Row, Publishers.

Eaton, S. B., et al.: Radiology of the pancreas and duodenum, Philadelphia, 1973, W. B. Saunders Co.

Engelhart, G., and Blauenstein, U. W.: Ultrasound in the diagnosis of malignant pancreatic tumors, Gut 11:443, 1970.

Felson, B., et al.: Echographic study of the pancreas, J.A.M.A. 232:287, 1975.

Ferrucci, J.: Radiology of the pancreas, 1976: sonography and ductography, Radiol. Clin. North Am. 14:543, 1976.

Filley, R. A., et al.: Echographic diagnosis of pancreatic lesions—ultrasound scanning techniques and diagnostic findings, Radiology 96:575, 1970.

Freimanis, A.: Echographic exploration of abdominal structures, Crit. Rev. Rad. Sci. 1:207, 1970.

Haber, K., et al.: Demonstration and dimensional analysis of the normal pancreas with gray-scale echography, Am. J. Roentgenol. Radium Ther. Nucl. Med. 126:624, 1976.

Hancke, S., et al.: Ultrasonically guided percutaneous fine needle biopsy of the pancreas, Surg. Gynecol. Obstet. 40:361, 1975.

Holm, H. H.: Ultrasonic scanning in the diagnosis of space-occupying lesions of the upper abdomen, Br. J. Radiol. 44:24, 1971.

Howard, J., et al.: Surgical diseases of the pancreas, Philadelphia, 1960, J. B. Lippincott Co.

Kahn, P. C.: Ultrasonic radionuclide scanning in pancreatic disease, Semin. Nucl. Med. 5:325, 1975.

King, D.: Diagnostic ultrasound, St. Louis, 1974, The C. V. Mosby Co.

Leopold, G. R.: Pancreatic echography: a new dimension in the diagnosis of pseudocyst, Radiology 104:365, 1974.

Leopold, G. R.: Echographic study of the pancreas, J.A.M.A. 232:287, 1975.

Leopold, G. R., and Asher, W. M.: Fundamentals of abdominal and pelvic ultrasonography, Philadelphia, 1975, W. B. Saunders Co.

Smith, E. H., et al.: Percutaneous aspiration biopsy of the pancreas under ultrasonic guidance, N. Engl. J. Med. 292:825, 1975.

Sokoloff, J., et al.: Pitfalls in the echographic evaluation in pancreatic disease, J. Clin. Ultrasound 2:321, 1974.

Stuber, J. L., et al.: Sonographic diagnosis of pancreatic lesions, Am. J. Roentgenol. Radium Ther. Nucl. Med. 116:406, 1972.

Walls, W. J., et al.: B-scan ultrasound evaluation of the pancreas, Radiology 114:127, 1975.

Walls, W., et al.: The ultrasonic demonstration of inferior vena cava compression: a guide to pancreatic head enlargement with emphasis on neoplasm, Radiology 123:165, 1977.

Weill, F., et al.: Ultrasonography of the normal pancreas, Radiology 123:417, 1977.

White, T. T.: Pancreatitis, Baltimore, 1960, The Williams & Wilkins Co.

Wolson, A., et al.: Ultrasonic characteristics of cystadenoma of the pancreas, Radiology 119:203, 1976.

Kidneys

Leopold, G. R.: Renal transplant size measured by reflected ultrasound, Radiology 95:687, 1970.

Leopold, G. R., et al.: Renal ultrasonography: an updated approach to the diagnosis of renal cyst, Radiology 109:671, 1973.

Morales, J., and Goldberg, B. B.: Combined use of ultrasound and nuclear medicine techniques in kidney disease, Semin. Nucl. Med. 5:339, 1975.

Pollack, H. M., et al.: A systematized approach to the differential diagnosis of renal masses, Radiology 113:653, 1974.

Rasking, M. M., et al.: Renal cyst puncture: combined fluoroscopic and ultrasonic technique, Radiology 113:425, 1974.

Sanders, R. C., et al.: B-scan ultrasound in the diagnosis of hydronephrosis, Radiology 108:375, 1973.

Pelvis (Chapters 27-30)
Obstetrics and gynecology

Bang, J., and Holm, H. H.: Ultrasonics in the demonstration of fetal heart movements, Am. J. Obstet. Gynecol. 102:956, 1968.

Barnett, B., and Morley, P.: Abdominal echography: ultrasound in the diagnosis of abdominal conditions, London, 1974, Butterworth & Co., Ltd.

Baum, G.: Ultrasound mammography, Radiology 122:199, 1977.

Beazley, J. M., and Underhill, R. A.: Fallacy of the fundal height, Br. Med. J. 4:404, 1970.

Calderon, C., et al.: Differences in the attenuation of ultrasound by normal, benign and malignant breast tissue, J. Clin. Ultrasound **4**:249, 1976.

Campbell, S.: An improved method of fetal cephalometry by ultrasound, J. Obstet. Gynaecol. Br. Commonwealth **75**:568, 1968.

Campbell, S., and Dewhurst, C. J.: Diagnosis of the small-for-dates fetus by serial ultrasonic cephalometry, Lancet **2**:1002, 1971.

Campbell, S., and Kohorn, E. I.: Placental localization by ultrasonic compound scanning, J. Obstet. Gynaecol. Br. Commonwealth **75**:1007, 1968.

Cochrane, W. J., and Thomas, M.: Ultrasound diagnosis of gynecologic pelvic masses, Radiology **110**:649, 1974.

Donald, I.: Sonar as a method for studying prenatal development, J. Pediatr. **75**:326, 1969.

Donald, I., and Brown, T. G.: Demonstration of tissue interfaces within the body by ultrasonic echo sounding, Br. J. Radiol. **34**:539, 1961.

Garrett, W. J., Grunwald, G., and Robinson, D. E.: Prenatal diagnosis of fetal polycystic kidney by ultrasound, Aust. N. Z. J. Obstet. Gynecol. **10**:7, 1970.

Garrett, W. J., and Robinson, D. E.: Assessment of fetal size and growth rate by ultrasonic echoscopy, Obstet. Gynecol. **38**:525, 1970.

Garrett, W. J., Robinson, D. E., and Kossoff, G.: Ultrasonic echoscopy in transverse lie, J. Obstet. Gynaecol. Br. Commonwealth **73**:679, 1966.

Goldberg, B. B., et al.: Ultrasonic fetal cephalometry, Radiology **87**:328, 1966.

Goss, C. M., editor: Gray's anatomy, Philadelphia, 1977, Lea & Febiger.

Gottesfeld, K. R.: Ultrasound in obstetrics and gynecology, Semin. Roentgenol. **10**:305, 1975.

Hall, A. J., et al.: Ultrasonic fetal cephalometry—some improvements and future developments, Ultrasonics **8**:34, 1970.

Hellman, L., and Pritchard, J. A.: Obstetrics, ed. 14, New York, 1971, Appleton-Century-Crofts.

Hibbard, L. T., et al.: Clinical applications of fetal cephalometry, Obstet. Gynecol. **29**:842, 1967.

Ianniruberto, A., et al.: Predicting fetal weight by ultrasonic B-scan cephalometry, Obstet. Gynecol. **37**:689, 1971.

Jellins, J., et al.: Ultrasonic visualization of the breast, Med. J. Aust. **1**:305, 1971.

Jones, G., and Jones, H.: Noviak's textbook of gynecology, Baltimore, 1975, Williams & Wilkins Co.

Kobayashi, M.: Illustrated manual of ultrasonography in obstetrics and gynecology, Philadelphia, 1975, J. B. Lippincott Co.

Kobayashi, T.: Grey scale echography for the diagnosis of early breast cancer. In de Vlieger, M., editor: Clinical handbook of ultrasound, New York, 1976, John Wiley & Sons, Inc.

Kobayashi, T., et al.: Differential diagnosis of breast tumors, Cancer **33**:940, 1974.

Kohorn, M. A., Walker, R. H. S., Morrison, J., and Campbell, S.: Placental localization: a comparison between ultrasound compound B scanning and radioisotope scanning, Am. J. Obstet. Gynecol. **103**:868, 1969.

Kossoff, G., et al.: Average velocity of ultrasound in the human female breast, J. Acoust. Soc. Am. **53**:1730, 1973.

Kossoff, G., and Garrett, W. J.: Intracranial detail in fetal echograms, Invest. Radiol. **7**:159, 1972.

Kossoff, G., and Garrett, W. J.: Ultrasonic film echography in gynecology and obstetrics, Obstet. Gynecol. **40**:299, 1972.

Kossoff, G., Garrett, W. J., and Radovanovich, G.: Grey scale echography in obstetrics and gynaecology, Australas. Radiol. **18**:62, March, 1974.

Lee, B. O.: Ultrasonic determination of fetal maturity at repeat cesarean section, Obstet. Gynecol. **38**:294, 1971.

Lunt, R. M., et al.: Reproducibility of measurement of fetal biparietal diameter by ultrasonic cephalometry, J. Obstet. Gynaecol. Br. Commonwealth **81**:682, 1974.

Morley, P., and Barnett, E.: The use of ultrasound in the diagnosis of pelvic masses, Br. J. Radiol. **43**:602, 1970.

Netter, F. H.: Ciba collection of medical illustrations. Vol. 2. Reproductive system, Rochester, N. Y., 1974, Case-Hoyt Color Printers.

Peery, T. M., and Miller, F. N.: Pathology, a dynamic introduction into medical and surgical diseases, ed. 2, Boston, Little, Brown & Co.

Perkins, R. P.: Antenatal assessment of fetal maturity. A review, Obstet. Gynecol. Surv. **29**:369, 1974.

Pystynen, P., Ylöstalo, P., and Järvinen, P. A.: Fetal cephalometry by ultrasound, Ann. Chir. Gynaecol. Fenn. **56**:114, 1967.

Robinson, D. E., Garrett, W. J., and Kossoff, G.: Fetal anatomy displayed by ultrasound, Invest. Radiol. **3**:442, 1969.

Romney, S. L., Gray, Little, Merrill, Quilligan, and Stander,: Gynecology and obstetrics: the health care of women, New York, 1975, McGraw-Hill Book Co.

Sauvage, J., Crane, J. P., and Kapta, M. M.: Difficulties in the ultrasonic diagnosis of hydatidiform mole, Obstet. Gynecol. **44**:546, 1974.

Taylor, E. S., Holmes, J. H., Gottesfeld, K. R., and Thompson, H.: Ultrasonic diagnostic procedures in obstetrics and gynecology, J. Obstet. Gynecol. **90**:655, 1964.

Thompson, H.: Ultrasonic diagnostic procedures in obstetrics and gynecology, J. Clin. Ultrasound **1**:160, 1973.

Watmough, D. J., et al.: A modified method of ultrasonic fetal cephalometry, Br. J. Radiol. **47**:352, 1974.

Willocks, J., et al.: Fetal cephalometry by ultrasound, J. Obstet. Gynaecol. Br. Commonwealth **71**:11, 1964.

Winsberg, F.: Echocardiography of the fetal and newborn heart, Invest. Radiol. **7**:152, 1972.

Other clinical applications (Chapters 31 and 32)
Thyroid

Beauqie, J. M., et al.: Primary malignant tumors of the thyroid: the relationship between histological classification and clinical behavior, Br. J. Surg. **63**:178, 1976.

Blum, M.: Enhanced clinical diagnosis of thyroid disease using echography, Am. J. Med. **59**:301, 1975.

Blum, M., et al.: Evaluation of thyroid nodules by A-mode echography, Radiology **101**:651, 1971.

Blum, M., et al.: Clinical applications of thyroid echography, N. Engl. J. Med. **287**:1164, 1972.

Blum, M., et al.: Improved diagnosis of nondelineated thyroid nodules by oblique scintillation scanning and echography, J. Nucl. Med. **16**:713, 1975.

Crile, G., Jr.: Aspiration biopsy of thyroid nodules, Surg. Gynecol. Obstet. **136**:241, 1973.

Crocker, E. F., et al.: Correlation of the caesium scan with the ultrasonic investigation of the solitary "cold" thyroid nodule. In AAEC Publication Abstracts of the Fifth Annual Scientific Meeting of the ANZ Society of Nuclear Medicine Sydney, Australia, 1974.

Crocker, E. F., et al.: The gray scale echographic appearance of thyroid malignancy, J. Clin. Ultrasound **2**:305, 1974.

Early, P., Razzak, M. A., and Sodee, D. B.: Thyroid. In Textbook of nuclear medicine technology, ed. 2, St. Louis, 1975, The C. V. Mosby Co.

Holmes, J. H., et al.: Practical improvements in thyroid imaging, J. Clin. Ultrasound **2**:235, 1974.

Jellins, J., et al.: Ultrasonic grey scale visualization of the thyroid gland, Ultrasound Med. Biol. **1**:405, 1974.

Means, J. H., et al.: The thyroid and its diseases, New York, 1963, McGraw-Hill Book Co.

Miller, J. M., et al.: The cystic thyroid nodule, Radiology 110:257, 1974.

Mishkin, M., et al.: B-Mode ultrasonography in assessment of thyroid gland lesions, Ann. Intern. Med. 79:505, 1973.

Mishkin, M., et al.: Ultrasonography of the thyroid gland, Radiol. North Am. 13:479, 1975.

Perlmutter, G. S., et al.: Ultrasound evaluation of the thyroid, Semin. Nucl. Med. 5:229, 1975.

Ramsay, I., et al.: Ultrasonics in the diagnosis of thyroid disease, Clin. Radiol. 26:191, 1975.

Rosen, I., et al.: The use of B-mode ultrasonography in changing indications for thyroid operations, Surg. Gynecol. Obstet. 139:193, 1974.

Rosenberg, I. N.: Newer methods of evaluating thyroid nodules, N. Engl. J. Med. 287:1197, 1973.

Shaub, M., et al.: The ultrasonic evaluation of nonfunctioning thyroid nodules, West. J. Med. 123:265, 1975.

Solgaard, S., et al.: Detection of thyroid cysts by ultrasonic examination, Acta Chir. Scand. 141:495, 1975.

Taylor, K. J., et al.: Gray scale ultrasonography in the diagnosis of thyroid swellings, J. Clin. Ultrasound 2:327, 1974.

Taylor, K. J., et al.: Comparison of radioisotope and ultrasound scans of the thyroid, Proc. R. Soc. Med. 68:381, 1975.

Thijs, L. G.: Diagnostic ultrasound in clinical thyroid investigation, J. Clin. Endocrinol. Metab. 32:709, 1971.

Thijs, L. G., et al.: Ultrasound examination of the thyroid gland: possibilities and limitations, Am. J. Med. 60:96, 1976.

Doppler techniques

Barnes, R., et al.: Thromboembolic complications of angiography for peripheral arterial disease: prospective assessment by Doppler ultrasound, Radiology 122:459, 1977.

Bone, G., et al.: Clinical implications of the Doppler cerebrovascular examination: a correlation with angiography, Stroke 7:271, 1976.

Fronek, A., et al.: Quantitative ultrasonographic studies of lower extremity flow velocities in health and disease, Circulation 53:957, 1976.

Johnson, W.: Ultrasonic flow detection for localization of splenic and renal veins, Arch. Surg. 3:1032, 1976.

Lye, C. R., et al.: The accuracy of the supraorbital Doppler examination in the diagnosis of hemodynamically significant carotid occlusive disease, Surgery 79:42, 1976.

O'Donnell, T. F., et al.: Doppler examination vs clinical and phlebographic detection of the location of incompetent perforating veins, Arch. Surg. 112:31, 1977.

Education requirements and guidelines
(Appendixes A and B)

Allied Medical Education Fact Sheet: A.M.A. Accredited Educational Programs in Allied Medical Occupations, Nov., 1974.

A.M.A. Council on Medical Education: Essentials of an accredited educational program for diagnostic medical sonographers, Sixth Draft, A.S.U.T.S., 1977.

A.S.U.T.S. Job Profile: Diagnostic ultrasound, 1975.

Baker, J.: Guidelines for the development of a new health occupation—diagnostic medical sonographer, A.M.A. Council on Health Manpower, June, 1974.

Cardiovascular technology, Community College of Philadelphia, March, 1976.

Carlsen, E. N., and Jansen, C.: The selection and education of an ultrasound technologist, Appl. Radiol. 3:41, Sept., 1974.

Chang, S.: Echocardiology training, Indiana University at Indianapolis, July, 1974.

Chang, S.: The creation of an echocardiographic technician, Sonix 1:32, Oct.-Nov., 1975.

Curriculum for cardiovascular technology, Indiana University at Indianapolis, June, 1976.

Feigenbaum, H.: Echocardiography, Philadelphia, 1972, Lea & Febiger.

Feigenbaum, H.: Educational problems in echocardiography, Am. J. Cardiol. 34:741, 1974.

Gramiak, R., et al.: Report of the Inter-Society Commission for Heart Disease Resources: optimal resources for ultrasonic examination of the heart, Circulation 51:A-1, 1975.

Guidelines for diagnostic ultrasound education, American Society of Ultrasound Technical Specialist, Education Committee. (In preparation.)

Hagen, S. L.: Regional questionnaire regarding ultrasound education, Episcopal Hospital, Philadelphia, Sept., 1974.

Hagen, S., et al.: The development of the ultrasound program, Appl. Radiol. 4:89, June, 1975.

Hagen-Ansert, S. L.: Analysis of the diagnostic ultrasound training programs, presented at the National Meeting of the American Society of Ultrasound Technical Specialists, San Francisco, Aug., 1976.

Kerber, R.: Errors in performance and interpretation of echocardiograms, J. Clin. Ultrasound 1:330, 1973.

Suggested readings

Barnett, E., and Morley, P.: Abdominal echography, London, 1974, Butterworth & Co., Ltd.

Bartrum, C.: Gray scale ultrasound: a manual for physicians and technical personnel, Philadelphia, 1977, W. B. Saunders Co.

Baum, G.: Fundamentals of medical ultrasonography, New York, 1975, G. P. Putnam's Sons.

Bechimol, A.: Non-invasive diagnostic technology in cardiology, Baltimore, 1977, The Williams & Wilkins Co.

Bock, J., and Ossoinig, K.: Ultrasonographia medica. Vols. I to III, Proceedings of the 1970 Congress, Vienna, Austria, 1971, Verlag der Weiner Medizinischen Akademie.

Bronson, Fisher, Pickering, and Trayner: Ophthalmic contact B-scan ultrasonography for the clinician, Westport, Conn., 1976, Intercontinental Publications, Inc.

Brown, B., and Gordon, D.: Ultrasonic techniques in biology and medicine, Springfield, Ill., 1967, Charles C Thomas, Publisher.

Brown, R. E.: Ultrasonography: basic principles and clinical applications, St. Louis, 1975, Warren H. Green, Inc.

Carlin, B.: Ultrasonics, 2, New York, 1960, McGraw-Hill Book Co.

Carter, B., et al.: Cross-sectional anatomy with CT and ultrasound, New York, 1977, Appleton-Century-Crofts.

Chang, S.: M-mode echocardiographic techniques and pattern recognition, Philadelphia, 1976, Lea & Febiger.

Dicken, W. N.: Diagnostic ultrasonics, Somerset, N.J., 1976, John Wiley & Sons, Inc.

Ensminger, D.: Ultrasonics, New York, 1973, Marcel Dekker, Inc.

Feigenbaum, H.: Echocardiography, Philadelphia, 1972, Lea & Febiger.

Feigenbaum, H.: Echocardiography, ed. 2, Philadelphia, 1976, Lea & Febiger.

Freeman, I.: Sound and ultrasonics, New York, 1973, Random House, Inc.

Freeman, L. M., and Blaufox, D. M.: Nuclear medicine and ultrasound, New York, 1976, Grune & Stratton, Inc.

Garret, W. J., and Robinson, D. E.: Ultrasound in clinical obstetrics, Springfield, Ill., 1970, Charles C Thomas, Publisher.

Gitter, K. A., Kenney, A. H., Sarin, L. K., and Meyer, D.: Ophthalmologic ultrasound, St. Louis, 1969, The C. V. Mosby Co.

Goldberg, B. B.: Diagnostic ultrasound in clinical medicine, New York, 1973, Medcom, Inc.

Goldberg, B. B., et al.: Abdominal gray scale ultrasonography, Somerset, N.J., 1977, John Wiley & Sons, Inc.

Goldberg, B. B., Kotler, M., Ziskin, M., and Waxham, R. D.: Diagnostic uses of ultrasound, New York, 1975, Grune & Stratton, Inc.

Goldberg, R. E., and Sarin, L. K.: Ultrasonics in ophthalmology, Philadelphia, 1967, W. B. Saunders Co.

Goldberg, S. J., Allen, H. D., and Sahn, D. J.: Pediatric and adolescent echocardiography, Chicago, 1975, Year Book Medical Publishers, Inc.

Gordon, D.: Ultrasound as a diagnostic and surgical tool, Edinburgh, 1964, E. & S. Livingstone, Ltd.

Gosink, B., and Squire, L. F.: Diagnostic ultrasound: exercises in radiology, Philadelphia, 1976, W. B. Saunders, Co.

Gottlieb, S., and Viamonte, M.: Diagnostic ultrasound, Chevy Chase, Md., 1975, The American College of Radiology.

Gramiak, R., and Waag, R. C., editors: Cardiac ultrasound, St. Louis, 1975, The C. V. Mosby Co.

Gregus, P.: Holography in medicine, Buildford, England, 1975, IPC Science & Technology Press, Ltd.

Grossman, C. C.: The use of diagnostic ultrasound in brain disorders, Springfield, Ill., 1966, Charles C Thomas, Publisher.

Grossman, C. C., Holmes, J. H., Joyner, C., and Purnell, E. W.: Ultrasound (diagnostic), New York, 1966, Plenum Press, Inc.

Harrison, D., Sandler, H., and Miller, H. A.: Cardiovascular imaging and image processing, Palos Verdes Estates, Calif., 1975. Society of Photo-optical Instrumentation Engineers.

Hassani, N.: Ultrasonography of the upper abdomen, New York, 1976, Springer Verlag.

Hildebrand, B. P., and Brenden, B. B.: An introduction to acoustical holography, New York, 1972, Plenum Press, Inc.

Hueter, T., and Bolt, R.: Sonics, New York, 1955, John Wiley & Sons, Inc.

Hussey, M.: Diagnostic ultrasound. An introduction to the interactions between ultrasound and biological tissues, Somerset, N. J., 1975, John Wiley & Sons, Inc.

IEEE: Proceedings of the Ultrasonics Symposium, 1973 (catalogue no. 73 CHO 807-8SU) New York, 1973, IEEE.

Joyner, C. R.: Ultrasound in the diagnosis of cardiovascular-pulmonary disease, Chicago, 1974, Year Book Medical Publishers, Inc.

Kazner, E., deVlieger, M., Muller, H. R., and McCready, V.: Ultrasonics in medicine, Proceedings of the Second European Congress, New York, 1975, American Elsevier Publishing Co., Inc.

Kazner, E., Schiefer, W., and Zulch, K. J.: Proceedings in echoencephalography, New York, 1968, Springer Verlag.

Kelly, E.: Ultrasonic energy: biological investigations and medical applications, Urbana, Ill., 1965, University of Illinois Press.

King, D. L.: Diagnostic ultrasound, St. Louis, 1974, The C. V. Mosby Co.

Kobayashi, M.: Illustrated manual of ultrasonography in obstetrics and gynecology, Philadelphia, 1974, J. B. Lippincott Co.

Kobayashi, M., Hellman, L. M., and Cromb, E.: Atlas of ultrasonography in obstetrics, and gynecology, New York, 1972, Appleton-Century-Crofts.

Leopold, G. R., and Asher, W. M.: Fundamentals of abdominal and pelvic ultrasonography, Philadelphia, 1975, W. B. Saunders Co.

Levi, D., and Donald, I.: Present and future of diagnostic ultrasound, Somerset, N.J., 1976, John Wiley & Sons, Inc.

Meyer, R. A.: Textbook of echocardiography, Philadelphia, 1977, W. B. Saunders Co.

Miskovitz, C., and Federici, E.: Echocardiography: a manual for technicians, Flushing, N.Y., 1977, Medical Examination Publishing.

Mostafawy, A., In cooperation with Nagle, J. B.: Pediatric sonoencephalography: the practical use of ultrasonic echoes in the diagnosis of childhood intracranial disorders, Heidelberg, Germany, 1971, Springer Verlag.

Rand, E.: Recent advances in diagnostic ultrasound, Springfield, Ill., 1971, Charles C Thomas, Publisher.

Reneman, R. S.: Cardiovascular applications of ultrasound, New York, 1975, American Elsevier Publishing Co. Inc.

Sanders, R.: Ultrasound, Radiologic Clinics of North America Symposium on B-scan, Philadelphia, 1975, W. B. Saunders Co.

Tenner, M. S., and Wodraska, G. M.: Diagnostic ultrasound in neurology (methods and techniques), New York, 1975, John Wiley & Sons, Inc.

Uematsu, S., and Walker, A. E.: A manual of echoencephalography, Baltimore, 1971, The Williams & Wilkins Co.

University of Texas M. D. Anderson Hospital and Tumor Institute: Radiologic and other biophysical methods in tumor diagnosis, Chicago, 1975, Year Book Medical Publishers, Inc.

de Vlieger, M., White, D. N., and McCready, V. R.: Ultrasonics in medicine, Amsterdam, 1974, Excerpta Medica Foundation.

Wainstock, M. A.: Ultrasonography in ophthalmology, Boston, 1969, Little, Brown & Co.

Wells, P. N. T.: Physical principles of ultrasonic diagnosis, New York, 1969, Academic Press, Inc.

Wells, P. N. T.: Ultrasonics in clinical diagnosis, Baltimore, 1972, The Williams & Wilkins Co.

Wells, P. N. T.: Biomedical ultrasonics, New York, 1977, Academic Press, Inc.

Wells, P. N. T.: Ultrasonics in clinical diagnosis, ed. 2, New York, 1977, Longman Group Ltd.

Williams, R. G., and Tucker, C. R.: Echocardiographic diagnosis of congenital heart disease, Boston, 1977, Little, Brown & Co.

Index